Kass

Handbook of Infectious Diseases

Obstetric and Perinatal Infections

Kass

Handbook of Infectious Diseases

Series Editors

JAY P. SANFORD, M.D.

Dean Emeritus
Uniformed Services University of the Health Sciences
Bethesda, Maryland

DAVID A. J. TYRRELL, M.D., F.R.S.

Formerly Director Medical Research Council
Common Cold Unit, Salisbury
Currently Adviser to MRC AIDS Directed Programme

THOMAS H. WELLER, M.D.

Richard Pearson Strong Professor of Tropical Public Health
Emeritus, Harvard School of Public Health
Boston, Massachusetts

SHELDON M. WOLFF, M.D.

Endicott Professor of Medicine
Chairman, Department of Medicine
Tufts University School of Medicine
Physician-in-Chief, New England Medical Center Hospital
Boston, Massachusetts

Obstetric and Perinatal Infections

DAVID CHARLES, M.D., FRCSC, F.R.C.O.G.

Formerly Professor and Chairman Of Obstetrics and Gynecology
Marshall University School of Medicine
Huntington, West Virginia

Memorial University of Newfoundland
St. Johns, Newfoundland

Boston University School of Medicine
Boston, Massachusetts

with 90 illustrations

Mosby
Year Book

St. Louis Baltimore Boston Chicago London Philadelphia Sydney Toronto

Mosby Year Book
Dedicated to Publishing Excellence

Publisher: George Stamathis
Developmental Editor: Leslie Fenton
Editorial Project Manager: Jolynn Gower
Project Coordinator: Pete Hausler
Book and Cover Design: Gail Morey Hudson

Printed in the United States of America

Mosby–Year Book, Inc.
11830 Westline Industrial Drive, St. Louis, Missouri 63146

Library of Congress Cataloging in Publication Data
Obstetric and perinatal infections / [edited by] David Charles.
p. cm.—(Handbook of infectious diseases)
Includes bibliographical references and index.
ISBN 1-55664-395-0
1. Communicable diseases in pregnancy. 2. Communicable diseases in the fetus. 3. Neonatal infections. I. Charles, David, 1924– II. Series.
[DNLM: 1. Infection—congenital. 2. Pregnancy Complications, Infectious. WQ 256 014]
RG578.O27 1992
618.3′2—dc20
DNLM/DLC
for Library of Congress 92-13137
CIP

92 93 94 95 96 GW/MY 9 8 7 6 5 4 3 2 1

This volume is dedicated
with much gratitude to
Jean
whose encouragement, support and
continued confidence make everything possible.

Both of us would like to respectfully inscribe this book
in honor and memory of the two distinguished physicians
Maxwell Finland and **Edward H. Kass**
who inspired and trained so many physicians
in the field of infectious diseases.

Contributors

JOHN G. BARTLETT, M.D.

Professor of Medicine, Johns Hopkins University School of Medicine; Chief, Infectious Diseases, Johns Hopkins Hospital, Baltimore, Maryland

ROGER E. BAWDON, Ph.D.

Associate Professor and Laboratory Director, University of Texas Southwestern Medical School, Dallas, Texas

DAVID CHARLES, M.D., FRCSC, F.R.C.O.G.

Formerly Professor and Chairman of Obstetrics and Gynecology, Marshall University School of Medicine, Huntington, West Virginia, Memorial University of Newfoundland Faculty of Medicine, St. Johns, Newfoundland, and Boston University School of Medicine, Boston, Massachusetts

JONATHAN CHARLES, M.D.

Clinical Professor, University of Hawaii John A. Burns School of Medicine, Honolulu; Pathologist, Kauai Medical Group and Wilcox Memorial Hospital, Lihue, Hawaii

JACQUES COUVREUR, M.D.

Associate Professor of Pediatrics, Saint Antoine Faculty of Medicine, Paris, France

SUSAN M. COX, M.D.

Associate Professor and Director of Maternal-Fetal Medicine, University of Kentucky College of Medicine, Lexington, Kentucky

MARINELLA CARDELLO CUMMINGS, M.S.

Staff, Department of Medicine, Division of Infectious Diseases, State University of New York Health Science Center at Brooklyn College of Medicine, Brooklyn, New York

F. GARY CUNNINGHAM, M.D.

Professor and Chairman, Obstetrics and Gynecology, University of Texas Southwestern Medical School; Chief, Obstetrics and Gynecology, Parkland Memorial Hospital, Dallas, Texas

FERNAND DAFFOS, M.D.

Chairman, Department of Obstetrics and Gynecology, Institut de Puericulture, Center of Prenatal Diagnosis, Paris, France

PATRICK DUFF, M.D.

Professor of Obstetrics and Gynecology, Division of Maternal-Fetal Medicine, University of Florida College of Medicine, Gainesville, Florida

DAVID A. ESCHENBACH, M.D.

Professor, Department of Obstetrics and Gynecology, University of Washington School of Medicine, Seattle, Washington

VIJAYA GANESH, M.D.

Associate Professor of Clinical Obstetrics and Gynecology, University of Medicine and Dentistry of New Jersey, New Jersey Medical School, Newark, New Jersey

RONALD S. GIBBS, M.D.

Professor and Chairman, Department of Obstetrics and Gynecology, University of Colorado School of Medicine, Denver, Colorado

DOUGLAS D. GLOVER, M.D.

Professor of Obstetrics and Gynecology, West Virginia University School of Medicine, Professor of Clinical Pharmacy, West Virginia University School of Pharmacy, Morgantown, West Virginia

LESLIE IFFY, M.D., FRCSC, FACOG

Professor of Obstetrics and Gynecology, University of Medicine and Dentistry of New Jersey, New Jersey Medical School; Director, Division of Obstetrics, University Hospital, Newark, New Jersey

DENNIS L. KASPER, M.D.

William Ellery Channing Professor of Medicine, Harvard Medical School; Chief, Division of Infectious Diseases, Beth Israel Hospital and Co-Director, Channing Laboratory, Brigham and Women's Hospital, Boston, Massachusetts

JEROME O. KLEIN, M.D.

Professor of Pediatrics, Boston University School of Medicine; Director, Division of Pediatric Infectious Diseases, Boston City Hospital, Boston, Massachusetts

BRYAN LARSEN, Ph.D.

Professor of Microbiology and Professor of Obstetrics and Gynecology, Marshall University School of Medicine, Huntington, West Virginia

WILLIAM J. LEDGER, M.D.

Professor and Chairman, Cornell University Medical College; Obstetrician and Gynecologist-in-Chief, New York Hospital, New York, New York

LAWRENCE C. MADOFF, M.D.

Instructor in Medicine, Harvard Medical School; Associate in Medicine, Beth Israel Hospital, and Associate Physician, Brigham and Women's Hospital, Boston, Massachusetts

WILLIAM M. McCORMACK, M.D.

Professor of Medicine and of Obstetrics and Gynecology and Chief, Department of Medicine, Division of Infectious Diseases, State University of New York Health Science Center at Brooklyn College of Medicine, Brooklyn, New York

HOWARD L. MINKOFF, M.D.

Professor of Obstetrics and Gynecology and Director, Maternal-Fetal Medicine, State University of New York Health Science Center at Brooklyn College of Medicine, Brooklyn, New York

GILLES R. G. MONIF, M.D.

Professor of Obstetrics and Gynecology, Creighton University School of Medicine, Omaha, Nebraska

RICHARD L. NAEYE, M.D.

Professor and Chairman, Department of Pathology, and Chief, Pathology Services, Milton S. Hershey Medical Center, Pennsylvania State University College of Medicine, Hershey, Pennsylvania

HEIN ODENDAAL, M.D., F.R.C.O.G., F.C.O.G. (S.A.)

Professor and Head, Department of Obstetrics and Gynecology, University of Stellenbosch and Tygerberg Hospital, Tygerberg, Republic of South Africa

RICHARD H. SCHWARZ, M.D.

Provost and Vice President for Clinical Affairs, State University of New York Health Science Center at Brooklyn College of Medicine, Brooklyn, New York

JOHN L. SEVER, M.D., Ph.D.

Professor of Pediatrics, Obstetrics and Gynecology, and Microbiology and Immunology, George Washington University School of Medicine and Health Sciences and Children's National Medical Center, Washington, D.C.

ANTONIO V. SISON, M.D.

Instructor, Department of Obstetrics and Gynecology, Georgetown University School of Medicine, Washington, D.C.

LEON G. SMITH Sr., M.D.

Director, Professor, and Chairman of Medicine, University of Medicine and Dentistry of New Jersey, New Jersey Medical School, Seton Hall School of Medicine, Newark, New Jersey

LEON G. SMITH Jr., M.D.

Director, Maternal-Fetal Medicine, Saint Barnabas Medical Center, Livingston, New Jersey

RICHARD L. SWEET, M.D.

Professor and Chairman, Department of Obstetrics, Gynecology, and Reproductive Sciences, University of Pittsburgh School of Medicine, Magee Women's Hospital, Pittsburgh, Pennsylvania

PHILIPPE THULLIEZ, M.D.

Chief, Laboratory of Toxoplasmosis, Institut de Puericulture de Paris, Paris, France

CHERYL K. WALKER, M.D.

Assistant Professor, Department of Obstetrics, Gynecology, and Reproductive Sciences, University of California San Francisco School of Medicine, San Francisco, California and Honorary Senior Lecturer, Department of Obstetrics and Gynecology, Makerere University, Kampala, Uganda; Project Director, Makerere University/University of California San Francisco School of Medicine Collaborative Health Project, San Francisco, California

Introduction: A Commemorative

The editing of this volume was undertaken after repeated requests from Ed Kass to produce an updated version of a book I edited with Maxwell Finland two decades ago. It now appears as the second volume in the Kass *Handbook of Infectious Diseases* series.

I first met Max in 1960. He was a recognized authority on infectious diseases as a result of his meticulous work in the 1930s. Max was one of the leading contributors to the basic science of microbiology and clinical bacteriology. Critical analysis of data and uncompromising standards of excellence were hallmarks of the man. His manner was understated, but the breadth of his knowledge of infectious diseases and his ability to solve any clinical problem were apparent to everyone who sought his aid. His compassion for the suffering and forebearance toward the weak are freely acknowledged by those who observed him administering to his patients.

I was particularly struck by Max's genuineness and honesty. He never affected a knowledge that he did not possess, but was modestly deferential to those he thought better informed than he. His nature was contemplative and his mind judicious.

Behind his searching eyes and austere look was a man who understood the forgotten people: tolerance, charity, and hope were by-words of his teaching. He loathed bigotry and fanaticism. This modest man might have been Kipling's prototype when he wrote:

Let us now praise famous men
Men of little showing
For their work continueth
Greater than their knowing!

Ed Kass had Max as his mentor, and under his tutelage he went from strength to strength. He had an incredibly wide range of interests, and he revealed an exceptional depth of knowledge in all of them, which never failed to amaze me. He was an expert in infectious diseases as well as a renowned clinical epidemiologist. He had the ability to assimilate new ideas as well as the capacity to query existing information in order to determine its ultimate nature. His example was one to emulate, owing to his great sense of purpose and attention to detail.

Ed believed that truth had many facets. He sought the truth in concepts that are beyond challenge, held by faith, or held to be self-evident. Yet he believed that even the highest truth is accessible to critical analysis:

"By doubting we are led to inquire, and by inquiring we perceive the truth"—this could have been the force driving his daimon.

He had strong convictions, but always kept an open mind. Ed practiced and preached precision, accuracy, and honesty in documenting all aspects of his work. Consequently, it is no surprise to anyone who worked with him that he inspired academic excellence by example and constructive criticism. He adhered to the words of Francis Bacon:

"Reading maketh a full man, conference a ready man, and writing an exact man."

My interaction with Max Finland and Ed Kass at both scientific and personal levels was the greatest honor to be granted anyone with an interest in infectious diseases. It is because of this experience that I accepted the task of editing this volume.

Preface

Life is a changing process, and the adaptation of the human body to infection involves numerous complex processes. Therefore, the outcome of any extraneous influence on the mother or her fetus or neonate cannot be predicted in precise quantitative terms. This volume is intended to be a trustworthy foundation for further progress in the research and understanding of perinatal infections.

The reader—whether obstetrician, infectious disease specialist, or perinatologist—will find this work to be a rich source of current knowledge regarding obstetric and perinatal infections. Their causes, prevention, recognition, and treatment—before, during, and after delivery—are presented by authorities on their respective topics.

William Blake wrote: "Art and science cannot exist but in minutely organized particles." This effort to so organize the body of knowledge of infectious diseases in the mother, fetus, and newborn has been made possible by the contributing authors. All are friends and colleagues who have been chosen for preeminence in their fields. Without them, this volume would not have been possible, and I am deeply grateful to them for their time and efforts.

I wish to express my thanks to Brian Decker, and to Mosby–Year Book, especially Leslie Fenton and Mary Mansor, who were my Developmental Editor and Sponsoring Editor, respectively. Finally, I would like to thank the Senior Editors, especially Drs. Jay Sanford and Thomas Weller, for their skillful editing of this volume.

David Charles

Contents

PART I

The Mother

CHAPTER 1

Normal Flora and Endogenous Infections

Bryan Larsen, Ph.D.

The recognition of the benign association of microorganisms with the human body dates back to Leeuwenhoek's early microscopic observations. He noted that little creatures visible only with the aid of the microscope he had invented were present in scrapings from his teeth. Since that time it has been learned that all skin and mucosal tissues having contiguity with the environment possess an indigenous microbiota. The composition and relationship of these microbial communities to the host have come more clearly into focus within the past few decades because of better methods of microbial identification, the use of electron microscopy to visualize relationships of organisms to tissues, and the application of the concept of microecology to explain the interactions between microorganisms and host. In this chapter, these concepts are discussed in relation to the microbial flora of the lower female genital tract and the infectious problems related to this flora. For the modern obstetrician-gynecologist, the genital microflora provides a unifying concept for various infections of endogenous origin. However, despite the usefulness of these concepts, there are misconceptions surrounding the microbial flora, and these are also addressed in this chapter.

Early Concepts of Vaginal Flora

The earliest studies of the flora of the vagina emphasized microscopic observations. Perhaps the greatest early impact was made by Döderlein, who did his work in the latter part of the nineteenth century and noted a typical dominance of large gram-positive organisms, which came to be called Döderlein's bacillus in his honor. The organisms that were microscopically designated as Döderlein's bacillus probably belonged to the genus *Lactobacillus*, although we now know that corynebacteria are also prevalent in asymptomatic women and may appear similar to lactobacilli on Gram's smears. The modern microbiologist recognizes that full identification of microorganisms requires isolation in pure culture and rigorous biochemical testing to establish the true identity of a bacterial species. Thus, the lactobacilli of the female genital tract have been shown to belong to a variety of species. The earliest investigators, however, expressed the concept that the vaginal flora was normally composed of gram-positive bacilli, it was quite homogeneous, and the presence of gram-negative organisms was indicative of a pathologic condition. Despite the limitations of this concept, it is still often recited today.

In the decade of the 1960s, dramatic improvements were made in the ability to isolate and identify strictly anaerobic microorganisms, and these techniques were applied to the vaginal flora, which was known to contain anaerobic species. Numerous surveys of vaginal flora, some of which focused on aerobic organisms and others that attempted to identify the full range of microorganisms, have demonstrated that the vaginal flora is far more diverse than the early classical studies indicated. Elsewhere the author has summarized in encyclopedic form the literature that reports on the microbial content of the lower genital tract,[5] and this extensive listing of microorganisms that have been isolated is not repeated here; however, Table 1-1 summarizes the results of the most reliable studies. The current state of our understanding of the flora is that each woman is host to several anaerobic and several aerobic species simultaneously. Carefully performed cultures may show 15 species of bacteria simultaneously present in samples taken from the posterior fornix. Among these bacteria are aerobic as well as anaerobic species, and by no means are these limited to gram-positive bacilli. It is important to discuss the principles that provide an understanding of how the flora can be the source of certain infectious complications.

Table 1-1 Typical Organisms Constituting the Normal Flora of Reproductive-Aged Women

Group	Organism	Typical Prevalence
Aerobic		
Gram-positive rods		
	Lactobacilli	45-88%
	Diphtheroids	14-72%
	Gardnerella vaginalis	2-58%
Gram-positive cocci		
	Staphylococcus epidermidis	34-92%
	Staphylococcus aureus	1-32%
	Group B streptococci	6-22%
	Group D streptococci	32-36%
	Nonhemolytic (non-group D) streptococci	14-33%
	Alpha-hemolytic (non-group D) streptococci	17-36%
Gram-negative rods		
	Escherichia coli	20-28%
	Others including *Proteus, Klebsiella, Enterobacter*	2-10%
Molicutes		
	Mycoplasma hominis	0-22%
	Ureaplasma urealyticum	0-58%
Yeast		15-30%
Anaerobic		
Gram-positive rods		
	Lactobacilli	10-43%
	Eubacteria	0-7%
	Bifidobacteria	8-10%
	Propionibacteria	2-5%
	Clostridia	4-17%
Gram-positive cocci		
	Peptococci	76%
	Peptostreptococci	56%
	Gaffkya anaerobia	5-31%
Gram-negative rods		
	Bacteroides bivius	34%
	Bacteroides melaninogenicus	18%
	Bacteroides fragilis group	0-13%
	Fusobacteria	7-19%
Gram-negative cocci		2-27%

Typical prevalence represents findings of various studies. Actual prevalence in a given population depends on the demographics of the population, microbiologic methods, and basis for naming organisms.

Nature of Microbial Pathogens

One of the lessons taught by Pasteur was that certain microorganisms predictably cause diseases. As an outgrowth of this very important tenet of microbiology the concept of pathogenic microorganisms was born. In Pasteur's time it was vitally important to understand that certain organisms like the anthrax bacillus caused a very predictable constellation of symptoms when introduced into a susceptible host. However, a common misuse of the concept of pathogenicity is the all-too-frequent attempt to categorize every microbial species as a pathogen or as a nonpathogen. In reality, many organisms that do not typically cause symptoms in human hosts are capable in some situations of behaving like a pathogen, eliciting symptoms of infection. The current experience with the acquired immunodeficiency syndrome (AIDS) has revealed that many organisms rarely associated with disease can cause symptoms in AIDS patients. In this example, a depression of the immune system is of primary importance in the genesis of infection. Yet many microorganisms have attributes shared by the so-called pathogens.

The microbial characteristics possessed by frank pathogens that enable them to consistently cause symptoms in susceptible hosts include the following.

First, these organisms are typically exogenous to the host. The symptoms of infection arise when the exogenous pathogen reaches a suitable locus in the host and becomes established. In contrast, normal flora organisms are endogenous, and their mere presence is not usually associated with symptoms unless the host is somehow altered.

The second characteristic of frank pathogens is their ability to survive in transit. Because these organisms are usually exogenous, natural methods for their transport and survival are necessary. *Neisseria gonorrhoeae*, for example, is an exogenous pathogen that despite its fragility overcomes the hostility of the environment by mucosa-to-mucosa transmission. This organism, therefore, does not leave the safety of the mucosal secretions in its movement from host to host.

The third attribute of highly virulent microorganisms is shared by the less virulent normal flora organisms. Specific attachment sites on susceptible tissues allow pathogenic microorganisms to avoid being washed away by mechanical processes and permit them to remain anchored in a microenvironment to which they are well adapted. Certainly, normal flora organisms also exploit tissue attachment sites for purposes of remaining in intimate association with the host at sites that are appropriate for their physiologic processes.

The ability of virulent organisms to initiate multiplication at the site of infection is an important feature of pathogenesis of infectious disease. In contrast to normal flora organisms, which multiply only sufficiently to maintain their numbers, pathogenic organisms tend to grow in a less controlled fashion. During the course of growth, the pathogenic organisms may elaborate metabolic end products that contribute further to their role as pathogens. Such products may include toxins and enzymes, which are a part of the fifth attribute of pathogens.

The fifth characteristic of typically pathogenic organisms is their invasiveness. The penetration of tissues by microorganisms is not completely understood on a molecular basis but may involve such processes as phagocytosis without intracellular destruction of the microbe. The production of enzymes that disrupt tissue architecture (collagenases, proteases, lipases, or silaidases) may allow the microorganisms to spread from their initial site of localization. The production of toxins may also cause damage to the tissue or destruction of leukocytes. In contrast, most normal flora organisms do not normally invade tissue or produce harmful end products that cause symptoms of infectious disease.

How Normal Flora Organisms Cause Disease

As indicated by the preceding discussion, there are some distinctions between frankly pathogenic microorganisms and members of the normal flora. Yet despite these distinctions, it is neither correct nor useful to persist in attempting to categorize all microorganisms as either pathogens or nonpathogens. Under certain circumstances the benign microorganisms of the normal flora may function in a way similar to classical pathogens and produce serious symptoms. There are three principal but not mutually exclusive ways in which normal flora organisms that colonize mucosal surfaces may produce symptoms of infection. First, a significant alteration in the host's immune system may result in normally benign organisms becoming the source of symptoms. In immunosuppressed individuals such as persons with AIDS, *Candida albicans*, which is a minor component of the normal flora of various mucosal sites, may produce thrush symptoms.

A second way in which normal flora organisms may cause symptoms is by undergoing a disruption of the normal ecologic interactions with other members of the normal flora. Recent findings of studies of bacterial vaginosis have indicated that such a disruption of the normal relationships among normal flora organisms may account for this condition. The organisms present in the vaginal milieu of the patient with bacterial vaginosis are not unique to the vaginal microenvironment. However, the numerical dominance of certain bacterial species and the diminished numbers of lactobacilli portray this condition as an alteration of the flora rather than the acquisition of organisms with unique pathogenic potential.

A third way in which normally benign members of the indigenous flora may function as pathogens is under circumstances that permit them to reach tissues other than the epithelial surfaces they usually colonize. This may be thought of as a dislocation of the normal flora. A common example is postsurgical infections, which are most commonly due to normal flora organisms that have been disseminated to deeper tissues by the operative procedure. Likewise, the ascending spread of lower-tract organisms to the upper genital tract in cases of pelvic inflammatory disease provides a further illustration of symptoms caused when ordinarily benign organisms reach an inappropriate anatomic location.

Microecology of Vaginal Flora

Because the bacterial flora of the lower female genital tract may undergo changes that can result in symptoms, it is as important to know what factors control the normal flora as it is to know which species comprise the flora. In the author's experience, one of the most powerful concepts for understanding the nature and control of the normal flora is the application of the science of ecology to the microbial communities that live in commensal relationship with the human host. Just as macrobiologists recognize that ecologic niches in nature provide habitats for visible flora and fauna, we are able to appreciate the relationship of the vaginal flora to the vaginal epithelium in much the same way. The vaginal epithelium represents the environment, and the microflora in intimate association with the underlying tissue forms an ecosystem. As we begin to discover the changes that occur in the epithelium, we can expect and indeed find that changes in the flora occur in response. The entire ecosystem is a dynamic entity responsive to a variety of microenvironmental conditions. These concepts, previously noted by Larsen and Galask,[7] have continued to provide a sound paradigm for endogenous infections.[6]

Vaginal Epithelium: Physicochemical Aspects

Microorganisms have minimum requirements for life, including the need for macronutrient supply, micronutrient supply, temperature, moisture, oxygen tension, and myriad other physicochemical aspects that allow them to flourish. The vaginal epithelium provides these necessities for the microorganisms indigenous to that site. For the most part, the nutrient conditions extant in the vagina have not been characterized, and research efforts are continuing in this regard. The vaginal epithelium consists of a squamous surface composed of cells that have matured from lower layers under the influence of estrogenic hormone. Studies in the author's laboratory have demonstrated the importance of estrogen stimulation in controlling vaginal flora in experimental animals.[10] In rats, the number of organisms present on the vaginal epithelium increased 10,000-fold after the animals were stimulated by estrogen.

The role of estrogenic hormone in controlling the vaginal flora of women has also been noted, although the profound changes seen in rats are not usually observed in women. This is probably due to the fact that the vaginal epithelium of humans is more or less estrogenized at all times during the reproductive years. The observations of Cruickshank and Sharman[1] in 1934 indicated that the lactobacillus colonization of the vagina is related to estrogenic effect on the vagina. Among female infants who still had transplacentally acquired estrogen, vaginal lactobacilli were abundant. Lactobacillus colonization diminished thereafter until menarche. During the reproductive years and particularly during pregnancy, lactobacilli increase, and once again decline in the menopause. This has been verified by culture observation on women serially evaluated during pregnancy and through the trimesters of pregnancy.[2] Specific findings included increased prevalence lactobacillus and yeast colonization and concomitant decreases in most other groups of microorganisms.

The sensitivity of lactobacillus colonization to estrogenic influences has often been explained as if a full explanation were well established, yet it should be recognized that the control of lactobacillus colonization is not necessarily properly understood. Based on histologic observation, it has been suggested that estrogen promotes glycogen deposition in the vaginal epithelium that is a substrate for lactobacillus growth. The lactobacilli produce acid from fermentation of the glycogen, and this in turn keeps vaginal pH low, thereby restricting the flora to primarily acid-tolerant species such as *Lactobacillus* species. Although these forces are probably to some extent operative in controlling the vaginal flora, several observations raise some questions regarding the bounds of this explanation. Not all lactobacilli from the vagina are able to utilize starch, and according to some of the older reports of Weinstein and colleagues[11,15,16] vaginal acidity may be produced without bacterial action. In studies of rat vaginal flora, we found that the changes in numbers of bacteria present occurred without significant changes in vaginal pH. Thus in the animal model at least, pH was clearly not the controlling factor. In addition, chemical measurement of vaginal glycogen did not reveal significant differences in glycogen deposition between premenopausal and postmenopausal women.[3]

Regardless of the controlling mechanism, estrogenic stimulation of the vaginal epithelium appears to play an important function in the normal colonization of the vagina. In addition to older studies, more recent studies that utilized contemporary microbiologic methods have demonstrated that the prevalence of *Bacteroides* colonization in women sampled during the proliferative phase of the menstrual cycle was 35 percent, whereas only 27 percent of women sampled during the secretory phase of the cycle were colonized with *Bacteroides*.[14] The same investigators also indicated a greater proportion of women undergoing hysterectomy during the proliferative phase experienced postoperative infection, compared to women undergoing operative procedures during the secretory phase. Interestingly, in this study the importance of the modification of the estrogen effect by progestin is implied rather than the presence or absence of estrogen being the essential difference between these individuals. Studies on postmenopausal women who were grouped according to use of replacement estrogen or no estrogen showed few differences except for a greater prevalence of some anaerobic species in the estrogen-treated group.[9] Despite the significance of estrogen in animal models of colonization, the role in humans seems less apparent, and the influence of progesterone in addition to other as yet undiscovered factors should be considered.

The importance of nutrients in the cellular components of the vaginal epithelium in supporting the nutritional requirements for bacterial growth provides some additional unresolved issues. Nutrients taken into microbial cells enter in solubilized form. Therefore, complex carbohydrates located intracellularly in vaginal epithelial cells may require extensive degradation before the nutrients would be available for bacterial growth. Other sources of nutrients may be present in the vaginal microenvironment apart from the intact vaginal tissue. Sloughed epithelium may be subject to enzymatic degradation, more so than attached squamous cells. In addition, serous transudates, menstrual fluid, secretions from endocervical glands, and other sources may provide for the nutrient needs of vaginal bacteria.

As noted in the discussion of pathogenic organisms, the epithelium provides anchorage sites for both pathogenic and normal flora organisms. The surface architecture and presentation of attachment sites is ultimately determined by the genetic constitution of the epithelial cells, but their state of maturity undoubtedly plays a role in their suitability for microbial attachment. It is well known that *Neisseria gonorrhoeae* is able to attach to and infect the vaginal tissue of prepubertal girls, but after menarche the estrogenized epithelium is resistant to colonization. The reverse is probably true of other microorganisms that are typically encountered in adult women.

Microbial Diversity

Because the vaginal epithelium is the habitat of microorganisms, and this habitat is subject to periodic changes with shifts in estrogenic and progestational hormone levels, changes in the concentration of solutes that reach the vaginal fluid by transudation, fluxes of cervical secretion and the local immunoglobulins contained in these secretions, and sundry other alterations, the vaginal flora must necessarily be affected by these changes in the microenvironment. The composition of the vaginal flora is not solely a reflection of the conditions provided by the vaginal tissue but also the result of complex interactions among the various microbial species that comprise the normal flora.

The microorganisms that are present in the vaginal flora are diverse. It is not unusual for a careful laboratorian using techniques for the cultivation of both aerobes and anaerobes to find 10 or even 15 different microbial species present simultaneously in vaginal cultures. This number of different species is not present in every subject, but in virtually every individual multiple aerobic and multiple anaerobic species are likely to be present. These microorganisms interact with each other in a variety of ways. For example, some organisms compete for nutrients and attachment sites on epithelial surfaces, whereas other organisms appear to have complementary or perhaps symbiotic relationships. One organism may produce pyruvic acid or acetic acid as an end product, and another organism utilizes these as substrates for growth. The proteolytic enzyme produced by one organism may provide amino acids that support the growth of a second organism. A reduced environment may be created by the metabolic activity of organisms that consume oxygen, thereby allowing obligate anaerobes to flourish in the presence of facultative organisms. Many other interactions among species may occur, although exactly which processes occur in a given patient is not well understood. These processes that allow cocolonization by multiple bacterial species are among the same metabolic collaborations that are involved in polymicrobial infections.

Effect of Microorganisms on Vaginal Epithelium

To this point we have reviewed the fact that the vaginal epithelium and its physicochemical composition provide a habitat for microorganisms. We have noted that the flora represents a mixed culture subsisting within the conditions provided by the vaginal surface and as modified by bacterial action. The third aspect of this microecosystem is the effect that the microorganisms have on the vaginal epithelium. In studies of gut flora, it is known that the rate of cellular maturation is influenced by the presence of the normal flora. Details of the effects of the vaginal flora on the vaginal epithelium are less well established than those that have been elucidated in the gut. Nevertheless, we know that the genital tract has a local immune system and that the normal flora organisms must provide antigens that interact with the local immunity. It is not known whether the function of a stable normal flora causes immunologic tolerance or some other effect on the immune system. It is notable that endotoxin, or lipopolysaccharide, which is produced by gram-negative bacteria, is mitogenic for B-lymphocytes. In the older literature, the presence of a predominantly gram-positive flora was equated with vaginal salubrity. Currently, the condition most conspicuously dominated by gram-negative organisms is bacterial vaginosis. As is discussed later, bacterial vaginosis has some rather sinister aspects, particularly during pregnancy. The normal flora is also generally considered to prevent the attachment and growth of frankly pathogenic microorganisms and thereby protects the tissue from invasion. The effects of bacterial end products are not limited to actions on the epithelium. *Bacteroides* spp. produce succinate, which is known to have antiphagocytic effects. The role of phagocytic cells on normal and unusual vaginal organisms may be a further important aspect of the vaginal microenvironment.

External Influences

It should be clear that the vagina and its bacterial flora are in a dynamic relationship and that alterations in either the tissue or the flora change the balance that exists in this ecosystem. Despite our lack of understanding of the details of these exceedingly complex processes, it is clear that the changes in balance between various species of microorganisms in the normal flora may result in some microorganisms causing symptoms. To this point we have limited the discussion to interactions that occur within the host, but it is appropriate to note that external influences may also disrupt the vaginal ecosystem, resulting in members of the normal flora producing symptoms.

The various external influences that may primarily affect the microorganisms or primarily affect the vaginal tissue are summarized here. Antimicrobial drugs, whether administered topically to the vaginal epithelium or systemically, are able to alter the vaginal flora. Interestingly, despite attempts some investigators made to try to eliminate the flora with antimicrobial douches or vigorous antimicrobial therapy, the normal flora is persistent, although it is clearly altered by such treatment. In addition to antimicrobials, the exposure of the vaginal epithelium to seminal fluid, which has a high pH, a high concentration of zinc, and a high concentration of fructose and also contains microorganisms, may have at least a transient influence on the ecology of the vagina. The introduction of tampons or pessaries may likewise have ill-defined effects. One of the alterations that may be related to vaginal tampons is the introduction of oxygen into the vaginal vault.

Finally, surgical trauma is known to alter the ecology of the vaginal flora. Several studies have cultured the vaginal flora before and after surgical procedures and found that an increase in the prevalence of various bacterial species occurs, but lactobacillus colonization typically declines.[4,12,13] Other conditions that cause breaches in the integrity of the vaginal epithelium, such as ulcerative infections (genital herpes), may result in secondary infection by normal flora organisms.

Summary

The normal flora is a dynamic entity that can be defined only within broad limits. The interactions of the vaginal microenvironment with the microbial flora have revealed that it is as important to understand influences that cause changes in the flora as it is to name the organisms present at any given time.

Conditions Arising from Normal Flora

Periodically, infectious conditions arise that directly or indirectly involve the normal flora. The purpose of this discussion is to briefly summarize conditions that appear to arise from the normal flora of the female genital tract. It should be emphasized, however, that any exogenous infectious process that involves the lower female genital tract must be superimposed on the normal flora or be in competition with the endogenous bacterial population. For the sake of space, only those infectious processes that are endogenous in nature and arise from the normal flora will be mentioned.

Several organisms associated with vaginitis are commonly found as members of the normal flora. Approximately 15 percent of women are colonized with *Candida albicans* but do not normally experience symptoms. Currently there is no known feature of those yeasts that is found in symptomatic cases of vaginal infection that distinguishes them from strains of yeast found as normal flora in colonized women. It is probable that in symptomatic cases the number of yeasts is greater than among women who are simply colonized. A frequently repeated scenario in yeast vaginitis is the development of symptoms after treatment with an antibacterial agent. This condition is consistent with a decrease in bacterial numbers coupled with increased growth and metabolism of the yeast. Certainly the symptoms of yeast vaginitis may be related to specific virulence factors produced by the fungal organism, but such factors may be in low concentration when the yeasts are in low concentration.

Gardnerella vaginalis was first described in 1955 as the single cause of nonspecific vaginitis. Since the early observations, many changes in nomenclature and changes in the understanding of this condition have occurred. Currently, the condition of bacterial vaginosis is attributed to a synergistic relationship between anaerobic microorganisms indigenous to the lower genital tract and *G. vaginalis*. The latter organism is also considered by most investigators to be a normal vaginal inhabitant. The collaboration of *G. vaginalis* and anaerobic bacteria has been extensively studied, and it appears that the condition of bacterial vaginosis may be considered the result of altered proportions among these members of the normal flora.

In the early 1980s infectious disease specialists became aware of toxic shock syndrome (TSS) and determined that this generalized toxic condition was the result of a specific factor elaborated by *Staphylococcus aureus*, namely, TSST-1 (toxic shock syndrome toxin-1). *Staphylococcus aureus* is not present in the vaginal flora of a large proportion of women, and it is debatable whether TSS represents an endogenous condition. However, clear evidence of an exogenous source for most cases of TSS is lacking. During the menstrual flow, cultures showed an increased prevalence of *S. aureus*[8] that did not seem to reflect an acquisition of new organisms but rather an increase in bacterial numbers to detectable levels. Pathogenesis of TSS could be the result either of bacterial numbers increasing to reach a critical level with toxin levels also reaching a critical level or of conditions that allow the organism to initiate toxin production. In either case, the microenvironmental conditions logically seem to have relevance to the process.

The mixed flora that contains anaerobic and aerobic species is associated with a variety of infectious complications, particularly surgical interventions involving the genital tract of women. Every surgeon is acquainted with the febrile morbidity that often complicates abdominal and vaginal hysterectomy. Although many factors relating to the surgical procedure are involved, it remains a fact that when an incision is made across a colonized epithelium, as occurs in gynecologic surgeries, the tissues are contaminated with normal flora organisms. In this context, as noted previously, these bacteria may not be benign. In most cases the normal defenses of the host are adequate to control the contaminating microorganism, and even when febrile morbidity occurs it is usually not life-threatening. Nevertheless, despite the use of antibiotics for prophylaxis, no method has been devised to obviate the contamination of the operative field by normal flora organisms, and occasionally very severe infectious complications develop. Most commonly involved in postoperative infections are the anaerobic bacteria, exemplified by *Bacteroides* sp. and the anaerobic gram-positive cocci, and the gram-negative facultative organisms, including *Escherichia coli, Enterobacter,* and less commonly *Klebsiella*. Knowledge of the kinds of organisms commonly involved in such infections helps to provide a rational approach to the selection of antimicrobial therapy.

Dissemination of lower-tract organisms to the upper genital tract occurs in several circumstances in obstetric and gynecologic patients. As with postoperative infections, the organisms frequently involved are the facultative gram-negative rods and various anaerobic species. Infectious complications may be polymicrobial, and therapy is usually instituted empirically on that basis. Specifically, it is now recognized that while acute salpingitis can be elicited by such exogenous pathogens as *N. gonorrhoeae* or *Chlamydia trachomatis*, lower genital microflora organisms may ascend to the upper tract and become involved in salpingitis, endometritis, and possibly tubo-ovarian abscesses. In the obstetric patient lower-tract organisms may be involved as causes of chorioamnionitis and in addition to the hazards to the fetus occasioned by such an infection, chorioamnionitis also predisposes the parturient woman to postpartum endometritis or endomyometritis. If cesarean delivery ensues in such patients, the likelihood of normal flora organisms being involved in uterine infection is enhanced.

Of particular interest to the obstetric patient is the carriage of group B beta-hemolytic streptococci in the vaginal or gut flora. This organism has a particular propensity to cause neonatal sepsis, although it represents a relatively minor hazard to the mother. It is certainly an arguable point whether this organism should be counted among the organisms that comprise the normal genital flora. However, in some asymptomatic women stable carriage of the organism has been reported. Like group B streptococci, *E. coli* may cause neonatal meningitis. The organism that appears most virulent in this context is the K1 serotype. The epidemiology of this organism is not entirely clear, and it may or may not be of endogenous origin.

Summary

The normal flora of the vagina and endocervix is more than a number of lactobacilli residing on an epithelial surface. This chapter has indicated that the vaginal epithelium and the microbial communities consist of a variety of different species with interlacing metabolic activities. The relationship of the colonized epithelium to the bacterial flora has been described as an ecosystem in miniature, which means that a balance exists among each of the components of the system, and a change in one part induces a change in other parts of the system. Therefore, the microbial flora of the female genital tract is dynamic in its response to various endogenous and exogenous influences. Although the organisms comprising the normal flora are distinguished from frankly pathogenic organisms, conditions may occur that allow these organisms to express greater virulence, blurring the distinctions between pathogen and nonpathogen. Because of these facts, the physician may utilize knowledge of the composition and mechanisms controlling the flora to understand the pathogenesis of endogenous infections and to select empiric therapy on a rational basis when such therapy is clinically warranted.

References

1. Cruickshank R, Sharman A. The biology of the vagina in the human subject. Journal of Obstetrics and Gynaecology of the British Empire 1934; 41:190–208.
2. Goplerud CP, Ohm MJ, Galask RP. Aerobic and anaerobic flora of the cervix during pregnancy and the puerperium. Am J Obstet Gynecol 1976; 126:858–868.
3. Gregoire AT, Kandil O, Ledger WJ. The glycogen content of the human vaginal epithelial tissue. Fertil Steril 1971; 22:64–68.
4. Grossman JH III, Adams RL. Vaginal flora in women undergoing hysterectomy with antibiotic prophylaxis. Obstet Gynecol 1979; 53:23–26.
5. Larsen B. Normal genital microflora. In: Keith LG, Berger GS, Edelman DA, eds. Infections in reproductive health. I. Common infections. 1985:3–31.
6. Larsen B. Ecological interactions in genital tract infections. International Journal of Feto-Maternal Medicine 1990; 3:229–235.
7. Larsen B, Galask RP. Vaginal microbial flora: practical and theoretic relevance. Obstet Gynecol 1980; 55:S100–113.
8. Larsen B, Galask RP. Vaginal microbial flora: composition and influences of host physiology. Ann Intern Med 1982; 96:926–930.
9. Larsen B, Goplerud CP, Petzold R, Galask RP. Effect of estrogen treatment on the genital tract flora of postmenopausal women. Obstet Gynecol 1982; 60:20–24.
10. Larsen B, Markovetz AJ, Galask RP. Role of estrogen in controlling the genital microflora of female rats. Appl Environ Microbiol 1977; 34:534–540.
11. Lewis RM, Weinstein L. The production of vaginal acidity by estrin, its importance in treatment of gonorrheal vaginitis. Surg Gynecol Obstet 1936; 63:640–643.
12. Ohm MJ, Galask RP. The effect of antibiotic prophylaxis on patients undergoing vaginal operations. II. Alterations of the microbial flora. Am J Obstet Gynecol 1975; 123:579–604.
13. Ohm MJ, Galask RP. The effect of antibiotic prophylaxis on patients undergoing total abdominal hysterectomy. II. Alterations of microbial flora. Am J Obstet Gynecol 1976; 125:448–454.
14. Thadepalli H, Savage EW Jr, Salem FA, et al. Cyclic changes in cervical microflora and their effect on infection following hysterectomy. Gynecol Obstet Invest 1982; 14:176–183.
15. Weinstein L, Howard JH. The effect of estrogenic hormone on the H-ion concentration and the bacterial content of the human vagina, with special reference to the Doderlein bacillus. Am J Obstet Gynecol 1939; 37:698–703.
16. Weinstein L, Wawro NW, Worthington RV, Allen E. The influence of estrogenic hormone on the H-ion concentration and bacterial flora of the vagina of the immature monkey. Yale J Biol Med 1938; 11:141–148.

CHAPTER 2

Epidemiology of Obstetric Infections

Leslie Iffy, M.D.
Vijaya Ganesh, M.D.

Historical Background

Although the art of helping the parturient is as old as humankind, obstetrics as a branch of medicine emerged only a few centuries ago. Andrew Baeder, a medical historian, quotes the tragic story of a Doctor Watt, who in 1522 was burned at the stake because, dressed as a woman, he attempted to help a mother during her childbirth.[6] Then and before, midwifery was practiced only by women. Besides the earlier exclusion of midwifery from the medical curriculum, it was considered unethical for a qualified physician to offer help to a woman in labor. It was not until the seventeenth century that surgeons, considered artisans rather than professionals, were permitted to assist mothers during childbearing. The most outstanding of these pioneers was Mauriceau, whose contributions to the science of obstetrics were important enough to survive until today.[52] Nonetheless, contemporary society perceived the activities of these men as scandalous at worst and ridiculous at best (Fig. 2-1).

The technical improvements introduced into midwifery by early accoucheurs generated interest within the medical profession; the new discipline eventually evolved into obstetrics. The scientific basis of the specialty gradually expanded, primarily as a result of contemporary interest in dissecting dead bodies and studying normal and pathologic anatomy. In the course of this evolution, the significance of the bony pelvis as a causative factor in protracted labor became recognized, a principle that had escaped the attention of generations of midwives. Nonetheless, the progress in understanding normal and abnormal labor processes was overshadowed by recurring evidence indicating that women were more likely to survive childbearing under the care of uneducated midwives than in the hands of highly trained physicians. Most women knew that their chances of living were better if they delivered on the kitchen table at home than if they gave birth in a well-equipped and adequately staffed hospital, a fact that the medical profession refused to acknowledge. This trend was demonstrated in England as late as the early 1930s.[42]

Puerperal Fever

The common denominator of the increased rate of maternal and neonatal deaths in institutions run by physicians was puerperal fever. This fact, as well as the inability of the medical profession to fight the contagium effectively, was documented by Arnold Lea[45] in 1910:

> In the 5 years 1851–5 the puerperal death rate from all causes was 4.9/1000 (births) and in the 5 years ending 1906 it still amounted to 4.2/1000. . . . We do no violence to the statistics if we put down the septic mortality in England and Wales as between 3000 and 5000/annum.

Puerperal fever remained the leading cause of maternal death worldwide until the early decades of the twentieth century. The medical profession offered a convenient explanation, namely, the "shame" suffered by women exposed to male attendings and the "humiliation" of unmarried mothers who took shelter in public hospitals. Although observations about the contagious nature of childbed fever were presented to the medical

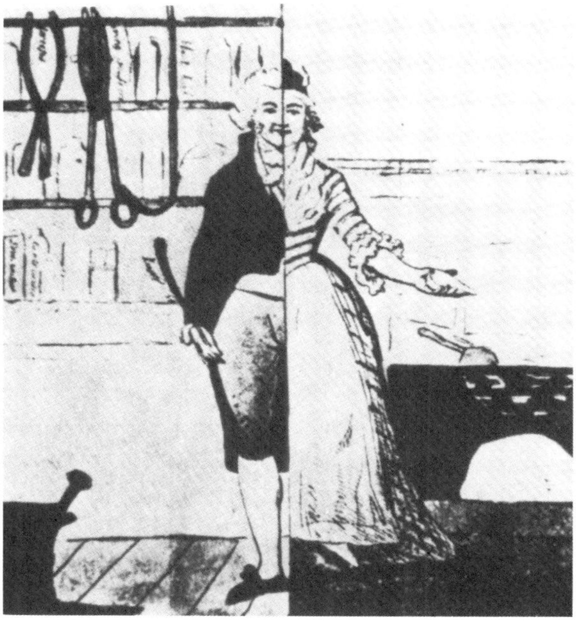

Figure 2-1 Male midwives and their instruments. (Cartoon by John Blunt, 1793.)

profession as early as 1768[15] and were reinforced by those of Leake,[46] White,[15] Hamilton,[31] and Gordon,[25] the profession ignored the "contagion theory." Effective infection control techniques were known and applied as far back as the days of the Roman Empire; however, hundreds of thousands of women paid with their lives for scientific pendantry between the first observations of the infectious nature of puerperal fever and Pasteur's discovery[58] of the offending microorganism in 1880. Had the medical profession considered circumstantial evidence and retrospective rather than prospective investigations, this disease could have been curbed more than two centuries ago. Gordon[25] documented the role of physicians as carriers of the contagion among patients: "It is a disagreeable declaration for me to mention that I myself was the means of carrying the infection to a great number of women."

Cederschjord in Sweden, 1839, achieved a measure of control over the spread of infection by providing each parturient with separate sponge and towel, based on the hypothesis that these objects, if shared, could transfer the offending material from infected mothers to uninfected ones.[15]

Oliver Wendell Holmes

Upon reviewing the contemporary literature, Oliver Wendell Holmes[34] concluded that the balance of evidence indicated that puerperal fever was transferred from one patient to another by inoculation of a "contagium." He recommended the implementation of effective preventive measures, such as the suspension of one's involvement in obstetric practice for 24 hours after participating in any postmortem examination or treating a patient suffering from puerperal fever or "erysipelatous processes."

Holmes's ideas were rejected by the leading American obstetricians of the time, such as Hodge[15] and Meigs.[54] The latter summarized his viewpoint as follows: "I prefer to believe that childbed fever is brought about by the will of Providence, which I understand, than that it is caused by some unknown contagium, which I don't."

Ignaz Semmelweis

The critical breakthrough with regard to the etiology of puerperal fever resulted from the retrospective studies of Ignaz Semmelweis,[64] conducted in the late 1840s. Working as an assistant in the department of Professor Klein at the Vienna Lying-in Hospital, he noted the marked difference in mortality rates from childbed fever between Division II, which taught student nurses (who did not participate in the performance of autopsies), and Division I, which provided education for medical students (who regularly performed postmortem examinations in the course of their studies). He acted on the hypothesis that the fivefold to tenfold higher rate of mortality in the medical students' division, which amounted at times to 15 percent of all parturients, derived from students carrying the contagion from the mortuary to the labor floor. He stipulated that personnel entering the obstetric area had to wash their hands thoroughly with chlorine of lime solution.[8] This measure resulted in a decline of the yearly mortality rates from more than 11 percent to less than 1.3 percent in the medical students' division, a result that, for the first time in decades (Fig. 2-2), was better than that observed in the nurses' service (Fig. 2-3).

Based on a careful analysis of the data he collected, Semmelweis outlined three important principles regarding the etiology of the disease:

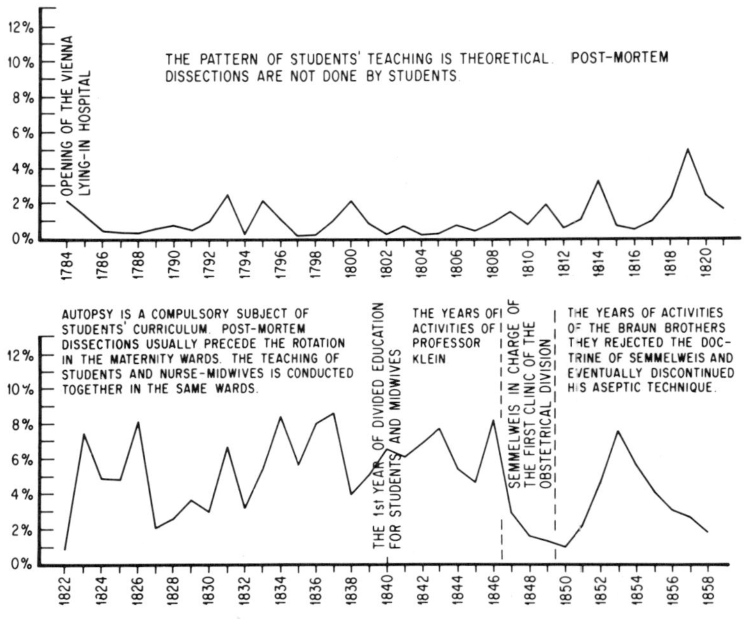

Figure 2-2 Maternal mortality statistics between 1784 and 1858 in the Vienna Lying-In Hospital, according to Semmelweis, 1861.[64] In the eighteenth and nineteenth centuries, the overwhelming majority of maternal deaths resulted from childbed fever.

1. Rather than being an entity of its own, puerperal fever is simply one manifestation of sepsis.
2. The spread of this and any other infection can be prevented by "aseptic" measures, involving the destruction of "organic animal matter" by appropriate chemical agents, such as chlorine solution, before the inoculation of the contagion into another patient.
3. Asepsis is an obligatory prerequisite for the practice of surgery as well as for that of obstetrics.

In keeping with these principles, Semmelweis "scrubbed up" before any operative procedure, thus establishing the new era of aseptic surgery.

In addition, Semmelweis implemented isolation techniques more rigorously than do most institutions in the Western world in the 1990s.

The success of his assistant in curbing the ravages of childbed fever failed to impress Professor Klein, who refused to extend his appointment beyond the year 1849. His departure from the institution was marked by a catastrophic increase in the maternal mortality rates of the hospital in the early 1850s (see Fig. 2-2).

Free of interference, Semmelweis set up his own maternity department in the crowded St. Rokus Hospital of Budapest. His results were unprecedented and included periods of time as long as 1 year without a single maternal death from childbed fever. Nonetheless, his reasoning failed to convince his contemporaries, who believed that "Controlled prospective studies are needed for a conclusion." Thus, epidemic outbreaks of childbed fever continued, decimating parturients in the leading medical centers of Paris, London, Vienna, Prague, and Berlin.

For experts who read the work of Semmelweis, in retrospect the evidence appears conclusive and the logic of his argument impeccable. However, his contemporaries preferred to believe that the conduct of his research was unscientific and the resulting evidence circumstantial. Therefore, to check the validity of his findings, Scanzoni,[65] then considered the leading European authority in obstetrics, set up a prospective experiment. He divided parturients into trial and control groups, handling some with and others without aseptic techniques. Because by its very design the experiment failed to control the environment, the study showed no difference between the two groups. Scanzoni therefore reiterated his own perception of the cause of puerperal fever: "Every busy physician makes observations in his practice which must convince him that the state of health in a puerpera is no more readily endangered by any noxious influence, than by a violently stimulating or depressing mental state."

With that statement, he and his contemporaries, including Virchow, sealed the fate of another generation of mothers until, in 1879, the discovery by Pasteur of streptococci in the uterus of a victim of puerperal fever established the infectious nature of the disease to everyone's satisfaction.[58]

Asepsis and Antisepsis

Acting on the notion that childbed fever could be contagious, beginning from 1870 Tarnier in the Maternité de Paris began to use isolation techniques. He supplemented them with an aseptic program from 1881. The respective impacts of these measures were reflected in the reduction of maternal mortality rates from 9.3 percent in the 1860s to 2.3 percent in the 1870s and to only 1 percent by the 1880s.[38]

Even at the end of the twentieth century, the prin-

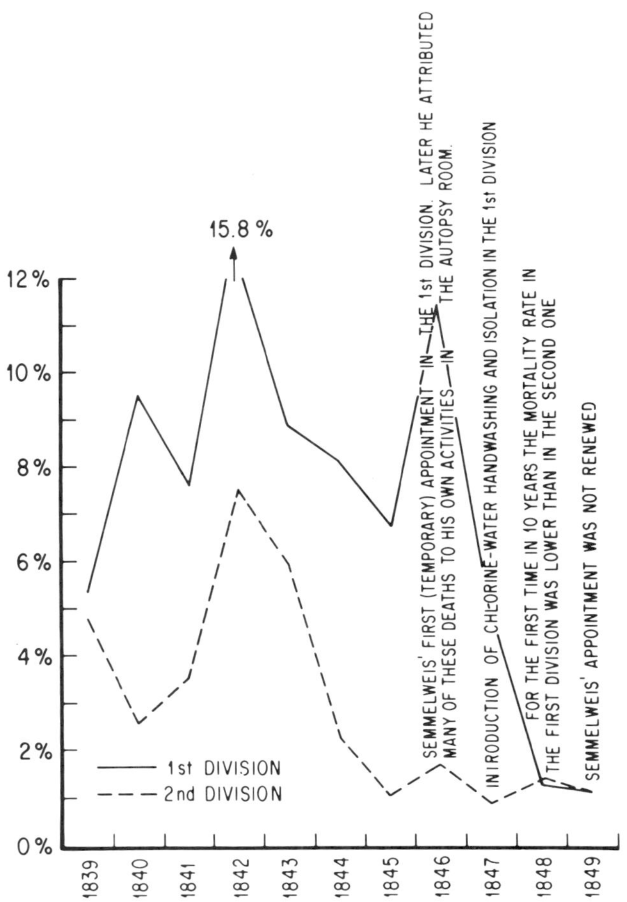

Figure 2-3 Mortality rates in the first and second divisions of the Department of Obstetrics in the Vienna Lying-In Hospital between 1839 and 1849, according to Semmelweis, 1861.[64] Note the precipitous fall of the mortality rates after the introduction of aseptic measures in the First Division.

ciples of "asepsis" often are mistaken for those of "antisepsis," an endeavor introduced and eventually abandoned by Lister.[48] He attempted to destroy the contagion by exposing the operative field to concentrated antiseptic solutions and vapors in the belief that it would destroy infectious material deposited there. Several years later Sir Almroth Wright, a famous physician of his time, concluded:[68] "Curious, indeed, is the failure of antiseptics. . . . Quite high were the expectations which were entertained with regard to what would be effected. What has actually been accomplished by antiseptics amounts in point of fact to almost nothing."

A contemporary physician, W. R. Hadwen, reflected years later upon the results in the Edinburgh Infirmary of "antiseptic surgery." It was practiced in the division of Sir John Lister where "surgeons were accustomed to go straight from the postmortem to the operating table," as compared to the division of Lawson Tait, who "would have no assistant's fingers in wounds he made, fingers whose dirt he had no means of gauging. . . ."[68]

The relevant recollections continue as follows:

Lawson Tait . . . mentions the results of abdominal operations in Edinburgh which he described as "truly awful,"—some 30 cases and not a recovery—all on the wrong side of the swing door (i.e., the division of Lister). But he himself in a long series of 1350 cases, of every degree of severity, only had a mortality of 5 percent, and yet he says: "At my hands there was no Listerism, no chemical antiseptics, nothing but soap and water and strict attention to detail.

Mortality Rates

It is generally agreed today that the cause of puerperal fever was correctly hypothesized by Gordon and Holmes and some of their predecessors, and accurately elucidated and conclusively documented by Semmelweis, and that the findings of the latter were further confirmed by the investigations of Pasteur. It is widely assumed that, the etiology having been established by the 1880s, the medical profession has resolved the problem within the boundaries of clinical practicalities; this widespread perception is far from correct. Although maternal deaths from puerperal fever declined dramatically by the early decades of the twentieth century in Scandinavia and the western part of continental Europe, mortality rates, pre-

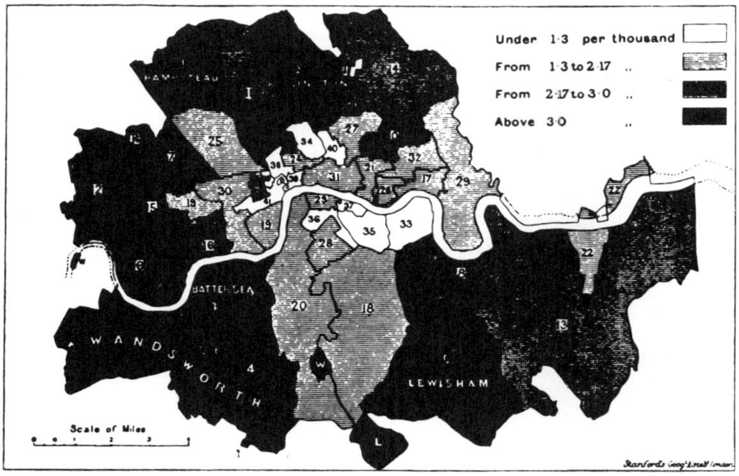

Figure 2-4 The incidence of puerperal fever in various districts of London during the years of 1891–1895, according to Kerr, 1933.[42] White areas, indicating the lowest infection rates, represent some of the poorest districts of the city, such as New Cross and Deptford. Black areas indicate the highest rates of maternal mortality from childbed fever; these areas were the high-class districts of London at the end of the nineteenth century. Similar trends were observed in others cities of England as late as the early twentieth century. (Reprinted with permission from Kerr JM. Maternal mortality and morbidity. Edinburgh: E&S Livingstone, 1933.)

Table 2-1 Maternal Mortality Rates in 1920

Denmark	2.35/1,000 births
Holland	2.42/1,000
Sweden	2.58/1,000
Uruguay	3.38/1,000
Italy	3.67/1,000
England and Wales	4.1/1,000
Ireland	5.53/1,000
Scotland	6.48/1,000
Chile	7.48/1,000
USA	7.99/1,000

Data from Loudon, 1987,[49] and Woodbury, 1926.[70]

dominantly from puerperal fever, remained high in many other countries. The most catastrophic statistics during and after the years of the First World War were reported from the United States (Table 2-1).[49,70] An almost equally unfavorable situation prevailed in Great Britain until Munro Kerr,[42] in an extensive retrospective study of maternal mortality statistics, pointed out the following trends in 1933:

1. The overall maternal mortality rates remained unchanged in the country during the preceding 50 years.
2. The maternal mortality rate from puerperal sepsis was twice as high in Britain as in the Netherlands across the English Channel.
3. Contradicting all at that time (and since) prevailing perceptions with regard to patients' predisposition for infection, maternal mortality rates were higher among high-socioeconomic-status suburbanites than among the poor living in the crowded, poverty-stricken areas of London (Fig. 2-4).

Munro Kerr pointed out that well-to-do patients, who could afford to buy medical care, were more likely to perish even in the 1930s from childbirth, as a result of the high incidence of puerperal fever in hospitals, than poor women who continued giving birth at home under the care of midwives. He attributed the difference to the role of physicians as carriers of the infection; a proposition that engendered no enthusiastic response from the medical profession at large. Accordingly, it was not until attention was drawn to this phenomenon by the lay press through an article in the London *Times*,[19] that the door to changes in the control of puerperal infection opened wide. Chassar Moir, the successor of Kerr in the professorial chair at Oxford, recounted that throughout the British Isles, rigid measures of isolation of infected patients and aseptic technology were implemented and enforced.[56] This effort resulted in a marked decline of maternal losses (Fig. 2-5). A significant drop in maternal mortality rates occurred before the introduction into the

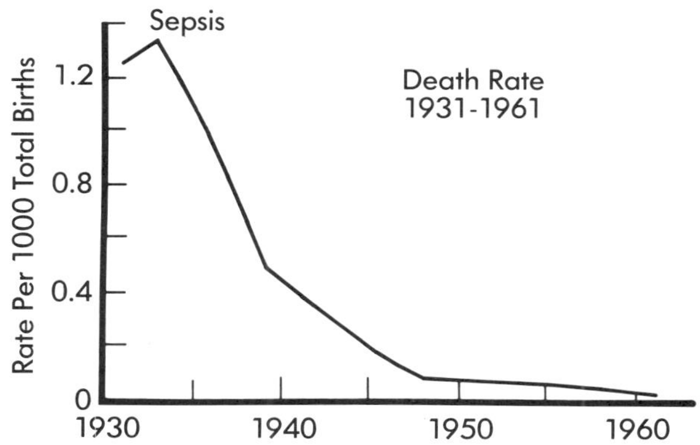

Figure 2-5 Maternal mortality rates from sepsis in Great Britain between 1931 and 1961, according to Moir, 1964.[56] The initial reduction of mortality rates in the mid-1930s is generally attributed to a nationwide effort, initiated by Munro Kerr, in implementing effective infection-control measures. The continued decline in the late 1930s Moir had largely attributed to the same effort, while Loudon, 1987,[49] suggested that the introduction of Prontosil (a sulfonamide) played a major role in the improved results at the end of the decade.

practice of medicine of chemotherapeutic and antibiotic agents.

Infection Control in the United States

The rapid improvement in Great Britain was not matched by comparable results in the United States. Based on statistics collected in 1941 and thus encompassing the last years of the preantibiotic era, the maternal mortality rate was still 17 per 1,000 in the Chicago Lying-In Hospital, 40 percent of which was attributable to puerperal infection.[15]

Some leading American obstetricians were in the front of the fight against the ravages of puerperal infection. Duly emphasizing that "To an obstetrician . . . is due the credit of pointing the correct way to modern . . . asepsis," DeLee and Greenhill presented in their textbook an extensive and precise description of the spread of infection and its prevention.[15] However, more recently, Duncan Reid[63] expressed his displeasure about infection control in America:

> With total confidence that puerperal infection can be controlled, the surgical conscience of those who care for the parturient is apt to become blunted and in some instances appears to be totally absent with respect to prevention of infection. Indeed, so flagrant are violations that one may wonder whether the laws governing infectious disease control no longer apply.

Similar exasperation was voiced by another outstanding expert with regard to the overall scene of infection control in America:[44] "Physicians behave as though Semmelweis and Oliver Wendell Holmes were shamans and the germ theory a mythical cult."

The senior author, having been educated in the infection-conscious Central European medical environment, was surprised to find grave shortcomings in elementary infection-control measures in reputable American teaching hospitals only two decades ago:

1. Patients with spiking fever from puerperal infection were kept in the same room with gravidas without any attempt at isolating them.
2. Nurses and physicians moved from the beds of patients with postoperative infection to those awaiting delivery without changing garments or wearing a glove and, as a rule, without washing their hands.
3. There was no thought given to assigning separate personnel to patients with discharging wounds and those awaiting the onset of labor at term.
4. In the absence of showers one single bathtub served the whole obstetric population, including patients preparing for cesarean section and those with discharging wounds.
5. Residents and attending physicians moved freely among delivery rooms, postpartum floors containing patients with infected wounds, and operating rooms.
6. Residents without apprehension would change the dressing with bare hands on a purulent wound minutes before moving to the operating room to perform a cesarean section.
7. Fully qualified surgeons would evacuate a pelvic abscess and move to handle the intestinal tract without changing gloves and without isolating the area of the abscess.

Epidemics of postcesarean infections were an everyday experience in these services, and the postoperative infection rates were at times as high as 90 percent. Despite the teaching of highly motivated and knowledgeable individuals, and even superbly organized institutions such as the Centers for Disease Control, the principles of infection control had apparently failed to impress the rank and file of medical practitioners in America. It appears that the antibiotic era arrived in this continent before the principles of asepsis and infection control could form deep roots. Furthermore, the rapidly growing and, on many accounts, well-deserved influence of American medical science removed the focus from puerperal and postoperative infections in many other parts of the world, including those that had been the cradle for the development of modern principles of infection control. As a result, against the background of a rapidly increasing number of effective antibiotics, by the second half of the century, maternal septic mortality and morbidity rates increased in many parts of Europe and America.[1,7,18,40] The magnitude of the setback suffered at the hands of the new "counterculture" is best said by an influential American expert of obstetric infection:[47]

> Successive editions of obstetric texts have promulgated the dogma that the risk of infection increases along with the duration of labor, the length of time for which membranes are ruptured, the length of time an internal uterine pressure catheter is in place, or the number of vaginal examinations during labor. . . . In fact . . . the only practical . . . approach to the prevention of infection is the use of prophylactic antibiotics.

If this opinion is correct, then Holmes, Semmelweis, and Kerr are to be forgotten and Klein, Scanzoni, and Meigs must be restored as the true heroes of the lost war against puerperal fever.

The acceptance by the leading medical authorities of the nature of puerperal and surgical infections and the discovery of antibiotics occurred within less than half a century. The conclusions derived from the discovery of the etiology of puerperal sepsis were implemented effectively in Great Britain only a few years before the discovery of penicillin and probably never in most parts of the world, many areas of the United States included. Thus, unlike continental Europe, prevention of infectious diseases in general, and that of puerperal sepsis in particular, moved from its prehistoric stages to the antibiotic era without a tangible transition. Therefore, it is necessary to reiterate the principles of infection control that proved highly effective before the discovery of the chemotherapeutic and antibiotic agents, thus permitting surgery to develop into a highly developed art by the 1930s.

Principles of Infection Control

It is often said that the rapid progress of medicine makes medical textbooks and publications obsolete within 4 to 5 years. The authors believe that this concept is erroneous in general and far removed from reality regarding the prevention of infectious diseases. In the preantibiotic era, the clinical manifestations of incurable infectious diseases facilitated the study of the pattern of transfer from one individual to the next. The infectious nature of leprosy, tuberculosis, smallpox, and plague were recognized before the beginning of the documented history of medicine. Currently, by contrast, immunization and early intervention and treatment introduce factors that hinder relevant studies, and the wide range of available antibiotics used both therapeutically and prophylactically makes the evaluation of infection-control measures extremely difficult.

The fact that the study of infections requires vastly different research protocols than other types of investigations is seldom understood, even by those engaged in infection-related research. The earlier mentioned experience of Scanzoni clearly established that in an infection-ridden environment the introduction or removal of one particular infection-control measure cannot have any tangible impact on the results of pertinent investigations. Apuzzio and Iffy wrote recently:[3]

> Numerous infection control measures, not proven in themselves effective in terms of statistical significance, have been abandoned in recent decades. As a consequence the consistency and rigidity of infection control measures have weakened, and the chain of events that are required for effective infection control is often broken. The concept that when one is in doubt, precautionary measures should be taken rather than ignored has lost support among many modern clinicians. . . . If infection control is to be effective and meaningful, any infection control measure must be proven to be unnecessary before being abandoned; it is not necessary to prove it useful for it to be utilized.

Hundreds of investigations have been undertaken with the naive idea of elucidating "whether" infectious agents can be transferred from one part of the body to another (for example, from the vulva into the uterine cavity), as if there could be any doubt. The very fact that a physician can introduce microorganisms from any part of the body (such as the upper vagina or the uterine surface) into a culture plate serves as unequivocal evidence that pathogenic microorganisms can, and are being, transferred to any site suitable for implantation (such as the amniotic cavity) by any agent, whether a cotton swab or the examining finger of the obstetrician.

The concept of asepsis being frequently ignored in modern hospitals, it appears necessary to reiterate the basic concepts that virtually eliminated puerperal fever from European obstetric units and led to spectacular progress in surgery well before the introduction of blood transfusion and antibiotics. More than stringent rules and protocols, comprehension of the manner by which infection spreads in an obstetric unit is the key to effective coordination and implementation of infection-control measures. Table 2-2 provides a list of those frequently observed attitudes that inevitably increase the risk of perinatal infection.

The success of infection-control measures hinges upon a coordinated effort of the medical, nursing, and paramedical personnel to prevent the transfer of infection. In general, meaningful participation in such an effort requires high standards of personal hygiene as well as a clear comprehension of the principles of asepsis. Regretfully, current educational patterns fail to provide an adequate basis for the latter, and some health care professionals, unexposed to the principles of hygiene in their early lives, tend to perceive measures directed at infection control as a cabalistic ritual rather than a purposeful course of action.

The terms *isolation, infection control, hygiene,* and *asepsis* are seldom, if ever, listed in the index pages of obstetric textbooks nowadays. Contemporary trends in nosocomial obstetric infections are closely related to this unfortunate situation. Scandinavian medical publications quote postcesarean infection rates in the range of 10 to 20 percent[27,62,66] and refer to American statistics conceding postcesarean infectious morbidity in excess of 50 percent[22,27,62,66] with apparent disbelief.

The fact that tuberculosis was far more prevalent among people living in underground dungeons than among those living in homes with good ventilation and sizable windows was known even to the lay public as early as the turn of the century. As a result of this recognition, homes with large windows came into vogue. Decades ago, numerous studies provided evidence that in an environment with access to sunlight, microorgan-

Table 2-2 Practice Patterns That Increase the Risk of Obstetric Infection

Failure to remove patients with chorioamnionitis, postpartum endometritis, or postoperative abscess from open floors
Allowing the same nurses to attend infected and noninfected patients in a random fashion
Failure on the part of medical and nursing staff to wash their hands before moving from patient to patient
Physicians handling wounds and changing dressings without wearing gloves or using instruments
Circulation of physicians between areas with and without patients suffering from infection
Using bathrooms or bathtubs for both healthy gravidas and infected parturients or puerperas
Wishful classification of broken-down infected wounds as "sterile separation"
Intrapartum vaginal examinations without washing hands thoroughly, without wearing two sterile gloves, or without disinfecting the vulva and separating the labia before the vaginal examination
Failure to isolate the skin with sterile towels in the course of cesarean sections
Failure to change scrubsuits inside and outside the obstetric unit
Failure to set aside septic operating room for surgery on infected patients
Failure to wear protective clothing in the labor and delivery area
Failure to change gloves during cesarean section after the removal of the fetus (the hand lifting the head from the pelvis becomes heavily infected by microorganisms of the lower segment and the upper vagina)
Emphasizing strict aseptic measures in the delivery rooms rather than in the labor rooms (the woman in labor is prone to infection, not the mother about to give birth)
Performing manual vaginal examinations in the presence of premature rupture of the membranes, prior to the onset of active labor
Using excuses for performing vaginal examination in the presence of premature rupture of the membranes (e.g. inserting prostaglandin tablets by hand rather than with speculum and forceps)
Unnecessary and frequent vaginal examinations in labor
Use of invasive procedures without strict indication (intrauterine pressure catheters, scalp electrode, scalp sampling)
Unnecessary rupture of the intact membranes for the sole purpose of utilizing invasive procedures
Shaving the operative field more than 1-2 hours before the performance of the operation
Antepartum or preoperative shower without the use of a potent antiseptic agent

isms are quickly destroyed, whereas they survive a long time in the dark. This simple expediency, which revolutionized modern architecture, soon became lost not only to hospital architects but to the medical profession as well. As a result, as late as 1979, a modern tertiary center with state-of-the-art obstetric facilities was opened in Newark, New Jersey, with all labor rooms windowless. In the same unit, one gets a scenic view of the neighborhood through two rows of huge windows from seldom-used corridors. This floor plan serves as a sad example of how the principles of "killing germs" have been buried under the ever-exploding number of scientific publications believed to reflect new advances in the science of medicine. At the same time, proper floor plans, depicting purposeful layout and ensuring smooth flow of patients into and out of the obstetric floor (Fig. 2-6), remain confined to the drawers of some well-informed architects.[23] Few obstetricians seem to know that the design of the obstetric unit largely determines one's ability to control infection in an often crowded environment. Apparently unaware that patients with infection must be isolated in their own environment, U.S. obstetric units have been built so that transfer of the patient from the labor area to the delivery area is inevitable. Although from the viewpoint of infection control this function has always been counterproductive, in a modern perinatal unit, this pattern is detrimental for a variety of other reasons:[59]

1. The fetal monitoring must be interrupted.
2. The chance of the patient giving birth in the corridor is considerable during her frantic transfer from the labor to the delivery room.
3. The personnel needs of the unit are increased.

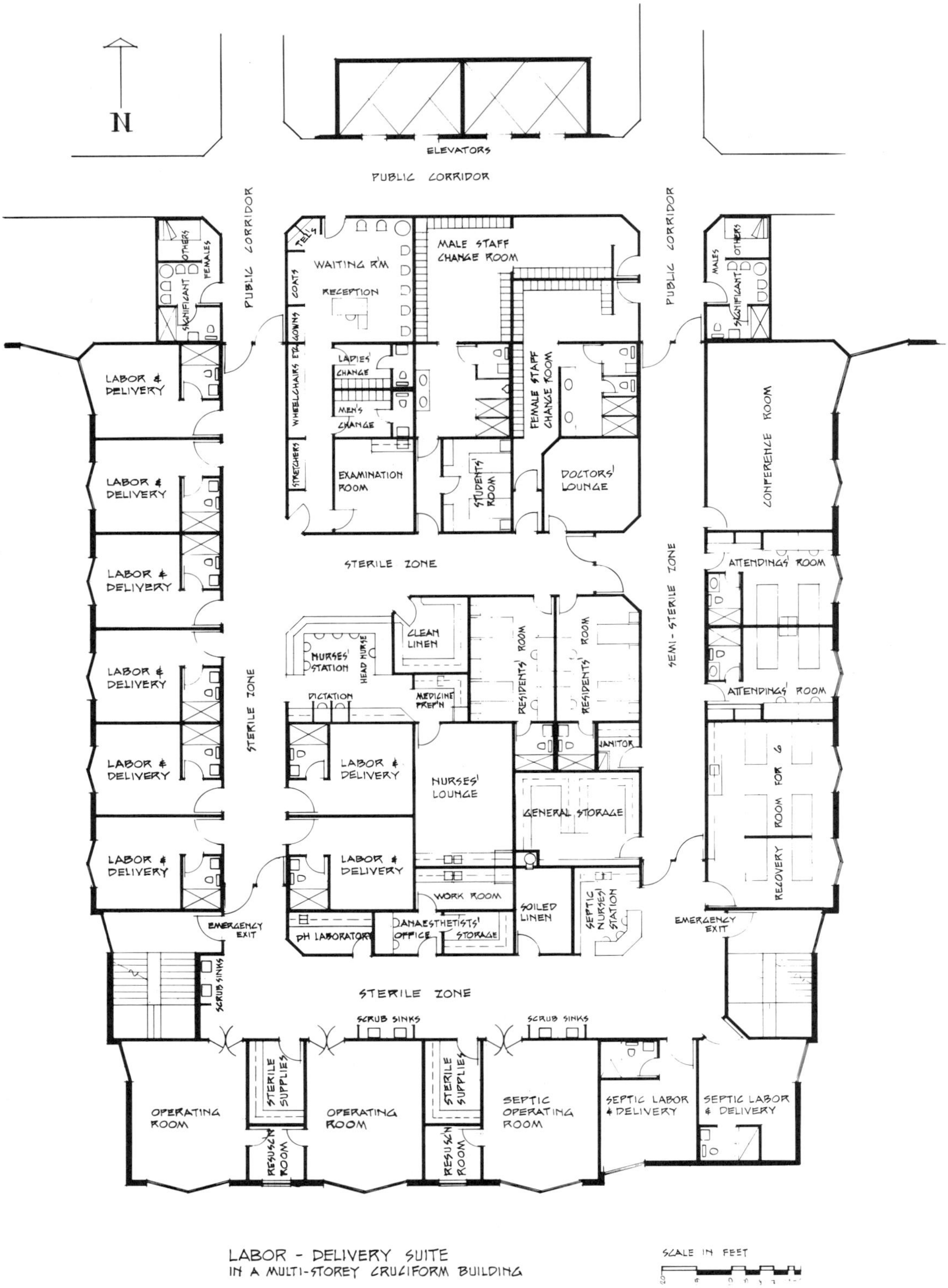

Figure 2-6 Architectural plan of a modern labor and delivery suite designed by Julian Gaspar (Hamilton, Ontario). The floor plan emphasizes traditional infection-control principles by separating sterile and semisterile areas, minimizing unnecessary movements in the obstetric unit by purposeful placement of various rooms with differing functions, and avoids the unnecessary transfer of potentially infected patients on the labor floor by offering adequate facilities, with self-contained shower and toilet facilities, for labor and delivery in the same room. Note that the flow of traffic is from sterile to semisterile to public areas whenever practical. Also note exposure to sunlight of operating and labor and delivery rooms. (Reprinted with permission from Iffy L, Apuzzio JJ, Vintzileos AM. Operative obstetrics. ed 2. New York: Pergamon Press PLC, 1992.)

The principles outlined earlier often are violated on the grounds that shortages in nursing and paramedical personnel make the implementation of infection-control measures impossible. In actual fact, insofar as effective control measures remove much of the burden associated with the care of severely ill patients, such as close surveillance and frequent dressing changes on infected wounds, rigid enforcement of infection control is extremely time- and cost-efficient.

Prevention of Obstetric Infections

In a leading 1947 textbook, the description of the epidemiology, mode of transfer, pathology, symptomatology, and prevention of puerperal fever occupied 22 printed pages. New developments induced the writers of more recent textbooks to reduce the space assigned to these subjects to a third or a fourth of what at that time had appeared essential. In this process, critically important relevant data vanished from the obstetric literature. Accordingly, some comments from DeLee and Greenhill's[15] 1947 textbook deserve reiterating:

> . . . Semmelweis distinguished two modes of inoculation: One from without, exogenous infection, and one from within, endogenous which he called autoinfection. . . . We limit the term autoinfection to those *rare* cases in which the bacteria of the genital tract, including the vulva, develop virulence and invade the tissues.
>
> . . . The [bacteria] . . . of the vulva, vestibule and vagina have the power to spread into the genital tract. . . . [However], if the woman is not molested by a meddling physician, she will almost always recover from her labor by the grace of the immunities provided by nature. While mild cases of autoinfection may occur occasionally, fatal cases are exceedingly rare.
>
> . . . exogenous infection is by far the most common and is always to be considered first when fever develops in a puerpera. . . . Most often the attending, the physician or the nurse infects the woman.
>
> . . . Some general hospitals are true cesspools of infection. . . . When an uninfected woman is taken from her home and placed in a hospital full of . . . suppurating wounds . . . the most extraordinary measures must be carried out to guarantee that she and her baby will not contract any of these infections. . .

Concerning the causes of puerperal infection, the same textbook says: "Prolonged labor, especially after rupture of the bag of waters, because of the frequent vaginal explorations. . . . Operative intervention, because of the wounds, contusions and the bacteria introduced from *without*, . . . Retention of pieces of placenta."

With regard to the preventability of puerperal infection, DeLee and Greenhill, well aware of the healing power of antibiotics presented the following opinions:

> Prevention plays a transcendently important role in puerperal infection. So much can be done by prevention that our efforts should be concentrated on asepsis and on a physiologic conduct of labor. . .
>
> Limit the number of internal examinations to an irreducible minimum [and] conduct labor as far as possible by external and rectal examinations. . . . Do not rupture the bag of waters until there is an indication for it. The membranes . . . mechanically prevent the access of bacteria to the uterus in prolonged labors.
>
> Avoid all measures to shorten the time of normal labor, such as manual dilatation of the cervix or having the woman bear down before the head has slipped through the cervix. Do not give pituitary extract to hasten delivery without a real indication.
>
> In a hospital the sick woman should be isolated . . . because of the danger of her infection causing . . . an epidemic of puerperal infection. . .

Some two decades ago, one of the authors had the opportunity of visiting the general hospital in the city of Dubrovnik, Yugoslavia, where, in a century-old building, the physicians still unfailingly maintained those infection-control measures emphasized by Semmelweis in Central Europe, Munro Kerr in Great Britain, and DeLee and Greenhill in America. In the course of rounds through the obstetric and gynecologic services, it transpired that throughout the 1960s the department maintained less than 5 percent postcesarean section and posthysterectomy infection rates. During the round, the visitor noted that not a single one of the temperature charts of approximately 20 postoperative patients displayed evidence of fever. At the same time, postoperative infections were rampant in the obstetric and gynecologic services of the hospital where he at that time worked.[36] Subsequently, to assess traditional infection-control measures in a modern perinatal unit in the same institution, with the enthusiastic participation of faculty members, a protocol was established that rigidly reintroduced the earlier described measures, all of which had been for several years abandoned. To eliminate any confounding factor, administration of prophylactic and perioperative antibiotics was discontinued in both services despite the alarming infection rate that was affecting about 80 percent of all patients who had been delivered abdominally. Unaware of the project implemented by the department, the hospital infection committee continued its regular surveillance of institutional infections and documented the ensuing results.

Although the overall effort began early in what we defined as the fifth study year, having used the previous four for comparison, all relevant actions could not be implemented at once. The enforcement of strict isolation techniques began immediately through the devoted efforts of Jeanette Lindsey, the head nurse who coordinated this effort, but the resident and nursing personnel were unfamiliar with the principles of infection control and even those of ordinary hygiene, and therefore effective implementation of aseptic techniques was delayed by 6 months or more. It required about the same length of time to convince the hospital administration to replace an old bathtub on the obstetric floor with a shower; until then, patients preparing for cesarean sections and those suffering from discharging postoperative wounds took their baths in this same tub in a random sequence, a state of affairs that would have driven Semmelweis into a rage 125 years earlier.

Reintroducing time-proven methods of infection control into a modern American perinatal center entailed overtones and undertones, some of them highly gratifying and others disappointing:

1. Through intellectual curiosity and honest interest in the welfare of the patients, almost invariably the

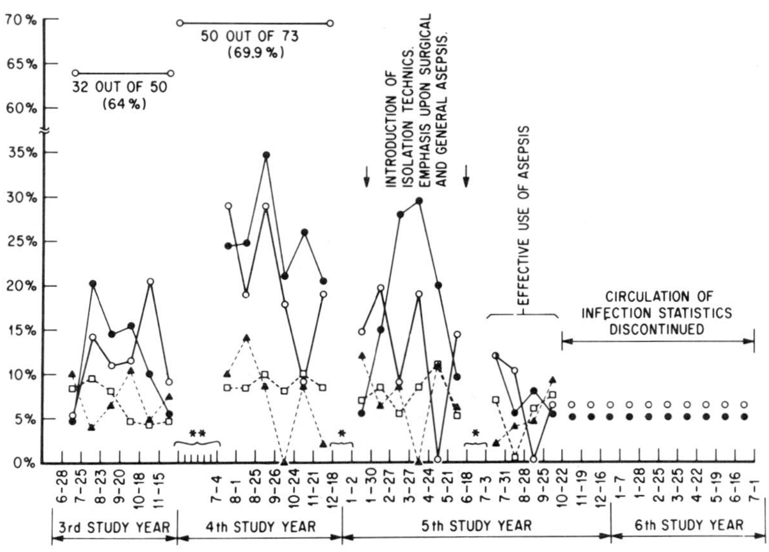

Figure 2-7 The impact of enforcement of asepsis and isolation techniques on infection rates in a department of obstetrics and gynecology. The horizontal lines in the left upper corner show "wound-related infection" rates, which include endometritis. The results are compared with infection rates in other departments (closed circles, gynecology; open circles, obstetrics; closed triangles, orthopedics; open squares, surgery; *, 2 weeks of data missing; **, no statistics available for the first 6 months of the year). Note the wide swings and opposing trends in obstetrics versus gynecology infection rates during the first half of the fifth study year. This peculiar phenomenon is attributed to the rotation of one senior resident who refused to adopt aseptic routines and infection control protocols. His rotation through the various services resulted in sharp increase in infection rates in the service that he joined and a precipitous decline in the service that he left. Infection rates remained low in both services when he finished his training in the middle of the fifth study year and left the department. (From Iffy, et al, 1979.[36])

attending and resident staff enthusiastically participated in the project and adhered to the agreed-upon infection-control measures.

2. Some physicians remained uninterested. A senior resident absolutely refused to cooperate. As a result, although the overall infection rates began to decline in both services during the fifth study year, the monthly statistics showed that infection rates abruptly increased in the service that he had joined and precipitously declined in the one that he had left. Leaving behind a dismal track record, this man left the service at the end of the academic year. From that day on, the infection rates remained low in both services (Fig. 2-7).
3. The importance of devoted and firm leadership was clearly reflected by the impact of the discipline maintained by the head nurse, who enforced the infection-control measures unfailingly.
4. The reluctance of some nurses to adjust to the new "time-consuming" requirements of infection control was a disheartening experience. However, even these nurses changed their attitude when they realized that the disappearance of postoperative infections reduced their work load.
5. There was no evidence that elimination of severe postoperative infections impressed the authorities of the institution more than those of the Lying-In Hospital in Vienna. Thus, within 2 years of the beginning of the project, for one reason or another, all key members of the infection-control project, including the head nurse, found reason to leave the hospital. As a result, postcesarean section infection rates returned to the pre-existing range (Fig. 2-8), as they did in Vienna after the departure of Ignaz Semmelweis (see Fig. 2-2).

The reduction of perinatal infections from the range of 80 percent to about 15 percent without the use of prophylactic antibiotics documented beyond a shadow of doubt that in the environment of a modern obstetric unit, traditional infection control measures were as effective as in the days of Semmelweis (see Fig. 2-3). Yet, even if the implications of this study were recognized by some,[69] the overall attitude of American obstetricians has remained unchanged. However well intended, the introduction of the concept of "universal precaution" drove the last nail into the coffin of effective infection control in the United States. The primary purpose for universal precaution was protection of medical and paramedical personnel, rather than prevention of the spread of infection from one patient to the next. Overall, the new measures aimed at the prevention of the propagation of the human immunodeficiency virus (HIV) and paid little attention to the fact that its usual transfer is different from those of most nosocomial infections. As a result, many hospitals have discarded isolation and asepsis routines and replaced them with what may be considered comparable to good general hygiene. While potentially useful for the prevention of acquired immunodeficiency syndrome (AIDS), the inability of general precaution to prevent the spread of hospital-based infections has al-

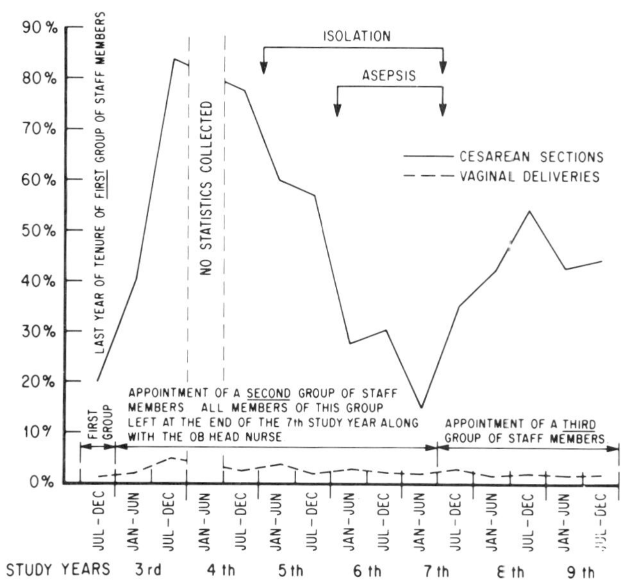

Figure 2-8 Postcesarean section infection rates in the course of eight study years projected against the major changes that occurred in the division of obstetrics of a major teaching institution. Implementation of isolation techniques and, subsequently, asepsis produced a sharp decline in postcesarean infection rates (continuous line). A similar but less dramatic decline occurred with regard to puerperal infections following vaginal deliveries (interrupted line). (From Iffy, et al, 1979.[36])

ready been documented through the unchanging infection rates in American hospitals. Indeed, against this background, prophylactic antibiotics may offer the only practical defense against life-endangering postoperative infections. This is an unfortunate state of affairs insofar as at the Statewide Perinatal Center of New Jersey we observed and documented the fact that traditional infection control measures and prophylactic use of antibiotics each have a separate and substantial impact upon the overall postoperative morbidity rates.[4] Of the two, infection control is the most important:

1. It prevents potentially dangerous and uncomfortable postoperative complications.
2. It avoids having the patient serve as a source of infection.
3. It removes the need for administering costly medication.
4. It precludes the development of antibiotic-resistant strains of microorganisms.
5. By all available data,[22,59,64] its overall impact is greater than that of prophylactic antibiotics.

Although effective infection control undoubtedly could reduce the costs of medical care nationwide by billions of dollars,[38] it does not serve the interests of the manufacturers of antibiotic agents. Accordingly, research directed at the evaluation of infection-control measures is unlikely to receive even minimal backing from pharmaceutical companies. Thus, whereas it is generally believed among both professionals and the lay public that the opportunities for infection control have been exploited fully by the medical profession, in actual fact infection control has been largely reduced to a ritualistic "scrubbing up" before operative procedures. Critically important measures such as isolation of the skin during the operation, clearly reflected in illustrations in traditional textbooks,[55] and changing of the glove following the removal of the fetus are seldom utilized by American obstetricians. The same is true for well-documented aspects of preoperative preparation.[2] Although violations are particularly prevalent among obstetricians, the concept of asepsis is also rapidly losing ground among representatives of other surgical specialties. Indeed, some of the best infection-control measures we observed in any operating room were those implemented by veterinary surgeons in facilities such as the New York Animal Hospital and the Animal Laboratory of the University of Illinois. In the latter, one of the authors performed a series of 10 extensive pelvic surgical procedures on monkeys without a single case of postoperative infection,[35] when at the same time in the gynecologic service infectious complication after abdominal surgical procedures was the rule.[36] This experience contradicts the generally voiced misconception, not shared by experts of the preantibiotic era,[15] that the usual source of infection following gynecologic surgery is the genital flora of the patient. This interpretation was clearly ruled out by the earlier quoted study concerning "traditional preventive measures."[36] It was found that throughout the several study years obstetric and gynecologic nosocomial infections ran a parallel course; each of them rapidly declining when infection-control measures were enforced and increasing again when effective preventive measures were abandoned (Fig. 2-9). From this, the following conclusion appears justified:

> The close parallel course of the infections in the two divisions, attended by the same medical personnel, suggests that throughout the 9 years of the review most nosocomial

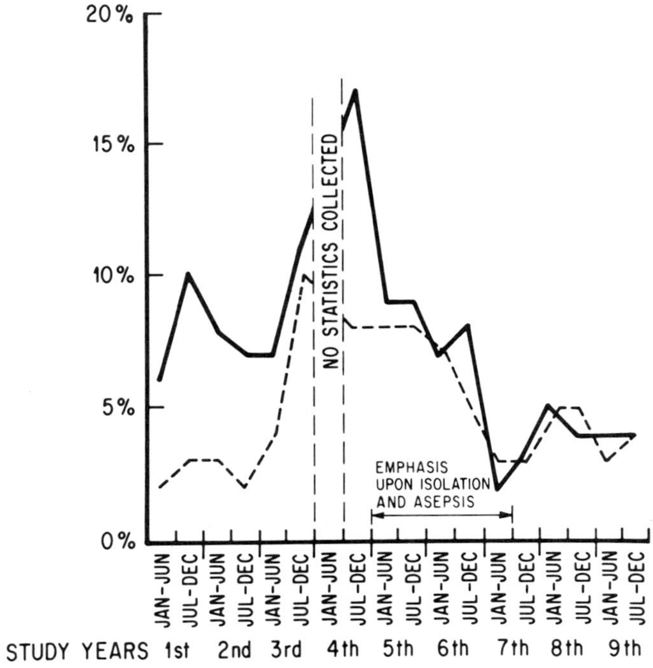

Figure 2-9 A 9-year review of all nosocomial infections in a department of obstetrics and gynecology (based on the statistics of the hospital infection committee). Note the parallel trends of the infection curves representing the obstetric (solid line) and the gynecologic (interrupted line) divisions. The similarity and the rapid decrease in infection rates during the time of emphasis upon isolation and asepsis suggest identical sources or spread by identical means of infection in the two services. The same finding contradicts the contention that obstetric and gynecologic infections, in general, are attributable to the endogenous bacterial flora of the patients. (From Iffy, et al, 1979.[36])

infections were caused by preventable [external] factors not unlike those in the Vienna-Lying-in-Hospital prior to 1840, when the students brought back the deadly contagium from the morgue to the second divisions of the obstetric service.

In the *Aetiologie,* Semmelweis strongly rejected the perception of contemporary physicians, namely, that the reason for the high rate of infection in city hospitals catering to poor patients resulted from the impaired state of health and inadequate standard of hygiene of the population.[64] His investigations indicated unequivocally that the high rate of infection was due to external factors under the control of the medical and paramedical personnel of the hospital.[8]

Role of Obstetricians in Nosocomial Infections

The magnitude of the problem created by nosocomial infections in American hospitals is indicated by the finding that by the 1970s, 5 to 7 percent of all hospitalized patients developed nosocomial infections.[1,28] Based on various calculations[1,65] the yearly costs of patients suffering from hospital-acquired infections could be anywhere between $5 and 30 billion. The rate of infections in obstetric practice has shown a sharper increase than those experienced in other surgical specialties.[1] By the 1970s, postcesarean section infection rates rose to disturbing proportions ranging between 20 and 80 percent in various teaching institutions.[1,4,14,20,24,26,38,60] Although more alarming in the United States than elsewhere, the phenomenon obviously is worldwide.[7,27,33,62,66,72] Because resistant strains of microorganisms almost invariably develop within a few years after the introduction of new antibiotics,[21] obviously prevention of puerperal, postoperative, and other nosocomial infections cannot rest on the use of prophylactic or therapeutic antibiotics. Conceptually, the use of prophylactic antibiotics resembles that of "antisepsis" insofar as it tends to destroy microorganisms that have already gained access to the wound rather than preventing the contamination. Although relatively effective in individual cases, the increasing number of wound infections throughout the world indicates that antibiotics do not provide an answer to the overall problem. The same conclusion derives from the recent epidemic increase of venereal infections that shows clearly that advocates of the sexual revolution in the 1960s erroneously assumed that antibiotics had solved the problem of venereal diseases.

Of all available infection-control measures, handwashing by medical and paramedical personnel is probably the most important.[51] Relevant investigations have shown that soap and water are only moderately effective when the hands are heavily contaminated. However, antiseptic agents such as chlorhexidine are eminently successful in suppressing pathogenic microorganisms, although disinfectant agents may be counterproductive if they damage the integrity of the skin through chemical irritation. In this eventuality, the likelihood of colonization by pathogenic microorganisms may actually increase.[10,30]

An important and often ignored principle is the exclusion from the care of obstetric patients of personnel suffering from tonsillitis, pharyngitis, boils, skin diseases, and other potentially contagious conditions. This rule also applies to cleaners, orderlies, delivery personnel, and visitors.

Critically important is the availability of separate bathrooms and toilets with appropriate handwashing facilities for patients. We have noted that when unexpected expenditures necessitate changing hospital building plans, predictably the financial difficulties are solved by eliminating toilets, showers, and bathrooms. This trend ensures that by the time of their opening, even modern and well-planned hospitals are reduced to uncontrollable cesspools of filth and disease.

Before the antibiotic era, it was documented conclusively that rectal examinations carried substantially less risk of contaminating the amniotic cavity than vaginal ones.[42] The profession has paid little attention to the fact that through properly controlled investigations the validity of this conclusion has been confirmed in the environments of modern perinatal units.[62] The same is supported strongly by the fact that at the hospital of the University of Debrecen in Hungary, where rectal examinations are routine, postcesarean infections were at the range of 5 percent in the early 1980s versus up to 50 percent at the Statewide Perinatal Center in Newark, where vaginal examinations were routine.[37] Results based on many decades of research indicating that vaginal examinations carried higher risks than rectal ones were dismissed in the United States on the ground of a modest study by Prystowsky,[61] who in 1954 in the low-risk environment of a U.S. Army hospital found no difference in infection risks between patients managed with vaginal versus rectal examinations. The acceptance of the results of this investigation rested upon obstetricians' unawareness of the fact that the documentation of statistical significance in infection control hinges upon certain preliminary conditions:

1. In order to show difference between two techniques of infection control, all other sources of infection must be effectively controlled.
2. In an environment where infection is not prevalent, there will be little if any difference between the effects of vaginal and rectal examinations.
3. When the environment is heavily contaminated and infection control measures are slack, the rate of infection is bound to be high, irrespective of the method of intrapartum examinations.

Indeed, when quoting the Debrecen-versus-Newark infection rates,[37] it is fair to concede that the difference cannot be attributed to methods of intrapartum examination alone. Most likely, vast differences in the overall standards of infection control are responsible for the diverse results, and the type of examination accounts for them only in part.

A series of investigations has provided unequivocal proof that the development of chorioamnionitis is directly related to the number of vaginal examinations and the time interval between the first examination and the eventual delivery.[5,22] Insistence on frequent vaginal examinations during the labor process ignores this well-recognized principle and exchanges a negligible advantage for a highly predictable danger in terms of intrapartum, puerperal, and postoperative infections.

It is not generally known to hospital personnel that an ordinary shower bath, if anything, increases rather than reduces the likelihood of postoperative infection. By contrast, use of a powerful antiseptic solution has been shown to reduce postoperative infections substantially.[9]

Surgical Aseptic Techniques

The fact that the overall process of labor seldom extends beyond 14 to 16 hours in modern institutions has reduced both the frequency and the severity of puerperal fever following vaginal deliveries substantially. With the ever-increasing rate of cesarean sections, the most frequent and most precarious infectious complications follow cesarean sections. Thus it readily follows that the development of postsurgical infections requires special attention.

Recent textbooks[60] disregard the long-established principle, still emphasized by Eastman and Hellman[17] some three decades ago, that the danger of peritonitis can be reduced substantially by covering the uterine incision wound (almost invariably the primary site of postoperative infection) by the bladder peritoneum. Surgeons before the antibiotic era were painfully aware of the dangers involved with the spread of infection into the peritoneal cavity. Reassured by the protection provided by prophylactic and therapeutic antibiotics, contemporary surgeons tend to ignore these time-proven preventive surgical methods.

The method of performance of the operation itself has a considerable bearing upon the likelihood of infection. The long-established method of draping the skin with sterile towels as early as practical during the operative procedure has never lost its importance. It has been documented that the use of plastic adhesive drapes is not useful in preventing infection.[13] It appears likely that the use of such a barrier generates heat, opens the pores, and by inducing sweating causes spread of microorganisms onto the skin and into the wound.

Preoperative skin preparation reduces the microbial count of the skin. Apart from facilitating the work of the surgeon, shaving serves no useful purpose; if it entails microinjuries to the skin, it is detrimental.

The time of shaving of the skin has considerable bearing upon the likelihood of postoperative wound infection. Ideally, it should be performed immediately before the operation and should be followed by gentle scrubbing of the skin with antibacterial solution for 5 minutes. Thereafter, the skin should be dried before the initial incision is made.

Available data show that the length of the hospitalization prior to the performance of an operation has a positive relationship with the likelihood of postoperative infection.[35]

Close attention to aseptic principles during the performance of the operative procedure is essential. The

Table 2-3 Care of Patients with Postoperative or Postpartum Infection

1. Before handling the patient or changing the dressing on the wound, wash your hands and put on sterile gloves.
2. Remove soiled dressings with instruments, and place them into disposable plastic bags.
3. Remove the soiled gloves, and wash your hands again.
4. Put on sterile gloves and clean the wound with sterile material, beginning at the center and moving outward.
5. Place sterile dressing onto the wound.
6. Discard gloves and place all waste material into sealed plastic bags.
7. Discard the gown worn during contact with the patient.
8. Wash your hands thoroughly with antiseptic solution.

Table 2-4 Postoperative and Postpartum Patients Requiring Isolation

Puerpera with recurrent episode of fever exceeding 100.4° F
Postoperative patients with cellulitis
Postpartum patient with odorous vaginal discharge or running fever of unknown origin postpartum
Patients with discharging wounds
Patients with drains
Patients with pulmonary infections involving productive cough

gloves of the surgeons should not touch the skin at any time, even after the disinfection of the skin with antiseptic solution. Spillage of amniotic fluid at the time of the uterine incision should be prevented, as far as practical, by placement of well-wrung wet towels into the gutters and, when the amniotic fluid is suspected to be infected, by placement of dry towels around the incision. After the removal of the fetus, the surgeon should change the glove that reached down to the lower uterine segment or the vaginal vault. Similarly, the glove that removes the placenta must be changed if the membranes have been ruptured for any length of time prior to the performance of the operation.

Whereas the draining of abscesses found during the operative procedure may be absolutely necessary, use of a drain in the absence of pre-existing infection increases the postoperative infection rate.[13]

Contamination of the air in the operating room is generally proportional to the number of people present. Obviously, unnecessary personnel and "significant others" should not be allowed in the operating room. Furthermore, contamination of the air is higher when members of the surgical team talk than when they are silent. Accordingly, unnecessary discussions in the course of the operation must be avoided.

The urinary tract is often the site of hospital-acquired infections. The most frequent reason for such infection is catheterization or prolonged use of an indwelling catheter. A dangerous and relatively frequent cause of infection is the elevation of the collecting bottle above the level of the bladder during the positioning of the patient on the operating table or her removal at the end of the surgery, thus creating a highly dangerous backflow.

Intravenous catheters are a recognized source of infection. The catheter and its site should be changed every 48 hours. In recent practice, a relatively frequent and dangerous source of infection is the catheter used for intravenous hyperalimentation. In related infections, the offending agent frequently is *Candida albicans*.

It is generally agreed that the number and thickness of sutures is directly related to the likelihood of wound infection. Natural fiber sutures appear to propagate infection more than synthetic material.

The postoperative patient displaying evidence of infection is a dangerous source of pathogenic microorganisms. Therefore special nurses with no duties in antepartum and intrapartum floors should be assigned to the care of such patients. The back-and-forth movement of resident physicians between postpartum floors and labor and delivery areas is an objectionable practice that carries substantial infection risks. Lack of attention to this important feature of infection control plays a substantial role in the high postcesarean infection rates in many hospitals.

The precautionary measures required during the care of infected postoperative patients is summarized in Table 2-3. The entities that require strict isolation on the obstetric floor are presented in Table 2-4.

Infectious Agents: Changing Trends

Recent data from the Centers for Disease Control (CDC) appear to indicate that the earlier observed national incidence of nosocomial infections remained essentially the same in the last decade.[29] Postpartum infection is one of the most important causes of hospital-acquired infections and a leading cause of maternal mortality and morbidity. In the past, group A streptococcus, the microorganism initially identified by Pasteur,[58] was the most common offender in puerperal sepsis. It has been long recognized that the infection was most often acquired in the hospital environment.[53] However, the relative frequency of puerperal sepsis due to the group

Table 2-5 Measures Utilized for the Prevention of Streptococcal Infections

Appropriate cultures must be obtained from affected mothers and neonates (lochia, blood, umbilical stump, etc.). The patients are to be isolated and treated aggressively with appropriate antibiotics.
Nasal and oropharyngeal cultures must be obtained from all hospital personnel in contact with obstetric patients and newborns.
Cultures must be obtained at regular intervals from hospital equipment, fomites, and the general environment.
Enforcement of aseptic protocols must be reviewed and reemphasized.
Elective procedures, such as circumcision of the newborn, must be canceled.
Evaluation of epidemiologic data for a common vector must be undertaken.

A streptococcus has declined. Women infected by this organism tend to develop high fevers, chills, and flushing of the skin usually within 24 to 48 hours after delivery. Accompanied by parametrial tenderness, the infection presents with copious amounts of odorless, serosanguinous lochia.

It was already known to Semmelweis that maternal infection often is replicated in the neonate, who exhibits signs and symptoms of sepsis and in severe cases septic shock. When a group A streptococcus infection is diagnosed, the measures outlined in Table 2-5 must be implemented vigorously.

In contemporary obstetric practice, group B streptococcus (GBS) and *Escherichia coli* are considered as the most important pathogens causing neonatal infections. GBS has been long known to exist in the gastrointestinal tract of cattle and was identified as a cause of bovine mastitis in 1937. Although the microorganism was cultured occasionally from human beings, only in the early 1970s did it emerge as a major cause of neonatal mortality and morbidity. Since then, numerous investigators have confirmed the role of GBS in both neonatal sepsis and maternal infections. Of the numerous varieties of GBS identified by Lancefield and others, type III is frequently associated with both early and late types of neonatal sepsis.[41] It is generally felt that the explosive increase in the rate of neonatal GBS infections is closely related to the explosive increase in the number of GBS-carrying mothers in the general population. According to current data, in many American communities as many as 10 to 20 percent of all pregnant women carry GBS in the lower genital tract, the anorectal region, or the urine, the exact rate depending on the number of sites cultured and the types of culture media used. The presence of GBS in the maternal genital tract exposes the fetus to the risk of colonization and, on some occasions, to the development of invasive disease. In the perinatal services of the Statewide Perinatal Center, Newark, we repeatedly encountered regretful neonatal losses in recent years from GBS infection. On more than one occasion, we had reason to suspect that the port of entry for the microorganism was the site of insertion of the internal scalp electrode.

Vertical transmission rates of GBS from mother to fetus range from 40 to 72 percent when the mother is culture positive, compared to 8 percent in neonates born to culture-negative mothers. The incidence of manifest neonatal disease is in the range of 0.2 to 0.4 percent with a mortality rate of 50 percent.[43] GBS can also be a nosocomial pathogen in neonatal nurseries. However, GBS rarely presents with an epidemic outbreak. Therefore, it is currently held that culture-positive infants do not need to be isolated in the neonatal nursery, a concept we consider dubious.

A recent report gave an account of an epidemic outbreak of puerperal sepsis caused by group C streptococci (GCS).[67] The microorganism was cultured from 23 puerperas in the course of 5 weeks. The relevant investigation concluded that the spread of the infection was largely attributable to the personnel in charge of the obstetric unit, many of whom carried GCS in the throat. Other sources of the infection were thought to be toilets and bathrooms. The epidemic ended only when the department was closed. Literary data indicate that a broad variety of microorganisms are capable of causing puerperal sepsis. Occasional reports quote a variety of previously unconsidered microorganisms, such as group G streptococcus,[32] *Mycoplasma hominis*,[71] *Chlamydia trachomatis*,[39] and others. Meanwhile, despite the increasing prominence of numerous alternative causative agents, occasional outbreaks of group A streptococcus epidemics in obstetric units are still reported.[12] There is every reason to believe that with increasing use of antibiotics and development of more and more resistant strains, the profile of causative agents will continue changing with increasing rapidity unless the medical profession interrupts the vicious circle by introducing effective preventive measures, as was done in many parts of the world during the preantibiotic era and is still done in some institutions in continental Europe.

Projections and Trends

Although the medical profession prefers to remember its history in terms of progress and achievements,[50] a comprehensive and well-balanced recollection must induce members of the profession to recall its failures and fallacies throughout the centuries. Contemporary authorities are readily willing to agree that some highly respected medical authorities of bygone ages were dangerous charlatans. It is not customary to concede, however, that shortsightedness and intellectual dishonesty are just as prevalent today as they were centuries ago.

We contend that abandonment of nineteenth-century discoveries concerning infection control by physicians of the late twentieth century is one of the greatest setbacks that the science of medicine has ever suffered. Blinded by the apparent security of new antibiotics and by a flood of misleading articles sponsored by their manufacturers, the medical profession has largely abandoned time-proven infection-control measures and tolerates postoperative and puerperal infection rates that were unheard of in the practices of self-respecting surgeons in the preantibiotic era.

It is amazing that in an age where exchange of information between continents occurs in seconds, the fact that many European centers have postcesarean and other postoperative infection rates under 5 percent virtually never reaches the pages of leading American journals and textbooks. The gratuitous notion that the catastrophic infection rate observed in hospitals derives from the poor hygienic habits of the patient population is widely voiced, despite the fact that the studies of Ignaz Semmelweis and Munro Kerr indicate unequivocally that the significance of this factor is modest.

Having failed to indoctrinate physicians and nurses about the overwhelming importance of traditional infection-control measures, the CDC elected to introduce a new concept,[11] "universal precautions." Regretfully, this approach fails to take into account that already established measures of isolation and asepsis have proven to be extremely effective. Thus they need to be supplemented, rather than replaced, by a new approach. Not surprisingly, after a few years of experience, it has already been noted that the technique of universal precautions, while extremely expensive, had only a marginal impact upon institutional infection rates.[16]

It is readily conceded that in the science of medicine there are no final words and that established principles inevitably lead to the discovery of new ones. It is not proposed, therefore, that isolation and asepsis represent the ultimate stage in infection control and that further progress is inconceivable. It is suggested, however, that any future effort directed at the elimination of infections must rest upon already established facts concerning infection control. The critical investigations with regard to this concept of necessity occurred before the antibiotic era. The research conducted at that time cannot be ignored or replaced by new investigations undertaken against the background of a widely conceded abuse of antibiotic agents. The public interest requires reduction of the use of antibiotics as far as possible, a concept that is not likely to obtain backing from the manufacturers. It is the task of physicians uncommitted to industrial research to reintroduce stringent preventive measures into the practice of medicine and the functions of hospitals.

The principles of infection control are not complicated. They require the perception that invisible pathologic microorganisms are everywhere in the hospital environment. Understanding this fact makes it possible for health care personnel at all levels of function to conduct their activities in a manner that does not expose their patients or themselves to the risk of infection. The implementation of effective infection-control measures requires no new research. In fact, relevant research is meaningless in an environment where the sources of infection are multiple and effective infection control is nonexistent.

The authors have opined in the past that the use of invasive procedures in a heavily contaminated hospital milieu is generally detrimental.[35,57] Only in an environment with impeccable infection-control measures can invasive techniques, such as intrauterine pressure monitoring, scalp electrodes, and scalp blood sampling, carry a favorable risk-benefit ratio. Emphasis upon such technology in heavily contaminated hospitals can only translate into catastrophic sequelae in terms of maternal and neonatal morbidity and mortality rates.

Given that cesarean sections and other surgical procedures are being performed with infection-control measures alone in many European institutions with negligible infection rates, it readily follows that the achievable target for American obstetric surgeons with the availability of prophylactic antibiotics is in the range of 2 to 3 percent. Acceptance of results that fall short of this target should be looked upon as a monumental failure on the part of late-twentieth-century perinatologists in achieving a goal that should be well within reach. The thought that future centuries are likely to look upon us as the professional brethren of Kline, Scanzoni, and Meigs rather than Holmes, Semmelweis, and Kerr should be a heavy burden on the shoulders of those of us who take pride in our professional reputation and standing.

References

1. Allen JR. Nosocomial obstetric infections and hospital epidemiology. In: Iffy L, Charles D, eds. Operative perinatology. New York: Macmillan, 1984.
2. Apuzzio JJ, Ganesh V. Principles of aseptic technique. In: Iffy L, Charles D, eds. Operative perinatology. New York: Macmillan, 1984:79–85.
3. Apuzzio JJ, Iffy L. Perinatal infection control. In: Keith LG, ed. Infections in reproductive health, common infections. Vol 1. Lancaster, England: MTP Press, 1988:171–184.
4. Apuzzio JJ, Iffy L, Cohen-Addad N. Relationship between changing obstetric philosophies and perinatal mortality rates. In: Gati I, ed. Recent progress in perinatal medicine. Vol 5. Budapest: Postgraduate Medical University Publication, 1987: 28–32.
5. Apuzzio JJ, Reyelt C, Pelosi M, et al. Prophylactic antibiotics for cesarean section: comparison of high- and low-risk patients for endomyometritis. Obstet Gynecol 1982; 59:693–698.
6. Baeder A. The roots of traditional midwifery. In: Iffy L, Kaminetzky HA, eds. Principles and practice of obstetrics and perinatology. New York: John Wiley & Sons, 1981:1797–1811.
7. Bernard A, Gimes G. Csaszarmetszes utani lazas lazas szovodmenyek okainak vizsgalata. Magyar Nöorvosok Lapja 1986; 49:146–150.
8. Bondiner E. Semmelweis: the lone rager against puerperal fever. Hosp Prac [Off] 1987; 22:194–210.
9. Brandberg A, Holm J, Hammarstem J. Post-operative wound infections in vascular surgery: effect of pre-operative whole body disinfection by shower bath with chlorhexidine soap. In: Newson SWB, Caldwell ABS, eds. Problems in the control of hospital infection. London: The Royal Society of Medicine, 1980:71–73.

10. Casewell MW. The role of hand disinfection in specific problems of today. In: Newson SWB, Caldwell ADS, eds. Problems in the control of hospital infections. London: The Royal Society of Medicine, 1980:23–27.
11. Centers for Disease Control. Recommendations for prevention of HIV transmission in health care settings. MMWR 1987; 36:535.
12. Claesson BEP, Claesson ULE. An outbreak of endometritis in a maternity unit caused by spread of group A streptococci from a showerhead. J Hosp Infect 1985; 6:304–311.
13. Cruse BJE, Foord R. A 5 year prospective study of 23,649 surgical wounds. Arch Surg 1973; 107:206–210.
14. D'Angelo LJ, Sokol RJ. Time-related peripartum determinants of postpartum morbidity. Obstet Gynecol 1980; 55:319–323.
15. DeLee JB, Greenhill JP. Principles and practices of obstetrics. Ed 9. Philadelphia: WB Saunders, 1947:775–814.
16. Doebbeling BN, Wenzel RP. The direct cost of universal precautions in a teaching hospital. JAMA 1990; 264:2083–2087.
17. Eastman N, Hellman LM. Williams Obstetrics. Ed 12. New York: Appleton-Century-Crofts, 1961:1190.
18. Editorial: Puerperal fever today. JAMA 1968; 206:367.
19. Editorial: London Times Literary Supplement, October 26, 1933.
20. Farrell SJ, Andersen HF, Work BA. Cesarean section: indications and postoperative morbidity. Obstet Gynecol 1980; 56:696–700.
21. Finland M. And the walls come tumbling down. More antibiotic resistance and now the pneumococcus. N Engl J Med 1978; 299:770–771.
22. Gaspar J. Architectural design of an obstetric perinatal unit. In: Iffy L, Kaminetzky HA, eds. Principles and practice of obstetrics and perinatology. New York: John Wiley & Sons, 1981:1729–1731.
23. Gaspar J, Kaminetzky HA, Powell J, Iffy L. Architectural design of labor and delivery unit and control of infection. In: Iffy L, Charles D, eds. Operative perinatology. New York: Macmillan, 1984: 73–78.
24. Goldner WL, Brown RB, Lundy LE, Bradley S. Infections in an obstetric and gynecological hospital. J Reprod Med 1980; 25:145–149.
25. Gordon A. Treaties of the epidemic puerperal fever of Aberdeen. London: Grant J. Robinson, 1795.
26. Green SL, Sorubbi FA. Risk factors associated with postcesarean section febrile morbidity. Obstet Gynecol 1977; 49:686–690.
27. Guldholt I, Espersen T. Maternal febrile morbidity after cesarean section. Acta Obstet Gynecol Scand 1987; 66:675–679.
28. Haley RW. Guideline for prevention of catheter-associated urinary tract infections and guideline ranking scheme. Springfield, VA: National Technical Information Service, US Department of Commerce, 1981:1.
29. Haley RW, Culver DH, White JW, et al. The efficacy of infection surveillance and control programs in preventing nosocomial infections in US hospitals. Am J Epidemiol 1985; 121:182–205.
30. Hall R. Degerming the hands of surgeons and nurses. In: Newson SWB, Caldwell ADS, eds. Problems in the control of hospital infection. London: The Royal Society of Medicine, 1980: 29–38.
31. Hamilton A. Treaties of midwifery. London, 1781.
32. Haynes J, Anderson AW, Spence WN. An outbreak of puerperal fever caused by group G streptococci. J Hosp Infect 1987; 9:120–125.
33. Hockuli E. Infektionen in der Geburtshilfe und Gynäkologie. Gynäkol Rundsch 1976; 16:S52–55.
34. Holmes OW. The contagiousness of puerperal fever. N Engl Quart J Med Surg 1842–1843; 1:503–550.
35. Iffy L, Caterini H, Arrata WSM, et al. Vaginal transposition of the ovary in primates. (Papio Cynocephalus and Macaca Arctoides) Australian and New Zealand Journal of Obstetrics and Gynaecology 1978; 18:76–81.
36. Iffy L, Kaminetzky HA, Maidman JE, et al. Control of perinatal infection by traditional preventive measures. Obstet Gynecol 1979; 54:403–411.
37. Iffy L, Lampe L, Mera Z. Infection control in obstetrics. In: Iffy L, Charles D, eds. Operative perinatology. New York: Macmillan, 1984:86–99.
38. Iffy L, Wecht CH. Medical-legal aspects of perinatal and surgical infections. In: Wecht CH, ed. Legal medicine. Philadelphia: WB Saunders, 1980:149–185.
39. Ismail MA, Moawad AH, Poon E, Henderson C. Role of *Chlamydia trachomatis* in postpartum endometritis. J Reprod Med 1987; 32:280–286.
40. Jewett JF, Reid DE, Safon LE, Easterday CL. Childbed fever: a continuing entity. JAMA 1968; 206:344–350.
41. Johnson GR, Galask RP. Group B streptococci disease. Clin Obstet Gynecol 1983; 10:105–121.
42. Kerr JM. Maternal mortality and morbidity. Edinburg: E & S Livingstone, 1933.
43. Kleun S, Cuna M. Nosocomial group B streptococcal infection control. Hospital Epidemiology 1989; 10 475–478.
44. Kunin CM. Hospital sepsis. Deerfield, Ill: Medcom, 1972.
45. Lea AWW. Puerperal infection. London: Henry Frowde, Oxford University Press, 1910.
46. Leake J. Practical observations in childbed fever, 1772.
47. Ledger WJ. Postpartum endomyometritis: contemporary clinical approaches. Perspectives and Problems in OB/GYN 1986; 2:2–9.
48. Lister J. On the antiseptic principle in the practice of surgery. Br Med J 1867; 2:246.
49. Loudon I. Puerperal fever, the streptococcus and the sulphonamides 1911–1945. Br Med J 1987; 295:485–490.
50. Lyons AS, Petricelli RJ. Medicine: an illustrated history. New York: HN Abrams, 1978.
51. Maki DG, Alvarado CJ, Hassemer CA, Zilz MA. Nosocomial infections. N Engl J Med 1983; 308:1540 (letter).

52. Mauriceau F. Traité dès Maladies des Femmes Grosses, et Accouchées. Paris, Chez l'Auteur, 1668.
53. McGregor J, Ott A, Villard M. An epidemic of child bed fever fetus. Am J Obstet Gynecol 1984; 150:385–388.
54. Meigs JG. Puerperal fever and 19th century contagionism: the obstetrician's dilemma. Trans Stud Coll Physicians Phila 1975; 42:273–280.
55. Merger R, Levy J, Malchior J. Precis d'obstetrique, Paris, Masson, 1977:555.
56. Moir JC. Munro Kerr's operative obstetrics. Ed 7. London, Balliere, Tindall & Cox, 1964.
57. Nimmo RA, Murphy GA, Adhate A, et al. Factors affecting perinatal mortality in an urban center. J Natl Med Assoc 1991; 83:127-152.
58. Pasteur L. Sur la fièvre puerperale. De l'extension de la theorie dès germes à l'etiologie de quelques maladies communes. Bull Acad Natl Med 1880; 9:435.
59. Pauerstein CJ. Clinical obstetrics. New York: John Wiley & Sons, 1987:752–756.
60. Pritchard JA, MacDonald PC. Williams obstetrics. Ed 16. New York: Appleton-Century-Crofts, 1980.
61. Prystowsky H. Is the danger of vaginal examination in labor overestimated? Am J Obstet Gynecol 1954; 68:639–644.
62. Rehu M, Nilsson CG. Risk factors for febrile morbidity associated with cesarean section. Obstet Gynecol 1980; 56:269–273.
63. Reid DE. Lethal intrauterine infection. In: Charles D, Finland M, eds. Obstetric and perinatal infections. Philadephia: Lea & Febiger, 1973:519–528.
64. Semmelweis IP. Die Aetiologie, der Begriff und der Prophylaxis des Kindbettfiebers. Pest, Wien und Leipzig, CA Hartleben Verlag 1861.
65. Spengler RF, Greenough WB. Hospital costs and mortality attributed to nosocomial infection. JAMA 1978; 240:2455–2458.
66. Suonio S, Saarikoski S, Vohlonen I. Risk factors for fever, endometritis and wound infection after abdominal delivery. Int J Gynaecol Obstet 1989; 29:135–142.
67. Teare EL, Smithson RD, Efstration A, et al. An outbreak of puerperal fever caused by group C streptococci. J Hosp Infect 1989; 13:337–347.
68. Thompson JC. Microbes or medicos? Kingston Health Chronicle 1949; 21:65–70.
69. Willson JR. The conquest of cesarean section-related infections: a progress report. Obstet Gynecol 1988; 72:519–532.
70. Woodbury RM. Maternal mortality. In: The risk of death in childbirth and from all diseases caused by pregnancy and confinement. Bull 158. Washington: US Dept of Labor, Children Bureau, 1926.
71. Young MJ, Cox RA. Near fatal puerperal fever due to *Mycoplasma hominis*. Postgrad Med J 1990; 66:147–149.
72. Zoltan I, Horvath S, Illei G. Lázas szövödmények császármetszés után. Orv Hetil 1975; 116:1532–1534.

CHAPTER 3

Pneumonia

John G. Bartlett, M.D.

Pneumonia is commonly considered the most serious acute infectious disease in industrialized and underdeveloped countries. Although it is a relatively uncommon complication of pregnancy, it may be a formidable problem in terms of determining the etiologic agent and the selection of appropriate antibiotic treatment. Incidence rates have been recently reported at 25 per 32,179 (1 per 1,400) deliveries; this infection was significantly associated with maternal medical complications and with preterm delivery. The majority of obstetric patients who acquire their infection in the community have the same spectrum of pathogens that are encountered by young, previously healthy adults with pneumonia. However, some pneumonic infections such as aspiration, influenza, and varicella pneumonia seem to be more frequent, more severe or both in this patient population. An increasing number of obstetric patients have the compounding problem of human immunodeficiency virus (HIV) infection, which requires consideration of the full spectrum of pulmonary complications in the host with compromised cell-mediated immunity in this population as well. The approach for this discussion is consideration of the obstetrical patient in four settings: (1) community-acquired pneumonia in the immunocompetent host, (2) patients with aspiration pneumonia complicating obstetric anesthesia, (3) hospital-acquired pneumonia, and (4) pneumonia in the obstetric patient with HIV infection.

Community-Acquired Pneumonia in the Immunocompetent Host

Clinical Presentation

The classic features of pneumonia are cough, dyspnea, fever, and sputum production. Findings with physical examination vary, depending on the pathologic changes and stage of disease in which the patient is evaluated. However, the usual findings with lobar pneumonia are tactile fremitus, percussion dullness, bronchial breath sounds, and whispered pectoriloquy. With bronchopneumonia, the findings for consolidation may be observed, but the most frequent finding is simply crackles. Laboratory studies considered fundamental in diagnostic evaluation of patients with suspected pneumonia include a chest x-ray and complete blood count. The chest x-ray is a pivotal exam because virtually all patients with pneumonitis have infiltrates and the etiologic agent in such cases is generally treatable with antimicrobial agents. By contrast, the same symptoms with a negative chest x-ray usually indicate a viral respiratory tract infection. The peripheral leukocyte count is usually 8,000 to 20,000 per cubic millimeter (mm^3), which does not help to distinguish likely agents or even with the separation of viral versus bacterial pathogens. Leukocyte counts of less than 4,000 per mm^3 or counts exceeding 25,000 per mm^3, x-rays showing multilobe involvement, and severe systemic toxicity are all viewed as indicators of severe or life-threatening pneumonia.

Microbiologic Studies

The utility of expectorated sputum samples for identifying common bacterial pathogens has been the subject of considerable controversy because of the frequency of both false-positive and false-negative results with routine methods to cultivate expectorated sputum.[26] The most realistic method to prove the quality of this work is with cytologic screening of specimens to ensure that the material obtained reflects secretions that originate in the lower airways without excessive salivary contamination.[2] The best specimens are physician-procured expectorated sputum samples obtained prior to antibiotic treatment. Once antibiotics have been started, the opportunity to obtain valid specimens from the respiratory tract is notably diminished. The utility of Gram's stain

Table 3-1 Community-Acquired Pneumonia in Previously Healthy Adults

	Common	Uncommon
Detected with routine culture of expectorated sputum	*Streptococcus pneumoniae* *Haemophilus influenzae*	*Moraxella catarrhalis* *Staphylococcus aureus* Group A beta-hemolytic streptococci Gram-negative bacilli *Neisseria meningitidis*
Atypical pneumonia	*Mycoplasma pneumoniae* Anaerobic bacteria *Chlamydia pneumoniae* Influenza virus *Legionella* sp. *Pneumocystis carinii*	*Coxiella* *Chlamydia psittaci* *Nocardia* Fungi Viruses: respiratory syncytial, parainfluenza, adenovirus Tuberculosis

for providing accurate and immediate information of diagnostic value is a separate issue. Most authorities feel that this exercise is useful, providing the specimens are carefully obtained and that interpretation is done by an experienced observer.[5]

Etiologic Agents

A list of microbes that are potentially responsible for community-acquired pneumonia in the healthy adult including pregnant women is legion, but the number that are implicated with frequency is a relatively short list (Table 3-1). For practical purposes, the approach here is based on microbiologic studies of expectorated sputum because this is the only specimen of diagnostic value that is obtained in the majority of cases. The organism that is most frequently detected with this specimen is *Streptococcus pneumoniae;* less frequent is *Haemophilus influenza*, and relatively rare pathogens are *Moraxella catarrhalis*, aerobic gram-negative bacilli; *Staphylococcus aureus, Neisseria meningitidis,* and group A beta-hemolytic streptococci. Previous experience indicates that a likely bacterial pathogen is recovered in approximately 50 percent of expectorated sputum samples from adult patients with community-acquired pneumonia who are sufficiently ill to require hospitalization.[9] The remaining patients, with no etiologic agent detected with this specimen source, may be referred to as "atypical pneumonia cases"; likely pathogens in this group are *Mycoplasma pneumoniae, Legionella,* anaerobic bacteria, *Chlamydia pneumoniae* (TWAR agent), and viral agents.

Streptococcus Pneumoniae

The pneumococcus is the most frequent pathogen responsible for bacterial pneumonia, although studies during the past two decades indicate a declining frequency that may represent either a true reduction in incidence or a decrease in the quality of bacteriologic studies.[11] Classical features of pneumococcal pneumonia include preceding upper respiratory tract infection, precipitous onset with a shaking chill and the rapid development of fever, dyspnea, pleurisy, and cough that is usually productive of purulent, blood-streaked, or "rusty" sputum. Chest x-rays invariably show a pulmonary infiltrate, and lobar consolidation specifically suggests this diagnosis. A pleural effusion is present in about 25 percent of cases, but fewer than 1 percent have empyema. In the majority of cases, the diagnosis is presumptive, based on direct examination of expectorated sputum, often utilizing the quellung reaction and cultures. Multiple antibiotics are active versus this organism, although virtually all authorities agree that penicillin G remains the drug of choice. Pneumococcal polysaccharide vaccine was licensed in 1977. It now contains antigens against the 23 serotypes that account for 85 to 90 percent of serotypes implicated in serious pneumococcal infections, and several studies suggest efficacy rates as high as 60 to 77 percent.[15] Pregnancy is not regarded as a risk factor for pneumococcal infection so that pneumococcal vaccine is not indicated on this basis alone.[6]

Haemophilus Influenzae

This organism is second only to the pneumococcus, with recovery rates in expectorated sputum of 5 to 10 percent of cases. Clinical features of *H. influenzae* pneumonia show the usual findings, including fever, cough, purulent sputum, leukocytosis, and a chest x-ray demonstrating a bronchopneumonia, with lobar consolidation seen in up to one-third of cases.[27] Pregnant women may be uniquely susceptible to infections with nontypeable strains.[25] Ampicillin and amoxicillin have traditionally been viewed as the drugs of choice, but 20 to 30 percent of type B strains and 10 to 20 percent of nontypeable strains are now resistant to this agent.[24] Preferred regimens include cephalosporins such as cefamandole, cefuroxime, or third-generation cephalosporins; for oral treatment, the preferred agents for ampicillin-resistant strains are amoxicillin plus clavulanic acid, cefixime, and cefaclor.

Mycoplasma Pneumoniae

This organism represents the most common form of mild, treatable infections of the lower airways afflicting young adults. The usual symptoms are headache, myalgia, cough, and fever, with pulmonary infiltrates on chest x-ray that generally show a bronchopneumonic pattern.[22] The cough is usually nonproductive; when sputum is obtained, it generally shows polymorphonuclear cells and mononuclear cells with no dominant organism.

Many cases are complicated by extrapulmonary manifestations including rashes, hepatitis, neurologic complications, myocarditis and pericarditis.[21] Pregnancy is not considered a predisposing condition. To establish the diagnosis, assays of blood for cold agglutins may be supportive, but this test lacks specificity. The usual diagnostic study is serology with paired sera separated by 4 weeks or more, but the information obtained is not available at the time diagnostic tests are required. These organisms lack a cell wall and consequently are not susceptible to cell-wall active antibiotics such as beta-lactams. The usual agents are tetracyclines or macrolides (erythromycin, clarithromycin, azithromycin); because tetracyclines are contraindicated during pregnancy, the options are limited to the macrolides.

Chlamydia Pneumoniae

This organism is a recently detected agent of pulmonary infections in young adults and is second only to *Mycoplasma* as the most frequent agent of pulmonary infections in university students.[12] The clinical presentation is similar to that of *Mycoplasma pneumoniae;* the difference is that it may be a more persistent infection, more likely to require hospitalization, and somewhat less responsive to treatment.[17] Available evidence suggests that *C. pneumoniae* accounts for 5 to 10 percent of both community-acquired and hospital-acquired pneumonia in adults. Unfortunately, the usual diagnostic test is a serologic assay that is not generally available and shows diagnostic titers only after week 5 or 6 of the illness. Preferred treatment is with erythromycin (2 g per day) for 10 to 14 days.

Legionella Pneumophila

The discovery of *Legionella pneumophila* following the epidemic of Legionnaire's disease in Philadelphia in 1976 had a profound effect on the management of community-acquired pneumonia because erythromycin became standard treatment for enigmatic pneumonia as a result of this work. *Legionella* actually accounts for a relatively small portion of cases, usually 2 to 6 percent of all cases among adults with community-acquired pneumonia.[23] It is an important cause of epidemics of pneumonia, especially outbreaks in hospitals and hotels, and sporadic cases show a distinct epidemiology pattern with high rates during the early fall. The usual host is over 30 years of age and smokes or has an immune deficiency with defective cell-mediated immunity. The diagnosis is established with culture or direct fluorescent antibody stain of respiratory secretions, serology, or a recently introduced urinary antigen assay.[7] The usual treatment for moderately or severely ill patients is erythromycin, 4 g per day intravenously until there is clinical improvement and then 2 g per day by mouth to complete a 3-week course. This organism is a relatively rare cause of pneumonia during pregnancy because it occurs primarily in older adults.

Viruses

A large number of viruses may cause upper respiratory tract infections, but only a small number are likely to cause pneumonia in adults. The major virus is influenza, an organism that has historically been responsible for severe cases of pneumonia in pregnant women during the epidemic of 1918–1919 and the Asian flu of 1957. These patients appeared to die with primary influenza pneumonia rather than with bacterial superinfections, as noted in other lethal infections in young adults. Epidemics during the past two decades have not resulted in major outbreaks with the high mortality encountered previously among pregnant women,[7] although this potential threat remains on the basis of epidemiologic patterns that have proven somewhat difficult to predict and anecdotal cases that continue to appear.[28] Pregnancy is not regarded as a specific indication for influenza vaccine; when requested, vaccination after the first trimester is preferred unless the first trimester corresponds to the influenza season.[7] The most serious disease is due to influenza A, the strain that is subject to the greatest antigenic variation. Amantadine has been used successfully both to prevent influenza A infection and to reduce symptoms after the infection is acquired. However, this drug is contraindicated during pregnancy. The major complication of influenza pneumonia is a bacterial superinfection, with the most common pathogen in this setting being *Streptococcus pneumoniae* and the most serious pathogen being *Staphylococcus aureus.* Antimicrobial agents should be selected accordingly.

Other respiratory tract viruses that may be implicated are respiratory syncytial virus (RSV) and parainfluenza virus, but these infections are usually restricted to the upper airways and bronchi; they seldom cause pneumonia in adults. The one virus worth mentioning in the context of pregnancy beyond influenza is varicella. The major complication in adults, especially pregnant women and adults with compromised cell-mediated immunity, is varicella pneumonia, in which case fatality rates may be as high as 30 to 40 percent. Approximately 95 percent of adults have serologic evidence of prior infection and are immune, although many have no recollection of an illness compatible with chickenpox. Susceptibility may be easily verified with serologic testing. Varicella-zoster immune globulin (VZIG) may effectively prevent infection following exposure, especially if given within 3 days. Pneumonia typically develops 2 to 5 days after appearance of skin lesions, and x-rays often reveal characteristic diffuse nodular lesions. Acyclovir is active in vitro versus this virus. Although no properly controlled study demonstrates benefit, a retrospective analysis of cases showed significantly more rapid reduction in fever among patients treated with acyclovir and anecdotal cases in pregnancy suggesting impressive responses.[13,16] When used for this indication, the usual regimen is 10 mg per kilogram intravenously every 8 hours for 7 days; for uncomplicated chickenpox the recommendation is for 800 mg by mouth 5 times per day for 10 days.[10]

Septic Emboli

This complication is relatively rare except in intravenous drug abusers with tricuspid valve endocarditis. The diagnosis is readily established when the susceptible host has a typical clinical presentation including fever, repeatedly positive blood cultures, and a chest x-ray showing typical embolic lesions. Treatment should be selected according to in vitro susceptibility studies. The usual pathogen is *S. aureus,* and the drugs of choice for initial treatment include either a penicillinase-resistant penicillin (nafcillin or oxacillin) or vancomycin. Concern regarding refusal to accept long-term hospitalization and the potential abuse of intravenous lines has prompted

Table 3-2 Treatment of Pneumonia in Pregnant Women

Agent	Usual Agent(s)	Alternatives	Comment
S. pneumoniae	Penicillin	Ampicillin, erythromycin, cephalosporins	
H. influenzae	Cefamandole, cefuroxime, amoxicillin-clavulanate	Cephalosporins, third generation	Ampicillin or amoxicillin for susceptible strains
Moraxella (Branhamella)	Erythromycin	Amoxicillin-clavulanate, cephalosporins	90–95% are resistant to penicillin and ampicillin
S. aureus	Nafcillin, oxacillin	Cephalothin, cefuroxime, cefamandole, clindamycin, vancomycin	Hospital-acquired strains are often methicillin resistant, requiring vancomycin
Anaerobes	Clindamycin	Penicillin G	It is likely that most beta-lactams are effective
Legionella	Erythromycin	—	Limited experience with imipenem suggests efficacy
Mycoplasma	Erythromycin	—	
C. pneumoniae	Erythromycin	—	
Influenza	—	—	Amantadine lacks established efficacy in influenza pneumonia and is contraindicated in pregnancy
Varicella	Acyclovir	—	Efficacy demonstrated

attempts at outpatient regimens with antibiotics given orally, such as cephalexin or ciprofloxacin.[8] Initial results with these studies appear to show satisfactory results.

Treatment

Antibiotics are optimally selected on the basis of microbiologic studies with clinical correlations to identify specific microbial agents. Drugs of choice are listed in Table 3-2 according to microbial pathogen. This list has appropriate respect for antimicrobial agents considered contraindicated during pregnancy. Thus tetracycline is not included in the listing despite its established efficacy in infections involving *M. pneumoniae* and *C. pneumoniae*, as well as potential benefit for infections involving *S. pneumoniae* and *H. influenzae*. The quinolones, including ciprofloxacin, are considered contraindicated during pregnancy but are generally avoided in community-acquired pneumonia anyway because they show reduced activity versus *S. pneumoniae* and are relatively expensive compared with alternative drugs. Sulfonamides, including trimethoprim-sulfamethoxazole, are also commonly used for patients with community-acquired pneumonias but are avoided in the listing because of their documented association with hyperbilirubinemia when they are given during the last 2 trimesters.

The studies cited indicate that the usual microbiologic studies—Gram's stain and culture of expectorated sputum—are likely to indicate a pathogen in approximately one-half of cases.[9] Therefore, the physician is required to make empiric decisions in about half of the cases. For outpatients who are not seriously ill, a common recommendation is erythromycin; alternative drugs that are sometimes preferred due to gastric intolerance of erythromycin include ampicillin, oral cephalosporins (cefaclor or cefixime), or amoxicillin-clavulanic acid. For patients who are more seriously ill and require hospitalization, a recommended regimen is erythromycin plus cefuroxime. This combination is active against virtually all nonviral agents of community-acquired pneumonia.

Aspiration Pneumonia

Aspiration pneumonia is described as the pulmonary sequelae reflecting abnormal entry of upper respiratory or gastric secretions into the lower airways.[3] Pregnant women are susceptible as a result of obstetric anesthesia, protracted vomiting, and possible distortion of the stom-

Table 3-3 Classification of "Aspiration Pneumonia"

Inoculum	Pulmonary Sequella	Clinical Features	Therapy
Acid	Chemical pneumonitis	Acute dyspnea, tachypnea tachycardia; ± cyanosis bronchospasm, fever Sputum: pink, frothy X-ray: infiltrates in one or both lower lobes Hypoxemia	Positive-pressure breathing Intravenous fluids Tracheal suction Corticosteroids
Oropharyngeal bacteria	Bacterial infection	Usually insidious onset Cough, fever, purulent sputum X-ray: infiltrate involving dependent pulmonary segment or lobe ± cavitation	Antibiotics
Inert fluids	Mechanical obstruction Reflex airway closure	Acute dyspnea, cyanosis, ± apnea Pulmonary edema	Tracheal suction Intermittent positive pressure breathing with oxygen and isoproterenol
Particulate matter	Mechanical obstruction	Dependent on level of obstruction, ranging from acute apnea and rapid death to irritating chronic cough ± recurrent infections	Extraction of particulate matter

ach by the gravid uterus. There are three different forms of aspiration pneumonia that are distinctively different in terms of pathophysiologic mechanism, clinical presentation, and therapy.[3] A classification of aspiration pneumonia, by inoculum, is shown in Table 3-3.

Infection

The most common complication of aspiration is an infection in the lower airways that involves the bacteria that normally reside in the upper airways, especially the gingival crevice or the stomach. The major pathogens are anaerobic bacteria, especially *B. melaninogenicus, Fusobacterium nucleatum,* and *Peptostreptococcus*. The natural history of this infection is a subtle onset of symptoms with cough, fever, and sputum production. X-rays in the early stage show infiltrates that are noted in the pulmonary segments favored by gravitational flow, including the posterior segments of the upper lobes or superior segments of the lower lobes that are dependent in the recumbent position or the lower lobes that are dependent in the upright position. When anaerobic bacteria are involved, the common late sequelae include necrosis of tissue with abscess formation or a bronchopleural fistula leading to an empyema. The usual treatment is clindamycin or penicillin G; other antimicrobial agents have not been extensively tested, but probably a wide range of drugs would prove satisfactory.

Chemical Pneumonitis

This disorder represents the pulmonary reaction to an inoculum that is toxic to the lung, the most common and best studied example being gastric acid pneumonitis. The classic description, published by Mendelson in 1946, includes observations of 66 obstetrical patients.[20] Subsequent animal studies indicated that the pH must be 2.5 or less and the volume should be large to produce the classical findings. The characteristic clinical feature was the precipitous onset of acute respiratory distress with cyanosis, cough productive of frothy and bloody secretions, and an x-ray showing infiltrates in one or both lower lobes. All of these patients in the original series survived, although more recent studies show that up to 30 percent of patients die from acute respiratory distress syndrome or pulmonary superinfections. The major form of therapy is respiratory support. Corticosteroids are commonly used but play no established role in treatment; antibiotic agents are commonly used and, although there is no evidence that infection plays a role in the early phases of this disease, bacterial superinfections late in the course are relatively common. This complication is now uncommon in obstetric practice because of improvements in the administration of anesthesia and other preventive measures.

Mechanical Obstruction

Aspiration of particulate matter or fluids that are not inherently toxic to the lung may cause pulmonary obstruction. With particulate matter, the severity of the disease is directly related to the extent or level of obstruction. Aspiration of fluids is readily cleared in the conscious patient with a cough reflex and is comparable to drowning in the absence of these protective mechanisms. The obvious therapeutic ploy is suction, bronchoscopy, or both measures to eliminate the obstruction.

Hospital-Acquired Pneumonia

Nosocomial pneumonia accounts for only about 15 percent of hospital-acquired infections, but it is the most common fatal form of these infections. Obstetric patients are not at particular risk unless they have severe associated conditions that necessitate intensive care. The bacteriology of hospital-acquired pneumonia is distinctly different from community-acquired pneumonia. The major pathogens are gram-negative bacilli, most frequently *Pseudomonas aeruginosa, Klebsiella* sp., and *Enterobacter* sp.; *S. aureus,* including methicillin-resistant strains and anaerobic bacteria, may also be implicated.[4] Culture of respiratory secretions usually yields the putative agent, and susceptibility tests provide a guideline to the selection of antimicrobial agents. For empiric treatment of seriously ill patients, common recommendations include an aminoglycoside combined with a third-generation cephalosporin or an antipseudomonad penicillin. With concern for ototoxicity to the fetus with aminoglycosides, an alternative regimen might be an antipseudomonad penicillin combined with a cephalosporin or vancomycin.

Patients with HIV Infection

The frequency of HIV infection is highly variable in different geographic areas. Many hospitals now report 5 to 10 percent of all pregnant women have positive serology for this virus. Such hospitals are now encouraged to do routine testing as a standard component of medical care.

The lung is an important organ of expression of HIV infection and may pose particular difficulty in the pregnant woman because many of the standard treatments must be given with extreme caution or avoided completely. In general, opportunistic infections of the lung are unlikely to occur until the T-4 cell count is reduced to 200 per mm^3. The occasional exceptions are pneumococcal pneumonia, tuberculosis, and influenza. All patients with HIV infection, including pregnant women, should have pneumococcal vaccine, influenza vaccine, and a purified protein derivative skin test for tuberculosis as part of their routine care. Persons who abuse intravenous drugs and others at high risk for tuberculosis should have anergy screening; those who are anergic should be treated with prophylactic isoniazid for at least 1 year. Patients with T-4 cell counts of less than 200 per mm^3 should receive prophylaxis for *Pneumocystis carinii* pneumonia. Although the safety of aerosolized pentamidine is not established, minimal amounts of this drug are actually absorbed and it is not likely to be problematic. An alternative and more realistic concern relates to the distribution of the drug in the presence of elevated diaphragms in the later stages of pregnancy. With regard to therapy, the major complications are *Pneumocystis* pneumonia and uncertainty regarding the safety of all regimens that are considered standard. One approach is to use the usual regimen of trimethoprim-sulfamethoxazole (15 to 20 mg per kilogram per day of trimethoprim by mouth or vein). An alternative oral regimen is dapsone (100 mg per day) plus trimethoprim (15 to 20 mg per kilogram per day). The alternative parenteral regimen is pentamidine (4 mg per kilogram per day by vein). All of these regimens are given for 3 weeks, and none has established safety during pregnancy. Nevertheless, these are the only drugs with established merit, and this disease inevitably progresses to death in the absence of treatment. The suggested approach is to provide the standard treatment with appropriate warning to the patient.

References

1. Bartlett JG. Anaerobic bacterial infections of the lung. Chest 1987; 91:901–909.
2. Bartlett JG, Brewer NS, Ryan KL. Laboratory diagnosis of lower respiratory infections. Washington, DC: American Society for Microbiology, 1978:1–15.
3. Bartlett JG, Gorbach SL. Triple threat of aspiration pneumonia. Chest 1975; 68:560–566.
4. Barlett JG, O'Keefe P, Tally FP, et al. The bacteriology of hospital-acquired pneumonia. Arch Intern Med 1986; 146:861–868.
5. Boerner DF, Zwadyk P. The value of the sputum Gram's stain in community-acquired pneumonia. JAMA 1982; 247:642–645.
6. Centers for Disease Control. Recommendations of the immunization practices advisory committee: pneumococcal polysaccharide vaccine. JAMA 1989; 261:1265–1266.
7. Centers for Disease Control. Prevention and control of influenza. MMWR 1990; 39 (RR-7):1–15.
8. Chambers HF. Right-sided *Staphylococcus aureus* endocarditis in intravenous drug abusers: two-week combination therapy. Ann Intern Med 1988; 109:619–624.
9. Dans PE, Charache P, Fahey M, Otter SE. Management of pneumonia in a prospective payment era. Arch Intern Med 1984; 144:1392–1397.
10. Feder HM Jr. Treatment of adult chicken pox with oral acyclovir. Arch Intern Med 1990; 150:2061–1065.
11. Fick RB Jr, Reynolds HY. Changing spectrum of pneumonia: new media creation or clinical reality. Am J Med 1983; 71:1–8.
12. Grayston JT, Kuo CC, Wang SC, Altman J. A new *Chlamydia psittaci* strain, TWAR isolated from acute respiratory tract infections. N Engl J Med 1986; 315:161–168.
13. Hankins GD, Gilstrap LC, Patterson AR. Acyclovir treatment of varicella pneumonia in pregnancy. Crit Care Med 1987; 15:336–337.
14. Heilman CA. Respiratory syncytial and parainfluenza viruses. J Infect Dis 1990; 161:402–406.
15. LaForce, FM. Pneumococcal vaccine: an emergency consensus. Ann Intern Med 1988; 108:757–758.
16. Landsberger EJ, Hager WD, Grossman JH. Successful management of varicella pneumonia complicating pregnancy. J Reprod Med 1986; 31:311–314.
17. MacFarlaine JT, Finch RG, Ward MJ, Macrae AD. Hospital study of adult community-acquired pneumonia. Lancet 1982; 2:255–258.
18. Madinger NE, Greenspoon JS, Ellrodt AG. Pneumonia during pregnancy: has modern technology

improved maternal and fetal outcome? Am J Obstet Gynecol 1989; 161:657–662.
19. Medical Letter. Drugs for anaerobic infections. 1987; 29:61–64.
20. Mendelson CL. The aspiration of stomach contents into the lungs during obstetric anesthesia. Am J Obstet Gynecol 1946; 52:191–205.
21. Murray HW, Masur H, Senterfit LB, Roberts RB. The protean manifestations of *Mycoplasma pneumoniae* infection in adults. Am J Med 1975; 58:229–242.
22. Phansel JK, Rosenow EC, Smith TF, Martin JW Jr. *Mycoplasma pneumoniae* pneumonia. Chest 1989; 95:639–646.
23. Ruf B, Schurmann D, Horbach I, et al. Prevalence and diagnosis of *Legionella* pneumonia: a 3-year prospective study with emphasis on application of urinary antigen detection. J Infect Dis 1990; 162:1341–1348.
24. Takala AK. Spectrum of invasive *Haemophilus influenza* type b disease in adults. Arch Intern Med 1990; 150:2573–2576.
25. Wallace RJ Jr, Balcer CJ, Quinones FJ, et al. Nontypable *Haemophilus influenzae* (biotype 4) as a neonatal, maternal and genital pathogen. Rev Infect Dis 1983; 5:123–136.
26. Washington JA. Noninvasive diagnostic techniques for lower respiratory infections. In: Pennington JE, ed. Respiratory infections: diagnosis and management. New York. Raven Press, 1989:52–68.
27. Weinstein L. Type B *Haemophilus influenzae* infections in adults. N Engl J Med 1970; 282:221–226.
28. Wells DL, Hopfensperger DJ, Ardea NH, et al. Swine influenza virus infection. JAMA 1991; 265:478–481.

CHAPTER 4

Viral Hepatitides

Gilles R. G. Monif, M.D.

Acute viral hepatitis is caused by a number of viruses. Viral infection of the liver manifests a spectrum of involvement ranging from subclinical infection to progressive fatal disease.

Etiology

There are at least four etiologically and epidemiologically distinct forms of hepatitis (Table 4-1): hepatitis A (infectious hepatitis); hepatitis B (serum hepatitis); hepatitis C (non-A, non-B hepatitis), which includes two epidemiologically distinct subtypes; and delta hepatitis.

Other viral agents, such as the Epstein-Barr virus, cytomegaloviruses, herpes simplex viruses, and yellow fever virus, among others, can cause an acute viral hepatitis. Their viscerotropism is described elsewhere.

Hepatitis A Virus

Hepatitis A virus (HAV) is a 27-nm ribonucleic acid virus that belongs to the picornavirus group (Table 4-1). It is primarily transmitted by person-to-person contact through fecal contamination and oral ingestion. Common source epidemics result from contaminated food and water. The incubation period of hepatitis A is 15 to 50 days (average 28 days). The virus reaches its highest concentration in the feces late in the incubation period and the early prodromal phase of illness and diminishes rapidly once symptoms appear. The period of greatest infectivity is the 2 weeks immediately before the onset of jaundice. A viremia occurs when the virus is shed in the feces. As a consequence, in rare instances HAV may be transmitted by a blood transfusion.

Hepatitis B Virus

Hepatitis B virus (HBV) is a 42-nm, double-shelled deoxyribonucleic acid (virus that belongs to the Hepadnaviridae group of viruses) (Table 4-1). The incubation period of hepatitis B is 45 to 160 days (average 120 days). Percutaneous and peroral contacts with infective body fluids are the principal modes of dissemination. Because of current screening procedures for HBV, transmission by transfusion of blood is rare.

Hepatitis C Virus (Non-A, Non-B Hepatitis Virus)

Recombinant technology has led to the identification of non-A, non-B hepatitis virus, now termed *hepatitis C virus* (HCV) (Table 4-1). The viral agent has been characterized as having a positive strand of RNA containing approximately 10,000 nucleotides. The virus has an 80-nm diameter and is presumed to have a lipid coat. The current presumptive classification places HCV within the Pestivirus family. Hepatitis C virus (HCV) accounts for approximately 20 to 40 percent of acute viral hepatitis in the United States and has an epidemi-

Table 4-1 Hepatitis Nomenclature

	Abbreviation	Term	Definition/Comments
Hepatitis A	HAV	Hepatitis A virus	Etiologic agent of "infectious" hepatitis; a picornavirus; single serotype
	Anti-HAV	Antibody to HAV	Detectable at onset of symptoms; lifetime persistence
	IgM anti-HAV	IgM class antibody to HAV	Indicates recent infection with hepatitis A; detectable for 4-6 months after infection
Hepatitis B	HBV	Hepatitis B virus	Etiologic agent of "serum" hepatitis; also known as Dane particle
	HB_sAg	Hepatitis B surface antigen	Surface antigen(s) of HBV detectable in large quantity in serum; several subtypes identified
	HB_eAg	Hepatitis B e antigen	Soluble antigen; correlates with HBV replication, high titer of HBV in serum, and infectivity of serum
	HB_cAg	Hepatitis B core antigen	No commercial test available.
	Anti-HBs	Antibody to HB_sAg	Indicates past infection with and immunity to HBV, passive antibody from HBIG, or immune response from HB vaccine
	Anti-HBe	Antibody to HB_eAg	Presence in serum of HBsAg carrier indicates lower titer of HBV
	Anti-HBc	Antibody to HB_cAg	Indicates prior infection with HBV at some undefined time
	IgM anti-HBc	IgM class antibody to HB_cAg	Indicates recent infection with HBV; detectable for 4-6 months after infection
Hepatitis C (non-A, non-B hepatitis)	PT-NANB	Parenterally transmitted	Diagnosis by exclusion; at least two candidate viruses, one of which has been proposed as hepatitis C virus; shares epidemiologic features with hepatitis B
	ET-NANB	Enterically transmitted	Diagnosis by exclusion; causes large epidemics in Asia, Africa, and Mexico; fecal-oral or waterborne
Delta hepatitis	HDV	Delta virus	Etiologic agent of delta hepatitis; can cause infection only in presence of HBV
	HDAg	Delta antigen	Detectable in early acute delta infection
	Anti-HDV	Antibody to delta antigen	Indicates present or past infection with delta virus

ologic characteristic somewhat similar to hepatitis B virus. Although the disease is transmitted primarily through parenteral contact involving blood and blood products, another distinct type of non-A, non-B hepatitis acquired by the oral route, hepatitis E virus, occurs. It is thought to be largely responsible for waterborne epidemics, particularly in developing countries. The probability that HCV can be sexually transmitted is suggested by the observation that 50 percent of individuals intimate with or sexually exposed to someone who had hepatitis in the past are serologically positive.

Delta Virus (Hepatitis D Virus, HDV)

Delta virus is a unique hepatotropic virus (Table 4-1). It is composed of a single strand of RNA, of low molecular weight, and has an internal protein core. The delta virus is 35 to 37 nm in size and is coded with the hepatitis B surface antigens. Its uniqueness comes from the fact that it, in itself, is incapable of attaching and hence infecting hepatocytes. Infection of the liver requires concomitant presence of the hepatitis B virus. The delta virus must borrow hepatitis B surface proteins, which permit attachment and subsequent infection of liver parenchymal cells. Without this critical step of attachment, there can be no infection. The routes of transmission of HDV are similar to those for HBV, and consequently patients at high risk for HBV infection are similarly at risk for HDV infection. Delta virus infection may occur concomitantly with HBV infection or may occur as a superinfection.

Epidemiology

Hepatitis A, B, C, and delta viruses all have differing incubation periods (Table 4-2); however, the degree of overlap is so great that this information is of little diagnostic value unless one is dealing with an early onset of disease relative to point of exposure.

Hepatitis A and probably hepatitis E are primarily transmitted by the fecal-oral route. HBV, HCV, and HDV are disseminated primarily by parenteral inoculation or some equivalent thereof.

Table 4-2 Incubation Period of the Principal

Causes of Viral Hepatitis

AGENT	INCUBATION PERIOD
Hepatitis A virus	2-5 weeks
Hepatitis B virus	4 weeks to 6 months
Hepatitis C virus	4 weeks to 6 months
Delta virus	2-20 weeks

Hepatitis A is subject to significant yearly fluctuations. With improved public health measures, there has been a progressive decrease in the number of cases occurring in the United States from 1970 to 1990 (Fig. 4-1); however, an increase in the number of cases of hepatitis B and recognition of hepatitis C have caused a plateau in the total number of cases of acute viral hepatitis identified by the Centers for Disease Control. Regional differences in prevalence exist for hepatitis A and B (Fig. 4-2). Hepatitis A is the principal cause of disease in childhood and early adolescence (Fig. 4-3). The main age of occurrence for hepatitis B is 6 to 8 years later.

Clinical Illness

Hepatitis A

Clinically overt disease caused by HAV characteristically has an abrupt onset of symptoms including fever, malaise, anorexia, abdominal discomfort, dark urine, and jaundice. Disease is significantly influenced by age. Most infections in childhood are asymptomatic or anicteric, whereas the disease in adulthood is more prone to be symptomatic and clinically overt. The case fatality rate is approximately 0.6 percent.

Hepatitis B

The onset of acute disease due to HBV is generally insidious. Clinical symptoms and signs include anorexia, malaise, nausea, vomiting, abdominal pain, and jaundice. Extrahepatic manifestations such as skin rashes, arthralgia, and arthritis occur. The case fatality rate for reported cases is approximately 1.4 percent. A variable proportion of individuals affected with HBV become chronically infected with the virus. Carriers and persons with acute infection have the highest concentration of

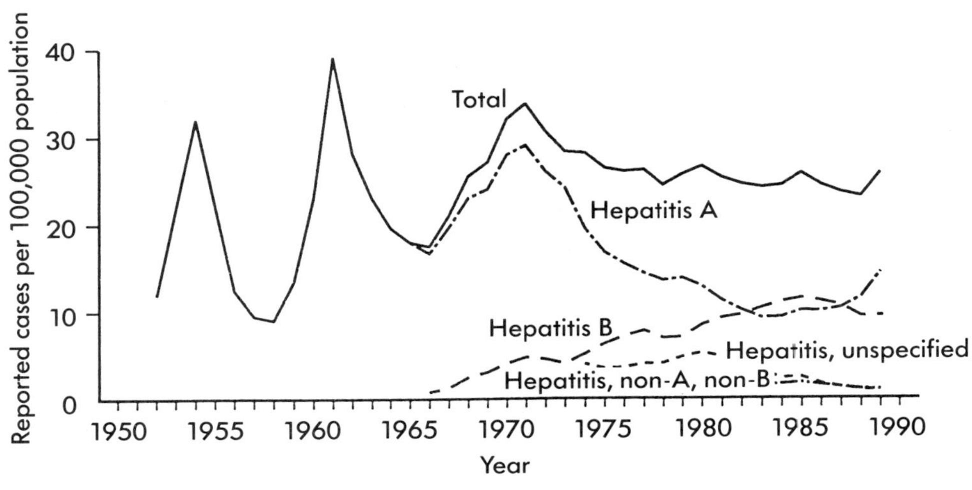

Figure 4-1 Reported cases of hepatitis, by year: United States, 1952–1988. (From Centers for Disease Control Surveillance Report 53, 1990.)

HBV in blood and serous fluids. Lower concentrations are present in saliva and semen.

A small percentage of patients go on to become chronic carriers of HBV. Twenty-five percent of the carriers develop chronic active hepatitis, which often progresses to cirrhosis. HBV carriers have the added risk (12 to 300 times that of other individuals) of developing a primary liver carcinoma. It is this group of patients with chronic viral synthesis that is of greatest concern to obstetricians and gynecologists.

Hepatitis C (Non-A, Non-B Hepatitis)

In the United States, hepatitis C is responsible for more than 90 percent of post-transfusion hepatitis infections. About 75 percent of all HCV infections are anicteric. The most common presenting complications are fatigue and anorexia. Later symptoms include malaise, fever, headache, generalized muscular aching, fatigue, loss of appetite, nausea, abdominal pain, and joint pain, sometimes followed by the presence of dark urine and jaundice.

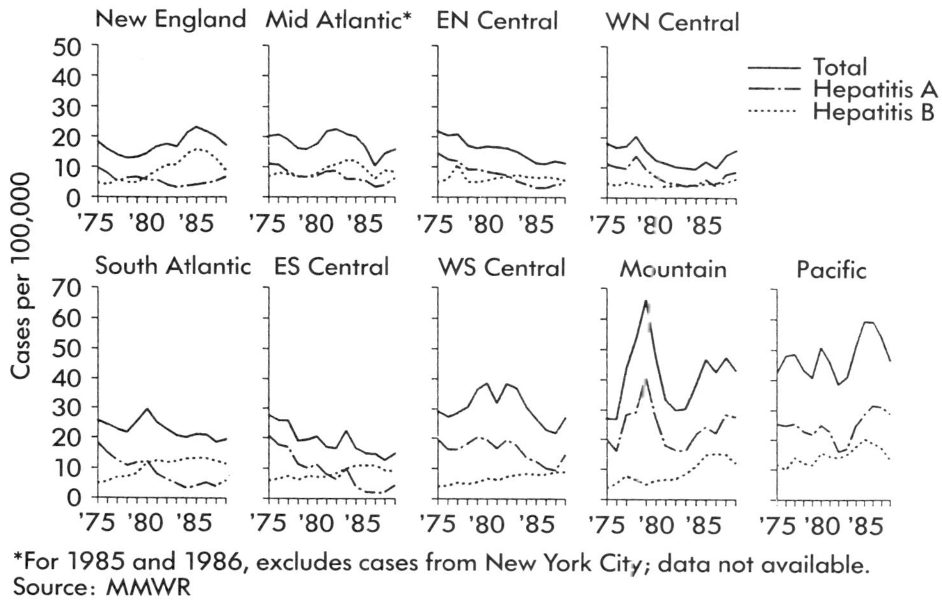

Figure 4-2 Reported cases of viral hepatitis, by region: United States, 1975–1988. (From Centers for Disease Control Hepatitis Surveillance Report 53, 1990.)

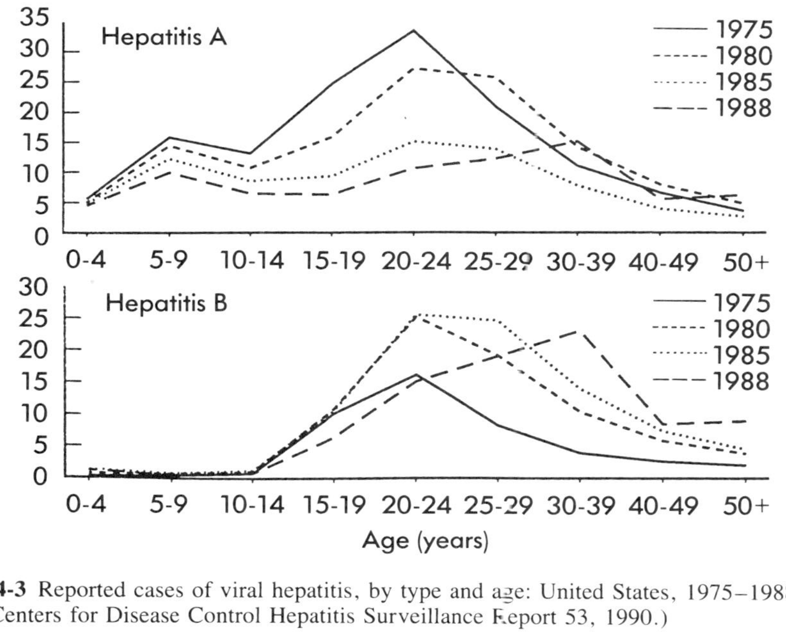

Figure 4-3 Reported cases of viral hepatitis, by type and age: United States, 1975–1988. (From Centers for Disease Control Hepatitis Surveillance Report 53, 1990.)

At least 50 percent of acute HCV infections lead to chronic hepatitis, and 20 percent of these chronic carriers develop cirrhosis and possibly hepatocellular carcinoma.[2]

Hepatitis D

The diagnosis of delta hepatitis requires the documentation of HBV infection plus demonstration of IgM antidelta virus antibodies. Immunoglobulin M (IgM) anti-HDV tests are available only in research laboratories.

Infection with delta virus causes acute hepatitis. Co-infection usually resolves, whereas a superinfection frequently causes chronic HBV infection and chronic active hepatitis. Both types of infection, co-infection and superinfection, may cause fulminant hepatitis.

Impact on Mother and Fetus

The impact of overt maternal disease depends on the duration of gestation. Disease in the third trimester tends to be more severe than that which occurs in the first two trimesters of gestation. This tends to be true for all of the hepatitides.

Morbidity that is due to direct involvement of the fetus has been documented for HBV only.

Perinatal transmission is one of the most efficient modes of spread of HBV. Infants born to mothers who are positive for both hepatitis B surface antigen (HB_sAg) and hepatitis B e antigen (Hb_eAg) have a 70 to 90 percent risk for HBV infection; 85 to 90 percent of infected infants remain chronically infected. For infants born to HB_sAg-positive, HB_eAg-negative mothers, the risk for chronic infection is as great as 31 percent. Children born to HB_sAg-positive mothers not infected at birth have a 30 to 60 percent risk for acquiring infection during the first 5 years of life (depending on the HB_eAg status of the mother).

The advent of sophisticated immunoserology has confirmed the occurrence of in utero acquisition of HBV infection. In utero hematogenous transmission from mother to fetus occurs in 5 to 15 percent of the cases. The probability of intrauterine transmission is directly related to the presence or absence of HB_eAg.

Diagnosis

Definitive diagnosis is based upon serologic exclusion and presumed probability. The criteria for serologic diagnosis of the various hepatitides are summarized in Table 4-3.

Hepatitis A

Diagnosis of acute hepatitis is made by the finding of IgM anti-HAV in the serum collected during the acute or early convalescent phase of disease. IgG anti-HAV develops in the convalescent phase of the disease and confers subsequent immunity against this form of hepatitis.

Table 4-3 Laboratory Criteria for Diagnosis of the Viral Hepatitides

Hepatitis A:	IgM anti-HAV positive
Hepatitis B:	IgM anti-HBc positive or HB_sAg positive, and IgM anti-HAV negative
Hepatitis C:*	IgM anti-HAV negative, and IgM anti-HBc negative (if done) or HB_sAg negative, and Serum aminotransferase levels greater than 2½ times the upper limit of normal
Hepatitis D:	HB_sAg or IgM anti-HBc positive and anti-HDV positive

*A serologic test for IgG antibody to the recently described hepatitis C virus is available, and many cases of non-A, non-B hepatitis can be demonstrated to be due to infection with the hepatitis C virus. With this assay, however, a prolonged interval (6 to 12 months) between onset of disease and detection of antibody may occur.

From Monif GRG. Infectious diseases in obstetrics and gynecology. Ed 3 Gainesville, Florida: Infectious Diseases Incorporated, 1991.

Hepatitis B

A number of well-defined antigen antibody tests identify HBV or its components. The HB_sAg is present in the serum 30 to 60 days after exposure to HBV and persists for a variable period of time. Anti-HBs develops after resolution of infection, and it is responsible for long-term immunity. Antibody to the core antigen (anti-HB_c) develops in the course of HIV infection and persists indefinitely. IgM anti-HB_c appears early in infection and persists for 6 months. It is a reliable marker of acute or recent HBV infection. A third antigen hepatitis B e antibody (HB_eAg) detected in individuals with both acute and chronic HBV infection correlates with high infectivity. Antibody with HB_eAg (anti-HB_e) develops in most HBV and correlates with the loss of replica in virus and lower infectivity.

Hepatitis C (Non-A, Non-B Hepatitis)

The Food and Drug Administration recently licensed two blood-screening tests that detect the presence of antibody to HCV (anti-HCV) in serum or plasma.

The HCV tests analyze binding between the patient's serum and the recombinant viral proteins. This procedure forms the basis of RIA and ELISA for antibody in test sera.

The presence of anti-HCV in human serum or plasma does not necessarily indicate ongoing hepatitis C but may be a remnant of a past infection with HCV. Levels of antibody are usually undetectable in early stages of an infection (the "window period").

Anti-HCV antibodies appear as early as 4 weeks and as late as 1 year after infection. The mean delay between onset of hepatitis symptoms and seropositivity is 15 weeks. In acute post-transfusion hepatitis, the mean delay between transfusion (infection) and appearance of anti-HCV is 22 weeks. Once the antibodies develop, they persist for years. Unlike hepatitis B, the "window period" with hepatitis C is variable. When the diagnosis of hepatitis C is strongly suspected, sequential repeat testing for anti-HCV antibodies is recommended. The major usefulness of the test is to screen out blood donors who could transmit HCV. A positive test for the presence of anti-HCV assists in the diagnosis of individuals with recent or prior signs and symptoms and/or biochemical evidence of hepatitis. A negative test is of limited value.

Hepatitis D

Currently there is no readily available serologic test for the detection of HDV.

Therapy

Hepatitis A: Passive Immunotherapy

The efficacy of immune serum globulin (ISG) for the prevention or modification of hepatitis A depends on the following:

1. Degree and type of exposure
2. Dose of ISG and its antibody content
3. Time interval between exposure and the administration of ISG

Optimal passive immunization following presumed exposure requires the use of high-titered, HB_sAG-negative ISG, administered as soon as possible after exposure. Different lots of ISG may vary as much as 16-fold in anti-HAV content. It will be imperative in the future for licensed lots of ISG to be marked as to anti-HAV titer.

Administration of ISG early in the incubation period of hepatitis A is capable of modifying or arresting the infection. A dose of 0.02 ml per kilogram of body weight affords effective protection for short-term exposure.

Hepatitis B

Two types of vaccines for hepatitis B are currently licensed in the United States:

1. Plasma-derived vaccine consisting of inactivated 22-mg HB_sAg particles
2. Recombinant hepatitis B vaccine produced by *Saccharomyces cerevisiae*

The current recommendation is that a series of three intramuscular doses of hepatitis B vaccine be given. This schedule induces a significant antibody response in more than 90 percent of healthy adults and in more than 95 percent of children.

The vaccines licensed in the United States are 80 to 95 percent effective in preventing infection or clinical hepatitis among susceptible individuals.

Prenatal Screening of All Pregnant Women for HB_sAg (CDC Recommendations)

All pregnant women should be routinely tested for HB_sAg during an early prenatal visit in each pregnancy. If a serum specimen is positive for HB_sAg, the same specimen should be tested again, and then the test results should be confirmed by neutralization. Although it is unnecessary to test for other HBV markers during maternal screening, each HB_sAg-positive mother should be evaluated for HBV-related acute or chronic liver disease.

Because more than 90 percent of women found to be HB_sAg positive on routine screening are HBV carriers, routine follow-up testing in later pregnancy is not necessary. In special situations, such as when the mother is thought to have acute hepatitis, when there has been a history of exposure to hepatitis, or when particularly high-risk behavior such as parenteral drug abuse has occurred during the pregnancy, an additional HB_sAg test should be ordered during the third trimester. Few women in populations at low risk for HBV infection have a change in HB_sAg status during subsequent pregnancies.

Management of Infants Born to HB_sAg-Positive Mothers

Infants born to HB_sAg-postive mothers should be given HBIG (0.5 ml) intramuscularly once they are physiologically stable but within 12 hours after birth. There is diminishing efficiency with time. Seven days or more after birth, no efficiency can be demonstrated.

The HB vaccine is administered in three doses as follows:

First dose:	HB vaccine (0.5 ml) intramuscularly (plasma-derived vaccine, 10 μg per dose; recombinant vaccine 5 μg per dose) concurrently with HBIG but at a different site. The first dose should be given within 7 days after birth.
Second dose:	Repeat initial dose at 1 month.
Third dose:	Repeat initial dose at 6 months.

The vaccinated infant should be tested for HB_sAg and anti-HBs at 12 to 15 months to monitor the effectiveness of immunization. Delay in the administration of HBIG to the infant of a carrier mother decreases the efficacy of therapy.

Hepatitis C (Non-A, Non-B Hepatitis)

There is no evidence that U.S.–manufactured IgG prevents infection due to HCV.

Hepatitis D

Because HDV is dependent on HBV for replication, prevention of hepatitis B either before or after exposure will prevent HDV infection.

References

1. Alessandro ZR, Elisabetta T, Pierino F, Enrico M. Vertical transmission of the HBV associated delta agent. Prog Clin Biol Res 1983; 143:127–132.
2. Alter MJ Coleman PJ, Alexander WJ, et al. Importance of heterosexual activity in the transmis-

sion of hepatitis B and non-A, non-B hepatitis. JAMA 1989; 262:1201–1205.
3. Arevalo JA, Washington AE. Cost-effectiveness of prenatal screening and immunization for hepatitis B virus. JAMA 1988; 259:365–369.
4. Beasley RR, Hwang LY, Lee GC, et al. Prevention of perinatally transmitted hepatitis B virus infections with hepatitis B immune globulin and hepatitis B vaccine. Lancet 1983; i:1099–1102.
5. Beasley RR, Hwang L, Stevens CE, et al. Efficacy of hepatitis B immune globulin for prevention of perinatal transmission of the hepatitis B virus carrier state: final report of a randomized double-blind, placebo-controlled trial. Hepatology 1983; 3:135–141.
6. Beasley RR, Linn CC, Wang KY, et al. Hepatitis B immune globulin (HBIG) efficacy in the interruption of perinatal transmission of hepatitis B virus carrier state. Lancet 1981; i:388–393.
7. Centers for Disease Control. Recommendations of the Immunization Practices Advisory Committee (ACIP): recommendations for protection against viral hepatitis. MMWR 1985; 34(22):313–335.
8. Centers for Disease Control. Recommendations of the Immunization Practices Advisory Committee: prevention of perinatal transmission of hepatitis B virus: prenatal screening of all pregnant women for hepatitis B surface antigen. MMWR 1988; 37:341–351.
9. Centers for Disease Control. Hepatitis surveillance report 52. Atlanta: US Department of Health and Human Services, Public Health Service, 1989:25.
10. Centers for Disease Control. Protection against viral hepatitis: recommendations of the Immunization Practices Advisory Commmittee (ACIP) MMWR 1990; 39:1–17.
11. Choo Q-L, Kuo G, Weiner AJ, et al. Isolation of a cDNA clone derived from a blood-borne non-A, non-B viral hepatitis genome. Science 1989; 244:359–362.
12. Crumpacker CS. Hepatitis. In: Remington JS, Klein JO, Eds. Infectious diseases of the fetus and newborn. Philadelphia: WB Saunders, 1983:591–618.
13. Delaplane D, Yogev R, Crussi F, Shulman ST. Fatal hepatitis B in early infancy: the importance of identifying HB_sAg-positive pregnant women and providing immunoprophylaxis to their newborns. Pediatrics 1983; 72:176–180.
14. Hadler S, DeMomzon M, Ponzetto A, et al. Delta virus infection and severe hepatitis. Ann Intern Med 1984; 100:339–344.
15. Krawczynski K, Bradley DW. Enterically transmitted non-A, non-B hepatitis: identification of virus-associated antigen in experimentally infected *Cynomolgus macaques*. J Infect Dis 1989; 159:1042–1049.
16. Krugman S. Hepatitis B infection and pregnancy. Infectious Disease Letters for Obstetrics and Gynecology 1980; 2:25–30.
17. Kumar ML, Dawson NV, McCullough AJ, et al. Should all pregnant women be screened for hepatitis B? Ann Intern Med 1987; 190:273–277.
18. Kuo G, Choo Q-L, Alter HJ, et al. An assay for circulating antibodies to a major etiologic virus of human non-A, non-B hepatitis. Science 1989; 244:362–364.
19. Monif GRG. Hepatitis B. In: Monif GRG, Osbourne NE, eds. TORCH agent. Omaha: IDI Publications.
20. Ramalingaswami V, Purcell RH. Waterborne non-A, non-B hepatitis. Lancet 1988; 1:571–573.
21. Redeker AG. Delta virus and hepatitis B. Ann Intern Med 1983; 98:542–543.
22. Rizzetto M. The delta agent. Hepatology 1983; 3:729–737.
23. Robinson WS. Hepatitis B virus and the delta virus. In: GL Mandell, RG Douglas, JE Bennett, eds. Principles and practice of infectious diseases. Vol 2. New York: John Wiley & Sons, 1985:1002–1029.
24. Stevens CE, Neurath RA, Beasley RP, Szmuness W. HB_eAg and anti-HBe detection by radioimmunoassay: correlation with vertical transmission of hepatitis B virus in Taiwan. J Med Virol 1979; 3:237–241.
25. Stevens CE, Toy PT, Ton MJ, et al. Perinatal hepatitis B virus transmission in the United States. JAMA 1985; 253:1740–1745.
26. Summers PR, Biswas MK, Pastorek JG II, et al. The pregnant hepatitis B carrier: evidence favoring comprehensive antepartum screening. Obstet Gynecol 1987; 69:701–704.
27. Wong VCW, Ip HMH, Reesink HW, et al. Prevention of the HB_sAg carrier state in newborn infants of mothers who are chronic carriers of HB_sAg and HB_eAg by administration of hepatitis-B vaccine and hepatitis-B immunoglobulin: double-blind randomized placebo-controlled study. Lancet 1984; 1:921–926.
28. Xu Z-Y, Liu C-B, Francis DP, et al. Prevention of perinatal acquisition of hepatitis B virus carriage using vaccine: preliminary report of a randomized, double-blind placebo controlled and comparative trail. Pediatrics 1985; 76:713–718.

CHAPTER 5

Tuberculosis and Pregnancy

Leon G. Smith, Jr., M.D.
Leon G. Smith, Sr., M.D.

Few beliefs regarding infectious diseases have changed as much as those about the effect of pregnancy on tuberculosis. Beginning with Hippocrates in the fifth century BC,[35] pregnancy was believed to be beneficial for a woman who had tuberculosis. Then, during the early part of this century, the opposite opinion was vigorously proposed.[41] However, several clinical studies, which were completed before the ubiquitous use of antituberculosis agents, firmly established the principle that pregnancy has little or no effect on the course of tuberculosis.[14,19]

Even though pregnancy has little effect on tuberculosis, active tuberculosis in the preantibiotic era was associated with an infant and maternal mortality rate of 30 percent.[34] Today, pregnancy outcome is excellent among women who are treated appropriately for tuberculosis.[20] Cases of maternal tuberculosis are often asymptomatic, and unrecognized disease can still produce devastating effects in a newborn infant.[3,22] Despite its lethal potential, this infection is relatively uncommon in both pregnant women and the general population of the United States at the present time.[10] Thus, if timely therapy is to be initiated, physicians must maintain a high level of suspicion for tuberculosis in high-risk mothers.

Some authors have recommended that all women who register for prenatal care be screened for tuberculosis by tuberculin skin testing,[6,9] but few clinics routinely screen all prenatal patients in this manner.[31] The American Thoracic Society and the Centers for Disease Control (CDC) have made recommendations for tuberculin testing in the general population; these also apply to the pregnant population.[17] They recommend tuberculin screening for (1) all members of a household where there is a patient who has an active case of tuberculosis; (2) patients with medical conditions that increase the risk of tuberculosis (for example, human immunodeficiency virus [HIV], gastrectomy, diabetes, or immunosuppressive therapy); (3) women who have symptoms compatible with tuberculosis; (4) immigrants from areas endemic for tuberculosis; (5) employees of hospitals, nursing homes, or prisons; and (6) recent immigrants from Asia, Latin America, and Oceania. If the tuberculin test is negative, no further evaluation is necessary; if positive, a chest radiograph (with the abdomen shielded) is performed. Further evaluation and management are dependent upon the patient's symptomatology, the radiographic findings, the stage of pregnancy, and the suspected strain of the organism. Isoniazid (INH), ethambutol, and rifampin are the three primary therapeutic agents; active disease requires the administration of two of these medications. Most antituberculosis therapies are not teratogenic; INH is considered the safest and has been studied the most extensively.[45] Streptomycin has been observed to cause vestibular and auditory impairment in the children of treated women.[42] Ethionamide is rarely needed in the treatment of tuberculosis, but it is a known teratogen; its use is contraindicated in pregnancy. Therapeutic abortion is seldom indicated unless the tuberculosis has disseminated or cardiopulmonary function has been severely compromised.[50] Fortunately, congenital tuberculosis is rare, even in mothers in whom the disease is advanced.[41] The main options for protection of the newborn who does not have active disease are either INH chemoprophylaxis or bacillus Calmette-Guérin (BCG) vaccination. Breast feeding is not contraindicated if adequate maternal treatment and neonatal prophylaxis can be implemented.[43]

Epidemiology

Despite the capability of modern medicine to prevent and cure tuberculosis, the disease persists as a worldwide health problem. An estimated 1 billion people in the world are infected annually with a resultant 1 to 3 million deaths.[10] In 1989, an estimated 10 to 15 million persons in the United States were infected with tuberculosis.[10] According to the CDC, active disease in the United States has a case rate of 9.3 per 100,000.[11]

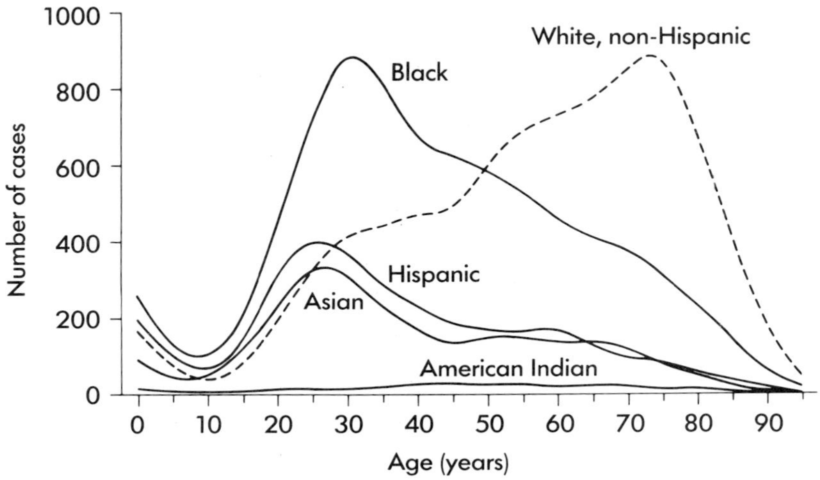

Figure 5-1 Epidemiology of tuberculosis in the United States, 1986: Centers for Disease Control. (From Smith MHD, Teele DW, 1990.[41])

Table 5-1 Persons in Whom Tuberculin Testing Is Indicated

1. Persons with signs (e.g., radiographic abnormality) and/or symptoms (cough, hemoptysis, weight loss, etc.) suggestive of current tuberculosis disease
2. Recent contacts with known tuberculosis cases or persons suspected of having tuberculosis
3. Persons with abnormal chest roentgenograms compatible with past tuberculosis
4. Persons with medical conditions that increase the risk of tuberculosis (silicosis, gastrectomy, diabetes, immunosuppressive therapy, lymphomas, etc.)
5. Persons with HIV infection
6. Groups at high risk of recent infection with *M. tuberculosis,* such as immigrants from Asia, Africa, Latin America, and Oceania; some inner city and skid row populations; personnel and long-term residents in some hospitals, nursing homes, mental institutions, and prisons

From American Thoracic Society Ad Hoc Committee to Revise Diagnostic Standards. 1975.[1]

Despite a 40-year overall decline in the number of tuberculosis cases, rates of infection have risen in certain groups.[13] The evidence strongly suggests that the recent increase in tuberculosis may be attributable to the increased prevalence of AIDS-associated *Mycobacterium tuberculosis,* and *M. avium,* and *M. intracellulare,* the influx of recent immigrants, and an increase in the number of citizens who live in impoverished, overcrowded conditions.[23,41] HIV infection has increased the incidence of tuberculosis by causing immunosuppression, which in turn allows latent tuberculosis infection to become a clinically apparent disease.

The incidence of tuberculosis differs greatly among races (Fig. 5-1). In 1985, the tuberculosis rate for nonwhites (Hispanics, Native Americans, and blacks) in the United States was four times that of the white population.[11] Nearly two-thirds of cases now occur among nonwhites. In eight major American cities that have large indigent communities, the infection rate is at least three times the national average.[8] Almost 40 percent of cases among minorities occur before the age of 35, that is, during childhood and the childbearing years. The rate of active tuberculosis infection among the homeless is 150 to 300 times higher than the nationwide rate.[12,48] Although specific data are not available, the higher risk in minority groups may be related primarily to socioeconomic conditions, such as poor housing and nutrition.

Tuberculosis is also common in immigrants from countries where the disease is prevalent. In these patients, organisms responsible for disease are frequently resistant to commonly used antituberculosis drugs, especially INH. Asians and Pacific Islanders were found to have a rate of 49.6 per 100,000, as compared with 5.7 per 100,000 in the white population of the United States.[12] Foreign-born persons at risk include not only immigrants (legal and illegal) and refugees, but also workers and students.

Mass screening of the inner city pregnant population for tuberculosis is inefficient; the false-positive rate is high. For example, the incidence of reaction to a tuberculin skin test, which cannot distinguish previous from active disease, is approximately 10 percent in most inner city clinics.[26] Yet in 1975, Schaefer and associates[34] estimated the incidence of tuberculosis infection at the New York Lying-In Hospital after 1965 to be between 0.6 and 1 percent, and only 3.2 percent of those infected had active disease during pregnancy. Bailey and colleagues in 1975 estimated a 4.8 percent incidence of tuberculosis infection in the population at Charity Hospital in New Orleans.[4] Therefore, to qualify as a good candidate for tuberculin testing, a pregnant patient must fulfill one or more of the criteria listed in Table 5-1.

The infectious agent, *M. tuberculosis,* is carried on airborne droplet nuclei. Droplet nuclei are produced when persons with pulmonary tuberculosis cough, sneeze, or speak. Droplet nuclei are so small (1 to 5 μm) that air currents normally present in any indoor space can keep them airborne for long periods of time.[16]

Once released from the host, they are dispersed throughout the room. The most significant source of infection is the person who has pulmonary tuberculosis but has not yet been diagnosed or treated; the closer the contact to the host and the younger the age of the recipient, the greater the risk.

Although patients with tuberculosis also generate larger particles containing bacilli, these particles do not serve as effective vehicles for transmission of infection because they do not remain airborne; if they are inhaled, they do not reach the alveoli.[28] Organisms that are deposited on intact mucosa or skin are not able to invade tissue. When large particles are inhaled, they come to rest on the wall of the upper airway or trachea, where they are trapped in the mucous blanket, carried to the oropharynx, and swallowed or expectorated.

Extrapulmonary spread of tuberculosis, although less common, has been well documented. Rarely, infected urine may be contagious in persons using the same toilet facilities.[16] Transmission of tuberculosis by the genital route is exceedingly rare but has been observed in prostatic tuberculosis.[39] Inoculation of abraded skin by contaminated tissues at autopsy examination may produce a primary skin infection in tuberculin-negative individuals (prosector's wart).[29] In some underdeveloped regions of the world, bovine tuberculosis, *M. bovis*, remains a problem; infection occurs by ingesting infected milk. *Mycobacterium bovis* penetrates the gastrointestinal mucosa or invades the lymphatic tissue of the oropharynx. Airborne transmission of *M. bovis* occurs rarely.

Tuberculosis in the fetus and newborn can be acquired in several ways: transplacental transmission, contamination via infected secretions at the time of birth, swallowing of amniotic fluid in utero, acquisition after delivery via human milk, or, more commonly, via the airborne vector mentioned above.[41]

Because of the development of excellent chemotherapeutics against the tubercle bacillus, tuberculosis patients need no longer be isolated. It is recommended that patients who have active disease should be admitted to a hospital initially, so that diagnostic studies and patient education may be undertaken.[32] The period of hospitalization is usually short, after which care is continued on an ambulatory basis. When respiratory embarrassment is present, intensive care may be required. Prenatal counseling and level II ultrasonography should be offered to any patient who has had exposure to antituberculosis therapy during the first trimester of pregnancy.

Etiology

Mycobacteria are obligate, aerobic, nonmotile, nonsporulating bacilli. Their distinguishing features include a slow growth rate, resistance to chemical disinfectants, the ability to survive within phagocytic cells, resistance to elution of carbol-fuchsin stain by acid-alcohol ("acid-fast"), a lack of toxin production, and a lipophilic cell wall. *Mycobacterium tuberculosis* is the leading human pathogen of the family Mycobacteriaceae, followed by *M. leprae*, the cause of leprosy. *Mycobacterium bovis* is mainly a pathogen in animals, but when transmitted via unpasteurized milk it occasionally produces a disease in humans that is similar to tuberculosis. Some "atypical" mycobacteria can produce pulmonary and systemic disease that is indistinguishable from tuberculosis. Of particular note is *M. kansasii*, as well as *M. avium* and *M. intracellulare*, which are responsible for infecting mainly immunocompromised persons, including AIDS patients.[28]

An important distinction exists between tuberculosis infection and tuberculosis disease. According to the American Thoracic Society, infection is a state in which the tubercle bacillus has become established but the patient shows no symptoms or radiographic abnormalities, and no tubercle bacilli are recoverable from a culture of body fluids. This state is characterized by a positive reaction to the tuberculin skin test; the reaction develops 2 to 10 weeks after the initial exposure.[1,2] Approximately 10 percent of those infected develop active infection. If untreated, these persons are at risk to develop active disease at any point in their lives. The risk is about 4 percent for each of the first 2 years and diminishes with time.[26] As mentioned earlier, pregnancy does not alter the natural history of the disease.

The development of clinical disease after infection is influenced by a genetic component. This influence has been demonstrated in the American black population and in animals by a higher incidence of disease in those who have an HLA-BW15 histocompatibility antigen.[28,46] The development of the disease is influenced by age (high risk in infancy and at age 16 to 21 years), undernutrition, immunologic status, and the presence of coexisting disease (silicosis, diabetes).[15,28,41]

Differential Diagnosis

The tubercle bacilli can infect every organ system; clinical presentations are therefore protean. Many patients may first be aware of fatigue, anorexia, weight loss, or low-grade fevers that persist over weeks to months. (The frequent fatigue and anorexia of pregnancy can mask these early symptoms.) Other patients present with acute febrile illness and generalized influenza-like illness. Acute symptoms may be superimposed on a more chronic pattern. At times, nonspecific symptoms associated with fever of unknown origin may be the only manifestations of tuberculosis.[16,50]

Typically, in pulmonary tuberculosis, there is a gradual onset of a cough. Over weeks, a mucoid or bloody, mucopurulent sputum often becomes noticeable. Rarely, there is recurring, dull, aching pain or tightness in the chest. Dyspnea is uncommon and usually signals extensive parenchymal involvement, massive pleural effusion, or other cardiopulmonary disease. Findings may include rales or signs of lung consolidation.

Tuberculosis pleuritis is generally unilateral. It may be associated with acute or recurrent pleuritic pain. Most patients with pleuritis have mild constitutional symptoms, but it is not unusual for a patient to have an acute febrile toxic illness.[17]

Extrapulmonary tuberculosis is often obscure but must be considered whenever a review of systems reveals chronic symptomatology. Urinary tract tuberculosis most commonly presents with sterile pyuria and recurrent fevers.[39] The entire lymphatic system is susceptible to infection. Hilar or mediastinal lymphadenopathy is most frequently seen, but isolated cervical and supraclavicular lymphadenopathy is well described in the literature. Skeletal tuberculosis is usually accompanied by both arthritis and osteomyelitis. Fever and localized pain are common. Tuberculous peritonitis is characterized by ascites, fever, a doughy abdomen, and concurrent pleural effusions.[7] Pericarditis secondary to tuberculosis may present with symptoms of congestive heart failure. Laryngeal disease usually presents with hoarseness and/or a sore throat.[24] Adrenal involvement may result in symptoms of Addison's disease. Intestinal infection may cause abdominal pain and diarrhea. Tuberculosis meningitis is a subacute disease that presents with fever, malaise, and a progressively more severe headache. Personality changes (irritability, confusion, apathy) are often prominent. Vomiting and stiffness of the neck may be absent until later stages. Seizures and a variety of cranial nerve palsies, especially of the sixth and third nerves, develop as the patient becomes more obtunded.[18,25] Tuberculosis mastitis is more commonly noted in lactating mothers[21]; the typical presentation is a single nontender breast mass with or without sinus drainage. Axillary lymph nodes may be enlarged or matted.

The tuberculin skin test has been the traditional method of demonstrating infection with *M. tuberculosis;* the intracutaneous (Mantoux) test is considered the most accurate. It is performed by injecting 0.1 ml (5 tuberculin units) of purified protein derivative (PPD) into the skin of the forearm. The test is read at 48 to 72 hours in a good light. The result is considered significant if 10 mm or more of induration, not erythema, is noted.[2] Zero to 4 mm of induration indicates a negative result. Five to 9 mm of induration is a doubtful reaction, unless the patient is a member of a high-risk category. High-risk patients (see Table 5-1) are considered to have a positive test if an induration of 5 mm or greater is present. Despite its decreased cell-mediated immunity, pregnancy does not appear to affect the cutaneous tuberculin reaction.[27,30,49]

Another important aspect of tuberculin skin testing is that a weakly reactive, false-positive PPD may be secondary to BCG vaccine or AIDS-associated *M. avium* and *M. intracellulare*. HIV tests should be given to patients who have a weakly reactive PPD and no risk factors for tuberculosis. BCG vaccination, used in many developing countries, produces PPD reactivity in a majority of cases. Based on Snider's suggestions,[44] the following guidelines may be used to interpret PPD tests in patients who have previously been vaccinated with BCG: (1) patients vaccinated more than 10 years ago should have their tuberculin skin test interpreted like that of any other individual, and (2) patients vaccinated less than 10 years ago who have a positive PPD reaction should not be considered infected unless they are at high risk for tuberculosis. Any skin reaction 10 mm or greater in size warrants antibiotic prophylaxis, regardless of the interval from vaccine to skin testing.

Definitive diagnostic proof of tuberculosis in both pregnant and nonpregnant patients depends on demonstration of *M. tuberculosis* by culture. Most patients with active tuberculosis have the acid-fast bacilli in their sputum, and the first sputum in the morning has the highest yield for bacterial culture. At least three early morning samples should be obtained. When sputum is not spontaneously produced, respiratory secretions or culture can be obtained by chest physiotherapy and inhalation of an aerosol, such as hypertonic saline, that generates a productive cough. Transbronchial biopsies are useful for culture and histologic confirmation when a bronchoscopy is indicated for other clinical purposes.

Because this organism requires several weeks to grow on classic culture media, several tests have been developed to expedite the identification process. The Ziehl-Neelsen technique of staining is used to identify acid-fast bacteria. In sputum or sections of tissue, mycobacteria can be demonstrated by yellow-orange fluorescence after staining with fluorochrome stains (auramine, rhodamine). The BACTEC method uses rapid radiometric techniques to detect, differentiate, and test for drug susceptibility of mycobacteria.[38] Results usually can be obtained in several days. Sputum antigen identification has proven technically difficult. Currently, DNA probes to the cell wall of four species of *Mycobacterium* have been used; they may reduce the time required for identification to 2 to 8 hours.[37] Serologic measurements of IgG antibody to mycobacterial antigens using an ELISA technique are experimental.[33] This test may gain importance for diagnosing extrapulmonary tuberculosis. If there is evidence of extrapulmonary disease, appropriate biopsy specimens can be obtained for smear and culture. Phagetyping has been used to determine whether the origin of the infection was maternal or from the nursery.

Meningeal infection is typified by a low glucose content, increased protein, increased cells (commonly lymphocytes), and no growth of common bacterial pathogens. Differentiation from fungal infection requires identification of the organism on slide, by culture, by serologic study, or by a combination of the three methods.[25] Specific antigens can also be identified in tuberculosis meningitis by using an ELISA technique, latex particle agglutination, or radioimmunoassays.

Patients with a positive PPD should be further evaluated by chest radiograph (with abdomen shielded). Any patient with symptoms of active tuberculosis should also have a chest radiograph because the PPD has a false-negative rate of up to 30 percent. The risk from an abdominally shielded chest radiograph is considered negligible.[47] Radiographic signs of tuberculosis are most commonly seen in the apical and posterior segments of the upper lobes. Lesions may appear dense and homogeneous with lobar, segmental, or subsegmental distribution. Occasionally, multinodular infiltrates have been noted. Other findings include cavitation, atelectasis, medial retraction of hilar markings, and deviation of the trachea. Miliary tuberculosis is characterized by diffuse, finely nodular (2 mm diameter), uniformly distributed lesions. A unilateral pleural effusion with no other radiographic findings may also signify active tuberculosis.

The physician should order drug susceptibility testing of the tubercle bacilli in two circumstances: (1) when the patient has migrated from drug-resistant endemic regions, such as Asia, South America, or Africa; or (2) when clinical response to antibiotic therapy is not apparent.[17] Initial failure to respond to a clinical regimen is defined as lack of eradication of acid-fast bacilli on smear or culture after 3 months of antibiotics. It should be noted that noncompliance is a major cause of regimen "failure."

Congenital Tuberculosis

In 1935, Beitzki[5] established the criteria for the diagnosis of congenital tuberculosis: (1) *M. tuberculosis* must be present in the child, (2) a primary complex must be present in the liver via contaminated umbilical venous blood, and (3) if a primary hepatic complex is lacking, then tuberculosis may be considered congenital only if tuberculous lesions are seen within a few days of life or in an older child who lives in a tuberculosis-free environment. This definition is still useful clinically to confirm the mode of transmission and course of infection. Based on these criteria, approximately 200 cases of congenital tuberculosis have been documented.[41] In many other cases, however, the route of transmission is often vague. The degree of active maternal infection, especially miliary or endometrial involvement, correlates best with in utero transmission. Occasionally, however, both history and examination fail to reveal the slightest evidence of maternal tuberculosis.[3]

Although there are differences of opinion, most investigators have concluded that tuberculosis has little effect on fetal wastage unless congenital spread is evident. In one large study, 600 of 616 pregnancies resulted in the birth of normal, live infants.[36] There were only seven cases of first-trimester abortion and nine intrauterine fetal deaths. Good and coworkers[20] reported similar findings with little fetal wastage as a consequence of maternal infection.

The clinical manifestations of congenital tuberculosis vary in relationship to the site and size of caseous lesions. Symptoms are usually present by the second or third week of life. The most common are respiratory distress, fever, and hepatomegaly, which may cause abdominal distention. Approximately half the patients have anorexia, poor weight gain, lethargy, or irritability. Peripheral lymphadenopathy is noted in one-third of the cases. Ear drainage and a papulomacular umbilicated skin lesion have been described in case reports. Rare clinical occurrences include subcutaneous nodules, jaundice, croup, apneic episodes, tachypnea, pleural effusion, hypoadrenocortism, thrombocytopenia, seizures, and meningitis.

Almost all affected neonates have radiographic findings, the most characteristic of which are miliary lesions. Some infants have discrete pulmonary infiltrates that can progress to cavitary lesions. Neonates who have an acute febrile illness accompanied by pulmonary infiltrates unresponsive to standard antibiotic therapy should be evaluated for possible congenital tuberculosis.

Diagnosing congenital infection is difficult even when the mother has a history of tuberculosis. Because the immune system of a neonate is less developed than that of an adult, indirect methods of diagnosis are unreliable. The tuberculin skin test is virtually always negative during the first 6 weeks after birth.[41] Despite its insensitivity, however, a PPD should be given because a reaction can offer valuable information quickly. Aggressive management is often required to document acid-fast bacilli by smear or culture and to test for drug susceptibility. Common noninvasive culture sources include gastric aspirates, urine, and skin lesions. Direct smear of the gastric aspirate is not reliable. Other sites that have diagnostic potential include lymph nodes, tracheal aspirates, bone marrow, and middle ear fluid. Liver biopsies are highly sensitive and are an excellent diagnostic tool when congenital tuberculosis is suspected. Although the yield for tuberculosis meningitis is low, the cerebrospinal fluid should also be examined.[41]

Treatment

Because untreated tuberculosis poses a far greater threat to the mother and her fetus than does the most aggressive therapy, the guidelines for treatment of pregnant women are similar to those for women who are not pregnant. Immediate institution of antituberculosis therapy is recommenced for a pregnant woman who has active tuberculosis infection, regardless of the trimester of her pregnancy. The suggested initial therapy should combine INH (5 mg per kg^{-1} per day^{-1}, usually a total of 300 mg) and rifampin (10 mg per kg^{-1} per day^{-1}). A 9-month regimen of these two agents has been found to be highly effective (Fig. 5-2). Shorter regimens and protocols that reduce the INH dosage to twice weekly have been used in the general population, but they have not been proven efficacious in pregnant women. If INH resistance is suspected, ethambutol (15 mg per kg^{-1} per day^{-1}) should be added to the regimen.[45]

Studies indicate that the primary agents for use against tuberculosis (INH, rifampin, and ethambutol) are the safest. Isoniazid is considered safest overall because there has been more clinical experience with it. Even so, a 5 percent incidence of adverse reactions to INH has been reported, with rash, fever, jaundice, and peripheral neuritis most prominent. Prophylactic administration of vitamin B_6 (pyridoxine, 50 mg daily) prevents the development of peripheral neuritis. Although the incidence of INH-induced hepatitis is very low (0.3 percent) in the reproductive age group, as many as 12 percent of patients have elevated plasma transaminase activity. Women receiving INH should be monitored for signs of hepatitis, and serum glutamicoxaloacetic transaminase (SGOT) activities should be measured monthly. An elevation of SGOT to three times the normal level requires discontinuation of the drug. Isoniazid should probably be avoided in any patient with a history of liver disease.[50] Ordinarily, rifampin does not produce untoward effects. Rash, fever, gastrointestinal disturbances, thrombocytopenia, and jaundice, however, have all been described. Limb-reduction defects have been noted with higher frequency in offspring of rifampin-treated mothers. Patients should also be warned that their urine will turn orange-red while taking rifampin. Because rifampin interferes with the efficacy of oral contraceptives, alternative means of birth control should be used.[40] Ethambutol produces even fewer adverse reactions than INH or rifampin. The most important side effect is optic neuritis, resulting in blurred vision and loss of ability to see the color green. Therefore, it is imperative to test visual acuity before ethambutol administration and to monitor it on a regular basis. Once the ethambutol is discontinued, visual recovery occurs in most cases.

Fortunately, secondary agents for tuberculosis are rarely required. The concerns about the teratogenic properties of these agents are listed in Table 5-2. Streptomycin has the potential to cause bilateral hearing loss

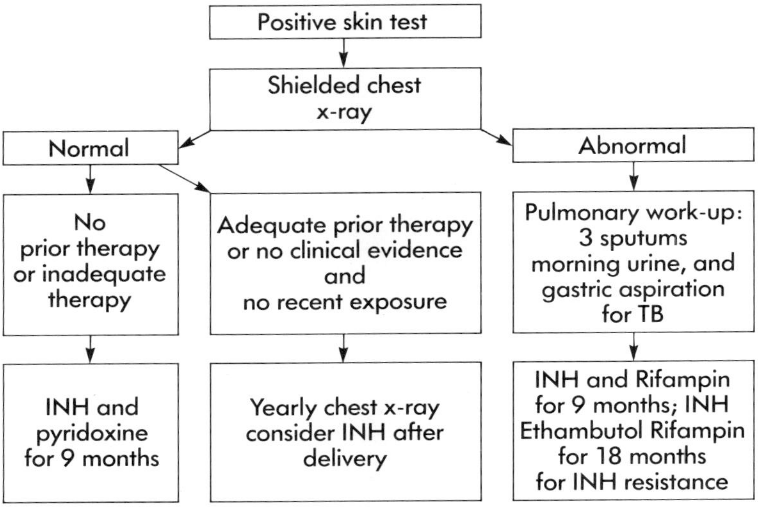

Figure 5-2 Algorithm for the treatment of tuberculosis during pregnancy. (Modified from American Thoracic Society. Control of tuberculosis. Am Rev Respir Dis 1983; 128:336–342.)

Table 5-2 Antituberculosis Drugs: Dosage and Adverse Effects

Drugs	Usual Adult Dosages and Route of Administration	Adverse Effect of Drug in Host	Teratogenic Effects
Isoniazid	300 mg/day PO	Gastrointestinal disturbances, peripheral neuropathy, hepatitis	Not teratogenic but may be embryocidal in rabbits and rats
Para-aminosalicylic acid (PAS)	10-12 g/day PO	Nausea, vomiting, diarrhea; rarely myxedema	Unknown
Ethambutol	25 mg/kg for 1 mo, then 10-15 mg/kg/day PO	Decreased visual acuity (optic neuritis)	Rats—decreased fertility; mice—cleft palate and exencephaly; rabbits—monophthalmia
Rifampin	600 mg/day PO	Gastrointestinal disturbances, headache; rarely hepatitis	Rodents—spina bifida and cleft palates; avoid use during embryogenesis
Streptomycin	0.75-1 g daily for 14 to 21 days, then 1 g 3 times/wk IM	Ototoxicity (vestibular and cochlear), headache, pain at site of injection; rarely nephrotoxicity	Unknown
Capreomycin	0.75-1 g/day for 60 to 120 days, then 1 g 3 times/wk IM	Nephrotoxicity and ototoxicity	"Wavy ribs" in litter of female rats
Viomycin	1-2 g/day for 2 to 4 wk, then 1-2 g 2 to 3 times/wk IM	Nephrotoxicity, ototoxicity	Unknown
Ethionamide	0.5-1 g/day in divided doses PO	Gastrointestinal disturbances, hepatitis, optic and peripheral neuritis	Teratogenic effects in rabbits and rats
Pyrazinamide	20-35 mg/kg/day PO	Hepatic toxicity, hyperuricemia	Unknown
Cycloserine	250 mg twice a day	Central nervous system psychoses, drowsiness, headache, convulsions	Unknown

From Good JT et al. 1981.[20]

and vestibular damage in both the adult and the fetus. Ethionamide is the only known teratogen of the group and therefore is contraindicated in pregnancy.

Today, surgical therapy is rarely needed in the treatment of tuberculosis. If chronic medical therapy fails, however, cavitary lesions in the lung may be resected. Therapeutic abortion is rarely advocated unless the patient is gravely ill with disseminated tuberculosis.[31]

Corticosteroids have been demonstrated to relieve the respiratory embarrassment and fever associated with acute, severe tuberculosis. A moderate dose of prednisone (30 to 35 mg daily) is recommended. The dosage can then be reduced by 2.5 mg every 3 days. When life-threatening adult respiratory distress syndrome is present, 60 to 80 mg of prednisone may be used. Steroids have not been clearly shown to have beneficial effects for a patient who has this syndrome. If an adequate tuberculosis treatment has been implemented, steroids do not affect the course of the infection.

If a mother has active disease, she and her newborn should be separated at delivery; separation should be maintained until the mother has a negative sputum culture. Isoniazid prophylaxis (10 mg per kg^{-1} per day^{-1}) should be given. If noncompliance appears to be an issue, then BCG vaccine can be administered. According to a recent study,[43] women taking antituberculosis drugs can safely breast-feed. Less than 0.75 percent of any antituberculosis agent given orally appears in a mother's milk. Such an amount is probably safe for the infant but inadequate for neonatal therapy. Routine monitoring of drug concentrations in milk and the infant's blood is not necessary.

Prevention

The term *prophylaxis* is misleading when used in reference to tuberculosis because it usually describes the treatment of subclinical infection, not the prevention of tuberculosis colonization. A pregnant patient who has had a PPD conversion within the past 2 years but who has no evidence of active disease should be given 300 mg of INH orally per day for 9 months after the first trimester. A patient who has had a PPD reactivity of unknown duration or who has been in close contact with a person who has tuberculosis should receive 300 mg of INH orally per day for 9 months after delivery.[17]

The BCG vaccine is a live attenuated strain of bovine tuberculosis that is often given to young children in endemic regions in an effort to produce immunity to tuberculosis. The efficacy of the vaccine, however, remains questionable. In several well-controlled studies, its efficacy ranged from 0 to 80 percent.[26]

The CDC has established the year 2010 as a target date for the elimination of tuberculosis (an incidence of less than 1 case per million population), with the year 2000 as an interim date for an incidence of 3.5 cases per 100,000.[10] Law requires that cases of tuberculosis be reported to local health departments. The reporter is vital to the identification of sources and contacts. Recent advances in biotechnology and computer networking should enable the selective diagnosis and treatment of high-risk populations. Socioeconomic factors such as overcrowding and homelessness, however, may be a significant obstacle to the elimination of tuberculosis.

In conclusion, there are four main caveats with regard to pregnant patients who have tuberculosis. First, prompt diagnosis and treatment are more critical in a pregnant patient because congenital tuberculosis is usually fatal to her infant. Second, preventive therapy of subclinical disease should be postponed until the second trimester. Third, most secondary antituberculin therapies have not been proven safe in pregnancy and should be avoided unless resistance to primary agents is evident. Fourth, women who continue to receive rifampin treatment after delivery cannot rely on oral contraceptives as a means of birth control. Despite these warnings, however, a woman who has been adequately treated for tuberculosis generally enjoys an uncomplicated pregnancy and may nurse her infant with little risk.

References

1. American Thoracic Society Ad Hoc Committee to Revise Diagnostic Standards. Diagnostic standards and classification of tuberculosis and other mycobacterial diseases. New York: American Lung Association, 1975.
2. American Thoracic Society and Centers for Disease Control. The tuberculin skin test. Am Rev Respir Dis 1971; 104:769–778.
3. Ascensi F, Otero MC, Perez-Tamarit D, et al. Pediatr Infect Dis J 1990; 9:223–224.
4. Bailey WE, Thompson DM, Greenberg HB. Indigent women of New Orleans require tuberculosis control measures. Health Service Report 1973; 87:737–740.
5. Beitzki H. Über die angioborne tuberkulose infektion. Ergeb Tuberk Fortschr 1935; 7:1–30.
6. Bowes WA Detection and treatment of tuberculosis. Contemporary Obstetrics and Gynecology 1975; 6:43–48.
7. Brooks JH, Stirrat GM. Tuberculous peritonitis in pregnancy. Case report. Br J Obstet Gynaecol 1986; 93:1009–1010.
8. Bush JJ. Protocol for tuberculosis screening in pregnancy. J Obstet Gynecol Neonatal Nurs 1986; 5:225-230.
9. Byrd R. Treating the pregnant tuberculous patient. Journal of Respiratory Diseases 1982; 4:27–30.
10. Centers for Disease Control. Screening for tuberculosis and tuberculosis infection in high risk populations. MMWR 1990; 39:1–7.
11. Centers for Disease Control. Tuberculosis in blacks—United States. MMWR 1987; 36:212–215.
12. Centers for Disease Control. Tuberculosis in minorities—United States. MMWR 1987; 36:77–79.
13. Centers for Disease Control. Tuberculosis, final data—US 1986. MMWR 1988; 36:817–820.
14. Cohen JD, Patton EA, Badger TL. The tuberculous mother. American Review of Tuberculosis 1952; 65:1–23.
15. Davies PD. A possible link between vitamin D

deficiency and impaired host defence to *Mycobacterium tuberculosis*. Tubercle 1985; 66:301–306.
16. Des Prez R. Tuberculosis. In: Wyngaarden JB, Smith LH, eds. Cecil textbook of medicine. Ed 16. Philadelphia: WB Saunders, 1982:1538–1542.
17. Diagnostic standards and classification of tuberculosis. Joint statement of the American Thoracic Society and the Centers for Disease Control. Am Rev Respir Dis 1990; 142:725–735.
18. Donaldson JO, ed. Neurology of pregnancy. Ed 2. Philadelphia: WB Saunders, 1989:103–125.
19. Edge JR. Pulmonary tuberculosis and pregnancy. Br Med J 1952; 2:845–847.
20. Good JT, Iseman MD, Davidson PT, et al. Tuberculosis in association with pregnancy. Am J Obstet Gynecol 1981; 140:492–498.
21. Gupta R, Gupta AS, Duggal N. Tubercular mastitis. Int Surg 1982; 67:422–424.
22. Hageman J, Shulman S, Schreiber M, et al. Congenital tuberculosis: critical reappraisal of clinical findings and diagnostic procedures. Pediatrics 1980; 66:980–984.
23. Hinman AR, Judd JM, Kolnick JP, Daitch PB. Changing risks in tuberculosis. Am J Epidemiol 1976; 103:486–497.
24. Jan A. Primary laryngeal tuberculosis. J Laryngol Otol 1986; 100:605–606.
25. Kingdom JCP, Kennedy DH. Tuberculous meningitis in pregnancy. Br J Obstet Gynaecol 1989; 96:233–235.
26. Medchill MT, Gillum M. Diagnosis and management of tuberculosis during pregnancy. Obstet Gynecol Surv 1989; 44:81–84.
27. Montgomery WP, Young RC, Allen MP, Harden KA. The tuberculin test in pregnancy. Am J Obstet Gynecol 1968; 100:829–832.
28. Mycobacteria. In: Jawetz E, Melnick JL, Adelberg EA, eds. Review of medical microbiology. Ed 16. Los Altos, Calif: Lange, 1984:228–234.
29. Mycobacterial diseases. In: Arnold HL, Odom RB, James WD, eds. Andrew's diseases of the skin. Ed 8. Philadelphia: WB Saunders, 1990:375–388.
30. Present PA, Comstock GW. Tuberculin sensitivity in pregnancy. Am Rev Respir Dis 1975; 112:413–417.
31. Pritchard JA, MacDonald PC, Gant NF. Medical and surgical illnesses during pregnancy and the puerperium. In: Williams obstetrics. Ed 17. Norwalk, Conn: Appleton Century Crofts, 1985:561–640.
32. Rogge PT. Respiratory complications. In: Niswander KR, ed. Manual of obstetrics: diagnosis and therapy. Ed 3. Boston: Little Brown, 1988:72–79.
33. Sada E, Ruiz-Palacio GM, Lopez-Vidal Y, Ponce de Leon S. Detection of mycobacterial antigens in cerebrospinal fluid of patients with tuberculous meningitis by enzyme-linked immunosorbent assay. Lancet 1983; 2:651–652.
34. Schaefer G, Zervoudakis IA, Fuchs FF, David S. Pregnancy and pulmonary tuberculosis. Obstet Gynecol 1975; 46:706–715.
35. Schwabe KH, Dobstadt HP. Lungentuberkulose und Schwangerschaft. Beitr Klin Tuberk 1966; 134:75–96.
36. Seilikoff IJ, Dorfmann HL. Management of tuberculosis. In: Rovinsky JJ, Guttmacher, eds. Medical, surgical, and gynecological complications of pregnancy. Baltimore: Williams & Wilkins, 1965:111–119.
37. Shoemaker SA, Fisher JH, Jones WD Jr, Scoggin CH. Restriction fragment analysis of chromosomal DNA defines different strains of *Mycobacterium tuberculosis*. Am Rev Resp Dis 1986; 134:210–213.
38. Siddiqui SH, Hwangbo CC, Silcox V, et al. Rapid radiometric methods to detect and differentiate *Mycobacterium tuberculosis/M. bovis* from other mycobacterial species. Am Rev Respir Dis 1984; 130:634–640.
39. Simon HB, Weinstein AJ, Pasternak MS, et al. Genitourinary tuberculosis: clinical features in a general hospital population. Am J Med 1977; 63:410–413.
40. Skolnick JL, Stoler BS, Katz DB, Anderson WH. Rifampin, oral contraceptives, and pregnancy. JAMA 1976; 236:1382.
41. Smith MHD, Teele DW. Tuberculosis. In: Remington JS, Klein J, eds. Infectious diseases of the fetus and newborn infant. Ed 3. Philadelphia: WB Saunders, 1990:834–847.
42. Snider DE. Pregnancy and tuberculosis. Chest 1984; 86:10S–13.
43. Snider DE. Should women taking antituberculosis drugs breastfeed? Arch Intern Med 1984; 144:589–590.
44. Snider DE. Bacille Calmette-Guérin vaccination and tuberculosis skin tests. JAMA 1985; 253:3438–3439.
45. Snider DE, Layde PM, Johnson MW, Lyle MA. Treatment of tuberculosis during pregnancy. Am Rev Respir Dis 1980; 122:65–79.
46. Stead WW, Senner JW, Reddick WT, Lofgren JP. Racial differences in susceptibility to infection by *Mycobacterium tuberculosis*. N Engl J Med 1990; 322:422–427.
47. Swarz HM. Radiation risk from the chest examination. JAMA 1974; 228:696–702.
48. Tuberculosis control among homeless populations. MMWR 1987; 36:257–260.
49. Weinstein L, Murphy T. The management of tuberculosis during pregnancy. Clin Perinatol 1974; 1:395–416.
50. Willson JR. Diseases of the respiratory system. In: Willson JR, Carrington ER, Ledger WJ, eds. Obstetrics and gynecology, Ed 7. St Louis: CV Mosby, 1983:292–303.

CHAPTER 6

Vaginitis During Pregnancy: Consequences and Treatment

David A. Eschenbach, M.D.

Vaginitis is at least as common during pregnancy as when reproductive-age women are not pregnant. The prevalence of candidiasis even increases during pregnancy. The diagnosis of vaginitis is unaltered by the physiologic changes of pregnancy. However, treatment of bacterial vaginosis and trichomoniasis is altered in pregnancy because of concerns that medication might affect the fetus.

In the past several years, it has been recognized that genital tract microorganisms are associated with premature delivery and premature rupture of fetal membranes.[35] Bacterial vaginosis and, to a lesser extent, trichomoniasis have both been related to premature delivery and membrane rupture, and bacterial vaginosis has been related to upper genital tract infection. Pregnant patients will need to be screened for these two infections in the future if a cause-and-effect relationship is shown between these infections and prematurity.

When vaginitis is accurately diagnosed, the treatment of vaginitis becomes straightforward. Therefore, an accurate diagnosis is a most important feature of treating vaginitis. Details on diagnosis are beyond the scope of this chapter, but the systematic determination of the appearance, the pH, the amine odor, and the microscopy of the vaginal discharge is key to establishing an accurate diagnosis. These determinations are not appreciably altered in pregnancy except for an increase of white blood cells in vaginal fluid. A systematic diagnostic scheme has been developed and should be utilized.[11,14]

Bacterial Vaginosis

Bacterial vaginosis is one of the most frequent vaginal infections in pregnancy. Bacterial vaginosis has been found in 15 to 20 percent of pregnant women.[13,18,19,28] Complaints of an increased amount of a fishy odor to the discharge occurs in symptomatic women. However, at least half of patients with this infection have either no or only mild symptoms. Therefore, an accurate prevalence of bacterial vaginosis can be found only by combining both asymptomatic and symptomatic patients. Asymptomatic patients with bacterial vaginosis have similar increases in the concentration of bacteria in the vagina as symptomatic patients, and thus the same rate of untoward effects would be expected in both groups.

Patients with bacterial vaginosis have consistently had an increased prevalence of *Gardnerella vaginalis*, selected anaerobic bacteria (most notably *Bacteroides* and *Mobiluncus*), and *Mycoplasma hominis* and a decreased prevalence of facultative lactobacilli.[12,28,49] Perhaps more important, a 1,000-fold increase in the concentration of *G. vaginalis*[49] have been found using quantitative microbiology.

Diagnosis

The diagnosis of bacterial vaginosis can be made clinically or by using a direct Gram's stain of vaginal fluid. The standard clinical diagnosis of bacterial vaginosis has become well established and it includes the presence of at least three of the following four characteristics of the vaginal discharge: a thin homogeneous appearance, a pH greater than 4.5, the release of a fishy amine odor upon alkalinization of the discharge with 10 percent potassium hydroxide (KOH), and clue cells on wet mount.[1,15] Clue cells are vaginal epithelial cells so covered with bacteria that the cell border is obscured.

Table 6-1 Relationship Between Bacterial Vaginosis and Prematurity

STUDY (REF.)	**Bacterial Vaginosis Total Examined (%)** WOMEN DELIVERING PREMATURELY	WOMEN NOT DELIVERING PREMATURELY	**Univariate** OR (95% CI)*	**Multivariate** OR (95% CI)*
Eschenbach (13)	28/57 (49)	27/114 (24)	3.1 (1.6-6.0)	—
Gravett (18)	19/44 (43)	6/ 44 (14)	3.8 (1.2-11.6)†	—
Gravett (19)	24/77 (31)	78/457 (17)	2.2 (1.3-3.8)	2.8 (1.1-3.5)‡
Martius (28)	21/61 (34)	21/115 (18)	2.3 (1.2-4.7)	2.3 (1.1-5.0)§

*Odds ratio = 95% confidence interval.
†Matched to controls not in labor for gestational age, demographic, and obstetric factors. *C. trachomatis*, Group B streptococci, *G. vaginalis*, Herpes simplex virus, and genital mycoplasmas were also studied.
‡Multivariate analysis was used to control for demographic and obstetric factors and *C. trachomatis*.
§Multivariate analysis used to control for demographic and obstetric factors and *C. trachomatis*, *Lactobacillus* sp., black-pigmented *Bacteroides* sp., *Mobiluncus sp;., and Ureaplasma urealyticum*.

The Gram's stain method described by Spiegel and associates uses the identification of certain bacterial morphotypes in the Gram's stain.[50] The diagnosis of bacterial vaginosis made by Gram's stain compares favorably to the diagnosis using strict clinical criteria.[15,38,50] Quantitative vaginal cultures, gas-liquid chromatography (GLC), and proline aminopeptidase can also be used to diagnose bacterial vaginosis, but these tests do not offer the availability, ease, and accuracy of clinical criteria or the Gram's stain.

Prematurity

A relationship between bacterial vaginosis and premature labor and/or premature rupture of membranes has been reported in several case-control studies where bacterial vaginosis was present significantly more often among patients who delivered before 37 weeks' gestation than among control patients who delivered at term.[13,18,28] A cohort of patients with bacterial vaginosis were also found to deliver prematurely more frequently than those without bacterial vaginosis (Table 6-1).[6] In addition, *Bacteroides,* the anaerobe most highly associated with bacterial vaginosis, has been associated with preterm delivery and preterm rupture of membranes (ROM).[31,36]

In the first report,[13] bacterial vaginosis diagnosed by GLC was found in about half of women who delivered with a gestational age of 37 weeks or less and in about one-quarter of control women who delivered at term ($p = 0.001$). The influences of demographic and obstetric factors and of other genital infections on prematurity were not studied in this preliminary report. In the second report, bacterial vaginosis identified by GLC was present in 43 percent of 44 women with premature labor and in 14 percent of 44 matched control women without premature labor ($p = 0.02$). Other microorganisms (*Neisseria gonorrhoeae,* group B streptococci, *G. vaginalis,* Herpes simplex virus, and the genital mycoplasmas) did not significantly differ between the two groups in this small sample of patients, except for *Chlamydia trachomatis,* which was also associated with premature labor.[18]

The relationship between pregnancy outcome and four genital infections (bacterial vaginosis, *C. trachomatis, N. gonorrhoeae,* and group B streptococci) was then prospectively investigated among a cohort of 534 pregnant women. The mean birth weight of the neonates born of mothers with bacterial vaginosis was 2,960 g compared to 3,184 g in the group without bacterial vaginosis (p less than 0.01).[19] In this study, numerous obstetric, demographic, and infectious factors were examined for their possible influence on the relationship between prematurity and bacterial vaginosis. Bacterial vaginosis was detected in 31 percent of 77 patients delivering before 37 weeks' gestation and in 17 percent of 457 women who delivered at term (p less than 0.01).[19] Bacterial vaginosis remained significantly correlated to premature delivery at less than 37 weeks in a multivariate analysis in which nonmicrobiologic factors and *C. trachomatis* were controlled (odds ratio = 2.0, 95 percent confidence interval 1.1 to 3.5).[19] Premature rupture of membranes before 37 weeks' gestation was also significantly associated with bacterial vaginosis in this study.

Bacterial vaginosis was diagnosed using Gram's stain criteria in a third case-control study.[28] The data were controlled for demographic, behavioral, and pregnancy characteristics associated with either prematurity or bacterial vaginosis within this population. Cases with premature labor differed from control in several aspects. Women with premature labor were younger, had more prior premature births, and during the current pregnancy had a higher rate of preterm premature ROM and a higher rate of fever (both intrapartum and postpartum) than the controls. Bacterial vaginosis was diagnosed in 34 percent of the 61 women who delivered before 37 weeks' gestation compared to 18 percent of the 115 women who delivered at term (p less than 0.05). Bacterial vaginosis was independently associated with a delivery earlier than 37 weeks in the multivariate analysis (odds ratio 2.3, $p = 0.03$). Lactobacilli were negatively related to prematurity (odds ratio 0.2, $p = 0.002$). These four studies have all found bacterial vaginosis related to premature delivery with remarkably similar odds ratios. In contrast, one study reported no association between bacterial vaginosis and prematurity.[10] The gonorrhea and human immunodeficiency virus rate was high in this Kenyan population, which may have confounded the results, but the lack of an association of bacterial vaginosis with prematurity in this report is unclear.

The combined results of these studies indicate a fairly consistent association between prematurity and/or preterm premature ROM and bacterial vaginosis, defined either by GLC or Gram's stain criteria. The association between bacterial vaginosis and prematurity remained when adjustment was made for demographic or obstetric variables that are associated with either bacterial vaginosis or prematurity in multivariate analyses. The relationship between bacterial vaginosis and prematurity has also been independent of selected other genital flora. However, many vaginal-cervical microorganisms have been related to premature delivery in various prior studies,[35] and in none of the studies of bacterial vaginosis were enough subjects enrolled to exclude the possibility of a significant relationship between these other microorganisms (except *C. trachomatis*) and prematurity. More study is required of the importance of bacterial vaginosis relative to other genital infections.

In the meantime, data relating microorganisms to prematurity would be more convincing if microorganisms in upper genital tract sites, such as amniotic fluid or placenta, were related to prematurity. Recent information indicates that microorganisms, especially those associated with bacterial vaginosis, can be isolated more frequently from the amniotic fluid or chorioamnion of women who deliver prematurely than from those who deliver at term.

Amniotic Fluid Infection

Abdominal amniocenteses have been performed on women in premature labor with intact membranes. The majority of women enrolled into these studies had no clinical signs of infection at the time of amniocentesis. A positive amniotic fluid culture has been present in about 15 percent of over 200 women in premature labor who underwent amniocentesis. Of those with a positive culture, 37 percent had anaerobic bacteria recovered from their amniotic fluid. Microorganisms commonly associated with bacterial vaginosis (*Bacteroides* sp., *M. hominis,* and *G. vaginalis*) were isolated from 49 percent of the women with a positive amniotic fluid culture.[27]

Women with a positive amniotic fluid culture usually deliver within 24 hours of the amniocentesis, despite the fact that most patients received tocolytic agents. In contrast, women with sterile amniotic fluid had a mean pregnancy prolongation of between 25 and 50 days.[27] The amniotic fluid infection, the presence of bacterial products, or the presence of cytokines from microorganisms and inflammation either initiates labor, further increases the likelihood of delivery among women already in premature labor, or both. The finding that half of the microorganisms isolated from the amniotic fluid are related to bacterial vaginosis suggests that this infection may play a substantial role in amniotic fluid infection among women with premature labor and intact membranes.

Placental Infection

Histologic chorioamnionitis is highly related to preterm birth.[20,22,41,46] Further, the highest prevalence of chorioamnionitis occurs in the most premature pregnancies.[22,46] It is now clear that the majority of histologic chorioamnionitis is caused by microorganisms in the chorioamnion. The recovery of microorganisms from the placenta and chorioamniotic membranes is highly correlated with histologic chorioamnionitis.[22,41] A very consistent 70 percent positive chorioamnion culture rate has been present among placentas with histologic chorioamnionitis.[22,41] Significantly lower chorioamnion positive culture rates (15 to 20 percent) are found in placentas without histologic chorioamnionitis.[22,41] The combined weight and consistency of these studies provide clear evidence that microorganisms cause histologic chorioamnionitis.

In a case-control designed study, the interrelationships were examined between histologic chorioamnionitis, chorioamnion infection, prematurity, and bacterial vaginosis.[22] Chorioamnion infection was demonstrated by the recovery of microorganisms between the divided amnion and chorion in 61 percent of 38 placentas of women who delivered before 37 weeks' gestation and from 21 percent of 56 placentas of control women who delivered at term (p less than 0.001).[22] Bacteria (any microorganism other than *M. hominis* or *Ureaplasma urealyticum*) were isolated from 45 percent of those who delivered prematurely and only 7 percent of controls who delivered at term (p less than 0.001).[22] The majority of bacteria isolated from the membranes were those associated with bacterial vaginosis. Multivariate analysis was used to control for factors that could otherwise explain the microbiologic findings, including demographic variables, duration of labor, duration of ROM, premature ROM, and fever in labor. Both a positive chorioamnion culture (odds ratio 3.8, p less than 0.01) and histologic chorioamnionitis (odds ratio 5.0, $p = 0.001$) were significantly related to prematurity in the multivariate analysis. Bacterial vaginosis diagnosed by Gram's stain was also related to a positive chorioamnion culture (odds ratio 3.5, p less than 0.006) and to histologic chorioamnionitis (odds ratio 2.6, $p = 0.05$) in the multivariate analyses.

Data from studies of the placentas demonstrate a strong, consistent relationship between the isolation of microorganisms from the placenta and histologic chorioamnionitis, with rare exceptions. Histologic chorioamnionitis has a well-established relationship with premature delivery, and recent evidence confirms a relationship between the isolation of microorganisms from the placenta and premature delivery. In some studies, potentially confounding variables such as duration of labor, duration of ROM, premature ROM, and maternal fever have been controlled to add further weight and confidence to a cause-and-effect relationship between these associations. Microorganisms associated with bacterial vaginosis are commonly isolated from the placenta. Further, bacterial vaginosis has been related both to infection of the chorioamnion and to chorioamnionitis in a multivariate analysis, which provided added strength to these associations.

Postpartum Infection

With a large concentration of virulent bacteria in the vagina of patients with bacterial vaginosis, it would not be surprising to find bacterial vaginosis related to postpartum infection. In fact, women with bacterial vaginosis undergoing cesarean section have a 5.8-fold increased risk of postpartum endometritis compared to women with normal vaginal flora.[53] In this report, a multifactorial analysis was used to study the effect of other labor variables on postpartum endometritis. A young maternal age and the duration of ROM were also related to postpartum endometritis. However, the relative risk of bacterial vaginosis in postpartum endometritis changed little when adjustment was made for these variables. Bacterial vaginosis appears related to postpartum endometritis independently of other variables. Patients with bacterial vaginosis and postpartum endometritis also had an increased rate of recovery of *G. vaginalis* and anaerobic bacteria from the endometrium.[53] Flora found in the vagina of patients with bacterial vaginosis can be recovered from about 60 percent of endometrial cultures obtained from women with postpartum endometritis.[52] Thus bacterial vaginosis is one of the more important risks for the development of postpartum endometritis, especially following cesarean section. An increased rate of abdominal wound infection was also related to bacterial vaginosis.[52] In a similar example, patients with bacterial vaginosis undergoing abdominal hysterectomy have a threefold increased risk of postoperative infection compared to patients with normal flora.[48]

Treatment

At this point controlled studies are in order to demonstrate whether treatment of bacterial vaginosis during pregnancy will reduce the prematurity rate. Tetracycline given to abacteriuric women led to a reduction of prematurity.[9] The effect of erythromycin given to patients with *U. urealyticum* to reduce prematurity has had mixed results.[16,30,32] Thus one needs to be cautious before concluding that effective therapy of bacterial vaginosis would necessarily reduce prematurity without well-designed and controlled studies. None of the antibiotics in these studies have been specifically given to treat bacterial vaginosis, and tetracyclines or erythromycins are not particularly effective against bacterial vaginosis. Treatment of bacterial vaginosis with effective antibiotics versus placebo is necessary to clarify further the role of bacterial vaginosis in prematurity, preterm premature ROM, and postpartum endometritis.

At present, treatment of bacterial vaginosis during pregnancy should be confined to symptomatic patients until controlled studies are available on whether treatment of bacterial vaginosis reduces adverse pregnancy outcomes and postpartum endometritis. Metronidazole 500 mg orally twice daily for 2 days is the regimen recommended for nonpregnant patients. The Centers for Disease Control recommends that metronidazole not be used in the first trimester of pregnancy.[37] Clindamycin 300 mg given orally twice daily for 7 days is recommended for the treatment of bacterial vaginosis at any time during pregnancy.[37] Amoxicillin does not effectively treat bacterial vaginosis during pregnancy, and erythromycin, tetracycline, Betadine douching, triple sulfa vaginal cream, and acidifying agents are either contraindicated or ineffective. There are no data to suggest that the treatment of male sexual partners prevents recurrent bacterial vaginosis, and it cannot be recommended at present. It is important for the clinician to remain alert to possible changes regarding the treatment of bacterial vaginosis in pregnancy.

Trichomoniasis

Trichomonas vaginalis infection is also common. Trichomoniasis accounts for approximately 25 percent of symptomatic vaginitis. *Trichomonas vaginalis* is a sexually transmitted parasite present in 12 to 30 percent of pregnant women.[6,36,45] One-half of women with trichomoniasis are asymptomatic. The parasite infects the vagina, urethra, bladder, and Bartholin's glands. The bacterial flora in the vagina of patients with *T. vaginalis* infection has not been extensively studied, but many of the clinical findings present in patients with trichomoniasis are those found in patients with bacterial vaginosis. A pH greater than 4.5, an amine odor with the addition of 10 percent KOH, and clue cells are frequently present in women with trichomoniasis. Thus the flora present in many women with trichomoniasis may be disturbed and high concentrations of anaerobes are common. Further, some of the pregnancy complications described in patients with bacterial vaginosis may also be present in patients with trichomoniasis.

Diagnosis

Asymptomatic women tend to have lower concentrations of *T. vaginalis* and hence need to be identified by culture rather than by wet mounts. Nonpregnant women with trichomoniasis have complaints of a yellow vaginal discharge and vulvar itching. Signs of trichomoniasis include colpitis mascularis (maculoerythematous ectocervical lesions), a purulent and frothy vaginal discharge, and erythema of the vagina and vulva.[55] Patients with these symptoms or signs should be scrutinized for trichomoniasis.

The pH of the vaginal discharge is usually greater than 4.5. An amine odor of the vaginal discharge is often present after the addition of 10 percent KOH. On wet mount, a varying but usually increased number of white blood cells (WBCs) are identified. Motile trichomonads vary in size, but they are usually slightly larger than WBCs. Trichomonads are identified by the rapid, jerking movement under a 400-power microscopic objective. Stationary trichomonads inhibited by WBCs can also be identified by the beating flagellar motion. A substantial proportion of women with trichomoniasis have an abnormal flora similar to that seen in bacterial vaginosis with clue cells, a decrease of lactobacilli, and an increase in the prevalence and concentration of other bacteria.

The diagnosis of trichomoniasis based only on a positive wet mount examination underestimates the prevalence of the infection by approximately 50 percent. The trichomonad can be identified by wet mount only with high concentrations of the microorganisms. About 50 percent of culture-positive women have low concentrations of *T. vaginalis* and hence have negative wet mounts.

Trichomoniasis is important to recognize in pregnancy because the presence of this infection is highly associated with the presence of other sexually transmitted diseases, particularly *N. gonorrhoeae*. *Trichomonas vaginalis* may support the transmission or the growth of *N. gonorrhoeae* or both. Up to a third of patients with *T. vaginalis* have *N. gonorrhoeae* and vice versa.

Prematurity

Trichomoniasis may also be associated with premature delivery. *Trichomonas vaginalis* identified by culture in the third trimester has been associated with statistically significant reduction in the mean age of delivery (38.2 weeks for culture-positive patients and 39.5 weeks gestation for patients without *T. vaginalis*).[21] The rate of low birth weight (less than 2,500 g) was 18 percent in those with and 7 percent in those without *T. vaginalis* (not a significant difference). This adolescent inner city population had a high prevalence of other sexually transmitted microorganisms, but none of the other five microorganisms, including *C. trachomatis* and genital mycoplasmas, correlated with abnormal pregnancy outcomes.[21] *Trichomonas vaginalis* was found to be related to premature ROM at term (relative risk [RR] less than 1.4, p less than 0.03).[36] *Bacteroides* species were related to preterm premature ROM, preterm delivery, or low birth weight, but *T. vaginalis* was not related to any of these other abnormal obstetric outcomes in this study.[36] In a recent large multicenter study of 7,073 women, *T. vaginalis* identified by culture at 23 to 26 weeks' gestation was examined for an association with abnormal pregnancy.[6] Multivariate analyses were used to control potentially confounding variables, including maternal age, demographic factors, and the recovery of many microorganisms previously associated with prematurity (*N. gonorrhoeae, C. trachomatis, Bacteroides* spp. genital mycoplasmas, and *Candida* sp.). *Trichomonas vaginalis* in the second trimester remained significantly associated with preterm premature ROM (RR = 1.4), premature delivery at less than 37 weeks' gestation (RR = 1.5), and low birth weight under 2,500 g (RR = 1.4).[6]

Trichomonas vaginalis has not been associated with prematurity in small studies,[29,45] but this could be related to the small relative risk noted in the large study.[6] However, *T. vaginalis* has not been associated with upper genital tract invasion in the nonpregnant patient, and *T. vaginalis* is infrequently isolated from the chorioamnion of patients who deliver prematurely.[22] The association between *T. vaginalis* and prematurity is further confounded by the very close association between *T. vaginalis* and bacterial vaginosis. To date, the effect of *T. vaginalis* on pregnancy has not been sufficiently separated from an effect of bacterial vaginosis to know whether *T. vaginalis* exhibits an independent effect upon pregnancy.

Treatment

Treatment of trichomoniasis in pregnancy presents difficulties. At present, treatment in pregnancy would be justified only for symptomatic maternal infection. In a study of limited size, treatment of trichomoniasis had no effect on adverse pregnancy outcome.[45] Treatment trials of trichomoniasis are needed to study further the effect of treatment on pregnancy outcome.[39] Metronidazole is the only effective drug available for the treatment of trichomoniasis in the United States. Oral therapy provides adequate levels of medication not only for vaginal but also for periurethral, urethral, and bladder infection. As mentioned, metronidazole is considered contraindicated in the first trimester of pregnancy.[37] Metronidazole has been administered to a large number of pregnant women, but neonatal effects are available for only a modest number of patients. In general, metronidazole has not been associated with recognized teratogenic or other adverse neonatal effects except for two small reports. Congenital anomalies were found in some women who took metronidazole during the first trimester.[2,42]

Mutagens associated with a carcinogenic potential have been identified in the urine of women taking metronidazole.[44] At present, metronidazole must be considered a weak carcinogen capable of producing DNA damage. This has given concern that an increase in rates of cancer may occur among those exposed to metronidazole. Two relatively small retrospective studies in adults have been held to show no relationship between metronidazole and cancer.[2,17] Rates of some cancers in fact were slightly increased among metronidazole and cigarette users compared to controls but with relative risks less than 2.[2] However, the studies were too small to detect an effect at less than a twofold increased risk. Weak carcinogens often are associated with risk ratios lower than 2. Data are also incomplete because of short 3- to 11-year follow-up, compared to up to a 30-year latency period for clinical cancer. Thus, studies of the relation of cancer to metronidazole are too small and of too short a duration of follow-up to address this issue with certainty in adults. There are no follow-up studies of infants exposed to metronidazole during pregnancy. The magnitude of this effect is uncertain in adults, but one must remain concerned about the potential carcinogenic effect of metronidazole in pregnancy, when the fetus is particularly susceptible to carcinogens.

Several modifications of therapy are possible to use during pregnancy. Treatment should be avoided in the first trimester when the neonate is most susceptible to the effects of drugs. Treatment can be considered for patients with moderate or severe symptoms in the second and third trimester of pregnancy. Clotrimazole has an inhibitory effect on *T. vaginalis* in vitro, although most clinicians find symptomatic infection quickly recurs and an actual microbiologic cure is rare. Asymptomatic or minimally symptomatic patients should not receive treatment during pregnancy, but rather they can be given a 2-g dose of metronidazole on the day of delivery. Levels of drug in breast milk are equal to serum levels. Breast feeding should be delayed for 24 hours so that limited levels of drug would be present in breast milk. In summary, because of concerns over the weak carcinogenic potential of metronidazole, at present its use should be limited during pregnancy. However, treatment trials of

T. vaginalis are required to resolve the issues of prematurity and safety.

Recommended treatment in pregnancy consists of 2 g of metronidazole given as a one-time dose.[37] Cure rates of over 95 percent are usually reported for nonpregnant women, particularly when male sexual partners also receive treatment. Nausea, the most common side effect, occurs in 5 to 25 percent of patients. A metallic taste is another common side effect. Cephalagia, dizziness, and dark urine also occur with metronidazole use. Patients should be advised to not drink alcohol for 24 hours after the last metronidazole dose because of a disulfuran-like effect that produces nausea when alcohol is concomitantly ingested.

Concomitant male sexual partner therapy is recommended to treat this sexually transmitted infection effectively. About three-quarters of male contacts of women with trichomoniasis acquire the microorganism. Approximately one-third of infected males seemingly undergo a spontaneous cure of their trichomoniasis urethral infection, but there is clear evidence that male sexual partners of women with trichomoniasis should be treated. Female cure rates are increased 10 to 25 percent when the male is also treated.

Candidiasis

Candida albicans causes 80 to 90 percent of vaginal fungal infections; other *Candida* species and *Torulopsis* cause the remaining infections. These saprophytic fungi can be isolated in small numbers from 5 to 20 percent of asymptomatic nonpregnant women. Asymptomatic pregnant women have a similar prevalence of *Candida* as nonpregnant patients.[31,36] Symptomatic infection usually results only when these organisms proliferate in large numbers. Possibly related to the increased levels of steroids, the prevalence of symptomatic candidiasis is increased during pregnancy.

Patients with diabetes, on immunosuppressive drugs, with acquired immunodeficiency syndrome, or on antibiotic therapy have particularly high rates of candidiasis. Most women with occasional sporadic candidiasis and even those with frequently recurrent candidiasis usually have none of these risk factors. However, recurrent candidiasis is more frequent when a patient is pregnant.

Diagnosis

Women with candidiasis usually experience vulvar and vaginal pruritus. External dysuria caused by vulvar inflammation is also common. A nonodorous or even a "sour milk" smelling vaginal discharge may occur, but a vaginal discharge is not a common complaint.

Patients with candidiasis have a variety of vaginal findings from patchy dry plaques to vaginal erythema without discharge to a normal appearing discharge and a normal vaginal mucosa. The pH of the vaginal discharge is invariably less than 4.5, reflecting a predominance of *Lactobacillus* bacterial flora in the presence of *Candida* spp. Usually only a few WBCs are present.[14] Hyphae are typically present when *Candida* becomes infectious. Hyphae are identified in a 10 percent KOH wet mount preparation using a 100-power objective. However, a small number of patients with infection are identified only by culture because of either a low number of microorganisms or the presence of non–*C. albicans* species (that do not form hyphae). Cultures for *Candida* should be performed for patients suspected to have candidiasis on the basis of symptoms or signs in whom hyphae are not identified on the KOH smear.

Prematurity

Candida albicans in the vagina has not been related to premature delivery, preterm premature ROM, or low birth weight.[21,28,31,36] However, *C. albicans* is occasionally isolated from the amniotic fluid of patients in preterm labor.[18] Rarely, an infant develops an overwhelming systemic *C. albicans* infection and succumbs from this infection. Thus *C. albicans* is a frequent vaginal isolate, but it has a low potential for invasion of the upper genital tract. Therapy of vaginal candidiasis would be expected to have virtually no impact, and it cannot be recommended to prevent the unusual occurrence of amniotic fluid infection or the rare occurrence of systemic neonatal infection.

Treatment

Systemic absorption of either azoles or nystatin from the vagina is so limited that both can be safely used during all trimesters of pregnancy. Boric acid and ketoconazole should not be used during pregnancy. Compared to nonpregnant women, candidiasis in pregnancy is more resistant to treatment, is more likely to relapse, and thus responds better to more prolonged 7 or even 14 days of therapy than to 1- to 3-day therapy regimens.

Topical azole therapy remains the first choice for the treatment of infrequent acute candidiasis. Azoles inhibit ergosterol (and membrane) synthesis and produce a fungistatic effect. *Candida* are in turn killed by the host lymphocytes through cell-mediated immune mechanisms. In high concentrations, azoles can produce direct membrane damage, resulting in a limited fungicidal effect. The topical azoles are effective, well tolerated, and relatively inexpensive. Products currently marketed include butoconazole (Femstat), clotrimazole (Lotrimin, Mycelex), miconazole (Monistat), and terconazole (Terazol). A wide range of doses and forms is available including, both creams and suppositories. For some preparations, the dosing was increased to twice daily or the dose was increased from 100 mg to 200 mg, while the length of medication was concurrently reduced from 7 to 3 days. Cure rates of the 3-day course have been reported equal to longer courses in nonpregnant patients. Short term 7- to 30-day cure rates with topical azoles used for 3 to 7 days are usually 80 to 90 percent in nonpregnant patients[4,8,43] and in pregnancy.[33] There is no suggestion that the cure rates differ between various azoles or between the suppository versus the cream form of azoles. Occasionally, vaginal irritation results from "inactive" compounds in the cream vehicle. Local *Candida* therapy is otherwise well tolerated, and systemic reactions are unusual.

However, a word of caution is in order for the use of short-term therapy. Single or short, three-dose therapy should not be used in pregnancy, when treatment failure is high even with 7-day regimens. Investigators usually study only nonpregnant patients and only patients with mild symptoms of short duration who have had no prior candidiasis. Usually only short-term (7 to 30 days) cure rates have been reported, and higher mycologic failure rates occur at or beyond 30 days for patients given a single dose as opposed to a longer course of therapy.[26] The clinical relevance of higher rates of *Candida* recovery at this time is unclear, but, of course, it could be associated with higher long-term failure rates.

Topical polyene therapy with nystatin has been largely replaced by topical azole treatment. Nystatin is well tolerated and inexpensive, but cure rates (50 to 80 percent) are lower than those of azoles, particularly in pregnancy or with recurrent infection.[7,33] Thus, nystatin is a second-line choice in treating vaginal candidiasis. Gentian violet treatment is effective for the treatment of candidiasis, but the staining of clothing and skin limits its use to the rare case unresponsive to other medication. Boric acid capsules[51] and orally administered ketoconazole and fluconazole are not to be used in pregnancy. Boric acid has unproven fetal safety data. Although boric acid absorption cannot be shown in nonpregnant patients, increased absorption from the vagina is possible during pregnancy. Ketoconazole is teratogenic in high doses in animals. Fluconazole produced structural defects in very high doses, perhaps related to an inhibition of estrogen synthesis. No controlled studies exist on the use of either ketoconazole or fluconazole in pregnancy.

Rapidly Recurrent Symptoms

Symptoms may recur within a few days of completing medication. Common reasons for the return of symptoms include a failure to properly take medication and a reaction to compounds in the vehicle. Patients with rapid recurrences should be examined to document the presence of *Candida* by a potassium hydroxide wet mount preparation and a culture for *Candida*. Medication should be changed to eliminate the possibility of a reaction to the vehicle. Patients without objective evidence of candidiasis but with persistent symptoms after these corrective measures should be scrutinized for neurodermatitis, lichen planus, lichen sclerosis, burning vulvar syndrome, and minor vestibular gland inflammation.

Drug resistance is a rare cause of rapidly recurrent candidiasis. Patients with drug-resistant candidiasis usually have reduced symptoms on therapy but a rapid recurrence of symptoms when medication is stopped. *Candida albicans* is almost uniformly sensitive to all azoles. Drug resistance is more common among unusual fungi such as *C. glabrata, C. torulopis,* and *C. tropicalis*.[23] Terconazole therapy may be tried because it has greater activity than other azoles against *C. glabrata* and *C. tropicalis*. Gentian violet therapy may also be of benefit. In rare instances none of the topical medications is effective in eliminating vaginal fungi, and azoles or nystatin has to be given every 2 to 3 days to suppress rather than eliminate resistant microorganisms.

Treatment failures have been so infrequent for candidiasis that systematic studies have not been performed to determine the relative cause of treatment failure. Additionally the follow-up period is usually too short (30 days or less) to assess accurately the frequency of failures. Compliance failure, pseudofailure due to a reaction to the vehicle, and drug resistance have been mentioned. Recurrent vaginal candidiasis has been postulated to result from gastrointestinal tract *Candida*. Although rates of oral and gastrointestinal *Candida* are increased in patients with candidiasis,[24,34] most patients carry gastrointestinal *Candida* without developing vaginal candidiasis. Oral nystatin has not dramatically reduced clinical cure rates, although a slight but statistically significant reduction in subsequent *Candida* vulvovaginitis was associated with oral nystatin administration.[39] Male sexual partners of patients with vaginal candidiasis have an increased rate of genital colonization as compared to controls.[24] Sexual transmission is probably limited to the small number of 10 to 15 percent of males who have *Candida balanitis* concurrent with candidiasis in their female partner.[40] However, treatment of males has not decreased subsequent rates of vaginal candidiasis in the female.[5]

The use of loose, well-ventilated clothing may help to prevent recurrence. Dietary measures to reduce high carbohydrate levels has been of some benefit to a subset of patients. These patients usually give a history of developing candidiasis shortly after ingesting large amounts of sugar. The concomitant treatment of uncontrolled diabetes is usually necessary to treat successfully the diabetic with candidiasis. The avoidance of foods made from yeast has been popularized, but scientific documentation of effectiveness does not exist. In fact, the yeast present in foods have not been associated with vaginitis. Oral yogurt ingestion has also been popularized to prevent vaginal candidiasis. The oral ingestion of yogurt can influence vaginal *Candida* colonization,[25] but scientific data do not exist on whether yogurt prevents vaginal candidiasis. High vaginal concentrations of lactobacilli are normally already present in patients with candidiasis. Cessation of antibiotic therapy can be considered, when possible, in a small number of patients taking chronic antimicrobials.

Frequently Recurrent Candidiasis

Recently, a significant subset of patients have been identified with chronic or frequently recurrent (at least four annual) episodes of vaginal candidiasis. These patients cumulatively represent a significant number of patients with vaginal candidiasis attending certain clinics. It is not clear whether these patients have a limited immunologic defect due to lymphocytes incapable of killing *Candida*[54] or some other reason for the recurrence. Recurrence does not seem to be related to unusual or drug-resistant strains. Human immunodeficiency virus (HIV) testing could be considered for patients with frequent recurrences of vaginal candidiasis or candidiasis that does not respond to treatment. However, almost none of these women have any other commonly recognized risk factors for candidiasis or HIV infection.

Frequently symptomatic disease is difficult to manage. An important breakthrough in the treatment of frequently recurrent candidiasis has been the recognition that suppressive rather than curative therapy is in order. Suppressive antimicrobial therapy has been successfully used in the treatment of chronic recurrent urinary tract infection, and this principle has been applied to chronic recurrent candidiasis. In nonpregnant patients, an initial therapeutic dose of 400 mg of oral ketoconazole or a standard intravaginal antimycotic agent was utilized daily for 14 days.[47] This was followed by a maintenance dose of 100 mg of oral ketoconazole daily for 6 to 12 months. The 6-month recurrence rate of 70 percent among those given placebo was reduced to 5 percent among those given daily ketoconazole maintenance.[47] Ketoconazole is not indicated for use in pregnancy. Suppressive therapy has not been studied in pregnancy, but maintenance regimens could include biweekly topical azole administration. Recurrence of vaginal candidiasis may resume at the same rates as was present prior to suppression when maintenance therapy ceases.

References

1. Amsel R, Totten PA, Spiegel CA, et al. Nonspecific vaginitis. Diagnostic criteria and microbial and epidemiologic associations. Am J Med 1983; 74:14–22.
2. Beard CM, Noller KL, O'Fallon WM, et al. Lack of evidence of cancer due to use of metronidazole. N Engl J Med 1979; 301:519–522.
3. Bradbeer CS, Mayhew SR, Barlow D. Butoconazole and miconazole in treating vaginal candidiasis. Genitourin Med 1985; 61:270–272.
4. Brown D, Binder GC, Gardner HL, Wells J. Comparison of econazole and clotrimazole in the treatment of vulvovaginal candidiasis. Obstet Gynecol 1980; 56:121–123.
5. Buch A, Christensen ES. Treatment of vaginal candidosis with natamycin and effect of treating the partner at the same time. Acta Obstet Gynecol Scand 1982; 61:393–396.
6. Cotch MF for Vaginal Infections and Prematurity Study Group. Carriage of *Trichomonas vaginalis* (TV) is associated with adverse pregnancy outcome. Paper presented at the thirtieth Interscience Conference on Antimicrobial Agents and Chemotherapy, October 21-24, 1990, Atlanta (abstract 681).
7. Davis JE, Frudenfeld JH, Goddard JL. Comparative evaluation of Monistat and Mycostatin in the treatment of vulvovaginal candidiasis. Obstet Gynecol 1974; 44:403–406.
8. Droegemueller W, Adamson DG, Brown D, et al. Three-day treatment with butoconazole nitrate for vulvovaginal candidiasis. Obstet Gynecol 1984; 64:530–534.
9. Elder HA, Santamarina BAG, Smith S, Kass EH. The natural history of asymptomatic bacteriuria during pregnancy: the effect of tetracycline on the clinical course and the outcome of pregnancy. Am J Obstet Gynecol 1971; 111:441–445.
10. Elliot B, Brunham RC, Haga M, et al. Maternal gonococcal infection as a preventable risk factor for low birth weight. J Infect Dis 1990; 161:531–536.
11. Eschenbach DA. Lower genital tract infections. In: Galask RP, Larsen B, eds. Infectious diseases in the female patient. New York, Springer, 1986: 163–186.
12. Eschenbach DA, Davick PR, Williams BL, et al. Prevalence of hydrogen peroxide producing *Lactobacillus* species in normal women and women with bacterial vaginosis. J Clin Microbiol 1989; 27:251–256.
13. Eschenbach DA, Gravett MG, Chen KCS, et al. Bacterial vaginosis during pregnancy. An association with prematurity and postpartum complications. In: Mardh P-A, Taylor-Robinson D, eds. Bacterial vaginosis. Stockholm, Almquist and Wiksell, 1984:213–222.
14. Eschenbach DA, Hillier SL. Advances in diagnostic testing for vaginitis and cervicitis. J Reprod Med 1989; 34:S555–565.
15. Eschenbach DA, Hillier S, Critchlow C, et al. Diagnosis and clinical manifestations of bacterial vaginosis. Am J Obstet Gynecol 1988; 158:818–828.
16. Eschenbach DA, Nugent RP, Rao AV, et al. A randomized placebo-controlled trial of erythromycin for the treatment of *Ureaplasma ureatylicum* to prevent premature delivery. Am J Obstet Gynecol 1991; 164:734–742.
17. Fredman GD. Cancer after metronidazole. N Engl J Med 1980; 302:519 (letter).
18. Gravett MG, Hummel D, Eschenbach DA, Holmes KK. Preterm labor associated with subclinical amniotic fluid infection and with bacterial vaginosis. Obstet Gynecol 1986; 67:229–237.
19. Gravett MG, Nelson HP, DeRouen T, et al. Independent associations of bacterial vaginosis and *Chlamydia trachomatis* infection with adverse pregnancy outcome. JAMA 1986; 256:1899–2005.
20. Guzick DS, Winn K. The association of chorioamnionitis with preterm delivery. Obstet Gynecol 1985; 65:11–16.
21. Hardy PH, Nell EE, Spence MR, et al. Prevalence of six sexually transmitted disease agents among pregnant inner-city adolescents and pregnancy outcome. Lancet 1984; 333–337.
22. Hillier SL, Martius J, Krohn MJ, et al. Case-controlled study of chorioamniotic infection and chorioamnionitis in prematurity. N Engl J Med 1988; 319:972–978.
23. Horowitz BJ, Edelstein SW, Lippman L. *Candida tropicalis* vulvovaginitis. Obstet Gynecol 1985; 66:229–232.
24. Horowitz BJ, Edelstein SW, Lippman L. Sexual transmission of *Candida*. Obstet Gynecol 1987; 69:883–886.
25. Isenberg H, Alperstein P, France K, et al. Use of ingested yogurt as prophylaxis for chronic candidal vaginitis. Paper presented at the twenty-ninth Interscience Conference on Antimicrobial Agents and Chemotherapy, American Society for Microbiology, September 17-20, 1989, Houston (abstract 994).
26. Lebherz T, Guess E, Wolfson N. Efficacy of single- versus multiple-dose clotrimazole therapy in the management of vulvovaginal candidiasis. Am J Obstet Gynecol 1985; 153:965–968.
27. Martius J, Eschenbach DA. The role of bacterial vaginosis as a cause of amniotic fluid infection, chorioamnionitis and prematurity: a review. Arch Gynecol Obstet 1990; 247:1–13.

28. Martius J, Krohn MJ, Hillier SL, et al. Relationships of vaginal *Lactobacillus* species, cervical *Chlamydia trachomatis* and bacterial vaginosis to preterm birth. Obstet Gynecol 1988; 71:89–95.
29. Mason PR, Brown McLI. *Trichomonas* in pregnancy. Lancet 1990; 1025–1026.
30. McCormack WM, Rosner B, Lee YH, et al. Effect on birthweight of erythromycin treatment of pregnant women. Obstet Gynecol 1987; 69:202–207.
31. McDonald HM, O'Loughlin JA, Tolley P, et al. Vaginal infection and preterm labor. Br J Obstet Gynaecol 1991; 98:427–435.
32. McGregor JA, French JI, Reller LB, et al. Adjunctive erythromycin treatment for idiopathic preterm labor: results of a randomized, double-blinded, placebo-controlled trial. Am J Obstet Gynecol 1986; 154:98–103.
33. McNellis D, McLeod M, Lawson J, Pasquale SA. Treatment of vulvovaginal candidiasis in pregnancy: a comparative study. Obstet Gynecol 1977; 50:674–678.
34. Miles MR, Olsen L, Rogers A. Recurrent vaginal candidiasis: importance of an intestinal reservoir. JAMA 1977; 238:1836–1837.
35. Minkoff H. Prematurity: infection as an etiologic factor. Obstet Gynecol 1983; 62:137–144.
36. Minkoff H, Grunebaum AN, Schwarz RH, et al. Risk factors for prematurity and premature rupture of membranes: a prospective study of the vaginal flora in pregnancy. Am J Obstet Gynecol 1984; 150:965–972.
37. 1989 Sexually transmitted diseases treatment guidelines. MMWR 1989; 38:S1–42.
38. Nugent RP, Krohn MA, Hillier SL. The reliability of diagnosing bacterial vaginosis is improved by a standard sized method of Gram stain interpretation. J Clin Microbiol 1991; 29:297–301.
39. Nystatin Multicenter Study Group. Therapy of candidal vaginitis: the effect of eliminating intestinal *Candida*. Am J Obstet Gynecol 1986; 155:651–655.
40. Oriel JD, Partridge BM, Denny MJ, et al. Genital yeast infections. Br Med J 1972; 4:761–764.
41. Pankuch GA, Appelbaum PL, Lorenz RP, et al. Placental microbiology and histology and the pathogenesis of chorioamnionitis. Obstet Gynecol 1984; 64:802–806.
42. Peterson WF, Stanch JE, Ryder CO. Metronidazole in pregnancy. Am J Obstet Gynecol 1966; 94:343–349.
43. Proost JM, Maes-Dockx RM, Nelis MD, Cutsem M. Miconazole treatment of mycotic vulvovaginitis. Am J Obstet Gynecol 1972; 112:688–692.
44. Roe JFC. A critical appraisal of the toxicology of metronidazole. In: Phillips I, Collier J, eds. Metronidazole in pregnancy. Am J Obstet Gynecol 1966; 94:343–349.
45. Ross SM, Van Middelkoop A. *Trichomonas* infection in pregnancy: does it affect perinatal outcome? S Afr Med J 1983; 63:566–567.
46. Russell P. Inflammatory lesions of the human placenta. I. Am J Diagnost Gynecol Obstet 1979; 1:127–137.
47. Sobel JD. Recurrent vulvovaginal candidiasis: a prospective study of the efficacy of maintenance ketoconazole therapy. N Engl J Med 1986; 315:1455–1458.
48. Soper DE, Bump RC, Hurt WG. Bacterial vaginosis and *Trichomonas vaginalis* are risk factors for cuff cellulitis after abdominal hysterectomy. Am J Obstet Gynecol 1990; 163:1016–1023.
49. Spiegel CA, Amsel R, Eschenbach DA, et al. Anaerobic bacteria in nonspecific vaginitis. N Engl J Med 1980; 303:601–607.
50. Spiegel CA, Amsel R, Holmes KK. Diagnosis of bacterial vaginosis by direct Gram stain of vaginal fluid. J Clin Microbiol 1983; 18:170–177.
51. Van Slyke KK, Michel VP, Rein MF. Treatment of vulvovaginal candidiasis with boric acid powder. Am J Obstet Gynecol 1981; 141:145–148.
52. Watts DW, Eschenbach DA, Kenny GE. Early postpartum endometritis: the role of bacteria, genital mycoplasmas and *Chlamydia trachomatis*. Obstet Gynecol 1989; 73:52–60.
53. Watts DW, Krohn M, Hillier SL, Eschenbach DA. Bacterial vaginosis as a risk factor for postpartum endometritis. Obstet Gynecol 1990; 75:52–58.
54. Witkin SS. Inhibition of *Candida*-induced lymphocyte proliferation by antibody to *Candida albicans*. Obstet Gynecol 1986; 68:696–699.
55. Wolner-Hanssen P, Krieger JN, Stevens CE, et al. Clinical manifestations of vaginal trichomoniasis. JAMA 1989; 261:571–576.

CHAPTER 7

Postpartum Infection

Jonathan Charles, M.D.
David Charles, M.D.

Few entities have left so profound an imprint on human memory and human history as puerperal sepsis. This affliction has been described in the last century under a variety of terms, the most widely used of which were *puerperal fever* and *childbed fever*. When it occurred in its epidemic form, it fully deserved the epithet "scourge of the lying-in room." The mortality associated with the affliction was appalling; indeed, at one time, recovery from this fearful malady was the exception, and the rule was death.

Puerperal fever is one of the most striking examples of iatrogenic infection. Acceptance of this fact in both Europe and America was achieved only after much rancor and vitriolic utterances by leaders in the profession who were against such a concept. Any evidence that this entity could be transferred by the obstetrician to the maternity ward was inconceivable to those whose role was to benefit the parturient. Perhaps it was especially difficult for sincere physicians to comprehend the fact that, despite their noble intentions, they could unwittingly endanger the lives of their patients. The struggle to understand and control puerperal sepsis constitutes one of the most dramatic episodes of medical science and is punctuated by essays that endure as much for their learned expression as for their scientific merit (Table 7-1).

The essential development in this saga was the acceptance of puerperal fever as a communicable disease. In 1795 Alexander Gordon, a physician in Aberdeen, furnished a frank account of 28 cases of puerperal fever and declared:

> The infection was as readily communicated as that of the small pox or measles, and operated more speedily than any other infection with which I am acquainted. . . . It is a disagreeable declaration for me to mention that I myself was the means of carrying the infection to a great number of women.[46]

Such a candid pronouncement did not make for success in his practice, and Gordon found it expedient to enter the navy, where he contracted tuberculosis and died at the age of 48.

The same thesis, namely, the transmission of the infection from physician to patient, was expressed with great ability and similar frankness in 1842 by Thomas Watson, professor of medicine at King's College, London:

> The dreadful suspicion, that the hand which is relied upon for succour in the painful and perilous hour of childbirth, and which is intended to secure the safety of both mother and child, but especially of the mother, may literally become the innocent cause of her destruction: innocent no longer, however, if, after warning and knowledge of the risk, suitable means are not used to avert a catastrophe so shocking.[106]

Table 7-1 Historical Events in the Recognition of Maternal Postpartum Infection

Date	Event
1795	Alexander Gordon determined that puerperal fever was a communicable disease.
1842	Thomas Watson confirmed Gordon's realization and postulated that infection could be transmitted from physician to patient.
1843	Oliver Wendell Holmes's classic treatise, "The Contagiousness of Puerperal Fever" was published.
1846	Ignaz Semmelweis presented unequivocal proof that puerperal fever can be caused by the lack of cleanliness of attending physicians and set forth his findings in the treatise, "On the Etiology, Concept and Prophylaxis of Puerperal Fever" (published 1861).
1855	Oliver Wendell Holmes further postulated "Puerperal Fever as a Private Pestilence," in which he stressed the importance of taking all possible measures to prevent the iatrogenic spread of infection during pregnancy.
1867	Joseph Lister introduced and outlined the concept of antisepsis in surgery with his article "On the Antiseptic Principle in the Practice of Surgery."
1879	Louis Pasteur presented microscopic evidence of microbes "en chainettes" (now known as streptococci) in the blood and the lochia of women with puerperal fever and published these findings in "Septicemie Puerperale."
1904	William Osler acknowledged the wisdom of Holmes's dissertations and the profound impact they had had on shaping modern antiseptic medicine.
1935	Rebecca Lancefield isolated Group A streptococci from the lower genital tract of febrile puerperal patients.

The contagious nature of puerperal fever was a matter of much debate. The most passionate American protagonist was Oliver Wendell Holmes (Fig. 7-1), whose essay "The Contagiousness of Puerperal Fever," read before the Boston Society for Medical Improvement on February 13, 1843, has come to be regarded as a classic of logic and eloquence. Holmes, an anatomist, had had no personal experience of puerperal fever, but his interest was aroused following the death of a physician who had just conducted an autopsy on a female who had succumbed to childbirth fever. The deceased physician, before he took to his bed, had attended the deliveries of several other women, and some of these also contracted childbirth fever. With the acquisition of such information, Holmes could not rest until he had accumulated a series of similar cases, which he duly reported in his paper. After reviewing the evidence, he offered eight practical suggestions for the avoidance of this scourge of parturient women. He concluded his essay:

> Whatever indulgence may have been granted to those who have heretofore been the ignorant causes of so much misery, the time has come when the existence of a *private pestilence* in the sphere of a single physician should be looked upon not as a misfortune but a crime; and in the knowledge of such occurrences, the duties of the practitioner to his profession, should give way to his paramount obligations to society.[58]

This communication was received with great indignation by some of his medical colleagues, and they lost no time in trying to refute his views. The most emphatic advocates of the noncontagious nature of childbirth fever were Hugh Lenox Hodge and Charles Meigs, two leading personages in American obstetrics. Hodge, professor of midwifery at the University of Pennsylvania, in 1852

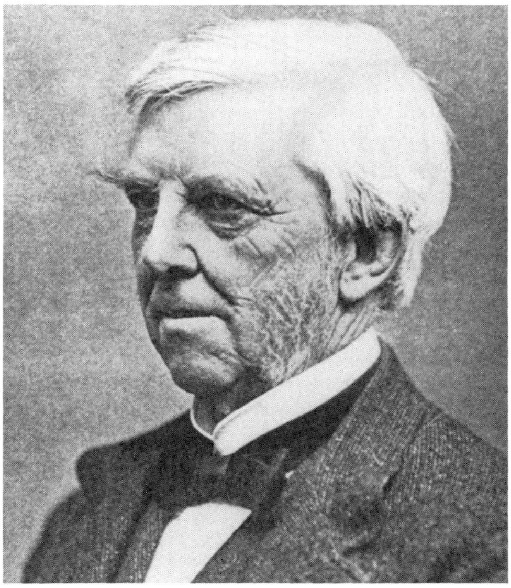

Figure 7-1 Oliver Wendell Holmes: 1809–1894.

denounced Holmes's accusation of the physician as a vector in the transmission of childbirth fever in no uncertain terms:

> The mere announcement of such an opinion must strike one with horror, and might induce you, at once to abandon a pursuit fraught with such danger and involving such terrible responsibilities; for what rewards can possibly compensate the obstetrician, who has reason to believe that he has actually poisoned one of those valued and lovely beings

who rested confidently and implicitly on him for safety and deliverance?[56]

A few years later in 1855, Holmes, now firmly established as dean of the Harvard Medical School, in a further epistle on this topic stated:

> *Persons* are nothing in this matter; better that twenty pamphleteers should be silenced, or as many Professors unseated, than that one mother's life should be taken. There is no quarrel here between men, but there is deadly incompatibility and exterminating warfare between doctrines. . . . If I am wrong, let me be put down by such a rebuke as no rash disclaimer has received since there has been a public opinion in the medical profession of America; if I am right, let doctrines which lead to professional homicide be no longer taught. . . . Indifference will not do here; our journalists and committees have no right to take up their pages with minute anatomy and tediously detailed cases, while it is a question whether or not the "Black Death" of childbed is to be scattered, broadcast by the agency of the mother's friend and advisor. Let the men who mold opinions look to it; if there is any voluntary blindness, any interested oversight, any culpable negligence, even, in such a matter and the fact shall reach the public ear; the pestilence carrier of the lying-in chamber must look to God for pardon, for man will never forgive him.[59]

Holmes's dissertations bestowed tranquility on the acrimonious arguments that had arisen pertaining to the contagiousness of childbed fever.

Almost half a century later, Osler commented on the literary efforts of Oliver Wendell Holmes in the following manner:

> A complete set of the writings of Oliver Wendell Holmes should be in every medical library. His Boylston prize essays on "Neuralgia," on "Malarial Fever" and on "Direct Explorations" can be hand bound in one volume. One of his writings is inestimable and will be remembered in the profession as long, I believe, as posterity will cherish his "Chambered Nautilus" or the "Lost Leaf." If you can find the original pamphlet on the "Contagiousness of Puerperal Fever," a reprint from the "New England Journal of Medicine and Surgery," 1843, have it bound in crushed levant—'tis worthy of it. The reprint of 1855 is more accessible. Failing either of these, get the journal and cut out and bind the article. Semmelweis, who gets the credit of introducing asepsis in midwifery, came some years later.[79]

Whether one views Osler's historical writing favorably or otherwise, it was a major event in nineteenth-century medicine. It not only proved an enduring and wide-ranging interpretation of the historical record but also came to the fore in the era of 1880 to 1920, after the concept that medicine as a biologic science had been accepted. This idea was in the main post-Darwinian, and it may indeed be dated from the time of Pasteur and his germ theory of disease or from Virchow with his "Cellular Pathology." Not to overlabor the distinction, but the metamorphosis of medicine from a craft to a science is distinctly modern, and the longstanding habit of sending for the physician is not much of an exception to our conclusion that the human appeal to biology is quite a recent development. There is no doubt that the elucidation of the causation and epidemiology of puerperal fever played a significant role in the evolution of the scientific basis of medicine.

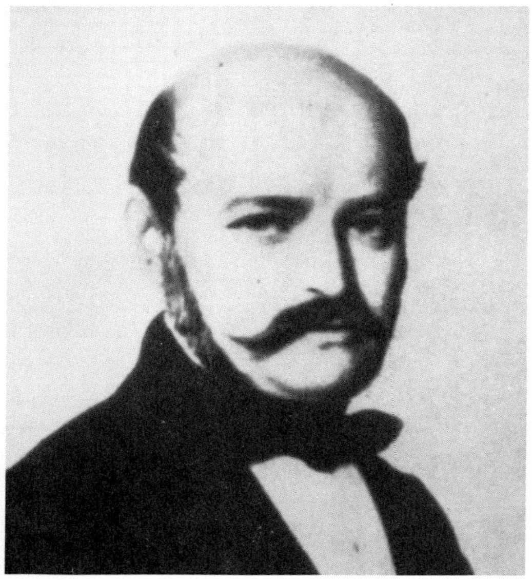

Figure 7-2 Ignaz Philipp Semmelweis: 1818–1865. (Watercolor by Agost Canzi, 1875, the Semmelweis Museum of Medical History.)

The progress of enlightenment in Europe was slower but no less colorful. A more clamorous alarm was sounded in Vienna, where in 1846 Ignaz Semmelweis (Fig. 7-2) was clinical assistant to the chief of obstetrics and gynecology at the Allgemeines Krankenhaus, which was at that time the largest maternity department in the world. The maternal mortality rate was appallingly high; in October 1843, one in three of the patients were victims of childbed fever. The authorities did not seem to be alarmed because the situation was not inferior to that in other European maternity hospitals. The fatalities were ascribed to "contagion" or mysterious meteorologic influences. This institution was organized as two separate units; one was used for the training of midwives and the other for medical students. In 1846, the mortality on the unit attended by medical students was 11.4 percent, and that where midwives were instructed was 2.7 percent. Semmelweis initiated a systematic study of the patient records to ascertain the cause of the high mortality on the medical student service, as the existing theories were of no help in explaining the large number of fatalities and the discrepant mortality rates between the two units. The medical students were almost, without exception, in the constant habit of assisting at autopsies, of which there were at least eight every day. The dissections were sometimes conducted by the students. If not, they at least handled the pathologic specimens and carefully examined them. The students then returned to the obstetric wards, where handwashing was by no means an established ritual. The midwives did not attend the pathology department. It was now clear to Semmelweis that something, which he referred to as "cadaveric particles," "decomposed animal organic matter," or "the harmful things," was probably being conveyed on the hands of

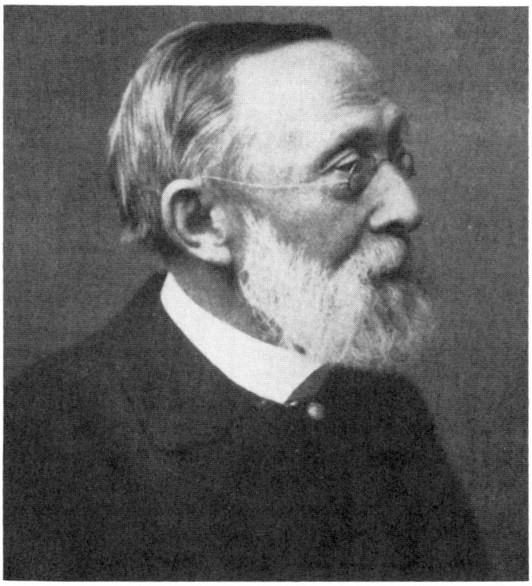

Figure 7-3 Rudolf Karl Virchow: 1821–1902.

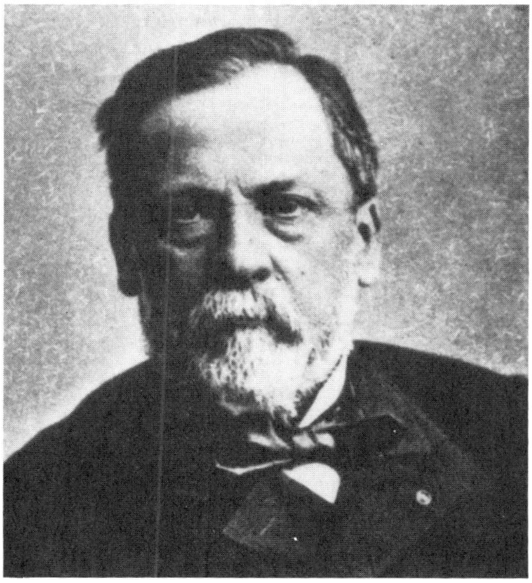

Figure 7-4 Louis Pasteur: 1822–1895.

the medical students to the women in labor. After great difficulty, he persuaded his colleagues to adopt a routine of washing their hands in chlorinated lime before entering the obstetric ward. His records show that by this simple measure, the mortality on the unit attended by the medical students was drastically reduced and was comparable to that in the unit attended by midwives. There is no doubt that his capacity for critical observation led him to discover the etiology of puerperal fever. Because of his opinions, Semmelweis incurred the opposition of the obstetric establishment. He paid heavily for his frank exposure of medical errors. Professor Klein, his superior, did not see fit to secure his reappointment, and Semmelweis's ideas were also opposed by Scanzoni, who was a towering figure at that time. The strongest opposition to Semmelweis was probably generated by Virchow (Fig. 7-3), the famous pathologist, who considered puerperal fever a thrombosis and stated that the Semmelweis theory was based on false premises.

Semmelweis left Vienna and returned to his native Budapest, where, at the age of 47, he infected himself while conducting an autopsy and died of septicemia. He died only a few years before the general acceptance of his views and Pasteur's isolation of the hemolytic streptococcus. Despite the defects of his classic work, "On the Etiology, Concept and Prophylaxis of Puerperal Fever"[94] (which has been rightly described as wordy, repetitious, and bellicose), there is no doubt that his advocacy of the doctrine of transmission of infection to the parturient by her attendants did more than anything else to eliminate the serious risks associated with puerperal sepsis in maternity hospitals in Europe in the last century.

It was a momentous event in civilization when Pasteur (Fig. 7-4) demonstrated the microbic nature of many diseases. We can hardly realize the change in the entire outlook—not only of physicians, but of ordinary citizens—when it was clearly depicted that disease is not a mysterious power suddenly emerging out of darkness and clutching a person by the throat but is, in many instances, due to invasion of the body by microbes, minute living organisms that can be contended with and often vanquished. Thus to Pasteur all credit is due for the modern recognition of the manifold role of bacteria and of the fundamental role that enzymes or ferments play in vital processes.

Pasteur in 1879 described the presence of microbes "en chainettes" in the lochia and blood of women with puerperal fever, which leaves no doubt that these were streptococci.[82] The close association of streptococci with puerperal infections was confirmed by many workers during the ensuing 50 years. In 1919, Douchez, Avery, and Lancefield initiated the serologic classification of the hemolytic streptococci, which led to the important question of whether one or more of the serologic groups of streptococci was responsible for puerperal sepsis.[19] Most of the strains obtained from human infections belonged to group A. It soon became apparent that the beta-hemolytic streptococci were of paramount importance in puerperal sepsis, but whether some or all of the various groups were involved was not certain.

The striking decrease in maternal mortality that accompanied the efforts of Holmes and Semmelweis implies that they were indeed dealing with iatrogenic nosocomial infections among the majority of women afflicted with puerperal sepsis. Nevertheless, some patients may have acquired the streptococcus from asymptomatic nasopharyngeal carriers or, as is usually noted today, from the microflora of the lower genital tract. There is probably no way today to gauge to what extent nosocomial infection with group A streptococcus was responsible for puerperal infections in the nineteenth cen-

Table 7-2 Most Common Bacterial Commensals of the Cervicovaginal Biota

Aerobe	Anaerobe
Gram-positive cocci	
Staphylococcus aureus	*Peptostreptococcus* spp.
S. epidermidis	
Group B Streptococcus	
Group D Streptococcus	
Streptococcus viridans spp.	
Enterococcus spp.	
Gram-positive rods	
Lactobacillus spp.	*Clostridium* spp.
Corynebacterium spp.	*Propionibacterium* spp.
	Eubacterium spp.
	Bifidobacterium spp.
Gram-negative cocci	
Moraxella spp.	*Veillonella* spp.
Gram-negative rods	
Enterobacteriaceae family	*Bacteroides* spp. (including *B. fragilis* group)
Acinetobacter spp.	*Mobiluncus* spp.
Gardnerella vaginalis	*Fusobacterium* spp.

tury as opposed to endogenous infections by this organism. The success of the doctrine of Semmelweis implies that the majority of the infections were of exogenous origin.

While all the work on the aerobic streptococci was in progress, evidence that was gradually collected indicated that anaerobic cocci were also involved in puerperal sepsis. For years these organisms were overlooked because the technical methods for culturing them in the absence of oxygen had not been developed. Anaerobes are now recognized as common causes of infection, often occurring in combination with aerobic bacteria. Genital tract infections in females are usually the result of a variety of facultative and strict anaerobic bacteria that combine to produce a polymicrobial infection. The cervicovaginal biota plays an important role in postpartum infections. The bacteria involved in postpartum infection reflect the normal microflora of the cervix and vagina, with such notable exceptions as group A beta-hemolytic streptococci and certain sexually transmitted pathogens. This flora is complex and includes anaerobes of the *Peptostreptococcus* and *Bacteroides* species, aerobic gram-negative bacilli of the Enterobacteriaceae family, and aerobic as well as microaerophilic streptococci (Table 7-2).

Current Status of Group A Streptococcus

A decade after the introduction of sulfonamides, Leonard Colebrook told the Royal College of Obstetricians and Gynecologists:

> It has been suggested that these streptococci are likely to die out under the influence of the new chemotherapeutic drugs. That seems to me improbable for several reasons:
>
> 1. This streptococcus is particularly well adapted for growth in the blood and tissues of human beings.
>
> 2. Although its virulence for man has been declining during the past forty to fifty years, as shown by the mortality of scarlet fever, there is no assurance that this phase will inevitably continue. We know too little about what determines periodic changes in virulence. . . .
>
> Finally, before I leave this aspect of the matter, may I urge the importance of maintaining our vigilance against these unseen enemies of the parturient woman? If we do not go forward in our preventive procedures, we shall probably go backward.[11]

Even before the availability of chemotherapeutic agents, major epidemics of puerperal sepsis were rarely encountered. This state of affairs could in part be ascribed to the introduction of antiseptic surgery by Joseph Lister.[72] Although Lister was, because of his inborn scientific curiosity, interested in physiology and in microbes, it was, he tells us, the tragedy of the high mortality in the hospital wards that urged him toward his antiseptic methods. The curtailment of the epidemicity of puerperal sepsis may possibly have resulted from better standards of obstetric care and from changes in the virulence of the organism. The spontaneous decline in virulence of group A beta-hemolytic streptococci is exemplified by the decreased mortality rate from scarlet fever and erysipelas that occurred prior to the introduction of the sulfonamides. Fluctuations in the virulence of these organisms for humans have occurred before, and they may recur in the future. Virulence may be looked upon as the ability of a pathogenic organism to:

1. Gain access to and parasitize a mucous membrane.
2. Produce demonstrable cell and tissue damage that may be secondary to the host's inflammatory response.
3. Protect itself against phagocytosis and other host protective systems.

Group A beta-hemolytic sepsis is currently a rare cause of puerperal infection, although sporadic outbreaks have been described. Blanco and associates in 1981 reported that 4 of 123 isolates (3.3 percent) from the blood of patients with puerperal endometritis were group A streptococci and 24 (19.5 percent) were group B organisms.[7] In 1989 Stevens and associates described 20 patients who were seen between 1986 and 1988 with serious group A streptococcal infections.[95] Two of the patients had postpartum sepsis. The investigators noted that many of the patients had a toxic shock–like syndrome, and they commented on the fact that in this series pyrogenic exotoxin A (scarlet fever toxin type A) was produced by many of the streptococcal isolates. Such a finding, together with the complication of adult respiratory distress syndrome and shock, supports the role of the toxin as a mediator in the streptococcal toxic shock syndrome. From their observations, the investigators suggest that the frequency of severe group A streptococcal infections may increase. Mastro and associates investigated an outbreak of 20 postoperative wound infections caused by group A streptococcus that occurred in a hospital between April 1985 and August 1988.[74] Two of the patients had had a cesarean section. In the epidemiologic studies, it was found that the individual responsible for the infections in the operating room had scalp lesions from which the organisms were isolated. The investigators state that the majority of outbreaks of postoperative wound infections are attributed to the presence of group A streptococcus in the vagina or rectum. They emphasize the need to evaluate all operating room personnel possibly infected with group A streptococcus in such an outbreak. Dan and associates reported the presence of clinically significant group A streptococcal bacteremia in 26 patients, of whom 2 had acquired the infection postpartum and were considered cases of nosocomial puerperal septicemia.[15] They emphasize that although, at the present time, group A streptococcal bacteremia is an uncommon condition, the clinician should be conversant with the entire spectrum of this entity in order to furnish optimal care to patients so afflicted.

The occasional reappearance of group A streptococcal infections should serve as a sober reminder that this pathogen is still with us, and we should not be complacent because the major epidemics are part of history. Failure to recognize what has become an uncommon disease could be detrimental to the health of the patient and also allow sporadic cases of group A streptococcal infections to assume epidemic proportions.

Significance of Puerperal Infections

Puerperal infection is synonymous with postpartum endometritis, which still is the most common infectious complication following parturition. Terms such as *myometritis, endomyometritis,* and *endomyoparametritis* have been used for this entity and attempt to define the extent of the infectious process that is preceded by puerperal endometritis. The diagnosis is suspected whenever postpartum fever occurs in the absence of other possible sites of infection.

The resulting morbidity of such an infection can be significant, especially following cesarean section. Pelvic abscess and septic pelvic thrombophlebitis are two serious sequelae of such an infectious process.

It is not always appreciated that the microbiology of puerperal endometritis is identical in many respects to wound infections in other areas of the body. On completion of the third stage of labor, a larger abraded area exists at the placental site that is analagous to any other wound. Also, there is the risk of autogenous infection from the patient's skin, nose, and throat, in addition to endogenous bacterial infection from the lower genital tract during parturition. Although the placental site is much less vulnerable to exogenous bacterial colonization than is a cutaneous wound, it allows greater opportunity for endogenous infection from the biota of the cervix and vagina. As a result of sound surgical asepsis and antisepsis, the placental site is nowadays far less susceptible to bacterial contamination during and after a normal vaginal delivery. In addition, there is a natural defense barrier of phagocytes at the placental site to counter bacterial invasion. Consequently, only highly virulent and invasive bacteria can become established after an uneventful labor. Nevertheless, retained placental tissue or fetal membranes, blood clot, or traumatized tissue allows bacteria of low virulence to replicate freely before encountering the host's defenses.

Although puerperal sepsis has been almost eliminated as a lethal disease, postpartum infectious morbidity is experienced by about 5 to 7 percent of puerperal patients. Various reports have indicated a marked disparity between the rates of infection following natural delivery and those following abdominal delivery. Sweet and Ledger in 1973 reported the presence of infectious morbidity in 155 patients of a total of 5,972 vaginal deliveries (0.26 percent), whereas among 464 cesarean sections 167 patients experienced febrile morbidity (36 percent).[100] Gibbs has stated that puerperal infection is more severe after cesarean section, as measured by such serious complications as abscess formation or death.[36] It is gratifying to note that the maternal mortality has markedly decreased in the last quarter century. Maternal mortality has been described as the yardstick of obstetric practice. Indeed, over the years only the statistics of maternal deaths have made it possible to compare the results of the practice of one obstetrician to another, of one hospital to another, and of one country to another, as well as the figures of one year to another. Despite improvements in the planning of obstetric units and in the nursing of puerperal patients, infection, as evidenced by the report of Gabel, still accounts for approximately 15 percent of the maternal mortality in recent years.[33] Good obstetrics calls for conscientious practice, unremitting watchfulness, and a firm belief that no obstetrician should ever be satisfied with his or her own work.

There has been a significant increase in the cesarean section rate worldwide in the past two decades. Notzon and associates recorded a fivefold increase in abdominal delivery in the United States between 1965 and 1985.[77] Today it is the most common operative procedure in U.S. hospitals.

Taffel in 1989 recorded the trends in the cesarean section rate of the United States from 1970 to 1987.[102] In the report, which was compiled from data from the National Center for Health Statistics, the estimated total births for 1987 were 3,809,000 and the number of cesarean sections 929,000, which means 24.4 percent of deliveries were by the abdominal route (Table 7-3). In a more recent communication, Taffel and associates reported that the cesarean section rate was 24.7 per 100 births for the year 1988 and the rate of primary section was 15.7 per 100.[103] Such figures indicate that approximately one of four births is by the abdominal route. The recognition that postpartum endometritis is associated with significant morbidity necessitates from both the medical and economic perspectives in-depth studies for lowering the high incidence of cesarean sections and for seeking methods of predicting patient risk with respect to puerperal endometritis.

A significant aspect of puerperal infection, which is often overlooked, is the possible separation of mother and child to prevent spread of infection to the latter. Also, the mother may not be able to breast-feed, depending on the class of antibiotics she is receiving.

Febrile Morbidity in the Puerperium

The development of fever on the first or second day postpartum should alert the physician to the presence of puerperal infection. The presence of fever is often the basis for instituting antimicrobial therapy and evaluating the response to the prescribed course of treatment. As

Table 7-3 The Continued Swing of the Pendulum to Cesarean Section in the 1980s

	1980	1985	1986	1987
Estimated total births	3,612,000	3,761,000	3,757,000	3,809,000
Estimated number of cesarean sections	596,000	854,000	905,000	929,000
Cesarean section rate	16.5%	22.7%	24.1%	24.4%

From Taffel SM. 1989.[102]

fever and infection are not synonymous, some form of standardization of the definition of febrile morbidity is required. A commonly used definition is based on "standard febrile morbidity" as established in the 1930s by the Joint Commission on Maternal Welfare. It is defined as an oral temperature of 38°C (100.4°F) or greater on any 2 of the first 10 days postpartum excluding the first 24 hours after parturition, and the temperature is to be recorded at least four times a day. There are many inherent fallacies in such a definition. As the definition is based strictly on temperature elevations and not on other clinical findings or microbiologic data, it is nonspecific and of unknown sensitivity. Ledger and associates in 1971 stated that fewer than one-third of their patients with a clinical diagnosis of puerperal endometritis satisfied this definition.[71] When the definition initially was prepared, the first 24 hours were excluded because the febrile response to most infections introduced during labor occurred after the first day, whereas fever on the first day was suggestive of an infection that was present before labor. However, this is not always the case. Filker and Monif monitored 1,000 postpartum patients for a temperature of at least 38°C in the first 24 hours following delivery.[31] They found that of 858 vaginal deliveries, 33 were febrile and of these 7 required antibiotic therapy. Of the 142 patients who had an abdominal delivery, 32 (44.4 percent) were febrile and 23 of them required antibiotics. They concluded from their study that a temperature of greater than 38.4°C was indicative of ensuing infection.

Although every postpartum woman who is febrile requires careful evaluation for any source of infection, many individuals with postpartum sepsis do not satisfy a definition of morbidity that is determined solely on the basis of fever. Stevenson and associates, in a 16-year review of maternal deaths from puerperal sepsis following cesarean section, found that a persistent low-grade temperature that never attained 38°C resulted in diagnostic and therapeutic delays in a significant number of women.[97] A small group of women are infected for several days before they exhibit a temperature of 38°C. Such infections, if neglected or not recognized, may proceed to a fulminant suppurative condition.

Bacteremia is just as likely to proceed to septic shock in the first 24 hours postpartum as later on in the puerperium. It cannot be too strongly emphasized that febrile episodes in the initial 24 hours after parturition require thorough investigation and must not be ignored.

Underestimates of the incidence of puerperal endometritis in current obstetrics can also be ascribed to the continued reliance on an outdated definition of morbidity. Today in many hospitals physicians prescribe potent systemic antibiotics to postpartum women whenever they note an elevation in temperature. Usually such therapy yields a good clinical response as illustrated by a rapid and persistent defervescence of the fever. If, in these circumstances, the obstetric service adheres to the outmoded temperature-defined morbidity standards, the patient is not included in the puerperal morbidity statistics. The latter partially accounts for the frequent discrepancy between the low incidence of puerperal morbidity and the high utilization of potent antibiotics in many obstetric units.

Standard febrile morbidity as currently defined does not take into account the site of the nidus of infection, and this fact also limits its utility.

Rates of infection in different hospitals vary on account of such factors as the intrinsic risk of the patient population, which is modified by their socioeconomic status; the character and frequency of specific operative procedures; and the quality of care provided by individual physicians and hospital personnel.

Postcesarean uterine infection is currently the most common hospital-acquired infection in obstetrics. Postpartum febrile morbidity in these cases usually results from an infection of, but not necessarily confined to, the uterine cavity. The infection may be present before delivery in the form of chorioamnionitis, which would then progress to puerperal endometritis. Postpartum pelvic infection may extend to the myometrium, parametrium, and adnexa. In some instances, septicemia occurs, and it is therefore essential to halt the progression of such an infectious process as early as possible.

Conversely, the obstetrician should not have the misconception that all individuals with puerperal fever have uterine sepsis. Except for the indigent population, uterine sepsis is rarely encountered after a vaginal delivery, and in such cases the physician must rule out other causes of fever. In fact, between 5 and 10 percent of postpartum women with a fever either have no infectious process or have an infection at a site other than the genital tract. Although fever is the cardinal sign of puerperal sepsis, it may be caused by a urinary tract infection, mastitis, pneumonia, atelectasis, episiotomy, or surgical wound infection.

Table 7-4 depicts the infectious complications that may be encountered in the postpartum patient. Each of these entities are discussed later in the chapter.

Table 7-4 Conditions Associated with Postpartum Fever

Endometritis
Wound infection
Episiotomy
Vaginal laceration
Cervical laceration
Paravaginal hematoma
Post pudendal block anesthesia
Post paracervical block anesthesia
Abdominal incision
Necrotizing fasciitis
Respiratory problems
Aspiration pneumonia
Atelectasis
Breast
Breast engorgement
Mastitis
Breast abscess
Drug fever
Contaminated intravenous infusion
Surgical misadventure
Swab or foreign body
Urinary tract infection
Thrombophlebitis

Differential Diagnosis of Puerperal Infection

As previously stated, some women develop postpartum fever without any evidence of infection. Filker and Monif in their study found that about 20 percent of postpartum patients have a temperature equal to or greater than 38°C (equal to or greater than 100.4°F) in the first 24 hours after parturition.[31] These women present no clinical evidence to suspect an infection, and the fever resolves by the second postpartum day. A diagnosis of puerperal endometritis should be considered when the patient is febrile and has general malaise, lower abdominal pain, and uterine tenderness. In such instances, the uterus is subinvoluted and the lochial flow may be scant and foul-smelling. If such features are present 48 hours after a vaginal delivery, the physician must always consider the possibility that a swab has been left in the vagina following the repair of a cervical or vaginal laceration or episiotomy.

Infections arising from an episiotomy or cervicovaginal laceration can present with a similar clinical picture. An infrequent but potentially serious infection may occur subsequent to pudendal or paracervical anesthesia. A delay in formulating a diagnosis and instituting therapy may allow the formation of a subgluteal or subpsoas abscess with extensive soft tissue destruction. Although such complications are rarely encountered in obstetric practice, they illustrate how an infectious process may spread along pelvic tissue planes.

Infection following utilization of a paracervical or pudendal block usually occurs after a vaginal delivery of an otherwise healthy patient and is manifested by an elevated temperature and local pain. The most striking features are the development of severe hip pain and the limitation of movement of the joint, which occur within hours or a few days after delivery. In some instances, pain occurs before the onset of a temperature elevation or other symptom. The hip pain is readily explained by the fact that the infectious process spreads in the loose areolar tissue at the base of the broad ligament to involve the lumbosacral nerve plexus and, if there is downward extension through the greater sciatic foramen, the capsule of the hip will be also infected. Early diagnosis and therapy are of utmost importance.

As in all branches of medicine, a diagnosis can be attained only after a review of the patient's history and a complete physical examination. The obstetrician must also remember that fever in the first 48 hours postpartum can result from the administration of contaminated intravenous infusions.

Fever is a common manifestation of drug allergy; although usually associated with other symptoms and signs of allergy, it may be the only clinical manifestation of drug toxicity. Drug fever may be present with or without rash or eosinophilia. Although certain drugs are more likely to cause fever than others, any drug has the capacity to produce a febrile response if it is given to a person who is hypersensitive to the compound. In the hospital, it is a good practice to examine carefully the order sheets and nursing notes of any patient who has an unexplained fever. Adverse reactions to antimicrobial agents are not uncommon. Obstetricians who prescribe one of the beta-lactam antibiotics as prophylaxis for an elective cesarean section are likely to encounter a patient with drug fever on the first postpartum day. The diagnosis of drug fever should be entertained only when the possibility of an infectious process has been excluded.

In patients delivering by the abdominal route, respiratory complications (such as aspiration pneumonia or atelectasis) result in fever within 24 hours of the surgical procedure. Aspiration pneumonia associated with obstetric anesthesia is an infrequent cause for early postpartum fever, yet as recently as 1972 Crawford stated that this complication was associated with half the obstetric deaths in Great Britain.[14] The measures that are widely adopted as prophylaxis against the occurrence of aspiration pneumonia include fasting prior to anesthesia, ingestion of antacids before anesthesia, skillful intubation, extubation only when the patient is fully awake, and lying on her side with the head lowered.

Atelectasis is another common complication; it develops in about 10 percent of women who undergo pelvic surgery. It is the most common cause of postoperative fever in the absence of uterine sepsis. Ninety percent of all postoperative respiratory complications are related to atelectasis.[97] Women with nasogastric tubes have a higher incidence of atelectasis, usually related to a decrease in deep breathing rather than to aspiration of stomach contents. Clinical manifestations customarily observed are elevated temperature, tachypnea, and tachycardia, most often occurring within the first 12 to 24 hours following completion of the operative procedure. On physical examination, decreased breath sounds, tubular breathing, and moist respiratory rales may be elicited on auscultation. These findings are most prominent at the lung bases. Frequently, however, there are few or no auscultatory or other physical findings. The diagnosis may then be substantiated in many instances by chest x-ray, which reveals an area of increased opacity, displacement of the mediastinum, and elevation of the diaphragm. Atelectasis usually resolves spontaneously by the third to fifth postoperative day. If the atelectasis does not resolve, the patient should receive chest physical therapy, intermittent positive pressure breathing, and aerosol therapy or intermittent continuous positive airway pressure by mask.

Frequently patients on the second or third postpartum day complain of swollen, tender breasts and exhibit a mild to moderate febrile response. This entity, which is associated with a sudden increase in milk volume that produces distention of the lactiferous ducts, is known as *breast engorgement*. The fever that may be associated with breast engorgement is of considerable interest and clinical significance. With currently available antimicrobial agents and knowledge of the consequences of sepsis, obstetricians tend to treat any febrile postpartum episode with antibiotics, even when the only complaint is mastalgia and no other cause of the pyrexia is discernible. Pyrexial episodes associated with breast engorgement usually abate in a few hours. Because antibiotic therapy is not without risk, it may be prudent to do without such medication when clinical and laboratory investigation reveal only breast engorgement.

The term *mastitis* denotes any inflammatory process involving the breast. As the majority of cases of acute mastitis occur during the puerperium, the term *puerperal mastitis* is used to denote this painful and distressing clinical entity. Mastitis and its possible consequence—breast abscess—represent the most serious complications of lactation and are dealt with in Chapter 8.

Operative obstetrics has become progressively less empirical and more selective; circumstances rather than conditions now determine the procedure. The outstanding successes from cesarean section not only have been responsible for the fact that almost 25 percent of pregnancies are terminated by the abdominal route but also have brought the practice of obstetrics into ever closer association with surgery. Obstetricians should, like surgeons, pay due heed and attention to wound closure and postoperative wound care. It is not easy today to appreciate the opposition to Lister's initiation of the art of antisepsis and particularly to his use of catgut as opposed to silver wire, silk, and thread, which in those days hung like setons out of every incisional wound. Infections of the abdominal wound are serious complications following cesarean section that can result not only in extended hospitalization but, on occasion, wound dehiscence.

A wound infection after cesarean section is often associated with endometritis, and more than a few Cassandras protest that the pendulum has swung too far to cesarean section. Personally, one would not venture to predict where this tendency may lead, despite the opinion of Taffel and associates, who believe that the cesarean section rate has now reached its zenith.[103] Both maternal morbidity and mortality are increased after cesarean section, compared to deliveries per via naturalis.

In the early stages, puerperal infections are frequently insidious in onset and can furnish the clinician with the predicament of diagnosis by exclusion. On occasion, endometritis may occur in the absence of any localizing signs or symptoms. The early clinical manifestations of postpartum infection are malaise, anorexia, and fever. When such features are present in association with wamble and pelvic or abdominal pain, it cannot be emphasized too strongly that the diagnosis of a surgical condition should be considered in the differential diagnosis. Liberal consultation with a surgical colleague is of prime importance if there is any doubt about a finite diagnosis. The obstetrician must recognize the acute episode, utilize obstetric experience, and blend it with that of the surgeon. In the best interest of the patient, the obstetrician must think as a surgeon and the surgeon as an obstetrician. Confusion of intra-abdominal disease with pulmonary or urinary tract infection is possible, and these should be considered and evaluated.

Physicians are reluctant to resort to surgical intervention during the puerperium; all too frequently they consider pelvic or generalized peritonitis as sequelae of puerperal sepsis. Abdominal distention, caused by laxity of the abdominal wall subsequent to parturition, is a normal accompaniment of the postpartum state. Therefore, its significance as a sign of existing pathology is often overlooked. In general, the obstetrician should realize that the presence of a silent, distended, tender abdomen is indicative of peritonitis originating from extension of an infectious process involving one of the abdominal viscera. Attention by the obstetrician to early symptoms of intra-abdominal disease and the initiation of appropriate consultation and surgical therapy should preclude the development of the serious and often lethal problems associated with diffuse peritonitis.

Appendicitis is the most common surgical condition encountered in the puerperium. Acute appendicitis in the postpartum patient has acquired notoriety associated with a high mortality rate, primarily because of delay in diagnosis, as it can be readily confused with puerperal endometritis by the obstetrician. The more protracted the delay, the graver the patient's condition and the more difficult the differential diagnosis. To temporize in order to attain an absolute diagnosis may jeopardize the patient's life. The acute surgical abdominal conditions encountered in the puerperium (Table 7-5) are discussed in detail in Chapter 23.

In the majority of cases, fever following childbirth should be ascribed to genital tract infection until proven otherwise. The prerequisite aerobic and anaerobic cultures should be obtained before the initiation of antibiotic therapy. Whenever a fluctuating fever is associated with rigors, blood cultures must be obtained. Treatment must, however, be instituted without awaiting laboratory reports. Any patient who has pyrexia that persists beyond 10 days should be suspected of having a polymicrobial infection, including anaerobic species, even in the absence of laboratory substantiation.

Host-Parasite Relationships in the Etiology of Puerperal Infections

Puerperal sepsis, like any clinical infection, depends on the defense mechanisms of the host and the nature of the infectious agent. Many aspects of host resistance are cell-mediated. The first cells involved in host defense

Table 7-5 Surgical Conditions That May Cause Diagnostic Problems in the Postpartum Patient

Acute appendicitis
Acute cholecystitis
Cholelithiasis
Perforated peptic ulcer
Acute pancreatitis
Intestinal obstruction
Strangulated hernia
Acute volvulus
Torsion of an ovarian cyst

when bacteria invade tissues are components of the phagocytic system. The latter is comprised of the circulating polymorphonuclear leukocytes, monocytes, and the free and fixed macrophages of the reticuloendothelial system. These phagocytes are often aided by antibodies and complement in the disposal of microorganisms.

Puerperal endometritis is frequently due to bacteria with minimal intrinsic virulence. Normally, many of the organisms are denizens of the lower genital tract. Postpartum endometritis results from the dissemination of these organisms in an area where tissue trauma has occurred. The greater the trauma, the greater the risk of infection, which is in accord with the fact that the more serious infections occur after cesarean section.

When the mucosal barrier is breached—as exemplified by the endometrium at the completion of labor—the tissue macrophage and humoral factors of the interstitial spaces impede the invasive potential of any contaminant bacteria. If there is bacterial invasion of the blood stream, the sessile macrophages of the reticuloendothelial system assist in their eradication. Many organisms may escape this defense mechanism unless antibodies and complement have been attached to the pathogen.

Initially the phagocytes, by chemotaxis, move toward bacterial products, leukocytes, and tissue cellular components as well as complement fragments. Bacterial adherence to the surface of a phagocyte results in phagocytosis, which is greatly augmented by the presence of immunoglobulin G or the complement component C3b attached to the bacterial cells. Both polymorphonuclear leukocytes and macrophages have specific receptors for immunoglobulin G and complement component C3b, which are the opsonins responsible for phagocytosis. One of the most important functions of complement appears to be the promotion of the phagocytosis of microorganisms.

The classic features of inflammation as enunciated by Celsus in the first century—rubor, calor, dolor, and tumor—are the result of increased vascular permeability, chemotaxis, phagocytosis, and lysosomal enzyme activity. All these aspects of the inflammatory response involve both humoral and cellular factors.

Table 7-6 Risk Factors in the Development of Postpartum Uterine Sepsis

Low socioeconomic status
Poor nutrition
Iron deficiency anemia
Decreased host resistance
Vaginal delivery
Traumatic delivery
Paravaginal hematoma
Retained placental tissue
Swab or other foreign body
Cesarean section
Amniorrhexis for more than 24 hours
Protracted labor
Amniotic fluid infection
Chorioamnionitis
Increased intrauterine manipulation
Necrotic tissue at suture line
Invasive electronic fetal monitoring
Intrauterine pressure catheter
Excessive number of pelvic examinations
Bacterial vaginosis

The host utilizes any mechanism available in an attempt to eliminate a nidus of infection. Some of the mechanisms do not succeed, but the desired effect—antigen elimination—requires that only a single mechanism be effective. At the same time, it is to be expected that bacteria will continue to adapt in their efforts to evade these mechanisms. The latter is in accord with the fact that antibiotics are antimicrobial agents that are produced naturally by microorganisms. The synthesis of antibiotics by microbes and the resistance of microbes to antibiotics are two sides of the evolutionary coin. In order to use antimicrobial agents in a rational manner, the physician must have information about the host, the infecting organisms, and the available agents, including their spectrum of activity.

Despite the limited information pertaining to host defense mechanisms in the uterus, it is essential to identify the various risk factors associated with the development of postpartum uterine sepsis.

Risk Factors in the Evolution of Puerperal Infections

Numerous risk factors have been associated with the development of postpartum uterine sepsis (Table 7-6). Many of them could be related to the socioeconomic status of the patient, as it is well recognized that the indigent are at increased risk of postpartum infection whether they have vaginal or abdominal delivery. It has long been realized that the standard of living has an important influence upon the pattern of morbidity, but the magnitude of the influence is difficult to assess. The concept of socioeconomic status is complex and imprecise, encompassing such influences as nutrition, education, housing, recreation, and health care. Family income provides a good index of material prosperity and has provided much valuable information about the association between disease and social circumstances. Patients from the socioeconomically deprived sections of the population are more prone to infection because of differences in host defense response, hygiene, and nutritional status.

Martius and associates found that bacterial vaginosis and *Chlamydia trachomatis* were related to preterm birth.[73] Furthermore, they noted that women in their study group who had preterm deliveries were more liable to have rupture of the fetal membranes, intrapartum fever, and postpartum sepsis. Gravett and associates from their studies concluded that approximately 20 percent of gravid patients have bacterial vaginosis.[47] They studied the relationship between prematurity, selected cervicovaginal organisms, and 30 demographic socioeconomic and obstetric variables. The results correlated premature labor with the presence or absence of bacterial vaginosis: early labor of less than 36 weeks gestation occurred in 25 percent of patients with bacterial vaginosis, yet in 13 percent of women without such an infection. These investigators also noted that amniotic fluid infection was associated with bacterial vaginosis. Recently, Eschenbach reported that there was a fivefold higher rate of endometritis following abdominal delivery in women with bacterial vaginosis than in women exhibiting no evidence of a vaginal infection.[25]

The socially deprived sections of the community, regardless of race, have a greater risk of puerperal infection due, in large part, to a lack of adequate education and nutrition. These communitites often receive suboptimal medical care from physicians who are "moonlighting," such as those who supplement their income by working a few hours a week in an inner city clinic. Continuity of care is thus compromised.

The studies of Rehu and Nilsson substantiate the fact that many of the indigent receive medical care from less experienced physicians.[88] They document the low number of pelvic examinations performed during labor, blood loss in excess of 800 ml at abdominal deliveries, and surgical procedures that frequently took longer than 60 minutes. Such facts imply that the physicians delivering care to the parturients were inexperienced.

Postpartum uterine infections have been kept under close scrutiny during the past 15 years because of the increased cesarean section rate, which seems to continue unabated, and before long it appears that in the United States 1 million of these procedures will be performed each year. Cesarean section is currently the predominant predisposing factor for the evolution of postpartum sepsis.

Sweet and Ledger in their study on puerperal morbidity found that the incidence of endometritis following abdominal delivery was sevenfold that following vaginal delivery.[100] Ledger and associates reported that bacteremia postpartum was increased tenfold following cesarean section compared to delivery per via naturalis.[70]

Whereas in the first half of this century physicians were trained to consider that the majority of infections were caused by one virulent organism, physicians nowadays recognize that postpartum uterine infections are due to a mixture of species including aerobic and anaerobic bacteria acting in synergy. Individually they have minimal intrinsic virulence and consequently are considered to be opportunistic organisms.

Parturients with prolonged rupture of the membranes in protracted labor are candidates for postpartum infections. If such women are delivered by cesarean section, the presence of intra-amniotic bacteria may play an important role in the evolution of postpartum sepsis. Poor progress in labor increases the number of vaginal examinations and ipso facto there is increased contamination and colonization of the lower uterine segment. Because many of the obstetric risk factors are interrelated, there has been no consensus as to which of them is most important. In fact, such factors as prolonged rupture of the membranes, ineffectual or protracted labor, and the number of pelvic examinations may all act in a synchronous manner to allow access of bacteria to the uterine cavity. In such circumstances, if the pregnancy is terminated by a traumatic delivery or cesarean section, postpartum sepsis ensues.

There has been concern about the role of internal fetal monitoring and intrauterine pressure transducers in postpartum uterine sepsis. Both measures are more often utilized when the labor is associated with uterine dysfunction, and abdominal delivery is often mandated for the concomitant fetal distress. There is little evidence to imply that the use of electronic intrauterine fetal heart monitoring produces an increased incidence of postpartum morbidity. Hagen found no difference in febrile morbidity in monitored women compared to unmonitored socially deprived women who had their pregnancies terminated by cesarean section.[51] This investigator did note that puerperal morbidity was increased following abdominal delivery in private patients who had been monitored as compared to patients of identical social standing who had not had internal fetal heart rate monitoring during labor. One must tend to agree with the views of Gibbs and his associates that it is the high-risk category of the patients (who often require a monitor) that is the important variable, not the intrauterine fetal monitoring itself.[41]

The length of time that has elapsed since the fetal membranes have ruptured is, in the opinion of some obstetricians, a factor in the development of postpartum sepsis. First of all, some statement is required as to the definition of premature rupture of the membranes. The patient is considered to have premature rupture of the membranes if amniorrhexis occurs before the onset of labor. It can be difficult, in some instances, to ascertain with certainty either when the membranes ruptured or when uterine contractions commenced. Following amniorrhexis and before the commencement of labor, a latent period must exist before the case can be termed premature rupture of the membranes.

The fetal membranes may rupture spontaneously prior to the commencement of labor in about 10 percent of pregnancies, and consequently intra-amniotic contamination by organisms from the lower genital tract is liable to occur. Gilstrap and Cunningham reported that all amniotic fluid cultures obtained from women with ruptured membranes for more than 6 hours' duration contained pathogenic bacteria, and 95 percent of the women developed postpartum endometritis.[43] Apuzzio and associates considered that patients who had ruptured membranes for more than 8 hours before delivery, had undergone more than three pelvic examinations, and whose labor lasted longer than 12 hours were at risk for postpartum endometritis.[2] They indicated that the low socioeconomic status of the patients evaluated was an important determinant in the development of postpartum sepsis.

Gibbs in 1980 reported that in his study of a socially deprived group of patients delivered by cesarean section the incidence of puerperal infection before amniorrhexis and prior to labor was 11 percent, but if labor was established and the membranes were intact, then it was 20 percent.[35] However, if abdominal delivery was performed after the membranes had ruptured and labor was established, then 43 percent of the patients had postpartum endometritis.

D'Angelo and Sokol from their studies concluded that duration of labor, and not the length of time after amniorrhexis, correlated best with an increase in postpartum morbidity.[16] They emphasized that the major risk factor was cesarean section. In their communication, they documented the relationship between potentially pathogenic organisms in the amniotic fluid and subsequent puerperal morbidity. Samples for microbiologic evaluation were obtained from the amniotic sac within 1 hour of delivery. Failure to incorporate such a temporal relationship in the collection of bacteriologic samples would not allow for an accurate assessment of the role of the bacteria in the evolution of postpartum sepsis.

Bobitt and Ledger were the first to present microbiologic data that suggested that unrecognized amnionitis is causally related to preterm labor and delivery.[8] They also found a positive relationship between the development of amnionitis and bacterial counts equal to or greater than 1,000 bacteria per milliliter.

Gibbs and associates suggested that the particular bacterial species responsible for the intra-amniotic infection was important, although no specific criterion of pathogenicity was included in their report.[38] The presence of multiple bacterial species in the amniotic fluid at the time of cesarean section may be of greater import than the presence of a single species in terms of postpartum infection. There is therefore a positive correlation between the likelihood of the development of amnionitis and the number of bacterial species present as well as the bacterial count itself.

Despite advances in perinatal medicine, prematurity remains the leading cause of perinatal mortality and morbidity. The premature birth rate has not shown any apparent alteration during the past 25 years. There is, however, accumulating evidence indicating that preterm labor is causally related to intra-amniotic infection. Hillier and associates, in a case-control study, found both clinical and histologic evidence of chorioamnionitis that was associated with premature delivery.[55] The microorganisms isolated from the placenta included facultative and anaerobic species, which are present in the vagina, as well as genital mycoplasmata. They noted an inverse ratio between gestational age and the frequency of microorganisms in the chorioamnion. In their multivariate analysis, they found that bacterial vaginosis was an independent risk factor for chorioamnionitis. The report made no comment on the incidence of postpartum infection in their patients under study.

Guzick and Winn found histologic evidence of chorioamnionitis in 20.9 percent of patients who had premature deliveries in the absence of premature rupture of the fetal membranes.[50] The latter implies that one of five preterm births in women with premature labor and intact membranes is associated with intra-amniotic infection. This report also failed to indicate whether such women have an increased risk of postpartum infection.

Romero and associates reported a study they conducted to ascertain if cachectin-tumor necrosis factor was present in infected amniotic fluid as an index of host response to infection.[91] The factor was not present in amniotic fluid from 54 patients with no intra-amniotic infection. It was present in 11 of 15 samples obtained from women in preterm labor with intra-amniotic infection. These investigators also state that interleukin-1 is more potent than tumor necrosis factor in stimulating prostaglandin synthesis by intrauterine tissues. Interleukin-1 is more frequently present than tumor necrosis factor in amniotic fluid from patients with intra-amniotic infection and preterm labor. These investigators consider that the fetal immune system is activated by infection of the amniotic sac and labor is initiated through the complex relationship between cytokines and prostaglandins.

In a previous communication, Romero and Mazor reviewed the data that portrays intrauterine infection as a major etiologic factor in preterm delivery.[90] No mention is made concerning the incidence of postpartum infection in such cases. If delivery is vaginal, fewer than 2 percent of such patients develop postpartum uterine sepsis, despite the contamination by microorganisms of amniotic fluid during parturition. In the absence of fulminant chorioamnionitis and once vaginal delivery has been achieved, the uterus is capable of eradicating any bacterial contaminants. When cesarean section is performed, however, the stage is set for possible postpartum uterine sepsis. This is so because of the intrauterine manipulation inherent in the operative procedure as well as necrosis of tissue at the suture line and hematoma formation. If the abdominal route is adopted as the method of delivery after prolonged rupture of membranes (with or without protracted labor), there is an increased liability of bacterial contamination of the abdomen from infected amniotic fluid. It is obvious from this discussion that the performance of a cesarean section in a parturient is the most important predisposing risk factor for postpartum infection.

Microbiology of Postpartum Infections

The bacteria involved in postpartum genital tract infections reflect the microflora of the cervix and vagina with a few possible exceptions, most notably group A beta-hemolytic streptococci and certain sexually transmitted pathogens.

Larsen and Galask have indicated that alterations in the ecosystem can stimulate the overgrowth of opportunistic bacteria, which then can behave as pathogens.[66] They found that the indigenous vaginal flora is fairly homogeneous and consists of aerobic and anaerobic bacteria. The aerobic components include lactobacilli, group B and D streptococci, *Staphylococcus epidermidis*, *S. aureus*, and several members of the family Enterobacteriaceae (see Table 7-2).

The recovery of anaerobes from the endogenous vaginal flora is highly variable, and Larsen and Galask point out that it depends on the adequacy of methods utilized for their isolation.[66] Improved anaerobic techniques, in conjunction with special media, have greatly helped to establish the presence of anaerobes as members of the endogenous human flora and to implicate them as the cause of many serious infections.

Larsen and Galask in a further report indicated that normal variations in the cervicovaginal ecosystem are related to puberty, reproductive life, pregnancy, and postmenopause states.[67] They found that the concentration of obligate anaerobes (in particular, the *Bacteroides* species) increased substantially in the puerperium.

The predominant anaerobic bacteria endogenous to the lower genital tract are various species of *Peptostreptococcus*, clostridia (including *Clostridium perfringens*, *Bacteroides*, *Mobiluncus*, and *Fusobacterium* (see Table 7-2).

A knowledge of the microbiology of postpartum infections allows the clinician to prescribe rational therapy. Bacterial isolates in the microbiology laboratory all too frequently fail to establish a diagnosis of puerperal endometritis because most culture techniques for obtaining samples from the postpartum endometrial cavity utilize a transcervical approach, which of necessity frequently involves contamination by the endocervical microflora. Furthermore, the bacteria isolated from the endometrial cavity in women with endometritis are identical with those encountered in the lower genital tract of sexually active women. These facts do not negate the value of microbiologic studies, which may directly contribute to the diagnosis or lack of diagnosis and furnish therapeutic guidance for treating postpartum endometritis.

It must be remembered that more than one bacterial species at the location of an infectious process represents a "mixed infection" but not necessarily a "synergistic infection." The bacteriology of postpartum infections of the genital tract may seem to many of little importance in the era of broad-spectrum antibiotics, but resistant strains of microorganisms continue to increase, making antimicrobial susceptibility studies mandatory in order to prevent serious infections. Likewise, empiric therapy may mask the presence of a streptococcal infection from an exogenous source that, if undetected, could persist as a reservoir of infection for other parturients. The incidence of group A beta-hemolytic infections may have been drastically reduced, but this microbe has not completely disappeared from the obstetric scene.

Aerobic Gram-Positive Cocci

Group A beta-hemolytic streptococcus is still an etiologic agent for the occasional case of postpartum endometritis. The organism may on rare occasions be cultured from the lower genital tract of asymptomatic women. The strains most likely to cause severe infections are usually derived from an exogenous source and are highly invasive and highly transmissible. A common mode of such exogenous bacteria involves direct transmission from asymptomatic carriers to the patient. Nursing personnel may become colonized after providing care to a patient with postpartum endometritis and may then in turn transmit these organisms to patients in labor. Claesson and Claesson described an outbreak of postpartum infection in an obstetric unit caused by group A streptococci.[10] Seven patients suffered from postpartum endometritis, and one infant had conjunctivitis. All the infections occurred in a 2-week period, and a thorough search was conducted to ascertain the source and the route of spread of the infection. Microbiologic studies suggested that the infection was probably spread by a hand shower. Infections caused by this organism are of such serious import that the discovery of one case of postpartum endometritis should be considered as a potential epidemic, and all measures should be adopted to delineate the source of the infection.

Lancefield and Hare in 1935 reported the isolation of group B streptococci from the lower genital tract of puerperal patients,[64] and in 1938 Fry recorded the presence of this species in vaginal cultures obtained from both asymptomatic patients and those who were febrile at the time of delivery.[32] Despite these early observations, group B streptococcus continued for many years to be regarded as primarily an organism that caused bovine mastitis and was consequently named *Streptococcus agalactiae*. Colebrook and Purdie first reported systemic maternal infection by this organism in 1937.[12] In 1964, prevalence surveys were instituted because Eickhoff and associates recorded that this bacteria was one of the most significant pathogens encountered in perinatal medicine.[23] Dillon and associates reported that group B streptococci have been isolated from the genital tract of between 8 and 30 percent of gravid patients.[18] These authors, as well as Baker and Edwards, indicate from their studies that this organism is the major cause of neonatal meningitis and sepsis in the United States.[4] In view of the high vaginal carriage rate among gravid women and because approximately 3 neonates per 1,000 live births have invasive group B streptococcal disease, various strategies have been explored to prevent such infections. Attempts at passive and active immunization during pregnancy may prove more efficacious than prophylactic antibiotics in the prevention of neonatal disease.[5,6] The nosocomial group B streptococcal infections are presented in Chapter 17.

The group B streptococci are one of the endogenous organisms that most frequently become pathogenic and result in postpartum endometritis. In fact, the greatest number of adult group B streptococcal infections occur in postpartum women. Pass and associates describe 21 cases of sepsis caused by this organism in parturient or postpartum women.[81] They noted a group B streptococcal sepsis rate of 1.85 per 1,000 deliveries. Cesarean section, which had been the method of delivery of 15 of the 21 cases, appeared to be a major factor in the development of group B streptococcal bacteremia.

Faro reported 14 cases of severe group B streptococcal infection in the puerperium of women who had had their pregnancies terminated by the abdominal route.[27] He also indicated that maternal group B streptococcal bacteremia appears to occur relatively frequently on an obstetric service and often develops within 24 hours of an operative delivery. These findings were further supported by the findings of Gibbs and associates[39] and Minkoff and colleagues.[76]

Recognition of the importance of group B streptococcus as a urinary tract pathogen is now well established. Wood and Dillon reported that more than 30 percent of significant bacteriurias in pregnancy were caused by this organism, a prevalence rate comparable to that of *Escherichia coli*.[108] Easmon and associates support these findings and note the association between the presence of group B streptococcus in the lower urinary tract and intrapartum pyrexia.[22]

Sutton and associates recorded the first case of extensive necrotizing fasciitis in an episiotomy site due to group B streptococcus and *Staphylococcus aureus*.[99] Backes and colleagues,[3] as well as Gallagher and Watanakunakorn,[34] have shown that group B streptococcus can cause infective endocarditis, which is an entity more often associated with *Streptococcus viridans* or group D streptococcus.

Aharoni and associates reported a rare case of postpartum group B streptococcal maternal meningitis.[1] To date, only five cases of this type of maternal infection in the postpartum patient have been recorded, and all occurred subsequent to a vaginal delivery. All patients were young and previously healthy, and no predisposing factors could be elicited. As shown in Table 7-7, there is a wide spectrum of nosocomial infections caused by the group B streptococcus.

Table 7-7 Nosocomial Infections Caused by Group B Streptococcus in the Postpartum Patient

Endometritis
Bacteremias
Wound infections
Pelvic cellulitis
Urinary tract infections
Endocarditis
Arthritis
Meningitis
Necrotizing fasciitis

During the past decade, group D streptococci and enterococci species have been increasingly associated with nosocomial infections and, as pointed out by Landry and associates, this organism should be regarded as an important blood stream pathogen.[65] Group D streptococci and enterococci are part of the biota of the lower genital tract in asymptomatic women but are found in the postpartum uterus in about 10 percent of patients with endometritis.

It has been widely accepted that the increasing use of antimicrobial agents is an important factor in the development of drug-resistant bacteria, although proving this hypothesis is difficult. Phelan and Pruyn, in a double-blind study using cefazolin as the prophylactic antibiotic for cesarean section, found group D streptococci to be the most resistant bacteria to this agent in postoperative cultures.[83] Gibbs and associates, in a study of wound abscess following cesarean section, came to similar conclusions and emphasized that this organism can be the causative agent for serious soft tissue infections.[37] Faro and associates reported that the bacteria isolated most frequently from the endometrium in patients with postpartum endometritis with unimicrobial infection were group D streptococci and enterococci.[30] Furthermore, they stated that the resistant organisms most likely in patients with postpartum endometritis treated with broad-spectrum cephalosporins are usually the enterococci.

In a recent communication, Faro and coworkers found that in patients undergoing cesarean section, 39 percent had group D streptococci and enterococci in vaginal cultures obtained before the operative procedure and prior to the administration of an antibiotic.[28] The day after the operative procedure and 24 hours following antibiotic administration, a further culture was obtained, and it was found that 62 percent of the patients were colonized by these bacteria. They noted significant differences in pretreatment and post-treatment isolation rates with a variety of broad-spectrum cephalosporins, but no differences were recorded in patients given ampicillin or piperacillin. Their study demonstrated that cephalosporin prophylaxis, even when administered in a single dose, exerts selective pressure on the vaginal biota. As demonstrated by the aforementioned studies, there is a firm belief that the three species of enterococci *(Enterococcus faecalis, E. faecium, E. durans)* assume a leading role in the cause of postpartum infections because of their overgrowth following the use of cephalosporins. Finally, as reported by Hoffman and Moellering, there are growing concerns about high-level gentamicin resistance by the enterococci.[57]

Streptococcus pneumoniae has always been considered a major respiratory pathogen and is not an organism that can be isolated from the biota of the lower genital tract. Darbas and colleagues recorded only seven isolates from 1,064 vaginal cultures (0.75 percent) and one isolate from 265 placentas.[17] Robinson recently reported a case of neonatal sepsis and puerperal endometritis where a serotype 3 pneumococcus was isolated from the mother and infant.[89] Westh and associates have reviewed the literature for the past 25 years and confirm that this organism is a rare cause of postpartum endometritis.[107]

Other streptococci—both alpha-hemolytic and nonhemolytic—are frequently found in the cervicovaginal flora of healthy women and consequently can be isolated in polymicrobial and postpartum infections. These bacteria are generally considered to have minimal virulence and so their importance in infectious processes is difficult to assess.

Staphylococcus aureus is frequently a primary pathogen and thus capable of causing serious disease in previously healthy people. The coagulase-negative staphylococci, with the possible exception of the urinary pathogen *S. saprophyticus,* are secondary opportunistic pathogens known to cause infection in association with the presence of an indwelling catheter. *Staphylococcus epidermidis* does not appear as the sole isolate in any puerperal infection reported and, when it occurs with other organisms, its role is obscure. It is, however, unwise to dismiss this organism as being of no importance because serious infections have been associated with the coagulase-negative staphylococci.

Staphylococcus aureus was reported by Stevens in 1927 to cause a staphylococcal form of scarlet fever and this entity is synonymous with an entity known as toxic shock syndrome which is a multi-system disease.[96] Certain strains of *S. aureus* produce a toxin that is now known as toxic shock syndrome toxin-1 (TSST-1). Coagulase-negative staphylococci that produce TSST-1 have also been incriminated in a few cases, as have group A beta-hemolytic streptococci. Blood cultures for the bacteria are apparently always negative. A latex agglutination test for TSST-1 is available. Therapy is predominantly supportive, and there is no evidence that antimicrobial therapy will alter the clinical course of the disease to a great extent. This entity was originally considered to be associated with the use of superabsorbent vaginal tampons by menstruating women. However, the large number of cases in nonmenstruating women as well as in males bear witness to the fact that toxic shock syndrome is not solely a tampon-related entity or even an exclusively female disease.

Guerinot and associates have recorded the occurrence of toxic shock syndrome in a postpartum patient,[49] and Green and LaPeter reported the disease in a postpartum woman and her infant.[48] Therefore, the obstetrician should be alert to the possible diagnosis of this disease in a postpartum patient who develops a sudden onset of fever followed by vomiting, diarrhea, and hypotension, with or without a scarlatiniform rash.

Aerobic Gram-Negative Bacilli

The gram-negative enteric bacilli are important etiologic agents in postpartum infections. The most commonly encountered are various types of the Enterobacteriaceae (most notably *Escherichia, Klebsiella,* and Proteus) and *Pseudomonas aeruginosa*. They are usually the offenders in urinary tract infections, and because of their presence in the cervicovaginal ecosystem they may easily become opportunistic pathogens.

Escherichia coli is isolated in approximately one-third of endocervical cultures from postpartum patients.[45,104] Postpartum endometritis caused by Enterobacteriaceae are usually polymicrobial; *E. coli* isolates may be found in a third and *Klebsiella* species in only a tenth of such cases. *Pseudomonas aeruginosa* is rarely isolated in cultures from patients with postpartum endometritis and in fact is more likely to be exogenously acquired when present in an obstetric unit.

Many Enterobacteriaceae, as well as other bacterial families, contain extrachromosomal self-encoding genetic elements termed *plasmids* or *resistance* (R) *factors,* which can encode resistance to several antibiotics. This resistance can be transmitted from one bacteria to another and also to other species via conjugation. Bacterial drug resistance can also involve inducible enzymes (e.g., beta-lactamases), genetic mutation, and transposons, the last being fragments of genetic material that can transmit resistance information between the chromosomes and the plasmids. Abuse of antibiotics in a hospital setting can produce selection pressure that favor R-plasmid–carrying strains, induce enzymes, and probably involve all modes of drug resistance by bacteria.

Gardnerella vaginalis has been isolated from blood cultures from puerperal patients. This organism is a gram-negative or gram-variable coccobacillus. Its more conventional setting is as a member of the vaginal flora or in association with bacterial vaginosis, which is characterized by a significant overgrowth of anaerobic bacteria, most noteworthy, *Mobiluncus*.[13] The apparent symbiotic relationship of *G. vaginalis* with anaerobic bacteria and its occasional appearance in blood cultures suggests that it may have a synergistic role with anaerobic organisms in puerperal endometritis. Rosene and coworkers reported that 20 percent of patients in their study who had postpartum endometritis and bacterial vaginosis had *G. vaginalis* and anaerobes in both their endometrial and vaginal cultures.[92] *Gardnerella vaginalis* alone or in conjunction with other facultative bacteria and anaerobes were cultured from vaginal cultures in a further 20% of patients with bacterial vaginosis without evidence of endometritis.

Anaerobic Bacteria

Anaerobic bacteria constitute a prominent component of the copious microbial flora of the human body. Approximately 10^9 anaerobes per ml are found in vaginal secretions, and they outnumber aerobic species by a factor of 10. Therefore, the physician who is aware of the nature of the normal vaginal flora can anticipate what infectious organisms may be encountered after an abdominal delivery. A clinical specimen from the genital tract of a patient with endometritis yields several bacterial strains, and so there are considerable difficulties in the evaluation of the relative pathogenic species isolated. Facultative species utilize oxygen, which in turn enhances the overgrowth of anaerobe species in polymicrobial infections. The anaerobic bacteria frequently encountered as a feature of the cervicovaginal flora are included in Table 7-2.

Peptostreptococci species are isolated from endometrial cultures from patients with postpartum endometritis, which is in accord with their high prevalence in the normal flora of the lower genital tract.

As noted by Gibbs and coworkers, *Bacteroides bivius* and *B. disiens* have been increasingly recognized in postpartum endometritis.[40] These and other anaerobic species have a propensity for infecting and replicating in necrotic decidual tissue, and as a result these infections are frequently associated with purulent and offensive lochia. A hallmark of established puerperal infections caused by these organisms is their chronicity, even after appropriate antibiotic therapy has been instituted.

As a class, the anaerobic organisms frequently lead a saprophytic existence on devitalized tissue including retained products of conception. Tissue that has a markedly reduced blood supply becomes progressively more anoxic, and an acidic environment develops with a concomitant reduction in the oxidation-reduction potential. Such an environment serves as an ideal site for the replication of anaerobic bacteria. These anaerobic bacteria may be best described as opportunistic pathogens in that they require some form of host compromise to allow initiation of the disease process.

Anaerobes may possess virulence attributes that enhance their role as pathogens. Kasper reported that *B. fragilis* and certain other gram-negative anaerobic bacilli produce a polysaccharide capsule that is antiphagocytic.[61] Onderdonk and coworkers demonstrated that this capsule can cause abscess formation in an animal model.[78] They also demonstrated that the success of *B. fragilis* in producing intra-abdominal abscess formation in their animal model depends on synergy with an aerobic species. Other factors may be important as virulence determinants within the *Bacteroides* species, including exoenzymes that degrade lipids, proteins, nucleic acids, and heparin.

Anaerobic organisms, such as the clostridia, possess several virulence factors and, growing in suitable conditions, they can have devastating results. *Clostridium perfringens* can be isolated from endocervical cultures of fewer than 5 percent of asymptomatic women. It is infrequently responsible for postpartum endometritis, which usually responds to prompt antibiotic therapy. *Clostridium perfringens* and the other histotoxic clostridia are further examples of anaerobic bacteria that rely on specific virulence factors for disease production. Fulminant clostridial infections are rarely encountered in puerperal patients. The isolation of *C. perfringens* from an endometrial culture should not automatically be assumed to constitute evidence of gas gangrene. Clinicians should, however, be alert to any evidence of clostridial myonecrosis. Failure to treat adequately nongangrenous anaerobic infections involving clostridia may lead to the serious sequelae of hemolytic anemia, as the infectious process extends beyond the endometrium and uterus. It is important to be aware of the propensity of *C. perfringens* to produce lethal infection. Once the pathologic process of gas gangrene is underway, death can ensue within 48 hours. Signs of progressive infection include gas gangrene, hyperbilirubinemia, disseminated intravascular coagulation, hypotension, and oliguria; it should be countered by prompt surgical intervention and extirpation of the infected uterus. One must emphasize that survival following a life-threatening infection due to *C. perfringens* is achieved only by prompt recognition and appropriate therapy instituted as expeditiously as possible; the latter is exemplified by the cases reported by Dylewski and associates.[21]

Genital Mycoplasmata

Mycoplasma hominis and *Ureaplasma urealyticum* are frequently isolated from the lower genital tract of gravid women. These organisms appear to serve as markers of sexual activity and can be correlated with the number of sexual partners of the patient. Mycoplasmata, as well as other components of the vaginal flora, gain access to the blood stream during parturition. McCormack and associates isolated mycoplasmata from the blood of 15 percent of 327 women immediately after parturition.[75] However, 10 minutes after parturition, only 8 percent of the blood samples were positive for mycoplasmata. Of this latter group (26 women), 10 of the isolates proved to be *M. hominis,* 15 were *U. urealyticum,* and in one patient both organisms were isolated. None of these patients with transient mycoplasmemia had any febrile morbidity.

The recovery of *M. hominis* after delivery has been associated with low antibody levels to this organism. Platt and associates reported that postpartum fever occurred in 40 percent of patients with an antibody titer of 1:8 and in 14 percent of women with higher antibody titers to *M. hominis*.[85] The association between this organism and postpartum fever is also supported by the finding of significant antibody titer elevations in patients with otherwise unexplained febrile morbidity. Young nulligravid patients may be especially susceptible to mycoplasma infections in the puerperium. Lamey and coworkers indicated that this was probably due to the fact that they lacked protective antibody.[63] They reported that 48 percent of the women who had an abdominal delivery and had mycoplasma recovered from the uterus or adnexa developed pyrexia of unknown origin in the puerperium. The patients were not seriously ill and had only mild abdominal discomfort. Bacterial cultures were not obtained so that a combined infection with a further bacterial species could not be excluded. *Ureaplasma urealyticum* was isolated from the blood of approximately 5 percent of febrile postpartum patients studied by Plummer and coworkers.[86]

Patients with postpartum septicemia caused by *M. hominis* and *U. urealyticum* are not seriously ill, and they recover uneventfully without antibiotic therapy. These organisms, whose potential as female genital tract pathogens is becoming increasingly recognized, are discussed in greater detail in Chapter 15.

Chlamydia Trachomatis

Chlamydia trachomatis is a strict intracellular bacterium that colonizes the squamocolumnar junction (including metaplastic epithelium) of the cervix. Currently, it is the most prevalent sexually transmitted disease pathogen in the Western world. Chlamydial infections may go totally undetected during pregnancy and may cause no complications. The incidence varies from area to area, as shown in the report of Heggie and associates, which demonstrated a cervical infection rate during pregnancy of between 2 and 37 percent.[54] Sweet and associates have shown that this organism can lead to an adverse pregnancy outcome by causing such maladies as prematurity, premature rupture of the membranes, chorioamnionitis, low-birth-weight infants, and perinatal mortality.[101] The latter topics are discussed in Chapter 14.

Sixty years ago, ophthalmologists recognized that postpartum infections occurred in a large number of mothers whose infants were seen by them for inclusion conjunctivitis. It is, however, only during the past decade that the relationship between *C. trachomatis* and postpartum endometritis has been documented. Wager and coworkers reviewed the postpartum course of patients who had chlamydial cervicitis prior to parturition.[105] They noted that an episode of endometritis occurred late in the puerperium in 22 percent of the women with a positive cervical culture and in 5 percent of patients whose cultures were negative. The latter studies, as well as those of Hoyme and associates, demonstrate that antepartum chlamydial infections are often followed by late postpartum endometritis, frequently occurring up to 6 weeks after vaginal delivery.[60] They only found limited evidence that *C. trachomatis* causes early postpartum endometritis after abdominal delivery. The increased frequency of chlamydial endometritis late in the puerperium as compared with early infection is in accord with the longer replication time and latency period of infectivity of this organism as compared to other pathogenic organisms.

Harrison and coworkers conducted a prospective study of chlamydia and mycoplasma infections during pregnancy and discovered that 2.9 percent of the patients developed postpartum endometritis or fever.[53] The prevalence among patients who had had vaginal deliveries was significantly lower than that among patients requiring abdominal deliveries (1.8 percent versus 9.0 percent). Among the patients who delivered vaginally, there was a positive correlation between black ethnicity and infection with *M. hominis,* postpartum fever, and endometritis. Although increased risks of fever and endometritis were associated with *C. trachomatis* and *U. urealyticum,* they were of a much lower magnitude and were not statistically significant.

Paavonen and coworkers noted that, despite the frequent occurrence of endometritis in postabortal and postpartum patients, pathologists found it difficult to identify the etiology in endometrial tissue.[80] There is some question as to the role of microorganisms that coexist in uterine infections. In their study, no patient in the group with chlamydial infections had mycoplasma isolated, whereas in the nonchlamydial group, *U. urealyticum* was isolated from four of the women. Chlamydia was the most common isolate in this study, and there were no significant differences between those with or without chlamydia in the presence of other organisms. Consequently, it is conceivable that any histologic differences in the endometrial studies between the two groups were due to *C. trachomatis*.

Chlamydia trachomatis is less frequently responsible for postpartum endometritis than are the conventional bacteria that represent the indigenous biota of the lower genital tract. Nevertheless, identification and specific therapy for *C. trachomatis* are necessary to prevent postpartum endometritis in patients with antepartum cervicitis as exemplified by a mucopurulent discharge. By this means it is possible to reduce the incidence of conjunctivitis or pneumonitis in their progeny. It is also important to the patient that identification and treatment be instituted prior to delivery, as the commonly prescribed therapy for early postpartum endometritis does not predictably eradicate *C. trachomatis*.

Future studies of the endometrium are required, both in the puerperium and during the various stages of the menstrual cycle, to assess the nature of the local host defenses against chlamydial infection.

Diagnostic Considerations

Fever is the cardinal sign of postpartum sepsis. It may occur before, during, or subsequent to parturition. Puerperal pyrexia occurring in the 48 hours subsequent to parturition may be caused by a urinary tract infection, which is only briefly discussed in this chapter as it is dealt with in detail in Chapter 18. Other entities producing postpartum fever are included in Table 7-4.

In addition to fever, the other clinical manifestations of puerperal endometritis are anorexia, malaise, abdominal pain, uterine subinvolution and tenderness, and purulent offensive lochia. Postpartum endometritis can be anticipated in patients who have had a nonelective cesarean section and who are from the socioeconomically deprived sections of society. Anorexia, nausea, malaise, and abdominal discomfort are, however, noted in the absence of any pathologic process in postpartum patients during the first 48 hours. However, one should not be lulled into thinking that no pathology is present; it is mandatory that the patient be evaluated for both possible pelvic and systemic infections.

As previously stated, the infectious process in postpartum uterine infections is not restricted to the endometrium and myometrium but can extend to the parametrium, cause pelvic cellulitis, and be accompanied by peritonitis. If a remittent fever is recorded within 24 hours of parturition, especially if it is accompanied by abdominal distention and tachycardia, a diagnosis of group B beta-hemolytic streptococcal or group A streptococcal endometritis should be considered. The patients appear critically ill with temperatures up to 39.5°C (104°F), and the purulent lochial discharge is replaced by a clear watery loss that on Gram's stain reveals the presence of numerous gram-positive cocci. The induration elicited on pelvic examination in the less severe forms of uterine sepsis is usually absent. If the obstetrician does not heed this evidence, pelvic cellulitis, peritonitis, and septicemia inevitably follow. A fever in excess of 39.5°C (104°F) with a discrepancy between the pulse rate and the fever is an ominous finding and is indicative of an infectious process that has spread beyond the uterus. Similarly, a pulse rate of more than 120 beats per minute is a sinister prognostic sign. Chills, high fever, and abdominopelvic pain are indicative of a severe infection, and when they are present, pelvic cellulitis, peritonitis, and bacteremia are inevitably present. In severe sepsis caused by beta-hemolytic streptococci, the pulse volume is small and the pulse tension is lowered. In the absence of severe blood loss or anemia, a persistently elevated pulse rate at any time in the puerperium should always raise suspicion of puerperal infection, even if the patient is afebrile.

The other organism that must be considered when a high fever associated with abdominal pain and uterine tenderness is present is *Clostridium perfringens*. Besides fever, pain is the most consistent symptom associated with the presence of this organism. If the possibility of clostridial infection is not considered, crepitation, hypotension, and oliguria occur despite volume replacement. In such cases, a Gram's stain of lochia reveals the presence of gram-positive rods. Although *C. perfringens* is rarely encountered in puerperal infections, it is important to recognize its propensity for lethal infection, as discussed earlier. As pointed out by Dylewski and associates, the manifestations of *C. perfringens* infection of the uterus are variable, ranging from endometritis to gas gangrene with fulminant septicemia.[21] Early diagnosis and therapy are critical to a favorable outcome.

Postpartum endometritis is usually insidious in onset and may be associated initially with minimal localizing signs. Uterine infections of polymicrobial etiology may be associated with low-grade pyrexia, a proportionate increase in pulse rate, malaise, anorexia, and frontal headache. The physician should be alert to the possibility of postpartum endometritis if the patient has a temperature of 38°C on the third or fourth day following parturition. Because of the low-grade pyrexia in many of these cases, Ledger and Kriewall introduced a "Fever Index" system that quantitates the number of degree hours that a patient has a febrile episode.[69] It has proven to be a valuable method of assessing febrile morbidity and response to therapy. Even in severe infections, uterine tenderness may not be elicited on abdominal examination. However, when present and associated with tenderness over the broad ligament areas, immediate microbiologic studies should be instituted. Depending on the microorganisms, the lochia varies from an offensive to an odorless serosanguineous discharge. It must be reiterated that postpartum pyrexia must be considered to be due to endometritis until proven otherwise. A decrease in the lochia has been noted in some patients 6 to 12 hours before the temperature is elevated, but it is not of diagnostic value.

The application of indirect hematologic measures of infection for the evaluation of postpartum uterine sepsis may be of little value. A physiologic leukocytosis occurs during parturition, and white blood cell counts up to 20,000 per cubic millimeter due to the mobilization of polymorphonuclear leukocytes may be observed in afebrile puerperal patients. Similarly, there is an elevation in the erythrocyte sedimentation rate. Consequently, such investigations are of limited value in the elucidation of postpartum pyrexia.

The greatest diagnostic challenge is identification of the organisms involved in the infectious process because a technique for obtaining cultures from the uterine cavity without contaminated intrauterine bacterial samples as proper controls does not exist. Furthermore, it is not known if the postpartum uterine cavity is sterile or transiently colonized, and this fact compounds the difficulties with respect to the interpretation of culture results derived from transcervical swabs or from the utilization of double- or triple-lumen cannulas.

These shortcomings do not mean that the laboratory is not of assistance, as it can in many instances indirectly contribute to the diagnosis and furnish therapeutic guidance for the treatment of postpartum endometritis. Attention should not be focused solely on the uterus; no potential sites of infection are overlooked. Positive urine or blood cultures aid in the differential diagnosis.

Regardless of which cultures are collected, they should be obtained before prescribing antibiotic therapy if at all feasible. Due consideration of the presence of anaerobic bacteria is important in both collection and transport of the specimens to the laboratory. The recovery of anaerobic species is dependent on the physician's efforts to reduce exposure of the specimens to atmospheric oxygen. Time is all important because exposure of a swab obtained from the site of infection to atmospheric oxygen for a few minutes markedly reduces or eliminates certain anaerobic bacteria. Many microbiology departments do not process vaginal or cervical specimens because they contain normal flora, and the significance of bacterial species present in the normal flora is impossible to establish. Consequently, if an endocervical culture is dispatched to the laboratory, it should be accompanied by an explanation of what is required. It is preferable that the physician discusses with laboratory personnel the reason why the specimen has been submitted; such a course of action is advantageous to both the physician and the patient.

Ledger and coworkers utilized transfundal needle aspiration in order to avoid contamination by endocervical microorganisms.[68] They did, however, state that on occasion negative cultures were obtained because the needle failed to enter the uterine cavity.

Considerable thought and effort have been expended by various groups of investigators and manufacturers to attain a culture device that will be protected in its passage through the endocervical canal and deliver uncontaminated bacterial cultures from the uterine cavity. To date, there have been concerted efforts to quantify the bacteria recovered, in a similar manner to the colony counts utilized in urine samples, which conceivably might separate vaginal and endocervical contaminants from the more numerous pathogens at the infected site.

Knuppel and coworkers asserted that cultures could be obtained from the uterine cavity by the transcervical route as the mean concentration of microorganisms in an infection of the uterine cavity is 1 millionfold greater than that in the nongravid woman or the woman who had had an elective cesarean section.[62] They utilized Teflon catheters containing a nylon-bristle brush and retractable wire in the inner cannula. The housing was a 40-cm number 10 French cannula containing a distal occluding polyethylene glycol plug. After the device was introduced into the uterine cavity, the brush was advanced to obtain a specimen for bacteriologic studies. It was retracted, transected from the wire, and placed into the appropriate media.

Gibbs and coworkers irrigated the uterine cavity with a solution of Ringer's lactate by means of a catheter that was introduced through the cervical canal.[42] They recorded no marked differences in the bacteriologic results in patients with or without clinical manifestations of postpartum endometritis.

Duff and associates evaluated four different techniques for acquiring intrauterine cultures from puerperal women.[20] Specimens for culture were obtained by transfundal aspiration, transcervical brush biopsy of tissue from the uterine cavity by means of a double-lumen catheter, transcervical endometrial lavage via a double-lumen catheter, and aspiration through a single lumen of the lower part of the uterine cavity. Quantitative cultures for aerobic and anaerobic species revealed that the largest number of organisms as well as the greatest variety of species was procured by aspiration via the single-lumen catheter. Double-lumen techniques employing a brush or lavage were equally efficacious in reducing, but not eliminating, endocervical bacterial contaminants.

Eschenbach and coworkers have provided some of the most lucid data pertaining to the microbiology of puerperal endometritis.[26] These investigators used a triple-lumen sampling method so as to avoid contamination by the bacterial flora of the endocervical canal. In their study of 55 febrile postpartum patients, 51 (93 percent) had at least one facultative and one anaerobic species isolated from cultures obtained from the uterine cavity. The bacterial isolates included *Gardnerella vaginalis*, *Peptostreptococcus* sp., *Bacteroides* sp., *Staphylococcus epidermidis*, group B streptococcus, and *Mycoplasma* sp. *Bacteroides bivius* was isolated from 11 patients, *P. asaccharolyticus* from 10, *Ureaplasma urealyticum* from 39, and *Mycoplasma hominis* from 11 of the women evaluated. As will be noted, 76 percent of the patients with endometritis had genital mycoplasmata. Only 16 percent had genital mycoplasmata alone without other isolates. Two percent of the cultures contained *Chlamydia trachomatis*. Of the study group with postpartum endometritis, 48 (87 percent) had had a cesarean section. These investigators also included a control group of 14 afebrile postpartum patients, among whom 43 percent had positive cultures, with few colony counts of low-virulence organisms. Not only is the acquisition of intrauterine cultures questionable but also their interpretation is a matter for concern. The tendency is to disregard such organisms as *S. epidermidis*, diphtheroids, and lactobacilli because they are not construed as pathogenic bacteria. When *Escherichia coli* or *Bacteroides fragilis* is isolated, it is assumed all too readily that they are the organisms responsible for the infection. The validity of this type of analysis is limited by the fact that organisms of low virulence may be involved in infections, and their role in polymicrobial infections must not be disregarded.

Culdocentesis has been attempted in women with a clinical diagnosis of postpartum endometritis as an indirect method to elucidate the causative agents. Platt and associates reported the recovery of anaerobic microorganisms from 87 percent of the transvaginal cul-de-sac aspirates from women with postpartum endometritis.[84] Such a high yield of anaerobic bacteria is a matter of concern because some of the bacteria may be the result of contamination by the vaginal flora. The availability of acceptable transcervical culture techniques will probably obviate the use of cul-de-sac aspirates for elucidating the pathogenic bacteria responsible for postpartum endometritis.

The most useful microbiologic studies, when positive, are those derived from blood cultures. A positive result immediately alerts the physician to the most significant microorganisms involved in the infectious process. The pathogenic organisms that invade the blood stream demand the physician's attention in order to make the correct therapeutic choice of antimicrobial agent. Positive blood cultures are found in more than 50 percent of febrile patients who have had a cesarean section.

Urinary Tract Infection

Haley and associates in their review of the nosocomial infection rate in acute care hospitals in the United States found that there were 5.7 nosocomial infections per 100 patient admissions and that urinary tract infections constituted 42 percent of such infections.[52] In some institutions, 2 percent of urinary tract infections were associated with catheterization. Between 1 and 5 percent of patients with single short-term catheterizations and 50 percent of patients with intermittent catheterizations develop bacteriuria. The assumption that the bacteriuria that follows catheterization is benign and will spontaneously resolve is erroneous, as many of the patients are liable to such complications as pyelonephritis or even septicemia.

Significant bacteriuria is defined as greater than 100,000 colony forming units per ml of a midstream specimen of urine collected by "clean catch." The definition serves to differentiate between inconsequential contamination and true urinary tract infection. A substantial number of cases of postpartum febrile morbidity are caused by significant bacteriuria. Sweet and Ledger consider it is one of the most common causes of puerperal fever.[100] The prevalence of postpartum bacteriuria varies according to past history of urinary tract infection, the level of intrapartum care, catheterization during labor, and type of delivery. In many patients who have an exacerbation of renal tract infection during the puerperium, a history of previous pyelonephritis is forthcoming or asymptomatic bacteriuria have been diagnosed during the prenatal period (see Chapter 18).

Women who undergo cesarean section, as well as those receiving epidural anesthesia, frequently require catheterization, and 15 percent subsequently develop bacteriuria without any evidence of a urinary tract infection. Although catheterization is necessary before cesarean section or a midforceps delivery, routine catheterization of all women in labor is inappropriate.

Stray-Pedersen and coworkers underscored the fact that in puerperal women one cannot rely on a single midstream voided urine specimen to assess the presence of bacteriuria.[98] They screened 6,803 puerperal women for bacteriuria by midstream specimens and found that 553 (8.1 percent) showed significant bacteriuria. Cultures of bladder urine aspirated from 483 of the 553 women only yielded positive isolates in 251 of the women, and from these results the frequency of true bacteriuria in their total study group was only 3.7 percent. These results demonstrate that midstream urine specimens yield a high percentage of false-positive results because of contamination by lochial discharge. They did, however, confirm by their studies that bacteriuria was most commonly associated with operative deliveries. They indicate that the physiologic urinary stasis, the dilation of the ureters, and vesicoureteric reflux observed during pregnancy can persist for several months after parturition with a concomitant risk of pyelonephritis if prenatal bacteriuria has persisted.

Postpartum pyelonephritis is an important cause of postpartum fever and is more common than at any time before delivery. Pyelonephritis does not usually occur before the end of the first week of the puerperium, and it is not always associated with costovertebral angle tenderness. Localizing signs are frequently absent; therefore, despite the fact that the lower urinary tract is also infected, there are often no symptoms referable to the urinary system by the patient.

It is important to consider a urinary tract infection in the differential diagnosis of postpartum fever. Particular attention should be paid to any puerperal patient who has had a history of previous urinary tract infection, epidural analgesia during parturition, catheterization during labor, and operative delivery. Such individuals, in the absence of symptoms referable to the urinary tract, warrant bacterial culture of their urine.

Pelvic Cellulitis

Pelvic cellulitis is one of the most important local inflammatory lesions to result from postpartum sepsis. It is an acute infective process involving the endopelvic fascia and fibroareolar tissue and results from lacerations of the vagina, cervix, or the lower uterine segment. When such lacerations become infected, a primary lymphangitis occurs in the adjacent soft tissue. Because loose connective tissue not only surrounds the blood vessels but also forms their sheaths, the inflammatory process may spread via the perivascular lymphatics to regions outside the true pelvis (Fig. 7-5). Similarly, the loose connective tissue of the pelvis is contiguous with that of the rest of the body, allowing infection originating in the pelvis to spread widely by lymphatic continuity. The cellular tissue lies immediately under the peritoneum; therefore, an acute cellulitis sets up a secondary peritonitis, and conversely a primary peritonitis secondarily involves the adjacent cellular tissue. A further fact that should be remembered is that the pelvic cellular tissue is related to the ureter in the same way as it is to the blood vessels. Consequently, postpartum uterine sepsis, having involved the pelvic cellular tissue, may track

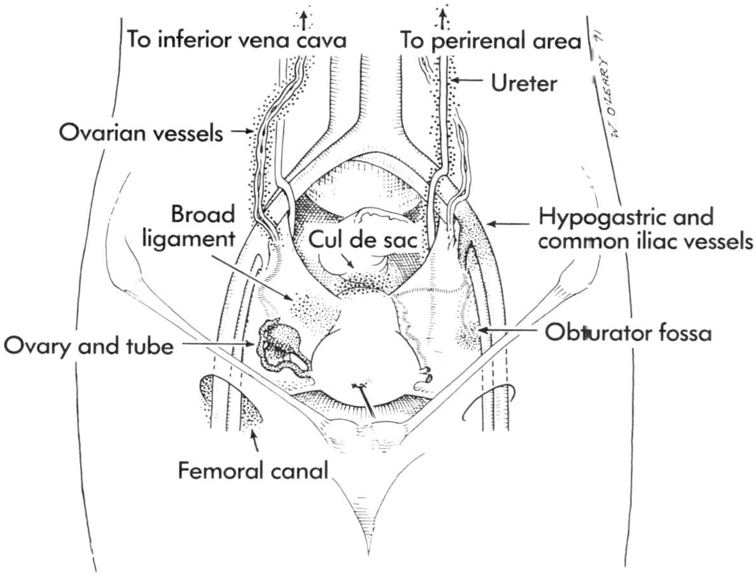

Figure 7-5 Modes and sites of spread of uterine sepsis.

along the ureter to the perinephric region or along the large vessels to reach the front of the thigh and buttock. From a purely anatomic perspective, the perimetrial tissue completely invests the supravaginal cervix but is almost nonexistent where the peritoneum covers the body of the uterus. Primary cellulitis is likely to occur when a cervical injury becomes infected, but it is unlikely to result solely from an infection confined to the uterine corpus. The cellular tissue that lies between the vaginal vault and the peritoneum measures one-third inch in thickness. In pregnancy, this is enormously increased; for instance, at term the broad ligaments lie above the pelvic brim, and the peritoneum does not dip into the lateral parts of the pelvis. This increase in size of the pelvic cellular space during pregnancy is readily appreciated when it is remembered that it accommodates a placenta that has been expelled through a rupture in the lower uterine segment; furthermore, it is possible to perform a cesarean section without opening the peritoneal cavity. This extensive increase of connective tissue in the pregnant state is of the greatest clinical importance. Pelvic cellulitis is similar to soft tissue infections in other parts of the body and can lead to abscess formation. The major symptoms are fever and lower quadrant and pelvic pain. As the infection increases in severity, the fever becomes spiking in character, the pain intensifies, and the patient develops a moderately elevated leukocyte count.

One of the earliest signs of cellulitis is fixity of the cervix accompanied by a tender unilateral swelling. Later the swelling extends laterally and becomes hard. It may obliterate the vaginal fornix and eventually become evident above the inguinal ligament. If the exudate opens up the folds of the broad ligament, the whole uterus is fixed and deviated to the opposite side. When the cellulitis has extended in a posterior direction, its presence is best defined by rectal examination, which usually reveals a horseshoe band of induration investing the bowel and contiguous with the induration in the uterosacral ligaments.

An entity that may simulate the rarer forms of cellulitis filling up the entire mesometrium is a hematoma produced by rupture of a uterine varicosity or of a broad ligament leiomyoma. The clinical history, if carefully evaluated, greatly assists the diagnosis of this clinical entity. In pelvic cellulitis, fever is a feature, but when a hematoma is present the history elicited is that of sudden pain, weakness, and perhaps vomiting. Pyrexia is slight and transient, unless suppuration has occurred.

Under favorable conditions, the exudation in cases of pelvic cellulitis subsides, recovery is complete, and the episode is so slight as to offer no impairment to future conception. When suppuration occurs, recovery may still be rapid if the purulent collection is evacuated; when the purulent process extends to areas distal from the uterus, however, convalescence may be prolonged and on occasion lasts for several months.

If the infectious process involving the uterus and pelvic cellular tissue is not halted by appropriate antibiotic therapy, abscess formation results, and the suppurative process extends to the pelvic veins and causes septic thrombophlebitis with the risk of septic emboli to the lungs.

When pelvic peritonitis is associated with inflammation of the endopelvic fascia, gaseous distention of the bowel due to a dynamic ileus is a concomitant finding. Vomiting, constipation, and urinary retention are also frequently noted in this setting. In the differential diagnosis—especially in the presence of such symptoms as abdominal pain, nausea, vomiting, and constipation—one must consider intestinal obstruction, perforation of a viscus, or appendicitis. The patient who has had protracted labor terminated by cesarean section is especially likely to develop a segmental colonic ileus. Abdominal distention is common in postpartum patients, and consequently it is often difficult to recognize the development of a bowel obstruction. Postpartum colon obstruction and volvulus are rare entities in the puerperal patient, but they must always be considered if the predominant symptom is abdominopelvic pain. These and other surgical problems that may be encountered in the puerperal patient are presented in Chapter 23.

Septic Pelvic Thrombophlebitis

Because of the contiguity of the major pelvic veins with sites of postpartum infection, thrombophlebitis is a common complication of protracted pelvic sepsis. Septic thrombophlebitis in the veins draining the pelvic organs may be the source of pyemic abscesses in the lungs owing to the embolization of fragments of infected clots. The pulmonary emboli that can occur in puerperal patients with septic thrombophlebitis are rarely fatal, the emboli being small because the clot in the involved venous channels is adherent to the inflamed vessel wall. The occurrence of thrombophlebitis and the liberation of small emboli can explain the intermittent fever and chills as well as the prolonged cause of some *Bacteroides* postpartum infections.

At one time, a single positive blood culture with subsequent negative cultures was considered to be indicative of bacteremia, and persistent positive blood cultures were thought to signify septicemia. This concept was found to be untenable, as serial positive blood cultures can be obtained from patients who have a localized nidus of infection that can be responsible for intermittent bacteremia. Final differentiation between bacteremia and septicemia must often be made retrospectively from an analysis of both the clinical and bacteriologic data. Many reports in the literature fail to differentiate between the two terms and many authors use *bacteremia* to denote overwhelming sepsis. Only by studying such reports can one discover that the patients have demonstrated evidence of septic embolic disease at sites distant from the pelvic organs. At the same time, it must be stated that bacteremia does not predict the severity of the clinical illness and does not imply a protracted clinical response to therapy.

Septic thrombophlebitis is to be suspected in a patient with pelvic sepsis who demonstrates wide temperature fluctuations, elevated pulse rate, and a failure to respond to antimicrobial therapy. This entity requires timely diagnosis coupled with aggressive management whenever antimicrobial therapy fails to ameliorate the postpartum infection. Septic thrombophlebitis is discussed in detail in Chapter 10.

Treatment

The cornerstones of treatment of postpartum uterine sepsis are probably uterine drainage and the administration of appropriate antibiotics. Uterine drainage and a pelvic examination must be performed to assess whether there are any retained secundines or swabs; at the same time, the obstetrician has an opportunity to evaluate the extent of the infection.

The aggressiveness of the infectious agents, their sensitivity to antimicrobial agents, and host resistance to the offending organisms determine the extent of the infection in puerperal sepsis. Both aerobic and anaerobic cultures must be ordered in a conscientious fashion and not merely as routine. Attention to detail is the only means at our disposal to abolish life-threatening sepsis, which always hovers in the wings of obstetric practice.

Ideally, therapy based on culture findings is the most rational approach; treatment, however, must be instituted prior to the identification of the offending pathogens and determination of their sensitivity to antimicrobial agents. When a clinical specimen yields several bacterial strains, there are often considerable difficulties in the evaluation of the relative pathogenic significance of the different species isolated. For these reasons, the initial therapy of infections involving anaerobes must be empiric. The initial choices reflect the obstetrician's philosophy of antibiotic use, which should be based on experience with previous patients. However, a foul-smelling discharge (which is pathognomonic of an anaerobic component to the infectious process) together with severe tissue necrosis (which can result when a cesarean section is performed after protracted labor in a socioeconomically deprived patient) mandates the administration of an antimicrobial agent that is effective against anaerobic species.

The availability of broad-spectrum beta-lactam antibiotics, which are effective against enteric and most of the aerobic species involved in postpartum sepsis, have gained popularity because in general they lack the ototoxicity and nephrotoxicity associated with the aminoglycosides. Nevertheless, such agents have been associated with hypersensitivity reactions, and not all possess adequate anaerobic coverage. There is no consensus as to the most efficacious antibiotic therapy for postpartum sepsis. In mild to moderately severe cases, parenteral administration of penicillin in a dosage of 10 to 20 million units per day or ampicillin 8 to 12 g per day has proven effective in cases with no gross operative trauma or prior exposure to antibiotic therapy. Such a regimen is usually adequate for the treatment of the majority of aerobic and anaerobic organisms (except for certain species of *Bacteroides* and enterococcus), and a dramatic response should be observed within 48 to 72 hours.

One of the major problems in the management of postpartum infections is the emergence of organisms that are resistant to penicillin. Such organisms can affect the success of penicillin therapy for these infections. Within the past decade, an increased resistance to the penicillins has been noted. In addition to bacteria known to be penicillin-resistant, such as *Staphylococcus aureus* and the Enterobacteriaceae, other previously susceptible bacteria now demonstrate an increased resistance because of their ability to produce the enzyme beta-lactamase. These bacteria include anaerobic organisms belonging to the *Bacteroides* species. Such beta-lactamase-producing bacteria may not only survive penicillin therapy but also may protect other susceptible bacteria from penicillin by releasing the free enzyme into their milieu.

Eschenbach summarized the role of beta-lactamase-producing bacteria in obstetric and gynecologic infections from 36 reports published between 1973 and 1986.[24] Aerobic and anaerobic beta-lactamase-producing bacteria accounted for 1,483 (22 percent) of the total 6,637 microorganisms isolated. The predominant beta-lactamase–producing bacteria were *S. aureus*, Enterobacteriaceae, *Neisseria gonorrhoeae*, *Bacteroides bivius*, and *B. fragilis*. The presence of these bacteria in polymicrobial infections warrants the administration of antimicrobial agents that will be effective in eradicating both beta-lactamase-producing bacteria and other pathogens.

Cefoxitin is still the most resistant cephalosporin to beta-lactamase produced by the *Bacteroides* species and as a result has been widely used for the therapy of postpartum endometritis. Since the introduction of newer broad-spectrum semisynthetic penicillins (such as piperacillin and mezlocillin) as well as cephalosporins, many studies have been reported in which single-agent therapy has been used for postpartum endometritis. Gilstrap and associates utilized piperacillin as a single-agent therapy for 20 patients with postpartum endometritis and compared the results obtained with 22 patients who received combined therapy with gentamicin and clindamycin.[44] They reported three clinical failures in the patients who received piperacillin alone but no failures in the group who had combined therapy. Clindamycin and an aminoglycoside, such as gentamicin, have been standard therapy for severe infections, and consequently all newer agents utilized for the treatment of postpartum uterine sepsis are compared with this antibiotic combination.

Faro and associates compared the efficacy of single-agent therapy of cefoxitin or mezlocillin with the combination of clindamycin and gentamicin.[29] These investigators noted that there were comparable cure rates between single-therapy agents and those obtained with combined therapy.

Calandra and associates emphasized that all too often therapeutic failures accrued from the use of antibiotics lacking a broad spectrum of activity.[9] They considered that imipenem or cilastatin was the first choice in monotherapy; otherwise, combination therapy in the form of a penicillin or cephalosporin plus metronidazole should be prescribed.

Poenaru and associates are in accord with the above findings and state that the mainstay of pharmacotherapy for serious intra-abdominal infection has been the use of an aminoglycoside to treat the gram-negative organisms, with either clindamycin or metronidazole for the anaerobes.[87] They reported that imipenem or cilastatin was a safe and efficacious alternative for treating patients who are seriously ill with intra-abdominal infection.

Cure rates, with these and other agents having a broad spectrum of activity against aerobic and anerobic species, are about 90 percent. Failure to demonstrate evidence of clinical improvement requires complete reassessment of the patient to rule out other sites of infection such as pyelonephritis or pneumonia or extension of the suppurative process, as is demonstrated by wound abscess, pelvic abscess, or thrombophlebitis. If the patient has had one of the cephalosporins as prophylaxis prior to abdominal delivery or has received one of this group of agents for treatment of postpartum sepsis, a persistent fever may be due to one of the enterococcus species.

The use and abuse of antibiotics in obstetric infections are presented in detail in Chapter 26. However, one must stress that prolonged antimicrobial therapy not only is unnecessary but also can be detrimental to the patient, leading to overgrowth of resistant bacteria or possible antibiotic resistance in the future because of plasmid or enzyme induction.

The propensity to have drug resistance developed against it is a quality shared by all classes of antimicrobial agents, the most recent being the fluoroquinolone antibiotics.[93] In order to control the spread of antibiotic resistance, we must focus on the employment of surgical precision in wound care in obstetrics and remember that every operation is a lesson in bacteriology. In addition, all physicians should focus on the use of prescribing restraints. It is essential for obstetricians to realize that short courses of antibiotics are effective for patients with bacteremic episodes as long as repeated blood cultures are obtained during and subsequent to antimicrobial therapy.

Likewise, the obstetrician must realize that one of the most important facts about antibiotic prophylaxis is that, regardless of the agent used, cases of postpartum sepsis will be encountered and will require further therapy. Antibiotics are obviously no substitute for meticulous care in the handling of tissue, securing hemostasis and aseptic technique during the operation, and vigilance for any evidence of infection during the postpartum course.

The continued development of new antimicrobial agents during the past decade has complicated therapeutic decisions. An antimicrobial agent must be chosen not only from a growing number of chemically unrelated compounds but also from many within the same chemical group. Genuine therapeutic advances must be distinguished from minor biochemical embellishments or etymologic distortions utilized by the pharmaceutical industry for sales promotion. Real progress should not be resisted, and when a new congener of a particular group of agents does what its predecessors could not accomplish, it should be made available. It should not, however, be introduced as a universal panacea for unrestricted use.

Future research is likely to be concerned with developing compounds capable of providing monotherapy for all infections: the Holy Grail of the pharmaceutical industry. Such compounds will need to have more predictable microbicidal activity against a wide range of pathogenic microorganisms than offered by currently available antimicrobial agents.

In conclusion, we still encounter serious infections in puerperal women, and we realize that history is reputed to repeat itself. In many ways, this has been true in the case of postpartum sepsis, although as knowledge of infectious disease has burgeoned, each repetition of history differs to some extent from the past. Emerging infectious disease problems are often seen in a different guise, resulting in the possibility that they may fail to be recognized. The experience of the past is crucial to progress in the future. We are therefore in accord with T. S. Eliot that: "Time present and time past are both perhaps present in time future, and time future contained in time past."

References

1. Aharon A, Potasman I, Levitan Z, et al. Postpartum maternal group B streptococcal meningitis. Rev Infect Dis 1990; 12:273-276.
2. Apuzzio JJ, Reyelt C, Pelosi M, et al. Prophylactic antibiotics for cesarean section: compari-

son of high and low risk patients for endometritis. Obstet Gynecol 1982; 59:693-698.
3. Backes RJ, Wilson WR, Geraci JE. Group B streptococcal endocarditis. Arch Intern Med 1985; 145:693-696.
4. Baker CJ, Edwards MS. Group B streptococcal infection. In: Remington JS, Klein JO ed. Infectious diseases of the fetus and newborn infant. Ed 3. Philadelphia: WB Saunders Co, 1990:742-811.
5. Baker CJ, Kasper DL. Group B streptococcal vaccine. Rev Infect Dis 1985; 7:458-467.
6. Baker CJ, Rench MA, Kasper DL. Response to type III polysaccharide in women whose infants have had invasive group B streptococcal infection. N Engl J Med 1990; 322:1857-1860.
7. Blanco JD, Gibbs RS, Castaneda YS. Bacteremia in obstetrics: Clinical course. Obstet Gynecol 1981; 56:621-625.
8. Bobitt JR, Ledger WJ. Amniotic fluid analysis and its role in maternal and neonatal infection. Obstet Gynecol 1978; 51:56-62.
9. Calandra GB, Ricci FM, Wang C, Brown KR. The efficacy results and safety profile of imipenem/cilastatin from the clinical research trials. J Clin Pharmacol 1988; 28:120-127.
10. Claesson BE, Claesson UL. An outbreak of endometritis in a maternity unit caused by spread of group A streptococci from a showerhead. J Hosp Infect 1985; 6:304-311.
11. Colebrook L. The control of infection in obstetrics. Br J Obstet Gynaecol 1946; 53:114-124.
12. Colebrook L, Purdie AW. Treatment of 106 cases of puerperal fever by sulphanilamide (Streptolide). Lancet 1937; 2:1237-1240.
13. Colmer J, Sodeman TM. Contemporary pathogens of the genitourinary system. Laboratory Medicine 1990; 21:730-735.
14. Crawford JS. Maternal mortality associated with anaesthesia. Lancet 1972; 2:918-919.
15. Dan M, Maximova S, Siegman-Igra Y, et al. Varied presentation of sporadic group A streptococcal bacteremia: clinical experience and attempts at classification. Rev Infect Dis 1990; 12:537-542.
16. D'Angelo LJ, Sokol RJ. Time-related peripartum determinants of postpartum morbidity. Obstet Gynecol 1980; 55:319-323.
17. Darbas H, Boyer G, Isolement DE. *Streptococcus pneumoniae* dans le prelevements genitaux. Pathol Biol (Paris) 1987; 35:177-180.
18. Dillon HC Jr, Khare S, Gray BM: Group B streptococcal carriage and disease: a six year prospective study. J Pediatr 1987; 110:31.
19. Douchez AR, Avery OT, Lancefield RC. Studies on the biology of the streptococcus. I. Antigenic relationships between strains of *Streptococcus haemolyticus*. J Exp Med 1919; 30:179-213.
20. Duff P, Gibbs RS, Blanco JD, St Clair PJ. Endometrial culture techniques in puerperal patients. Obstet Gynecol 1983; 61:217-222.
21. Dylewski J, Wiesenfeld H, Latour A. Uterine infection with *Clostridium perfringens*. Rev Infect Dis 1989; 11:470-473.
22. Easmon CSF, Hastings MJG, Neill J, et al. Is group B streptococcal screening during pregnancy justified? Br J Obstet Gynaecol 1985; 92:197-201.
23. Eickhoff TC, Klein JO, Daly AK, et al. Neonatal sepsis and other infections due to group B beta-hemolytic streptococci. N Engl J Med 1964; 271:1221-1228.
24. Eschenbach DA. A review of the role of beta-lactamase producing bacteria in obstetric-gynecologic infection. Am J Obstet Gynecol 1987; 156:495-503.
25. Eschenbach DA. Bacterial vaginosis: emphasis on upper genital complications. Obstet Gynecol Clin North Amer 1989; 16:593-610.
26. Eschenbach DA, Rosene K, Tompkins LS, et al. Endometrial cultures obtained by a triple lumen method from afebrile and febrile postpartum women. J Infect Dis 1986; 153:1038-1045.
27. Faro S. Group B streptococcus and puerperal sepsis. Am J Obstet Gynecol 1980; 138:1219-1220.
28. Faro S, Martens MG, Hammill HA, et al. Antibiotic prophylaxis: is there a difference? Am J Obstet Gynecol 1990; 162:900-909.
29. Faro S, Phillips LE, Baker JL, et al. Comparative efficacy of mezlocillin versus cefoxitin versus clindamycin plus gentamicin in the treatment of patients with postpartum endometritis. Obstet Gynecol 1987; 69:760-766.
30. Faro S, Phillips LE, Martens MG. Perspectives on the bacteriology of postoperative obstetric-gynecologic infections. Am J Obstet Gynecol 1988; 158:694-700.
31. Filker R, Monif GRG. The significance of temperature during the first 24 hours postpartum. Obstet Gynecol 1979; 53:358-361.
32. Fry RM. Fatal infection by haemolytic streptococcus group B. Lancet 1938; 1:199-201.
33. Gabel HD. Maternal mortality in South Carolina from 1970 to 1984: an analysis. Obstet Gynecol 1987; 69:307-311.
34. Gallagher PC, Watanakunakorn C. Group B streptococcal endocarditis: report of seven cases and review of the literature, 1962–1985. Rev Infect Dis 1986; 8:175-188.
35. Gibbs RS. Clinical risk factors for puerperal infection. Obstet Gynecol 1980; 55(Suppl):178-184.
36. Gibbs RS. Severe infections in pregnancy. Med Clin North Am 1989; 73:713-721.
37. Gibbs RS, Blanco JD, St Clair PJ. A case-control study of wound abscess after cesarean section. Obstet Gynecol 1983; 62:498-501.
38. Gibbs RS, Blanco JD, St Clair PJ, Castaneda YS. Quantitative bacteriology of amniotic fluid from women with clinical intraamniotic infection. J Infect Dis 1982; 145:1-8.
39. Gibbs RS, Blanco JD, St Clair PJ, Castaneda YS. Vaginal colonization with resistant aerobic bacteria after antibiotic therapy for endometritis. Am J Obstet Gynecol 1982; 142:130-134.
40. Gibbs RS, Forman J, St Clair PJ, Baseman JB. Detection of serum antibody response to *Bacteroides bivius* by enzyme-linked immunosorbent

assay in women with intraamniotic infection. Obstet Gynecol 1987; 69:208-213.
41. Gibbs RS, Jones PM, Wilder CJY. Internal fetal monitoring and maternal infection following cesarean section: a prospective study. Obstet Gynecol 1978; 52:193-197.
42. Gibbs RS, O'Dell TN, Macgregor RR, et al. Puerperal endometritis: a prospective microbiologic study. Am J Obstet Gynecol 1975; 121:919-925.
43. Gilstrap LC, Cunningham FG. The bacterial pathogenesis of infection following cesarean section. Obstet Gynecol 1979; 53:545-549.
44. Gilstrap LC, Maier RC, Gibbs RS et al. Piperacillin versus clindamycin plus gentamicin for pelvic infections. Obstet Gynecol 1984; 64:762-766.
45. Gopelrud CP, Ohm MJ, Galask RP. Aerobic and anaerobic flora of the cervix during pregnancy and the puerperium. Am J Obstet Gynecol 1976; 126:858-865.
46. Gordon A. A treatise on the epidemic puerperal fever of Aberdeen. London: GG and J Robinson, 1795.
47. Gravett MG, Nelson HP, DeRouen TA, et al. Independent associations of bacterial vaginosis and *Chlamydia trachomatis* infection with adverse pregnancy outcome. JAMA 1986; 256:1899-1903.
48. Green SL and LaPeter KS. Evidence for postpartum toxic-shock syndrome in a mother-infant pair. Am J Med 1982; 72:169-172.
49. Guerinot GT, Gitomer SD, Sanko SR. Patient with toxic-shock syndrome. Obstet Gynecol 1982; 59(Suppl):43-45.
50. Guzick DS, Winn K. The association of chorioamnionitis with preterm delivery. Obstet Gynecol 1985; 65:11-16.
51. Hagen D. Maternal febrile morbidity associated with fetal monitoring and cesarean section. Obstet Gynecol 1975; 46:260-267.
52. Haley RW, Culver DH, White JW, et al. The nationwide nosocomial infection rate: a new need for vital statistics. Am J Epidemiol 1985; 121:159-167.
53. Harrison HR, Alexander ER, Weinstein L, et al. Cervical *Chlamydia trachomatis* and mycoplasma infections in pregnancy. JAMA 1983; 250:1721-1727.
54. Heggie AD, Lunicao GG, Stuart LA, Gyves MT. *Chlamydia trachomatis* infection in mother and infants. Am J Dis Child 1981; 135:507-511.
55. Hillier SL, Martius J, Krohn M, et al. A case control study of chorioamnionic infection and histologic chorioamnionitis in prematurity. N Engl J Med 1988; 319:972-978.
56. Hodge HL. On the non-contagious character of puerperal fever: an introductory lecture. Philadelphia: TK and PG Collins, 1852.
57. Hoffman SA, Moellering RC. The enterococcus: "putting the bug in our ears". Ann Intern Med 1987; 106:757-761.
58. Holmes OW. Contagiousness of puerperal fever. N Engl Quart J Med Surg 1842-1843; 1:503-550.
59. Holmes OW. Puerperal fever as a private pestilence. Boston: Ticknor & Fields, 1855.
60. Hoyme UB, Kiviat N, Eschenbach DA. The microbiology and treatment of late postpartum endometritis. Obstet Gynecol 1986; 68:226-232.
61. Kasper DL. The polysaccharide capsule of *Bacteroides fragilis* subspecies *fragilis:* immunochemical and morphologic definition. J Infect Dis 1976; 133:79-87.
62. Knuppel RA, Scarbo JC, Mitchell GW, et al. Quantitative transcervical uterine cultures with a new device. Obstet Gynecol 1981; 57:243-248.
63. Lamey JR, Eschenbach DA, Mitchell SH, et al. Isolation of mycoplasmas and bacteria from the blood of postpartum women. Am J Obstet Gynecol 1982; 143:104-112.
64. Lancefield RC, Hare R. The serological differentiation of pathogenic and non-pathogenic strains of haemolytic streptococci from parturient women. J Exp Med 1935; 61:335-349.
65. Landry SL, Kaiser DC, Wenzel RP. Hospital stay and mortality attributed to nosocomial enterococcal bacteremia: a control study. Am J Infect Control 1989; 17:323-329.
66. Larsen B, Galask RP. Vaginal microbial flora: practical and theoretical importance. Obstet Gynecol 1982; 55(Suppl):100-113.
67. Larsen B, Galask RP. Vaginal microbial flora: composition and influences of host physiology. Ann Intern Med 1982; 96:926-930.
68. Ledger WJ, Gee C, Pollin PA. A new approach to patients with suspected anaerobic postpartum infections: transabdominal uterine aspiration for culture and metronidazole for treatment. Am J Obstet Gynecol 1976; 126:1-6.
69. Ledger WJ, Kriewall T. The fever index: a quantitative indirect measure of hospital-acquired infections in obstetrics and gynecology. Am J Obstet Gynecol 1973; 115:514-520.
70. Ledger WJ, Norman M, Gee C, Lewis W. Bacteremia on an obstetric-gynecologic service. Am J Obstet Gynecol 1975; 121:205-212.
71. Ledger WJ, Reite Am, Headington JT. A system for infectious disease surveillance on an obstetric service. Obstet Gynecol 1971; 37:769-778.
72. Lister J. On the antiseptic principle in the practice of surgery. Br Med J 1867; 2:246-248.
73. Martius J, Krohn MA, Hillier SL, et al. Relationships of vaginal *Lactobacillus* species, cervical *Chlamydia trachomatis* and bacterial vaginosis to preterm birth. Obstet Gynecol 1988; 71:89-95.
74. Mastro TD, Farley TA, Elliott JA, et al. An outbreak of surgical wound infections due to group A streptococcus carried in the scalp. N Engl J Med 1990; 323:968-972.
75. McCormack WM, Rosner B, Lee Y-H, Rankin JS. Isolation of genital mycoplasmas from blood obtained shortly after vaginal delivery. Lancet 1975; 1:596-599.
76. Minkoff HL, Sierra MF, Pringle GF, Schwarz RH. Vaginal colonization with group B streptococcus as a risk factor for post cesarean section febrile morbidity. Am J Obstet Gynecol 1982; 142:992-995.

77. Notzon FC, Placek PJ, Taffel SM. Comparison of national cesarean section rates. N Engl J Med 1987; 316:386-389.
78. Onderdonk AB, Kasper DL, Cisneros RL, Bartlett JG. The capsular polysaccaride of *Bacteroides fragilis* as a virulence factor: comparison of the pathogenic potential of encapsulated and unencapsulated strains. J Infect Dis 1977; 136:82-89.
79. Osler W. Aequanimitas, with other addresses to medical students, nurses and practitioners of medicine. Philadelphia: P Blakiston, 1904:p.305.
80. Paavonen J, Kiviat N, Brunham RC, et al. Prevalence and manifestations of endometritis among women with cervicitis. Am J Obstet Gynecol 1985; 152:280-286.
81. Pass MA, Gray BM, Dillon HCJ. Puerperal and perinatal-infections with group B streptococci. Am J Obstet Gynecol 1982; 143:147-152.
82. Pasteur L. Septicemie puerperale, Bull Acad Med (Paris) 1879; 2me serie—Tome VIII:8256-8260.
83. Phelan JP, Pruyn SC. Prophylactic antibiotics in cesarean section: a double blind study of cefazolin. 1979; 133:474-479.
84. Platt LD, Yonekura ML, Ledger WJ. The role of anaerobic bacteria in postpartum endometritis. Am J Obstet Gynecol 1979: 135:814-817.
85. Platt R, Warren JW, Edelin KC, et al. Infection with *Mycoplasma hominis* in postpartum fever. Lancet 1980; 2:1217-1221.
86. Plummer DC, Garland SM, Gilbert GL. Bacteremia and pelvic infections in women due to *Ureaplasma urealyticum* and *Mycoplasma hominis*. Med J Aust 1987; 146:135-137.
87. Poenaru D, De Santis M, Christou NV. Imipenem versus tobramycin: antianaerobic antibiotic therapy in intra-abdominal infections. Can J Surg 1990; 33:415-422.
88. Rehu M, Nilsson CG. Risk factors for febrile morbidity associated with cesarean section. Obstet Gynecol 1980; 56:269-272.
89. Robinson EN Jr. Pneumococcal endometritis and neonatal sepsis. Rev Infect Dis 1990; 12:799-801.
90. Romero R, Mazor M. Infection and preterm labor. Clin Obstet Gynecol 1988; 31:553-584.
91. Romero R, Manogue KR, Mitchell MD, et al. Infection and labor. IV. Cachectin-tumor necrosis factor in the amniotic fluid of women with intraamniotic infection and preterm labor. Am J Obstet Gynecol 1989; 161:336-341.
92. Rosene K, Eschenbach DA, Tompkins LS, et al. Polymicrobial early postpartum endometritis with facultatively anaerobic and anaerobic bacteria, genital mycoplasmas and *Chlamydia trachomatis:* treatment with piperacillin or cefoxitin. J Infect Dis 1986; 153:1028-1037.
93. Schaefler S. Methicillin-resistant strains of *Staphylococcus aureus* resistant to quinolones. J Clin Microbiol 1989; 27:335-336.
94. Semmelweis IP. The etiology, the concept and the prophylaxis of childbirth fever. Baltimore: Williams & Wilkins, 1941. (Translated by FR Murray; originally published in 1861).
95. Stevens DL, Tanner MH, Winship J, et al. Severe group A streptococcal infection associated with a toxic shock-like syndrome and scarlet fever toxin A. N Engl J Med 1989; 321:1-7.
96. Stevens FA. Occurrence of *Staphylococcus aureus* infection with a scarlatiniform rash. JAMA 1927; 88:957-958.
97. Stevenson CS, Beheny CA, Miller NF. Maternal death from puerperal sepsis following cesarean section: a 16 year study in Michigan. Obstet Gynecol 1967; 29:181-191.
98. Stray-Pedersen B, Blakstad M, Bergan T. Bacteriuria in the puerperium. Am J Obstet Gynecol 1990; 162:792-797.
99. Sutton GP, Smirz LR, Clark DH, Bennett JE. Group B streptococcal necrotizing fasciitis arising from an episiotomy. Obstet Gynecol 1985; 66:733-736.
100. Sweet RL, Ledger WJ. Puerperal infectious morbidity: a two year review. Am J Obstet Gynecol 1973; 117:1093-1100.
101. Sweet RL, Landers DL, Walker C, Schachter J. *Chlamydia trachomatis* infection and pregnancy outcome. Am J Obstet Gynecol 1987; 156:824-833.
102. Taffel SM. Cesarean section in America: dramatic trends 1970–1987. Stat Bull Metrop Insur Co 1989; 70:2-11.
103. Taffel SM, Placek PJ, Mohen M. 1988 US cesarean section rate at 24.7 per 100 Births: a plateau? N Engl J Med 1990; 323:199-200.
104. Thadepalli H, Chan WH, Maidman JE, Davidson EC Jr. Microflora of the cervix during normal labor and the puerperium. J Infect Dis 1978; 137:568-572.
105. Wager GP, Martin DH, Koutsky L, et al. Puerperal infectious morbidity: relationship to route of delivery and antepartum *Chlamydia trachomatis* infection. Am J Obstet Gynecol 1980; 138:1028-1033.
106. Watson T. Lecture on the principles and practice of physic, delivered at King's College Hospital, London: JW Parker, 1843.
107. Westh H, Skibsted L, Korner B. *Streptococcus pneumoniae* infections of the female genital tract and in the newborn. Rev Infect Dis 1990; 12:416-422.
108. Wood EG, Dillon HC Hr. A prospective study of group B streptococcal bacteriuria in pregnancy. Am J Obstet Gynecol 1981; 140:515-520.

CHAPTER 8

Mastitis and Antibiotic Concentrations in Breast Milk

Douglas D. Glover, M.D., R.Ph.

Mastitis is a nonspecific term that denotes any inflammatory process in the breast. Because the bulk of acute cases occur during lactation, the terms *lactational mastitis* and *puerperal mastitis* have logically evolved. Over the years, a multiplicity of other appellatives have been employed for breast infection that are largely descriptive in nature. Lack of nomenclature standardization has resulted in a hodgepodge of terms that has brought more chaos than order to the present state of confusion. "Acute puerperal mastitis," for example, indicates (more than an allusion) the abrupt onset of subjective symptoms. "Epidemic mastitis" suggests a contagious origin, whereas "sporadic puerperal mastitis," otherwise known as "nonepidemic mastitis," implies random occurrence in contrast to a nosocomial origin of the epidemic form. However, epidemic mastitis occasionally occurs in a sporadic manner in women who have had their babies at home, and it may make its appearance many weeks after delivery, negating the idea that this infection is a result of institutional care. Despite the perplexity of nomenclature the clinician encounters, milk stasis is a significant factor in the pathogenesis of either form of mastitis (Table 8-1).

Nearly four decades ago, Gibberd[17] characterized sporadic mastitis as a cellulitis of the breast principally involving the interlobular connective tissue, the pathogen gaining entry via a cracked or fissured nipple. The resultant cellulitis comprises a V-shaped wedge, the boundaries of which are demarcated by Cooper's ligaments that form septa between the lobes of the breast. Sporadic mastitis is a result of poor nursing technique, with breast engorgement resulting in milk stasis.

By contrast, epidemic mastitis is associated with mammary adenitis that is the result of infection of the ductal system of the breast. Evidence of nipple trauma is lacking, and pus can usually be expressed from the nipple of the involved breast. Several lobes of one or both breasts may be involved, suggesting multiple portals of entry for the infection as previously mentioned. Epidemic mastitis may be hospital acquired, although women who deliver at home may occasionally have acute puerperal mastitis. In contrast to the acute onset of fever associated with flulike symptoms that characterizes sporadic mastitis, inception of the epidemic form is usually insidious, and it has a more protracted course. The interval between delivery and onset of symptoms has been reported to vary from a few days to 5 months, although the largest number of cases occur in the second and third weeks.[14]

Prevalence

The prevalence of sporadic mastitis has remained relatively constant for the last 50 years, affecting 1 to 5 percent of lactating mothers.[43] This is in agreement with Marshall and associates,[25] who reported 2.5 percent of nursing women to be afflicted, of which 4.6 percent had abscess formation. In contrast, the prevalence of epidemic mastitis has declined from a peak of 20 percent of breast-feeding mothers in the 1950s and 1960s, when outbreaks of nosocomial infection were commonplace, to an infrequent occurrence today.

Symptoms

Milk stasis, often a result of a missed or delayed feeding, precedes the onset of symptoms in sporadic

Table 8-1 Mastitis

Sporadic Form	Epidemic Form
Random occurrence	Hospital acquired
Mammary cellulitis	Mammary adenitis
Nipple trauma	Fissure usually absent
Acute onset	Insidious onset
Pus not expressible from nipple	Pus expressible from nipple

Table 8-2 Bacterial Isolates in Order of Frequency

Staphylococcus aureus
S. epidermidis
Group B beta-hemolytic streptococci
Group A beta-hemolytic streptococci
Streptococcus faecalis
Escherichia coli
Haemophilus influenzae
Serratia marcescens
Klebsiella pneumoniae

From Charles D, Glover DD. Current Therapy in Obstetrics. Philadelphia: BC Decker, 1988.

mastitis. Nipple engorgement predisposes the woman to fissure formation from infant mastication. The resultant fissure serves as a portal of entry for bacteria to the ductal system, setting the stage for sporadic mastitis to develop.

Most women with sporadic mastitis experience a sudden onset of symptoms that include breast tenderness, chills, and fever. The temperature usually exceeds 101° F and may be as high as 105° F. General malaise, cephalalgia, and anorexia, suggestive of a flulike illness, are commonly experienced. In the lactating woman, influenza symptoms in the absence of respiratory changes should alert the clinician to early sporadic mastitis. Such women have developed toxic shock syndrome when only minimal evidence of mastitis is present.[15]

The symptoms of epidemic mastitis have an insidious onset and are similar to those of the sporadic form, albeit much less severe. Bacteria gain entry via the lactiferous ducts and periductal lymphatics and cause mammary adenitis. On occasion pus is expressible from the nipples. Most commonly the onset of symptoms is 2 to 3 weeks postpartum.

The clinician must carefully distinguish mastitis from focal breast engorgement. In the latter case, the lactiferous duct becomes blocked, and a segment of the breast is swollen. The affected area is firm and tender to the touch, but there is absence of both erythema and fever. Such a problem is remedied by promptly putting the baby to the breast and applying local heat.

Microbiology of Puerperal Mastitis

The predominant microorganism identified in either form of puerperal mastitis is *Staphylococcus aureus*. In a study by Marshall and coworkers,[25] *S. aureus* was isolated from the milk of 23 of 48 infected breasts. Furthermore, 73 percent of the women involved were found to have staphylococcal-contaminated milk in the contralateral breast. These investigators surmised that transmission from the infected to the noninfected breast was via the nursling.

Less commonly, *S. epidermidis* is isolated from the milk of an infected breast. A decade ago this organism was considered a skin contaminant and not a putative cause of breast infection, although today its role in mastitis is more clearly defined. *Staphylococcus epidermidis* ranks second to *S. aureus* as a pathogen in mastitis. However, investigations in laboratory animals imply that even though coagulase-negative staphylococci may cause breast infection, the mastitis that results is usually mild. These microorganisms may interfere with colonization of more virulent bacteria such as *S. aureus*.[21]

Group B streptococci, first recognized to cause mastitis in 1979, have recently been isolated from a breast abscess of a mother whose child also had mastitis, from which microorganisms of the same phage type were identified.[38] In contrast to mastitis caused by staphylococci involving only one breast, group B beta-hemolytic streptococci have a proclivity for bilaterality. When bilateral mastitis is encountered, group B streptococcus is generally the causative organism.

The vast majority of puerperal mastitis cases are caused by gram-positive aerobic microorganisms. Table 8-2 lists the various bacterial isolates in the order of frequency they are encountered in clinical practice. Although septicemia may complicate mastitis, its occurrence is considered a rarity. Likewise, toxic shock syndrome associated with lactational breast abscess has also been reported.[2,10,12,13,37]

Breast Abscess Formation

Blood flow to the mammary gland is 400 to 500 times the volume of milk produced.[24] It is a matter of conjecture that diminished mammary perfusion precedes abscess formation, although development of an abscess is rare in the woman who maintains lactation. The effectiveness of antimicrobial therapy is limited to the phase of active perfusion.[14] Should nursing be interrupted, the blood supply to the breast rapidly declines and tissue perfusion becomes compromised. If treatment is delayed beyond 24 hours, tissue ischemia is progressive and may be sufficient to preclude adequate delivery of antibiotic to the site of infection.[38] Tissue ischemia in conjunction with milk stasis sets the stage for abscess formation. The response of the lactating breast to the suppurative process is to wall off the infected area where pus accumulates to form an abscess cavity.[14] Further administration of antibiotics is to no avail and surgical management supersedes antimicrobial therapy

Diagnostic Modalities

Since the portal of entry for bacteria in the majority of breast abscesses is in the vicinity of the nipple, it logically follows that most collections of pus are subareolar in location. Diagnosis of the superficial abscess is by physical examination. Palpation of localized heat or fluctuation may identify a superficial or subareolar abscess, although skin changes other than erythema are usually absent in early abscess formation.

As previously mentioned, the ligaments of Cooper act as a barrier to restrict the infectious process to a single lobe. Septa formed by these ligaments preserve the normal architecture of the breast. An abscess located deep in the interlobular tissue may have its characteristic fluctuance masked by interceding breast parenchyma and thus may be difficult to detect. Likewise, a retromammary collection of pus may defy demarcation. In such cases, ultrasonographic or radiographic assistance may be required to arrive at a diagnosis.

For many years mammography has been employed to identify and localize abscess cavities, but this technique has certain disadvantages. Mammographic findings are nonspecific, and it may not be possible to distinguish among an abscess, a neoplasm, and an area of fibrocystic disease. Typically, an acute abscess is a poorly defined density[1] that may resemble a cyst unless gas-producing microorganisms are present. As time passes and the abscess matures, a capsule forms to make the margins of the cavity appear more distinct. Breast compression, which may be painful for the patient, is required for mammography.[1]

Likewise, ultrasonography also requires pressure and may be painful for the patient, albeit to a lesser degree than mammography. The ultrasonographic appearance of an abscess may vary from hypoechoic with a clean, smooth wall that resembles a cyst to a shaggy wall with variable amounts of debris that is characteristic of an abscess.[1]

Once the diagnosis of an abscess is established, prompt surgical intervention is indicated. Immediate incision and drainage is mandatory. The incision is made over the site of maximum tenderness and may be made in a radial or circumferential manner. Once the abscess cavity is opened, care is taken to disrupt all loculi that have formed. A biopsy should be performed to make sure that a carcinoma has not been missed, although neoplasia in the puerperal woman is uncommon. A dependent drain is inserted through a stab wound, and the abscess cavity is packed. Cavities of smaller abscesses may be closed with deep mattress sutures and perioperative antibiotic therapy used in lieu of a dependent drain.

A specimen of pus should be obtained for culture and sensitivity testing before perioperative antibiotics are started. Prior antibiotic treatment may negate a useful operative culture. Antibiotics are continued for 5 to 7 days after incision and drainage. Many surgeons select erythromycin as the antibiotic of choice pending identification of the putative organism and determination of whether it is penicillin resistant. Clindamycin, cephalosporins, and methicillin are also used.[4]

Once drainge is accomplished and antibiotic therapy established, there is no reason why lactation should not resume. Inhibition of lactation may actually hinder resolution by increasing breast engorgement. Should breast feeding not be possible, judicious use of a breast pump to prevent engorgement is indicated.

Treatment of Puerperal Mastitis

Devereux's classic report[14] on treatment of mastitis and abscess prevention has influenced the management of acute puerperal mastitis since 1969. A more recent investigation from Oslo[26] confirms most of Devereux's conclusions, but with slight modification.

There is agreement that the effectiveness of therapy regarding both the speed of recovery and prevention of abscess formation depends on the rapidity with which treatment is instituted. According to Devereux, fever usually subsides within 48 hours and objective signs of infection clear by the fifth day of antibiotic therapy. His study consisted of 71 mastitis cases, of which 47 women continued uninterrupted lactation. Infant weaning was avoided except when the nipples were severely fissured, lactation failed, or there was evidence of suppuration. None of the women who were persistent with breast feeding developed an abscess.

Of the nine women in this study with clinical evidence of mastitis more than 24 hours before treatment, six had abscess formation. These six represented 75 percent of all who developed abscess and were the basis for his conclusion that early antibiotic treatment is crucial to abscess prevention.

Six of Devereux's 71 patients had suffered mastitis in a previous gestation, and two of them had developed abscesses. Of the six, two had experienced multiple episodes of mastitis, supporting the concept that faulty nursing technique with breast engorgement is a major risk factor for mastitis.

Finally, Devereux concluded that the choice of antimicrobial agent is not as important as early initiation of therapy. The preponderance of mastitis patients in his study received sulfisoxazole, a bacteriostatic agent. He contended that host resistance factors are more important than the choice of antibiotic, provided sufficient tissue perfusion is maintained. The contribution of the antimicrobial agent is to halt replication of the microorganism and to shift the advantage to the host. Provided there is adequacy of both humoral and cellular defense mechanisms, the success of antibiotic therapy is likely.

Matheson and colleagues,[26] in a recent multicenter study conducted in Oslo, compared favorable versus unfavorable outcomes to treatment of 43 mastitis patients. These authors concurred with Devereux that delay between onset of symptoms and physician consultation is predictive of unfavorable outcome for mastitis. Women with poor treatment results had a mean delay of 4.1 days (± 3.6 days) versus 2.0 days (± 2.6 days) for those with a favorable outcome. Likewise, they reported that six of eight women in their study recovered quickly without antibiotic treatment and concluded that host defense mechanisms alone were sufficient in that cohort of

Table 8-3 Antibiotics Commonly Used to Treat Mastitis

Drug	Dose (mg)	Frequency	Duration (Days)	Cost ($)*
Amoxicillin–Clavulanate	500/125	q8h	5–7	40.62–56.87
Ampicillin	250–500	q6h	5–7	3.00–7.00
Cephalexin	250–500	q6h	5–7	13.00–33.60
Cloxacillin	250–500	q6h	5–7	8.00–22.40
Dicloxacillin	250–500	q6h	5–7	10.00–25.20
Erythromycin	250–500	q6h	5–7	5.19–10.76
Nafcillin	250–500	q4–6h	5–7	20.03–77.83
Penicillin V	250–500	q6–8h	5–7	2.80–5.60
Sulfamethoxazole-trimethoprim	800/160	q12h	5–7	5.00–7.00

*Cost = lowest dose, least frequent, and shortest duration of treatment *and* highest cost, most frequent, and longest duration of treatment.
Cost refers to prescription price to the consumer based on multisource availability of drugs in the United States.

patients. This is in agreement with a conclusion reached by Devereux two decades before.

However, Matheson and his associates reported that 70 percent of the coagulase-positive *S. aureus* strains isolated from breast milk were beta-lactamase producing and therefore resistant to phenoxymethylpenicillin. Four of the eight women who experienced unfavorable outcome were from this group. Phenoxymethylpenicillin was not able to prevent suppuration in these patients.

In addition to emphasizing the importance of early mastitis treatment and meticulous emptying of the breast, these authors advise restricting erythromycin treatment to those women known or suspected to be allergic to penicillin because staphylococci rapidly become resistant to this antibiotic. They recommend empiric treatment with 250 mg penicillin V four times a day and suggest that use of penicillinase-resistant penicillin be restricted to those failing to show clinical response after 48 hours as well as those who have pronounced symptoms when they initially present with mastitis.

The more commonly prescribed treatment regimens and their pharmacology are outlined in Tables 8-3 through 8-5. When a penicillinase-resistant penicillin is indicated, nafcillin or one of the isoxazolyl penicillins, such as oxacillin, cloxacillin, or dicloxacillin, should be effective therapy for infection caused by beta-hemolytic streptococci as well as penicillin G-resistant and penicillin G-sensitive staphylocci.

Clavulanic acid is a beta-lactam structurally related to the penicillins that inhibits some beta-lactamases that inactivate beta-lactam antibiotics. Clavulanic acid penetrates the bacterial cell wall and acts as an inhibitor of a wide variety of plasmid-mediated as well as some chromosomally mediated bacterial beta-lactamases. Complexing with penicillin-binding protein-2, it initially acts as a competitive inhibitor, although ultimately it becomes noncompetitive and irreversible. As a result of beta-lactamase inhibition, beta-lactam antibiotics are protected from enzymatic degradation. It must be emphasized that such agents are of no value once ischemia has developed.

Included in Table 8-3 is the combination bacteriostatic agent sulfamethoxazole-trimethoprim, which is infrequently employed in mastitis treatment. Its use is limited to those women with suspected or confirmed methicillin-resistant, coagulase-positive staphylococcal infection who are allergic to beta-lactam antimicrobials.[23] Whereas this agent is used in an outpatient setting, a therapeutic alternative is intravenous administration of vancomycin in a dosage regimen of 500 mg every 6 hours for 5 days, which requires hospital admission. Vancomycin is reserved to treat severe, potentially life-threatening staphylococcal infection that has not responded to other therapeutic modalities. On occasion, vancomycin is administered concurrently with an aminoglycoside, such as gentamicin, for therapeutic synergism.

Resolution of fever and pain are usually prompt following institution of antimicrobial therapy. Pain is caused by milk stasis and breast engorgement, and the treatment for both is to keep the breasts emptied. Continued lactation is to be encouraged, however. Should the nipple be fissured, a breast shield may permit the woman to continue nursing as the nipple heals. If pain proscribes nursing, a breast pump may be required to empty the breast satisfactorily and relieve pain.

Non-narcotic analgesics are useful adjuncts for pain control. Acetaminophen or aspirin in a dosage regimen of 650 mg every 4 hours is usually adequate. It must be emphasized that analgesics are not a substitute for emptying the breasts; elimination of pain is accomplished by relieving breast engorgement. Likewise, acetaminophen and aspirin are quite effective as antipyretic agents. Fever and pain subside within 24 to 48 hours in the majority of cases. Failure suggests suppuration that requires further evaluation.

A discussion of pharmacotherapy would be incomplete without mention of adverse effects to the drugs used in treatment. Obviously, the most common adverse

Table 8-4 Pharmacokinetics of Beta-Lactams Used to Treat Mastitis

Drug	Oral Absorption (%)	Effect of Food on Oral Absorption	Time to Peak Serum Concentration (Hours)	Half-Life (Hours)	
				NORMAL RENAL FUNCTION	IMPAIRED RENAL FUNCTION
Amoxicillin/Clavulanate	Well absorbed	None	1.0–2.0	1.3–1.0	—
Ampicillin	35–50	Slightly decreased	1.5–2.0	1.0–1.5	10–15
Cephalexin	Rapid	None	1.0	0.9–1.2	5–30
Cloxacillin	50	Decreased	1.0–2.0	0.5–11	0.8–1.0*
Dicloxacillin	37–50	Decreased	0.5–1.0	0.5–1.0	1.0–3.0
Nafcillin	Variable; poor	Decreased	1.0–2.0	0.5–1.0	1.2–1.5
Oxacillin	30–33	Decreased	1.0	0.5–0.7	1.0–3.0
Penicillin V	60	Minimal	0.5–1.0	1.0	0.5–1.0*

*Markedly increased with impaired hepatic and impaired renal function.
Abstracted from the USP DI, ed 12, Rockville, MD: The United States Pharmacopeial Convention, Inc. Copyright, The United States Pharmacopeial Convention, Inc. Permission Granted.

Table 8-5 Pharmacology of Beta-Lactams Used to Treat Mastitis

Drug	Protein Binding (%)	Hepatic Biotransformation (%)	Renal Elimination (% Unchanged)	Vd (L/kg)
Amoxicillin/Clavulanate	Low (both)	28–50	50–70/25–45	—
Ampicillin	17–20	12–50	25–60	0.28
Cephalexin	10–15	No	80/6	0.26
Cloxacillin	95–97	9–22	30–45	0.10
Dicloxacillin	95–97	9–10	60	0.09
Nafcillin	87–90	60	10–30	1.10
Oxacillin	90–93	49	40	0.20
Penicillin V	80	56	20–40	0.20

Abstracted from the USP DI, ed 12, Rockville, MD: The United States Pharmacopeial Convention, Inc. Copyright, The United States Pharmacopeial Convention, Inc. Permission Granted.

drug reaction (ADR) is pruritus, with or without rash, indicating hypersensitivity. The overall incidence of ADR in one prospective investigation[6] of hospital inpatients receiving antibiotic therapy was 4.4 percent. Specific drug reaction rates in this study revealed that 5.2 percent had adverse effects with cephalosporins, 5.7 percent with ampicillin, and 8.5 percent with methicillin. In general, such reactions are mediated either by immunoglobulin M or E, the latter characterized by urticaria, which places the woman at risk for anaphylaxis. The most serious ADR is pseudomembranous colitis, which is not uncommon although the precise incidence is unknown. It is characterized by abdominal cramps or pain, often associated with abdominal bloating; the woman may experience a watery or bloody diarrhea that may be severe. Likewise, she may exhibit fever and vomiting and complain of excessive thirst, an unusual tiredness, and weight loss. Amoxicillin, ampicillin, and these in combination with clavulanate or sulbactam are the usual culprits; however, pseudomembranous colitis may complicate any penicillin therapeutic regimen.

A much less common occurrence is cholestatic jaundice, characterized by dark or amber urine and pale stools in association with upper abdominal pain and icteric sclera. The actual frequency of cholestatic jaundice is unknown, and its association with antibiotic therapy is usually overlooked. Likewise, nausea and vomiting, muscle weakness (due to hypokalemia), and dizziness, each a nonspecific symptom, may be reported by patients taking any of the penicilloic acid derivatives, although they more commonly occur with amoxicillin, ampicillin, and penicillin G and V. Nevertheless, provided the clinician makes an early diagnosis and promptly prescribes effective therapy, mastitis is usually a benign process that can be effectively managed without hospital admission.

Transmammary Excretion of Drugs

Throughout this chapter emphasis has been placed on the importance of continued lactation during treatment for mastitis. The breast-feeding mother's concern about harm to her child from the antibiotic prescribed for her is certainly reasonable. Unfortunately, there is a paucity of data to aid the clinician in answering such a patient's queries, although knowledge of certain facts may assist the physician in this regard.

The amount of antibiotic ingested by an infant from its mother's milk depends largely upon three factors: the pH of the milk at the time of nursing, the degree to which the antibiotic is protein bound, and the lipid solubility of the drug. The pH of lacteal secretions varies widely from 6.35 to 7.65.[33] As a rule, the pH of breast milk is lower than the pH of maternal plasma.[3] Only the nonionized fraction of free antibiotic diffuses across the lipid membrane to enter the alveolar lumen where milk is formed. As equilibrium is established across the biologic membrane, the concentration of non-ionized drug in the milk should equal that of plasma. Drugs that are weak acids, such as the beta-lactam antibiotics, are highly ionized at plasma pH and enter milk slowly to achieve low concentration.[9] Weakly basic drugs, such as erythromycin, are highly ionized at the lower pH of milk and become "ion-trapped" in the lacteal secretions.[9,34] As the nonionized fraction of the drug in milk falls to levels below that of the maternal plasma, diffusion of the agent across the lipid membrane continues until equilibrium of nonionized substances achieves parity. In such a case, the concentration of the antimicrobial agent in milk exceeds that of maternal plasma and the milk/plasma ratio is greater than unity. However, should the drug be a weak acid that is highly ionized at plasma pH, only the nonionized fraction diffuses across the biologic membrane. Because that fraction is small, the concentration in milk is low and the milk/plasma ratio is less than unity.[35] Therefore, minor changes of pH on either side of the lipid membrane can significantly alter the concentration of drug in milk.

The magnitude of free drug in maternal plasma is an important determinant of the concentration attainable in the mother's breast secretions.[29] Alterations of protein-binding characteristics related to pregnancy have significant implications in transmammary passage of drugs. It is reported that binding of certain drugs to several albumin models progressively declines from the fourth month of gestation to term.[11] This change accompanies a decrease in plasma albumin and gamma globulin levels.[29] In the gravid woman, reduced binding capacity has been demonstrated for a number of drugs, including antimicrobial agents. The reason for this alteration in protein binding is unclear, although it is surmised that the increase in total plasma lipids and free fatty acids may be a factor.[5,36] Likewise, the binding capacity of albumin is further reduced in late pregnancy[42] and contributes to the higher levels of free drug observed near term. Protein binding begins to increase a week after parturition, but the binding capacity does not normalize until several weeks postpartum.[11,31]

The free fraction of drugs in milk protein is generally less than that for plasma protein,[33] but data on the binding properties of milk-specific protein fractions in the human are lacking. At birth, the unbound drug fraction in the newborn is elevated, increasing the quantity of pharmacologically active drug available to the baby.[20] Likewise, the lipid content of colostrum is low at a time when the binding capacity of a neonate's plasma is impaired. With passage of time, the fat content of milk rises and the free drug fraction declines in conjunction with progressive maturation of the nursling's hepatic and renal functions.[18] Such a reciprocal relationship serves to protect the newborn infant from drug intoxication.

Finally, the lipid solubility of a drug is an important determinant of the antibiotic content in the lacteal secretions. Despite the fact that a drug is nonionized, its passage through the lipid barrier is gradual if its lipid solubility is low.[33] This has a therapeutic implication regarding the penicillins, the mainstay of mastitis pharmacotherapy, that have low lipid solubility as well as low concentrations in breast milk.

The amount of drug ingested by an infant is less if the child nurses at times when the maternal plasma levels are low.[44] Most antibiotics appear in the lipid fraction that varies in accordance with the time of day. Rather than produced and stored in the breast between feedings, milk is formed as the infant suckles. Therefore, the plasma content of antibiotic at the time of nursing determines the concentration the agent achieves in milk. The lipid content of the lacteal secretions varies with a circadian rhythm that reaches a peak at 10 A.M. and a nadir between 6 and 10 P.M.[44] In general, the peak plasma concentration of a drug occurs about 1 to 2 hours after oral administration. By giving the first daily dose of a lipophilic antibiotic after the midmorning feeding and timing subsequent doses to follow feedings throughout the day, the amount of drug ingested by the infant can be minimized.

Beta-Lactam Antibiotics

The beta-lactam antibiotics are a class of highly ionized, weakly acidic antimicrobial agents that appear in low concentration in breast milk. They have a high degree of protein binding and low lipid solubility that limits transmammary passage. As a rule, the concentration of the beta-lactams in milk is less than 1 μg per milliliter, and the total amount a suckling infant can ingest is 3 to 4 percent of the maternal area under the curve of serum concentrations versus time.[22]

Although measurable levels of beta-lactams are higher at steady state than after a single dose, the maximum concentration in milk remains low. Likewise, concentrations in breast milk are higher after intramuscular or intravenous administration than when the antibiotic is given orally. As shown in Table 8-6, penicillin G achieves peak concentration 1 hour after IM administration, after which levels rapidly decline.[27] The isoxazolyl

Table 8-6 Beta-Lactam Concentrations in Maternal Serum and Breast Milk

Antibiotics	Route	Dose (mg)	Fluid	Hours After Dose: 1	2	4	6
Penicillin G	IM	360	Serum	0.92–1.00 (0.35)	0.35–0.48 (0.42)	0.35–0.37 (0.36)	Trace
			Milk	0.32–0.37 (0.35)	0.10–0.40 (0.20)	Trace–0.3 (0.10)	Trace
Penicillin V	IM	1,000	Serum	10.10–16.0 (13.40)	4.80–6.40 (5.50)	0.90–1.60 (1.30)	0.20–0.50 (0.40)
			Milk	0.19–0.23 (0.20)	0.20–0.30 (0.26)	0.20–0.30 (0.20)	0.19–0.39 (0.30)
Oxacillin	IM	500	Serum	3.00–4.80 (4.10)	0.70–1.30 (1.00)	Trace	0.00
			Milk	0.18–0.44 (0.30)	0.23–0.70 (0.50)	0.24–0.40 (0.30)	Trace
Cloxacillin	IM	500	Serum	3.40–3.70 (3.50)	1.70–2.70 (2.30)	0.40–0.60 (0.50)	0.10–0.30 (0.20)
			Milk	0.00–0.20 (0.10)	0.00–0.20 (0.10)	0.20–0.40 (0.30)	0.20–0.40 (0.30)
Dicloxacillin	PO	500	Serum	5.00–5.20 (5.10)	4.60–4.80 (4.70)	0.80–1.00 (0.90)	0.20–0.40 (0.30)
			Milk	0.00	0.20–0.30 (0.20)	Trace–0.30 (0.10)	0.00
Ampicillin	PO	500	Serum	4.00–7.00 (5.50)	4.60–4.80 (4.70)	0.80–1.00 (0.90)	0.20–0.40 (0.30)
			Milk	0–Trace	0.00–0.20 (0.10)	0.10–0.20 (0.14)	0.12–0.16 (0.14)
Mezlocillin	IV	1,000	Serum	13.20–16.50 (14.90)	6.60–7.00 (6.80)	0.60–0.90 (0.80)	Trace
			Milk	0.00	0.00	Trace	0.00
Cefoxitin	IV	1,000	Serum	12.60–18.00 (15.40)	4.50–5.20 (4.80)	0.80–1.10 (0.80)	0.00–Trace
			Milk	0.00	Trace	Trace	Trace
Cephalexin	PO	500	Serum	5.10–6.60 (5.80)	3.70–4.10 (3.90)	2.20–3.50 (2.80)	0.40–0.80 (0.60)
			Milk	Trace	0.20–0.40 (0.30)	0.60–0.80 (0.70)	Trace–0.20 (0.10)

Numbers in parentheses are means. Concentrations are expressed in μg per ml.
Modified from Matsuda S. Transfer of antibiotics into maternal milk. Biological Research in Pregnancy 1984; (2) 5:57-60.

penicillins attain even lower levels in milk and lack observable peak concentrations. Ampicillin achieves low concentration after oral dosage, at times insufficient for quantitation.[30]

More data are available for the cephalosporins than for any other category of antimicrobial agent. Largely a product of the last two decades of pharmaceutical research, cephalosporins originated in an era of unprecedented resurgence of interest in breast feeding. Only recently has drug clearance via breast milk been accepted as a pharmacodynamic principle. This comes at a time when the lactating woman is demanding protection for her breast-fed progeny. Such was not the case when penicillin was introduced nearly a half century ago. Additionally, most cephalosporins are still under patent and represent high-profit items for pharmaceutical companies. As a category, their content in breast milk is so small that the risk of toxicity to the suckling infant is negligible. Considering the predictability of limited milk content, it behooves the manufacturer to generate premarketing data that shows absence of apparent risk to the unintended recipient, the breast-fed baby. Recent entries into the cephalosporin market have had milk data available with the initial introduction of the product. It is noteworthy that drugs less safe lack such information.

Beta-Lactam Transfer to the Nursling

The increased albumin content of forming milk is the earliest observable change in acute mastitis.[7] Schalm attributed this to enhanced capillary permeability that leads to leakage of albumin and salt across the lipid membrane.[40] Likewise, increased transfer of sodium bicarbonate[8] causes the pH of milk to rise. Even minor pH changes can significantly alter ionization of the antibiotic therein. Thus, it is not surprising that the content of penicillin in the lacteal secretions increases in mastitic milk.[26a,30,45] Peak concentration of penicillin V has been reported to be 10- to 20-fold higher than the minimum inhibitory concentration of penicillin-sensitive *Staphylococcus aureus*.[16] Additionally, Matheson and coworkers have shown the time to peak concentration of penicillin to be shorter in both the infected and uninfected breast.[26a]

Nevertheless, the amount of ingested penicillin V by the suckling infant is very small. Matheson and associates[26a] calculated from average milk concentrations the relative dose of antibiotic ingested by the baby to be 0.14 percent of the weight-adjusted maternal daily dose. They demonstrated no accumulation of penicillin V in two women who received ongoing therapy for 4 and 10 days, respectively. The maximum dose to the infant would be 0.5 percent of the weight-adjusted maternal daily dose.

Caution must be exercised in interpreting the results of the Matheson study. Oxytocin nasal spray was given to the participants to expedite breast emptying, although controls did not use this agent. Intravenous administration of oxytocin to the parturient has been shown to reduce protein binding of certain drugs.[19] Levels of free salicylate and diazepam have been reported to rise; however, not all drugs appear to be affected. The effect of transnasal oxytocin administration on serum levels of unbound beta-lactam antimicrobials has not been investigated. Additionally, comparative penicillin serum levels in mastitic versus normal lactating women have not been studied. Antipyrine concentration in goats has been reported to rise when mammary blood flow is enhanced. The effect of drug interaction and inflammation is an area of human lactation research that has too long been neglected.

Peiker and Schröder[30] investigated oxacillin and ampicillin pharmacokinetics in 23 women treated for puerperal mastitis by making daily determinations of serum and breast milk concentrations of the antibiotics for 6 days. Thirteen of these women received 1 g ampicillin by mouth four times a day, and the other 10 received 3 g of oxacillin a day. In addition to noting considerable patient-to-patient variability of drug levels in milk, they observed considerably higher levels at steady state than after administration of a single bolus of drug.

Infant Factors

Our concerns regarding potential adverse effects from transmammary delivery of antimicrobial agents to the newborn baby are probably more fancy than fact. Intramuscular and intravenous administration of penicillin infrequently causes loose stools in the recipient and, when it does, the problem is rarely severe. Oral penicillin may alter the stools somewhat more frequently, but even this is not common. Penicillins are frequently used in treating lactating women; however, most infants are likewise unaffected.

Nursing behavior as a factor in limiting drug delivery is of paramount importance to the baby. As previously stated, by feeding her infant when maternal serum concentrations are low, a mother significantly reduces delivery of penicillin. If the mother's breasts are engorged when serum antibiotic levels are high, ingestion of the drug by the baby is minimal. Drug content of milk is determined by the maternal serum levels at the time of infant feeding. Should the infant suckle both breasts at a feeding, drug concentration in one breast may differ considerably from the other. Frequent feeding exposes the nursling to more drug than feeding it at 4-hour intervals. The mother should be encouraged to avoid frequent feeding. Meticulous attention to each of these details lessens the risk of antibiotic exposure to the child.

Absorption from the infant's gastrointestinal tract varies considerably among the various penicillins. Whereas penicillin G is readily absorbed by the newborn baby, uptake of ampicillin from the intestine is poor and highly variable. Peiker and Schröder[30] studied urinary clearance of eight nurslings whose mothers received oral ampicillin and compared the urine concentrations to those of the mother's milk. No ampicillin was recovered from the urine of four of the eight infants tested, whereas four had low but measurable quantities of the antibiotic. Urinary content of oxacillin was measurable and approximated the maternal milk concentrations in eight of nine specimens from babies whose mothers received 1 g oxacillin orally three times a day. Breast milk and infant pharmacokinetic data for the older penicillins such as penicillin G is not available.

In a recent communication, Smith and associates[41] determined the apparent bioavailability of dicloxacillin in 26 children with a wide range of ages by comparing the area under the serum concentration versus time curve following intravenous and oral administration of a standardized dose of drug. Whereas the overall average bioavailability was 59.89 percent, children under 6 months of age had a shorter time to peak concentration (1.39 ± 0.49 hours) and lower bioavailability (64.35 percent ± 13.62 percent) than those who were older. Likewise, variabilty in absorption was least in neonates and increased with age.

Presumably the presence of milk in the gastrointestinal tract somewhat impedes absorption of the penicillins and serves as a protective mechanism from excessive dosage. After absorption from the gut, the newborn organism must contend with immature hepatic and renal systems. Excretion of the penicillins is largely renal, and the liver plays a relatively minor role in drug metabolism.[28] Renal function in the neonate is underdeveloped, and penicillin clearance is slow but predictable. In the first week of extrauterine life of a term baby, the half-life of penicillin G is 3.3 hours. This falls to 1.4 hours by 2 weeks, compared to a half-life of 0.5 hours in older children.[35] The serum half-life of penicillin in babies correlates inversely with age.

Renal excretion of penicillin G in adults is principally tubular, with only 10 percent *dependent* upon glomerular function. However, in term neonates renal clearance correlates closely with creatinine clearance.[28] Presumably this is due to greater tubular immaturity as compared to glomerular function at birth. Despite this glomerular-tubular imbalance, the term neonate can clear 30 percent of an intramuscular dose of penicillin G in 8 to 12 hours. Values for orally administered penicillin G are unavailable.

Conclusions

Beta-lactams have a wide therapeutic index and a low risk of toxicity to the breast-fed baby via transmammary exposure to drug. Although adverse effects occur, they are relatively rare and usually not life-threatening. A common complication of antibiotic therapy in the neonatal period is oropharyngeal candidiasis. Twenty percent of nongravid women have vaginal carriage of yeast, and this number increases in pregnancy. A baby delivered to such a mother may likewise have yeast colonization, and florid infection may follow antibiotic treatment. Although exposure to antibiotics via breast milk is of a different magnitude, nevertheless the risk of clinical candidiasis exists.

As previously stated, the amount of antibiotic ingested by a neontate via transmammary passage is quite small. However, in theory this quantity may be sufficient to sensitize the baby to the antibiotic agent. Allergic reactions in newborns are extremely rare, but one such anecdote of a Herxheimer reaction in a case of congenital syphilis, albeit poorly documented, has been reported.[39] Development of hypersensitivity through such an exposure is probably more theory than fact.

A major advantage of breast-feeding one's progeny is the lower incidence of infectious diarrhea of the nursling. Breast-fed babies have an intestinal microflora consisting largely of *Bifidobacterium bifidum,* in contrast to predominately gram-positive anaerobes including enteropathogens in the gut of artificially fed infants. Despite the protection afforded a child by low concentrations of antibiotic in breast milk, these small amounts of antimicrobial agents can alter the intestinal microflora. Consideration of such an effect on the gastrointestinal ecosystem must always be given the nursing infant when antimicrobial therapy is contemplated.

Puerperal mastitis is and will continue to be a benign process, provided all of the rules are assiduously followed. Early diagnosis and prompt institution of effective pharmacotherapy are of cardinal importance. There exists a 24-hour window from the onset of symptoms to the start of treatment in which the woman must see her physician. To accomplish this, an effective education process must be in effect. Patient education begins in the third trimester of gestation and continues throughout lactation. New mothers must be taught to appreciate the importance of proper breast-feeding technique in order to avoid the pitfalls of nipple trauma and missed feedings. They must be educated in regard to signs and symptoms of mastitis and the consequence of failure to communicate with their health care practitioner. Additionally, both patients and the health care team must fully appreciate the need for continued lactation in a woman who complains of breast pain. However, such patient education is for naught unless the office staff is cognizant that prompt examination is a prerequisite to abscess prevention. All too frequently a young mother is told by the telephone receptionist that no appointment is available, and delay originates at the physician's office.

Delays have dangerous ends.

William Shakespeare

King Henry VI, Part I
act III, scene ii

References

1. Adler DD. Ultrasound of benign breast conditions. Semin Ultrasound CT MR 1989; 10:106–118.
2. Barnett A, Lavey E, Pearl RM, Vistnes LM. Toxic shock syndrome from an infected breast prosthesis. Ann Plast Surg 1983; 10:408–410.
3. Beeley L. Drugs and breast feeding. Clin Obstet Gynecol 1981; 8:291–295.
4. Benson EA. Management of breast abscesses. World J Surg 1989; 13:753–756.
5. Burt RL. Plasma nonesterified fatty acids in normal pregnancy and puerperium. Obstet Gynecol 1960; 15:460–464.
6. Caldwell JR, Cluff LE. Adverse reactions to antimicrobial agents. JAMA 1974; 230:77–80.
7. Carroll EJ, Jain NC. Bacterial activity of normal milk, mastitic milk, and colostrum against *Aerobacter aerogenes.* Am J Vet Res 1969; 30:1123–1132.
8. Carroll EJ, Schalm OW, Lasmanis J. Experimental coliform *(Aerobacter aerogenes)* mastitis: distribution of whey protein during the early acute phase. J Dairy Sci 1963; 46:1–7.
9. Catz CS, Giacoia GP. Drugs and breast milk. Pediatr Clin North Am 1972; 19:151–166.
10. Chesney PJ, Davis JP, Purdy WK, et al. Clinical

manifestations of toxic shock syndrome. JAMA 1981; 246:741–748.
11. Dean M, Stock B, Patterson RJ, Levy G. Serum protein binding of drugs during and after pregnancy in humans. Clin Pharmacol Ther 1980; 28:253–261.
12. Demey HE, Hautekeete ML, Bossaert LL. Case report: mastitis and toxic shock syndrome. Acta Obstet Gynecol Scand 1989; 68:87–88.
13. deSaxe MJ, Hawtin P, Wieneke AA. Toxic shock syndrome in Britain: epidemiology and microbiology. Postgrad Med J 1985; 61 (Suppl 1):5–21.
14. Devereux WP. Acute puerperal mastitis. Am J Obstet Gynecol 1970; 108:78–81.
15. Eschenbach DA. Acute postpartum infections: symposium on emergency management of infectious diseases, Emerg Med Clin North Am 1985; 3:87–115.
16. Garrod LP, Lambert HP, O'Grady F. Penicillins I. In Antibiotics and chemotherapy, Ed 5. Garrod LP, Lambert HP, O'Grady F (Eds). Edinburgh:Churchill Livingston, 1981.
17. Gibberd GF. Sporadic and epidemic puerperal breast infections. Am J Obstet Gynecol 1953; 65:1038–1041.
18. Hall B. Changing composition of human milk and early development of appetite control. Lancet 1975; 1:779–781.
19. Hamar C, Levy G. Factors Affecting the serum protein binding of salicylic acid in newborn infants and their mothers. Pediatr Pharmacol 1980; 1:31–43.
20. Hamar C, Levy G. Serum protein binding of drugs and bilirubin in newborn infants and their mothers. Clin Pharmacol Ther 1980; 28:58–63.
21. Holmberg O. Coagulase–negative staphylococci in bovine mastitis. In Màrdh PA, Schleifer KH (Eds). Coagulase negative staphylocci. Stockholm: Almquist & Wiksell Int, 1971.
22. Kafetzis DA, Brater DC, Fanourgakis JE, et al. Ceftriaxone distribution between maternal blood and fetal blood and tissues at parturition and between blood and milk postpartum. Antimicrob Agents Chemother 1983; 23:870–873.
23. Kalstone C. Methicillin-resistant staphyloccal mastitis. Am J Obstet Gynecol 1989; 161:120.
24. Linzell JL. Mammary blood flow and methods of identifying and measuring precursors of milk. In Larson BL, Smith VR (Eds). Lactation. Vol 1. New York: Academic Press, 1974.
25. Marshall BR, Hepper JK, Zirbel CC. Sporadic puerperal mastitis. JAMA 1975; 233:1377–1379.
26. Matheson I, Aursnes I, Horgen M, et al. Bacteriological findings and clinical symptoms in relation to clinical outcome in puerperal mastitis. Acta Obstet Gynecol Scand 1988; 67:723–726.
26a. Matheson I, Samseth M, Loberg R, et al. Milk transfer of phenoxymethylpenicillin during puerperal mastitis. Br J Clin Pharmacol 1988; 25:33-40.
27. Matsuda S. Transfer of antibiotics into maternal milk. Biological Research in Pregnancy 1984; 5:57–60.
28. McCracken GH Jr, Ginsberg C, Chrane DF, et al. Clinical pharmacology of penicillin in newborn infants. J Pediatr 1973; 82:692–698.
29. Mendenhall N. Serum protein concentrations in pregnancy: concentrations in maternal serum. Am J Obstet Gynecol 1970; 106:388–399.
30. Peiker G, Schröder S. Unterschungen zur Konzentration von Oxacillin und Ampicillin in Serum and Muttermilch bei der Mastitis puerperalis. Pharmazie 1986; 41:793–795.
31. Perucca E, Ruprah M, Richens A. Altered drug binding to serum protein in pregnant women: therapeutic relevance. J R Soc Med 1981; 74:422–426.
32. Rasmussen F. Mammary excretion of benzylpenicillin, erythromycin, and penethamate hydroiodide. Acta Pharmacol Toxicol 1959; 16:194–200.
33. Rasmussen F. Studies on mammary excretion and absorption of drugs. Copenhagen: Mortensen, 1966.
34. Rasmussen F. Excretion of drugs by milk. In Brodie BB and Gillette JR (Eds). Concepts in biochemical pharmacology. Berlin, Heidelberg, New York: Springer Verlag, 1971.
35. Rasmussen F. The mechanisms of drug excretion into milk. In Galli C, Jacini G, Pecile A (Eds). Dietary lipids and postnatal development. New York: Raven Press, 1973.
36. Reboud P, Groulade J, Groslambert P, Colombo M. The influence of normal pregnancy and the postpartum state on plasma proteins and lipids. Am J Obstet Gynecol 1963; 86:820–828.
37. Reingold AL, Hagrett NT, Dan BB, et al. Nonmenstrual toxic shock syndrome: a review of 130 cases. Ann Intern Med 1982; 96(Part 2):871–874.
38. Rench MA, Baker CJ. Group B streptococcal breast abscess in a mother and mastitis in her infant. Obstet Gynecol 1989; 73:875–877.
39. Rollier MR, Rollier M, Bellouchi M. Reaction d'Herxheimer au lait maternel dans une syphilis congenitale precoce. Bull Soc Franc Dermatol Syph 1967; 74:178–181.
40. Schalm OW. Pathologic changes in milk and udder of cows with mastitis. J Am Vet Med Assoc 1977; 170:1137–1140.
41. Smith AL, Meeks CA, Koup JR, et al. Dicloxacillin absorption and elimination in children. Dev Pharmacol Ther 1990; 14:35–44.
42. Stock B, Dean M, Levy G. Serum protein binding of drugs during and after pregnancy in rats. J Pharmacol Exp Ther 1980; 212:264–268.
43. Sweet RL, Ledger WJ. Puerperal infectious morbidity: a two year review. Am J Obstet Gynecol 1973; 117:1093–1100.
44. Wilson JT, Brown RD, Cherek DR, et al. Drug excretion in human milk: principles, pharmacokinetics and projected consequences. Clin Pharmacokinet 1980; 5:1–65.
45. Ziv G. Practical pharmacokinetic aspects of mastitis therapy: 1. parenteral treatment. Vet Med 1980; 75:277–290.

CHAPTER 9

Septic Shock

Richard H. Schwarz, M.D.

Sepsis is the third leading cause of shock, exceeded only by hemorrhagic and cardiogenic shock. The association between shock and infection was recognized before 1900,[12] but the attention of obstetricians and gynecologists was first focused on the subject by a classic paper by Studdiford and Douglas in 1956.[39] In their report they described a series of deaths in patients with septic abortion and shock that was unresponsive to vasopressor therapy. The deaths resulted from renal failure with fluid overload and pulmonary edema. This was at a time when illegal abortions were very common (estimated to be more than 1 million annually), as were hospitalizations for septic abortion and abortion deaths (more than 1,000 annually). Since then, there have been enormous advances in the understanding of the pathophysiology and management of septic shock. Many of the developments in treatment, particularly of shock lung, grew out of military medical experience in Korea and Vietnam, where this problem was very common.

The spectrum of obstetric and gynecologic pathology associated with septic shock has also changed. There has been a marked decrease in the incidence of septic abortion in the United States since the Supreme Court decision in 1973[37]; however, the problem persists in many parts of the world with restrictive abortion policies. Infection, although not common, is the most frequent complication of medical abortion. A unique syndrome of midtrimester septic abortion in pregnancies with intrauterine devices in place was described by Christian in 1974.[15] In these cases, the abortion was caused by the infection rather than the result of it, and the clinical course was often insidious, with shock or even shock lung as the initial manifestation; the source of infection was not obvious. Other causes of septic shock in the pregnant or recently pregnant woman include chorioamnionitis, pyelonephritis, and postpartum endometritis. Recent reports implicate chorionic villus sampling[2] and genetic amniocentesis[31] as precipitating events. In the gynecologic patient, pelvic inflammatory disease, postoperative pelvic infections, pelvic abscess, and pelvic infection associated with gynecologic malignancy are all potential causes.

Epidemiology

Septic shock is a relatively rare, albeit lethal, occurrence. There are in excess of 300,000 gram-negative bacteremias reported each year, and it is estimated that septic shock complicates about one-fourth of these cases.[25] Bacteremia and therefore septic shock are relatively uncommon on obstetric and gynecologic services. Bryan and coworkers[11] reported a rate of 2.0 episodes per 1,000 admissions on obstetric and gynecologic services as opposed to 11.5 per 1,000 admissions on all other hospital services in a 5-year survey. They also report a low mortality rate in those patients whose bacteremias were related to pregnancy (1 in 63). Ledger and colleagues,[27] Blanco and associates,[8] and Weinstein and coworkers[41] have reported similar low mortality rates.

Septic shock is relatively rare in individuals under age 40 except pregnant women, newborns, and immunocompromised people. Contributing to the latter group are chronic illnesses such as diabetes, malignant disease, chemotherapy, parenteral hyperalimentation, prolonged hospitalization, and, more recently, acquired immunodeficiency syndrome. The explanation for the low incidence in pregnant women likely rests on the generally healthy nature of this population. Other contributing factors to the lower incidence and lower mortality in the obstetric patient are the transient nature of the bacteremia; the type of organisms involved; the pelvic site of the infections, which makes them more amenable to surgical extirpation; and the absence of underlying disease.[22] Fried and Vosti[19] reported a significantly higher mortality when there was significant underlying pathology. Maternal mortality has become very rare, but when it does occur infection is among the leading causes.[20] By contrast, in gynecologic practice, the patients may have both a higher incidence and a poorer prognosis, particularly in older patients and those with malignancies.

Definitions

In approaching the subject of septic shock, it is well to establish definitions for several frequently used terms.

Bacteremia. Bacteremia is the situation in which bacteria can be isolated from blood. Bacteremic patients may or may not be seriously ill. Some have suggested that the definition should be based upon a minimum number of organisms per cubic millimeter or upon more than one positive culture. These requirements may fail to apply under certain circumstances, especially if the bacteremia is transient.

Septicemia. This is a less precise term that is generally used to imply that the patient is clinically ill as well as bacteremic.

Endotoxemia. This term is an exacting one that indicates the presence of endotoxin in the blood. It is limited in its application because of the relative impracticability of the endotoxin assay. It has been suggested that endotoxemia may be an early predictor of septicemia.[40] It should also be noted that not all patients with endotoxemia have positive blood cultures.

Shock. This term has been variously defined. At a gross level, the problem is a "low flow state" with reduced visceral perfusion and gradual multiorgan failure. Other definitions concentrate on the microcirculation and its derangements or the metabolic problems that occur with anaerobic glycolysis, organic acid accumulation, and metabolic acidosis. At the other extreme, one can focus on cellular events that are the same, regardless of the etiology of the shock. Cellular hypoxia and the lack of metabolic substrates are the basic problem. A decrease in the ATP production impairs protein synthesis, which in turn compromises the integrity of the cell membrane and ultimately leads to cell dysfunction and organ failure.

Etiology

Shock can accompany infection (septicemia) caused by a wide variety of microorganisms, including both gram-negative and gram-positive exotoxin-producing bacteria, and it has been reported, albeit rarely, with viral, fungal, and rickettsial infections as well. Far and away the most common clinically as well as the best studied are the gram-negative facultative endotoxin-producing bacteria. Among these enteric organisms, the most frequently implicated is *Escherichia coli*, followed by *Klebsiella*, *Proteus*, and *Pseudomonas*.[3] All of these organisms are part of the normal genital flora. *Bacteroides* species and other gram-negative anaerobes are also endotoxin producers that can produce septic shock.

Pathophysiology

A good deal has been learned about the physiologic derangements in septic shock, but there is still much to be clarified. For obvious reasons, most of the definitive studies have been done in animals; therefore, the results must be interpreted in light of species differences in response to endotoxin. Confusion in clinical studies often exists because of failure to differentiate gram-negative and gram-positive septic shock. The derangements also vary from patient to patient and even from time to time in the same patient. When all of this is coupled with the lack of a clinically practical endotoxin assay and the constraints of clinical research in desperately ill patients, it is understandable that there is much about septic shock and its pathophysiology yet to be understood. The following summarizes current thinking about the complex events that occur in response to endotoxin.

Endotoxin is a lipopolysaccharide complex that is protein bound in the cell wall of gram-negative bacteria and released upon the disintegration of the organisms. Endotoxin has no qualitative differences among the various gram-negative species. The lipid-A moiety of endotoxin appears to be the active fraction that induces the succession of pathophysiologic changes in laboratory animals. The association between endotoxin and gram-negative septic shock was first described in 1951 by Borden and Hall.[10] The first line of defense against endotoxin is the reticuloendothelial (RE) system. In experimental animals, inactivation of the RE system causes a normally tolerated dose of endotoxin to become lethal. Although there is no conclusive evidence in humans, several investigators[5,6,29] have found that in a number of species the fixed-dose response to endotoxin was more severe, with more profound metabolic acidosis and earlier cardiovascular collapse, in the pregnant animal than in others. The reasons for this difference are unclear. At the same time, the fetus and newborn are more resistant to endotoxin.

The release of endotoxin initiates a cascade of events brought about in part by the direct action of endotoxin and its active lipid moiety, as well as by the release of a variety of potent, physiologically active intermediary substances. The following describes some of the substances and specific actions; however, the clinical course of events is the net result of these actions.

Endotoxin. This substance can act directly on the hypothalamic thermoregulatory center to produce fever[7] or initiate the release of pyrogens from leukocytes and reticuloendothelial cells.

Complement system. When activated, this system can lead to granulocyte aggregation in the lung as well as the release of a variety of potent vasoactive substances, including histamine, serotoxin, bradykinin, and prostaglandins.

Factor XII. Activation of Factor XII leads to disseminated intravascular clotting. Factor XII triggers kallikrein production. This substance intensifies plasmin production and activates factors VII and XII and bradykinins, which cause vasodilation, pain, and swelling.

The *adrenal glands and the sympathetic nervous system*. Both are stimulated, with a resultant outpouring of catecholamines.

Heart. The mechanism of cardiac dysfunction in septic shock has been the subject of considerable study. For

Table 9-1 Clinical Phases of Septic Shock

	Hypotension	Temperature	Urine Output	Mental Status	Skin	Metabolic State
Warm hypotensive	Modest	Early hypothermia, then fever chills	Normal	Mild lethargy, confusion	Warm, dry	Respiratory alkalosis, hyperglycemia
Cold hypotensive	Increasing	Fever, later hypothermia	Reduced	Increased confusion, loss of consciousness	Cold, clammy	Metabolic acidosis
Irreversible	Severe	Hypothermia	Renal failure	Coma	Profound constriction	Severe acidosis, hypoxemia, hypoglycemia

some time a circulating myocardial depressant substance (MDS) has been postulated that is responsible for the changes, with a characteristic decreased left ventricular ejection fraction. Coronary circulation is normal or increased in these patients, and thus ischemia does not appear to be the cause of the cardiac changes.[17] The role of MDS seems now confirmed by the work of Parker and Parrillo.[34,34a] and associates. The changes are reversible with survival.

Endorphins. Animal studies have shown an increase in beta-endorphin levels in response to endotoxin. Some have postulated that endorphins may play a role in myocardial depression and consequently consider that a narcotic antagonist might be therapeutically helpful, although this has yet to be confirmed.

Cytokines. Recently experimental attention has been focused on the role of these compounds in mediating the effects of endotoxin. Specifically, *tumor necrosis factor* or cachectin, a protein produced in large quantities by endotoxin-activated macrophages, appears to be capable of inducing most if not all of the physiologic changes brought about by endotoxin.[28]

Prostaglandins. Although the prostaglandins are released in increased quantities in septic shock, their precise role is unclear. Thromboxane A is synthesized by platelets and is a vasoconstrictor and promoter of platelet aggregation. Prostacyclin is released from the vascular endothelium and is a vasodilator that prevents platelet aggregation. Obviously, the balance between the two is critical, and it is likely that these agents may play a role in the response to endotoxin because both platelets and the vascular endothelium are involved.

Kidneys. This is another primary target of endotoxin,[13] with the result that there is decreased renal blood flow and oliguria. Acute tubular necrosis appears to be more common following septic shock than with shock caused by postpartum hemorrhage. In animal studies,[35] damage to the peritubular capillaries seems to be central to the development of acute tubular necrosis.

Lungs. This is an area of critical change. As a result of diminished pulmonary blood flow, endothelial damage occurs, with extravasation into the interstitium, together with microthrombi as well as platelet and leukocyte aggregation and the destruction of type II cells, which produce surfactant. Consequently, there is markedly reduced compliance, atelectasis, and adult respiratory distress syndrome or shock lung, which has now become the leading cause of death in patients with septic shock.

All of these changes and undoubtedly many others yet to be defined contribute to the complex and rapidly evolving picture of septic shock (Table 9-1). Three clinical phases of septic shock have been described: warm hypotensive, cold hypotensive, and irreversible. One of the early manifestations may be a change in the mental status of the patient, such as lethargy, confusion, or disorientation. This is probably the result of decreased cerebral blood flow, and it increases as generalized hypoxia and metabolic acidosis develop. Early, the patient may be hypothermic as the result of the direct action of endotoxin on the hypothalamic thermoregulatory centers. Fever ensues subsequently and is most often present in the early "warm" phase. The patient's skin is warm and flushed from vasodilation, and there may be chills. Hypotension is modest, and urinary output is generally maintained. There is early leukopenia, followed by leukocytosis, and the manifestations of disseminated intravascular coagulation (DIC) may be apparent only in laboratory results and not clinically, with thrombocytopenia. Microangiopathic hemolytic anemia can occur because of the disrupted intravascular flow patterns produced by the fibrin thrombi and platelet aggregrates in the microcirculation.

The early metabolic manifestation is respiratory alkalosis, which is followed by a progressive metabolic acidosis as hypoxemia results in anaerobic glycolysis. The early outpouring of catecholamines causes breakdown of liver glycogen with hyperglycemia, but as stores are exhausted hypoglycemia occurs.

As the patient moves into the cold hypotensive phase, massive vasoconstriction leads to cold, clammy skin, and once again fever may be replaced by hypothermia. There will generally be a further decrease in blood pressure, with tachycardia and oliguria. This is the point in the clinical course where the diagnosis is often first made. If there is not aggressive intervention during this phase, the process inexorably moves to an irreversible stage. Irreversibility is the result of the progressive and prolonged cellular hypoxia, which causes irreparable cell damage, multiorgan failure, and death. Manifestations include severe metabolic acidosis with lactate accumulation, DIC, anuria, cardiac failure, and coma. Even though therapy appears to be successful in correcting the hemodynamic abnormalities, often patients are lost subsequently to shock lung, which can be extremely frustrating to treat.

Diagnosis and Evaluation

Although the manifestations of shock, such as hypotension and tachycardia, may be relatively easily recognized, the etiology of the shock may be less apparent. Often, there is a significant degree of hypovolemia accompanying the infectious process. For example, in the case of septic abortion, there may be blood loss; with peritonitis or ileus, there can be large fluid losses into the extravascular spaces. In the initial evaluation process, it is essential that the clinician not only establish the etiology of the shock but also define the precise nature of the physiologic disruption, that is, is there predominant vasoconstriction or vasodilation, is DIC present, or is there evidence of shock lung?

In most instances it is possible to glean much information from the patient's history, but this can be difficult in the severely ill patient whose level of consciousness may be reduced or, as is common in patients who have undergone illegal abortions, there is great reluctance on the part of the patient to divulge details. The timing and exact nature of an abortion attempt, along with an estimate of the blood loss and the sequence of symptoms, can be very helpful. A history of underlying serious illness, such as diabetes, hypertension, or renal disease, may not only help to clarify the diagnosis but also bring about modifications in treatment. In other cases, the etiology of the septic shock may be more obvious from the history, for example, in the case of pyelonephritis or chorioamnionitis.

The physical examination provides considerable information concerning the nature of the physiologic disturbance and thereby gives some evidence as to where in the clinical progression the patient stands.

Blood pressure and pulse pressure. Most patients with septic shock are hypotensive, although the blood pressure must always be assessed in relation to the patient's normal pressure and to the vascular tone. Blood pressure in the normal range may represent hypotension to the chronically hypertensive patient and can be accompanied by reduced perfusion. By way of contrast, there may be good perfusion in moderate hypotensive patients with extensive vasodilation and poor perfusion when patients are normotensive but markedly vasoconstricted. The pulse pressure is a rough guide to cardiac output, a reduced pulse pressure indicating reduced output.

Pulse. Tachycardia is generally the finding in septic shock, but the rate may be critical in management. Beta-agonists such as isoproterenol, which have a positive chronotropic effect on the myocardium, are contraindicated if the pulse rate exceeds 120 because of the risk of potentially lethal tachyarrhythmias.

Skin temperature. This can give a sense of the status of the peripheral circulation. Warm, dry, flushed skin indicates peripheral dilation and is most often found early in the process. Cold, clammy skin indicates peripheral constriction and most often a more advanced stage of septic shock. In the extreme, vasoconstriction can be so profound that tissue viability is compromised in vulnerable areas, such as the tip of the nose and the ear lobe.

Heart and lungs. This examination should be directed toward determining whether there is evidence of complications, such as congestive heart failure or pulmonary embolism. In the case of shock lung, although there may be tachypnea, the physical findings are minimal despite severe dysfunction.

Abdomen. The findings, of course, vary with the basic diagnosis but can be helpful in defining the extent of the process and thereby defining what is required therapeutically to control it. In the case of a patient with a septic abortion, signs of diffuse peritonitis suggest uterine perforation or a spreading inflammatory process that will probably require an aggressive and extensive surgical approach. This would be equally the case if the problem is pelvic inflammatory disease (PID), in which instance these diffuse signs would likely signal a ruptured abscess. In the case of chorioamnionitis, the pregnant uterus is obvious, but generally additional findings are modest at best and may include a degree of uterine tenderness and irritability.

Pelvic Examination

This, too, varies with the underlying pathology, but like the abdominal examination it can help to focus the management plan. In the case of a patient with a septic abortion, uterine size determines the propriety of evacuation by curettage, and the presence of adnexal masses suggests also that curettage will not suffice to control the source of endotoxin. There are similar implications in the management of the patient with septic shock and PID, in whom the presence of abscess means that an abdominal approach is likely required.

Laboratory Examination

A complete blood count including a platelet count is in order (Table 9-2). The hemoglobin and hematocrit may be reduced by concomitant blood loss, and the white blood cell count is usually elevated as the result of sepsis, although occasionally there may be an initial leukopenia. Thrombocytopenia may be the earliest indication of the development of disseminated intravascular clotting.

Urine analysis is critical if the underlying cause is pyelonephritis. Hemolysis may also be detected by urine examination. Perhaps the most critical evaluation, however, is the monitoring of urinary output.

A coagulation profile should be performed, even if there is no evidence of clinical DIC, to serve as a baseline; it should include, in addition to the platelet count, *prothrombin time (PT) and partial thromboplastin time (PTT)*, fibrinogen, fibrin split products, and thrombin time.

Arterial blood gases demonstrate an early respiratory alkalosis followed by a progressive metabolic alkalosis. An arterial line placed for blood pressure monitoring can provide ready access to serial measurements, and these values can serve as an excellent guide to the effectiveness of treatment. Serum lactate levels should be measured; some investigators indicate that these levels may be prognostic indicators.[14,32]

Table 9-2 Laboratory Findings in Pelvic Inflammatory Disease

Test	Finding
Hemoglobin/hematocrit	Often reduced due to blood loss
Leukocyte count	Early leukopenia followed by elevation
Platelet count	Thrombocytopenia an early sign of DIC
Urine analysis	Rule out pyelonephritis and hemolysis
Coagulation profile	Initial baseline then to detect DIC
Arterial blood gases and electrolytes	Early respiratory alkalosis followed by metabolic acidosis; excellent guide to adequacy of treatment
Serum lactate, blood urea nitrogen, and creatinine	Prognostic indicator for renal failure or prerenal causes
Microbiologic studies	Gram-stained smears and cultures; may only help retrospectively
Endotoxin assays	Not clinically useful
Imaging studies	Status of heart, lung, and bowel; foreign bodies
Electrocardiogram	Continuous monitoring

Blood urea nitrogen (BUN) and creatinine levels are generally elevated secondary to either prerenal or renal causes.

Microbiologic studies should be performed; however, often they are of only retrospective assistance because antibiotic therapy must be instituted empirically. Blood cultures are most likely to identify the specific offending organism(s), but cultures should also be obtained from the urine, operative site, endometrium, and peritoneal cavity, as applicable. Cultures from the vagina or cervix are less helpful unless they identify exogenous organisms (those not part of the normal genital flora). Gram-stained smears may be helpful as part of the initial evaluation.

Endotoxin assays would be of value if a practical, clinically usable, and reliable assay were available. However, this is not the case at this time.

Radiographic or other imaging studies provide useful information with regard to the status of the heart, lungs, and bowel and may detect foreign bodies, in the case of septic abortion, or gas, in the case of infections caused by gas-forming organisms.

The electrocardiogram is most often monitored continuously in patients in intensive care settings, but it can also be useful diagnostically in cases of pulmonary embolism or hyperkalemia related to renal failure. Tachycardia is almost always present, and these patients are particularly susceptible to serious tachyarrhythmias because of the presence of acidosis.

Blood volume can be measured by isotope dilution techniques, but this is generally not helpful because the circulating volume reflects a number of parameters including vascular tone and because deficits are generally calculated based on standards of height and weight or on surface area tables. Such calculations are likely to be erroneous in the face of massive vasoconstriction and, consequently, fluid replacement is best guided by a more dynamic measurement, such as pulmonary wedge or central venous pressure.

Treatment

The goals of treatment in a patient with septic shock can be summarized as follows:

1. To control and eliminate the infection that is the source of the endotoxin. This can be termed *primary therapy*, and without it all of the support measures cannot succeed.
2. To establish and maintain homeostasis until all of the endotoxin that has been released is cleared. This is supportive therapy, which takes many forms.
3. To be alert to and to treat early and aggressively the late complications of septic shock, such as renal failure and shock lung.

Primary Therapy

One of the factors that permits a somewhat lower mortality rate in obstetric and gynecologic patients with septic shock is that the focus of the infection and consequently the source of endotoxin are more amenable to surgical extirpation. This is true for most instances of septic shock in this discipline with the most noticeable exception of pyelonephritis. When surgery can be applied, antibiotic therapy becomes secondary.

Surgery

In the case of a patient with a septic abortion, the first goal—elimination of the source of endotoxin—can be accomplished usually by simple curettage, most often now using the suction technique. If an abscess is present, if there has been a uterine perforation, or occasionally if there is not much tissue obtained at curettage, all of which mean that the process has spread beyond the endometrial cavity, more extensive surgery, laparotomy, and hysterectomy may be required.

One important lesson learned early on in the management of patients with the combination of septic abortion and septic shock is that surgical management cannot be deferred to await complete stabilization. Deeming a patient too sick to have surgery often proves to be a lethal decision.

In the case of patients with chorioamnionitis, delivery is the key and, in fact, the therapeutic equivalent of draining an abscess. It is best accomplished by the vaginal route if it can be done expeditiously. If not, cesarean section is in order, as it also is if there is evidence of fetal distress. A low cervical technique should be used, if possible. If there is any question of myometrial involvement, hysterectomy should be considered, and some suggest this might be a wise choice in any case in older, high-parity women, given the gravity of the situation.

Patients with pelvic or tubo-ovarian abscess require either extirpation or, in selected cases, drainage. Rarely, in a patient with septic pelvic thrombophlebitis who fails to respond to the combination of heparin and antibiotics, venous ligation (vena cava and ovarian vein) may be required.

Antibiotics

Antimicrobial strategies must be empiric because the patients are desperately ill and the causative organisms are unidentified. Because the most common organisms involved are gram-negative facultatives of the Enterobacteriaceae group and because of the possibility of resistance, an aminoglycoside such as gentamicin or tobramycin is appropriate. Dosing may need to be modified because of impaired renal function; this is best accomplished by measuring serum levels. Gram-negative anaerobes such as *Bacteroides* species are endotoxin producers and therefore must be included in the antibiotic strategy. Clindamycin or metronidazole are the most appropriate choices. Most practitioners would add a third antibiotic, usually penicillin or ampicillin, to achieve more complete coverage. Although this addition fills in coverage for gram-positive aerobes, however, penicillins do not augment the activity against endotoxin producers. Some of the newer generations of cephalosporins approach the coverage of the combinations,[1] but most clinicians turn to the combinations with which they have greater experience. Occasionally the administration of a bolus of a bactericidal antibiotic, such as an aminoglycoside, to a bacteremic patient can precipitate septic shock by the sudden release of endotoxin. Although antibiotic strategies and broad coverage are important, for most instances of septic shock in obstetric and gynecologic patients, the surgical approach to the source of endotoxin is more critical. Pyelonephritis is an exception because there is no surgical approach to the problem.

Supportive Treatment

The purpose of supportive treatment is to maintain homeostasis until the endotoxin can be cleared. To determine the appropriate supportive approach, it is necessary to utilize the laboratory and physiologic measurements previously outlined.

Volume Replacement

Patients with septic shock commonly have hypovolemia because they may have lost blood and lost volume into the bowel or the peritoneal cavity. In the early stages of septic shock (warm phase) when vasodilation predominates, volume replacement alone may suffice to stabilize the patient. Volume must be appropriately replaced with blood, colloid or balanced electrolyte solutions, and the guide to the volume replaced should be the central venous pressure (CVP) or, better still, the pulmonary wedge pressure (PWP). The use of CVP monitoring may suffice in a young, otherwise healthy individual but because it requires extrapolation of right heart pressures to the left it is particularly subject to error in patients with pre-existing chronic pulmonary disease, valvular heart disease, or impaired myocardial function. However, utilization of the Swan-Ganz catheter to measure PWP requires greater sophistication than CVP measurement and is not without complications. If there is a question as to whether the patient can tolerate volume replacement, a volume stress test with the rapid administration of 100 to 200 ml of a balanced salt solution while the PWP or CVP is monitored will provide the answer.

Correction of Acidosis

Clearly, the optimal way to correct the metabolic acidosis is to correct the basic cause, hypoperfusion and hypoxia. However, this may take time and meanwhile the acidosis, if severe, can lead to serious tachyarrhythmias as well as to the inactivation of beta-adrenergic agents. Consequently, at least partial correction by the administration of sodium bicarbonate is indicated.

Corticosteroids

This continues to be one of the most controversial areas in the management of septic shock. Enthusiasts have suggested the use of large "pharmacologic" doses of corticosteroids, initially with little or no supporting data from human studies. The dose suggested is 30 mg per kilogram of methyl prednisolone as a single intravenous bolus. Repeat doses or tapering off is not suggested. Proponents suggest that mechanisms of action may include stabilization of liposomal membranes,[21] preservation of capillary integrity in the face of anoxia, reduction of peripheral resistance, reduction of oxygen affinity by increasing 2.3 diphosphoglycerate (2.3 DPG), improvement of cellular metabolism, and a positive inotropic effect on the myocardium.[30] Prospective as well as retrospective studies by Shumer[38] support steroid use and indicate improved outcome. Other studies, including a collaborative study from Veteran's Administration hospitals,[23] suggest no benefit to patients with sepsis who have a more normal sensorium at the time of treatment. A second placebo-controlled collaborative study involving 382 patients indicates that the early use of large doses of steroids provided no benefit in preventing or treating shock or in reducing overall mortality.[9] It must be noted that none of these studies focused on young obstetric patients.

Vasoactive Agents

These agents are best designated by the sympathetic nervous system actions that they either evoke or block. Alpha-receptors do not exist in the heart; consequently, alpha-mimetic agents produce peripheral vasoconstriction, and alpha-lytics or alpha-blockers cause peripheral vasodilation. Beta-agonists exert their primary effect on the myocardium, increasing the force of contractions (myotropic) effect of the use of these agents is guided by the physiologic alteration in a given patient.[24,33]

Digitalis

Digitalis is administered to stimulate the myocardium, which is working at less than optimal efficiency because of the direct effect of endotoxin on the circulating myocardial depressant substance (MDS). Specific indications include tachycardia with elevated CVP (greater than 15cm H_2O) or PWP (greater than 16 mm Hg). Caution must be exercised in view of the possibilities of hyperkalemia and renal function impairment. Digitalis may be less effective in the presence of endotoxin.

Heparin

It has been suggested that heparin be administered prophylactically to patients with septic shock because most will have at least laboratory evidence of disseminated intravascular clotting. However, no data show this approach to be clearly beneficial,[16] and consequently it would seem prudent to limit the use of heparin to those patients with clinically evident DIC.

Vasoactive Drugs

Although supportive treatment should be tailored to the individual patient, some guidelines can be suggested. The patient in the early "warm" phase (with hypotension; warm, dry skin; and perhaps reduced urinary output) can most often be stabilized by simple volume replacement as determined by CVP or PWP. Steroids and vasoactive agents are applied if volume replacement fails. In the patient with vasodilation, the agent of choice should produce vasoconstriction. It would be advantageous if the agent also stimulated the myocardium, and therefore an alpha-beta-mimetic agent such as metaraminol or ephedrine would be a good choice.

In the hypotensive patient who has reduced urinary output (indicating reduced central perfusion) and also has peripheral constriction with cold, clammy skin, fluid therapy alone will not suffice and indeed may not be tolerated because most such patients have an elevated CVP or PWP. Vasoactive drugs for such patients should not produce peripheral constriction, which is already maximal, but rather stimulate the myocardium (beta-agonists) and/or cause peripheral vasodilation (alpha-blockers). Digitalis may also be helpful. Agents of choice for this group of patients are isoproterenol, dopamine, and chlorpromazine.

Isoproterenol is a beta-agonist that has both inotropic and chronotropic actions on the myocardium. Because of the latter, it is contraindicated if there is significant tachycardia to begin with. Because the drug also inhibits peripheral constriction, its use must be accompanied by enough volume replacement to maintain adequate perfusion.

Dopamine has both alpha- and beta-adrenergic actions, but its most important effects are improving renal blood flow.[36] The dose is 2 to 5 mg per kilogram per minute, and an effort should be made to maintain the blood pressure at 20 to 30 mm Hg below normal to avoid excessive vasoconstriction.

Chlorpromazine has no central effect and therefore acts as a pure alpha-lytic. It is administered in small bolus doses of 2.5 to 5 mg intravenously.

Shock Lung

This poses a special and difficult therapeutic problem. All patients with septic shock must be carefully observed through the clinical course and for 24 to 48 hours after tachypnea. If it occurs, arterial blood gases should be measured and oxygen administered. A chest x-ray should be obtained as a baseline, even though it may show very little early in the course. If the Pao_2 remains stable, treatment should continue until the lungs clear. If the Pao_2 continues to drop, intubation or tracheostomy must be carried out with mechanical ventilation and positive end-expiratory pressure (PEEP) of 5 cm H_2O. If the Pao_2 remains below 60 mm Hg, the PEEP can be increased up to 15 cm H_2O. Fluid intake must be restricted, and steroids and furosemide may also be helpful. In severe cases, treatment response is often frustrating, with oxygen concentrations falling despite heroic measures. Shock lung is the most common cause of death in patients with septic shock.[18]

Experimental Therapy

There have been several reports[4,26,42] that early prophylactic use of human antibody to the lipopolysaccharide core of endotoxin can reduce the incidence of shock and death from sepsis. This approach has not gained clinical acceptance. Even more recently, primate studies indicate that antibodies to cachectin may also offer benefits in life-threatening sepsis.

Conclusions

The treatment of septic shock is not a simple matter that lends itself to a rigid protocol. Patients should be managed in an intensive care unit by or in consultation with the intensive care specialist. The major management steps (Fig. 9-1) can be summarized as follows:

1. Replace volume using the PWP or CVP as the guide.
2. Support respiration with early aggressive use of intubation and mechanical ventilation.
3. Initiate broad-spectrum combination antibiotic therapy.

Replace volume
(CVP or PWP)
↓
Support respiration
(intubation and ventilation)
↓
Broad-spectrum combination antibiotics
↓
High-dose corticosteroids (?)
↓
Surgical control of infection focus
(do not await complete stabilization)
↓
Supplemental vasoactive agents (as indicated)
↓
Digitalis, diuretics, and heparin (as indicated)

Figure 9-1 Flow chart showing steps for managing septic shock.

4. Administer a high-dose corticosteroid bolus (controversial).
5. Surgically control the focus of infection. This cannot await complete stabilization of the patient.
6. Use supplemental vasoactive agents as indicated.
7. Administer digitalis, diuretics, and heparin as indicated.

References

1. Appuzzio JJ, Pelosi MA, Landau IE. The new antibiotics and soft-tissue infections. Female Patient 1983; 8:51–52.
2. Barela AI, Kleinman GE, Golditch IM, et al. Septic shock with renal failure after chorionic villus sampling. Am J Obstet Gynecol 1986; 154:1100–1102.
3. Barnett JA, Sanford JP. Bacterial shock. JAMA 1969; 209:1514–1517.
4. Baumgartner JD, Glauser MP, McCutchan A, et al. Prevention of gram-negative shock and death in surgical patients by antibody to endotoxin core glycolipid. Lancet 1985; 1:59–63.
5. Beck-Jansen P, Brunkmann CR III, Johnson GH. Circulatory shock in pregnant sheep. Effects of endotoxin in utero-placental and fetal umbilical circulation. Am J Obstet Gynecol 1972; 112:1084–1094.
6. Beller FK, Schmidt EH, Holzgreve W: Septicemia during pregnancy: a study in different species of experimental animals. Am J Obstet Gynecol 1985; 151:967–975.
7. Bennett IL, Petersdorf RG, Keen WR. Pathogenesis of fever. Evidence for direct cerebral action of bacterial endotoxins. Trans Assoc Am Physicians 1957; 70:64–73.
8. Blanco JD, Gibbs RS, Castaneda YS: Bacteremia in obstetrics: clinical course. Obstet Gynecol 1981; 58:621–625.
9. Bone RC, Fisher CJ Jr, Clemmer TP, et al. (The Methylprednisolone Severe Sepsis Study Group). A controlled clinical trial of high-dose methylprednisolone in the treatment of severe sepsis and septic shock. N Engl J Med 1987; 317:653–658.
10. Borden CW, Hall WH. Fatal transfusion reactions from massive bacterial contamination of blood. N Engl J Med 1951; 245:760–765.
11. Bryan CD, Reynolds KL, Moore EE. Bacteremia in obstetrics and gynecology. Obstet Gynecol 1984; 64:155–158.
12. Cavanagh D, Rao PS, Comas MR. Septic shock in obstetrics and gynecology. In: Friedman EA: Major problems in obstetrics and gynecology, vol 7. Philadelphia. WB Saunders, 1977.
13. Cavanagh D, Rao PS, Sulton DMC. Pathology of endotoxin shock in the primate. Am J Obstet Gynecol 1970; 108:705–722.
14. Cefalo RC, Thiel GB. Hyperlacticacichemia patients with septic abortion. Am J Obstet Gynecol 1968; 102:21.
15. Christian CD. Maternal deaths associated with an intrauterine device. Am J Obstet Gynecol 1974; 119:441–444.
16. Corrigan JJ Jr, Kiernat JF. Effect of heparin in experimental gram negative septicemia. J Infect Dis 1975; 131:138–143.
17. Cunnion RE, Schaer GL, Parker MM, et al. The coronary circulation in human septic shock. Circulation 1986; 73:637–644.
18. Fishman AP. Shock lung: a distinctive nonentity. Circulation 1973; 47:921–923.
19. Fried MA, Vosti KL. The importance of underlying disease in patients with gram-negative bacteremia. Arch Intern Med 1968; 121:418–423.
20. Gibbs CE, Locke WE. Maternal deaths in Texas, 1969 to 1973. Am J Obstet Gynecol 1976; 126:687–691.
21. Glenn TM, Lefer TM: Role of liposomes in the pathogenesis of splanchnic ischemic shock in cats. Circ Res 1970; 27:783–793.
22. Gonik B. Septic shock in obstetrics. Clin Perinatol 1986; 13:741–754.
23. Henshaw L, Peduzzi P, Young E, et al. (The Veteran's Administration Systemic Sepsis Cooperative Study Group). Effect of high-dose glucocorticoid therapy on mortality in patients with clinical signs of systemic sepsis. N Engl J Med 1987; 317:659–665.
24. Knuppel RA, Rao PS, Cavanagh D. Septic shock in obstetrics. Clin Obstet Gynecol 1984; 27:3–10.
25. Kreger BE, Craven DE, McCabe WR. Gram negative bacteremias. IV. Re-evaluation of clinical features and treatment of 612 patients. Am J Med 1980; 68:344–355.
26. Lachman E, Pitsoe SB, Gaffin SL. Anti-lipopolysaccharide immunotherapy in management of septic shock of obstetric and gynecologic origin. Lancet 1984; 1:981–983.
27. Ledger WJ, Norman M, Gee C. Bacteremia on an obstetric-gynecologic service. Am J Obstet Gynecol 1975; 121:205–212.
28. Michie HR, Manogue KR, Spriggs DR, et al. Detection of circulating tumor necrosis factor after endotoxin administration. N Engl J Med 1988; 318:1481–1486.
29. Morishima HO, Newman WH, James LS. Effects of endotoxin on the pregnant baboon and fetus. Am J Obstet Gynecol 1978; 131:899.
30. Mostoy GJ, Alho A, Jaeger T. Effects of corticosteroids on the circulation in shock: experimental and clinical results. Fed Proc 1970; 29:1861.
31. Muggah HF, D'Alton ME, Hunter AGW. Chorionic villus sampling followed by genetic amniocentesis and septic shock. Lancet 1987; 1:867–868.
32. Oliva PB. Lactic acidosis. Am J Med 1970; 48:209–225.
33. Peters WP, Johnson MW, Friedman PA. Pressor effect of naloxane in septic shock. Lancet 1981; 1:529–532.
34. Parker MM, Shelhamer JH, Bachrach SL, et al. Profound but reversible myocardial depression in patients with septic shock. Ann Intern Med 1984; 100:483–490.

34a. Parillo JE, Burch C, Shelhamer JH, et al. A circulating myocardial depressant substance in humans with septic shock. J Clin Invest 1985; 76:1539–1553.

35. Richman A, Gerber LI, Bales JV. Peritubular capillaries: a major target site of endotoxin induced vascular injury in the primate kidney. Lab Invest 1980; 43:327–332.
36. Schwarz RH, Aviado DM. Drug action reaction and interaction III: dopamine for endotoxin shock. J Clin Pharmacol 1976; 16:88–98.
37. Seward PN, Ballard CA, Ulene AL. The effect of legal abortion on the rate of septic abortion at a large county hospital. Am J Obstet Gynecol 1973; 115:335–338.
38. Shumer W. Steroids in the treatment of clinical septic shock. Ann Surg 1976; 184:333–341.
39. Studdiford WE, Douglas GW. Placental bacteremia: a significant finding in abortion accompanied by vascular collapse. Am J Obstet Gynecol 1956; 71:842–858.
40. VanDeventer SJH, Buller HR, ten Cate JW, et al. Endotoxaemia: an early predictor of septicaemia in febrile patients. Lancet 1988; 159:605–608.
41. Weinstein MP, Murphy JR, Retter LB. The clinical significance of positive blood cultures: a comparative analysis of 500 episodes of bacteremia and fungemia in adults. Rev Infect Dis 1983; 5:54–70.
42. Ziegler EJ, McCutchan JA, Fierer J, et al. Treatment of gram-negative bacteremia and shock with human antiserum to a mutant *Escherichia coli*. N Engl J Med 1982; 307:1225–1330.

CHAPTER 10

Septic Pelvic Thrombophlebitis

Patrick Duff, M.D.

Septic pelvic vein thrombophlebitis is an uncommon but potentially life-threatening complication of soft tissue infections of the pelvis. The disorder must always be considered as one of the principal elements in the differential diagnosis of persistent puerperal or postoperative fever. This chapter reviews the pathophysiology of septic pelvic vein thrombophlebitis and provides practical guidelines for diagnosis and management of this unusual complication.

Pathophysiology

Septic pelvic vein thrombophlebitis may develop in gynecologic patients as a complication of severe pelvic inflammatory disease or as a sequela of pelvic cellulitis after hysterectomy. More commonly, however, the disorder occurs in women who have recently delivered. It usually presents in association with puerperal endometritis and affects approximately 0.5 to 1.0 percent of women with this condition.[9]

During delivery, particularly by cesarean, a series of pathophysiologic changes occur that predispose the patient to endometritis, bacteremia, and thromboembolism.[7,12] When the duration of labor and ruptured membranes is prolonged, large numbers of bacteria from the lower genital tract are introduced into the endometrial cavity. These pathogens include aerobic streptococci, such as group B streptococci, and enterococci; aerobic gram-negative bacilli, such as *Escherichia coli, Klebsiella pneumoniae,* and *Proteus* species; anaerobic streptococci; and *Bacteroides* species. When the hysterotomy incision is performed, the bacteria gain access to the vascular system and peritoneal cavity. Once inoculated into these sites, these microorganisms are well adapted to resist host defense mechanisms. For example, group B streptococci and *Bacteroides* species have well-defined capsules that impair the phagocytic function of host neutrophils and macrophages. Similarly, aerobic gram-negative bacilli have a complex cell wall that enhances the virulence of the organism. Most of these pathogenic bacteria produce a variety of proteolytic enzymes that interfere with host phagocytosis and facilitate dissemination of the organism through tissue planes. In addition, most of the pelvic pathogens also synthesize, or can be induced to synthesize, beta-lactamases. These enzymes may then degrade penicillin and cephalosporin antibiotics used to treat pelvic infections.

If the size of the bacterial inoculum introduced into the pelvic cavity is unusually high, host defenses may be overwhelmed, and infection then develops. Bacteria that colonize the pelvic veins draining the uterus may injure the vascular endothelium and create a nidus for thrombus formation. Thrombogenesis is accentuated by the hypercoagulable state of pregnancy and the marked venous stasis that occurs in the pelvic vasculature after delivery.[9,12] The right ovarian vein is more severely affected by stasis because of compression from the dextrorotated uterus and the underlying dilated ureter. In addition, the right ovarian vein follows a more horizontal course than the left, and stasis is more likely to occur at the sites of valve leaflets. Accordingly, thrombosis is much more common in the right ovarian vessel.[3,16]

Clinical Presentation

The published reports concerning septic pelvic vein thrombophlebitis can be quite confusing unless the clinician understands that the disorder occurs in two distinct forms. The most commonly described clinical presentation is that of acute thrombosis of one or both ovarian veins.[3,9,16] Because thrombosis occurs most commonly on the right side, most authors have termed this condition *right ovarian vein syndrome*.

Right ovarian vein thrombosis usually occurs within the first 4 days after delivery. Affected patients typically have high fever, chills, and unilateral lower abdominal pain. The pain may radiate into the groin, upper abdomen, or flank. Gastrointestinal symptoms such as nausea, vomiting, and bloating are common.

On physical examination, the patient usually is diaphoretic and tachycardic and appears seriously ill. Approximately one-third of women sustain septic pulmonary embolization and thus have findings such as tachypnea, stridor, and bronchospasm. The most striking findings are abdominal tenderness, guarding, and adynamic ileus, as well as a mid-quadrant mass that occurs in approximately half to two-thirds of patients. The mass typically is sausage-shaped and tender; it originates near the uterine cornua and extends cephalad toward the insertion of the ovarian vessel into the inferior vena cava on the right or the renal vein on the left.

The clinical manifestations of ovarian vein thrombosis are usually so prominent that they simulate an abdominal emergency such as acute appendicitis, nephrolithiasis, broad ligament hematoma or phlegmon, adnexal torsion, or pelvic abscess. Accordingly, in up to 50 percent of patients in earlier reports, the correct diagnosis was established at the time of exploratory laparotomy.

The second presentation of septic pelvic vein thrombophlebitis has been characterized as "enigmatic fever."[9-11] Initially, patients with this condition usually have clinical findings suggestive of endometritis. In response to antibiotics, affected women often show some improvement with the exception of persistent fever. The temperature curve may demonstrate an intermittent spiking pattern or a prolonged plateau. These individuals usually do not have a significant degree of abdominal or pelvic pain or tenderness or a palpable periumbilical mass. Presumably they have multiple thrombi in the smaller vessels of the pelvis rather than a single large thrombus. Because these patients usually do not have impressive physical findings, they rarely undergo exploratory laparotomy. Rather, as is discussed later, the diagnosis is established by exclusion and by an apparent therapeutic response to anticoagulation.

Table 10-1 summarizes the principal clinical features of ovarian vein thrombosis and enigmatic fever. Table 10-2 highlights the disorders that should be considered in the differential diagnosis of these syndromes.

Table 10-1 Clinical Manifestations of Septic Pelvic Vein Thrombophlebitis

Finding	Ovarian Vein Thrombosis	Engimatic Fever
Fever	Present	Present
Abdominal or pelvic pain	Moderate to severe	Mild or absent
Abdominal or pelvic tenderness	Moderate to severe	Mild or absent
Palpable mass	50–70%	Uncommon
Diagnosis at exploratory laparotomy	Common	Uncommon
Diagnosis by radiographic examination or ultrasound	Probable	Unlikely

Table 10-2 Differential Diagnosis of Septic Pelvic Vein Thrombophlebitis

Ovarian Vein Thrombosis	Enigmatic Fever
Pyelonephritis	Drug fever
Nephrolithiasis	Viral syndrome
Acute appendicitis	Collagen vascular disease
Broad ligament phlegmon	Persistent endometritis
Adnexal torsion	Pelvic abscess
Pelvic abscess	Factitious fever

Diagnosis

The diagnostic approach to septic pelvic vein thrombophlebitis varies, depending on whether the patient is suspected of having ovarian vein syndrome or enigmatic fever (Table 10-3). In patients with the former disorder, the diagnosis has been established by performing an intravenous pyelogram and observing concentric narrowing of the proximal ureter and dilation of the renal collecting system.[6] These findings result from compression of the ureter, usually on the right side, by the enlarged ovarian vein. In such individuals, conventional venography may demonstrate large thrombi in the ovarian vessels and identify extension of the clot into the inferior vena cava or renal veins.[9]

Less invasive techniques such as a phleborrheogram, doppler flow measurements, radiolabeled platelet scan and gallium scan have not been of consistent value in diagnosing ovarian vein thrombosis. Rudoff and associates[17] have reported successful diagnosis of this condition by ultrasound examination. On longitudinal scan of the abdomen, they noted a large echogenic mass within the inferior vena cava. Although experience with ultrasound examination in this condition is limited, its ready availability, low risk, and relatively low expense make it worthy of more systematic evaluation.

The two noninvasive tests of greatest value in evaluating patients with suspected ovarian vein thrombosis are computed tomography (CT) and magnetic resonance imaging (MRI).[2,14] On CT scan, the principal positive finding is a distinct lucent area in one or both ovarian vessels (Figs. 10-1 and 10-2). An axial scan is the preferred view for observing this abnormality. In an MRI scan, occlusive thrombi usually appear as bright areas, in contrast to the dark, patent vessels. This abnormality is usually most easily observed on a coronal scan.

The clinician must realize that each of these diagnostic tests is of principal value in detecting thrombi in large vessels such as the ovarian veins. In patients with enigmatic fever, CT and MRI scans are likely to be negative. Accordingly, a brief trial of anticoagulation may be necessary to establish the correct diagnosis.[9]

Septic pulmonary embolization is a potentially life-threatening complication of septic pelvic vein thrombophlebitis. Josey and Staggers[13] documented this se-

Table 10-3 Tests of Value in Evaluating Patients with Suspected Septic Pelvic Vein Thrombophlebitis

Test	Principal Application: Ovarian Vein Thrombosis	Principal Application: Enigmatic Fever	Positive Finding
Intravenous pyelogram	+		Concentric narrowing of proximal ureter Dilation of renal pelvis
Venogram	+		Intravascular thrombus
Ultrasound	+		Echogenic mass within major vessel
Computed tomographic scan	+		Lucency within major vessel
Magnetic resonance image	+		Echogenic density in major vessel
Therapeutic response to heparin	+	+	Defervescence within 48 to 72 hours of start of anticoagulation

quela in 15 of 46 patients (32 percent). If pulmonary embolus is suspected, the patient should have a chest x-ray and ventilation-perfusion scan. In addition, pulmonary status should be assessed by analysis of arterial blood gases and pulse oximetry. If these tests are equivocal, consideration should be given to performing a pulmonary arteriogram to identify the presence of thrombi in the lungs.

Management

Patients with septic pelvic vein thrombophlebitis should be treated with full anticoagulant doses of heparin.[4,9] The drug should be administered by continuous or intermittent intravenous infusion. The initial loading dose should be in the range of 5,000 to 7,500 units, followed by an infusion of approximately 1,000 units per hour. The maintenance infusion should then be titrated until the partial thromboplastin time is 1.5 to 2.0 times normal or the serum heparin concentration is 0.2 to 0.7 IU per milliliter. Some patients may require surprisingly high doses of heparin because of the effect of heparinases that are produced by infecting bacteria.

In previous clinical reports, anticoagulation usually has been continued for 7 to 10 days.[3,10,13,16,18] There are no data indicating that long-term anticoagulation with oral agents or subcutaneous heparin is necessary in patients with septic pelvic vein thrombophlebitis. The one exception to this general rule is the patient who has a documented pulmonary embolism. In such patients, strong consideration should be given to continuation of therapeutic anticoagulation for 8 to 12 weeks. Doses of coumarin (Coumadin) can be adjusted by maintaining the prothrombin time at approximately 1.5 times the control value. Subcutaneous heparin therapy may be monitored in the same manner as intravenous administration.

No published experience describes use of thrombolytic agents in septic pelvic vein thrombophlebitis. Such agents, of course, are contraindicated in patients who recently have had a major surgical procedure such as cesarean delivery.[18]

In addition to receiving anticoagulation, patients with septic pelvic vein thrombophlebitis also must be treated with antibiotics that are effective against the polymicrobial flora that causes soft tissue infections of the pelvis.[7-9] Table 10-4 lists several regimens of proven effectiveness in the treatment of seriously ill patients with mixed aerobic-anaerobic infections. These regimens have been highlighted because they provide virtually complete coverage against all potential pelvic pathogens. As noted, the only single agent listed is imipenem-cilastatin. Although many extended-spectrum cephalosporins and penicillins have been used to treat pelvic infections, all have at least some minor deficiencies in their coverage of aerobic gram-negative bacilli and *Bacteroides* species. Accordingly, as a general rule, these drugs should not be used by themselves to treat patients who are very seriously ill.

Parenteral antibiotics should be continued for the same length of time as intravenous heparin. At the conclusion of 7 to 10 days of therapy, antibiotics may be discontinued, provided that the patient is afebrile and asymptomatic. There is no justification for an extended course of oral antibiotics once the patient has been discharged.

Once antibiotic and anticoagulation therapy is initiated, most patients show a clear response to treatment within 48 to 72 hours.[9,13] If no improvement occurs within this interval, two possibilities must be considered. The first is that of an incorrect diagnosis. Assuming that septic pelvic vein thrombophlebitis is not present, the most likely alternative explanations for the patient's persistent febrile course are undiagnosed wound infection, pelvic abscess, or drug fever.[7,8,16]

The second major consideration is that the thromboembolic process is so extensive that anticoagulation and antibiotics alone are insufficient to effect a complete response and that surgical intervention is necessary.[4,9] If this diagnosis is considered likely, the patient should be explored through a lower midline incision that can be

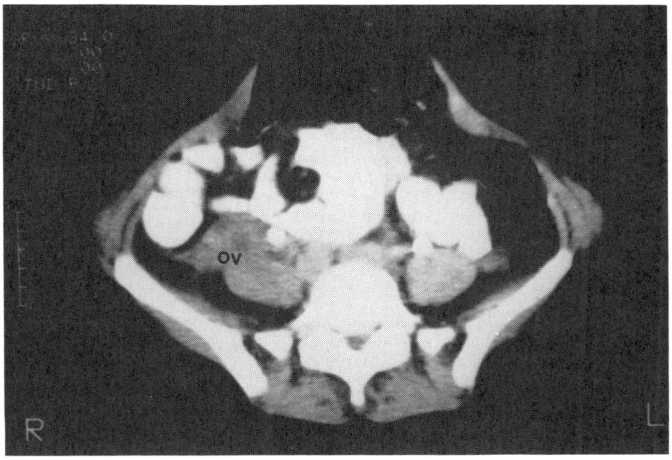

Figure 10-1 CT scan of mid-pelvis shows lucency within center of ovarian vein (OV) in a patient with right ovarian vein thrombosis.

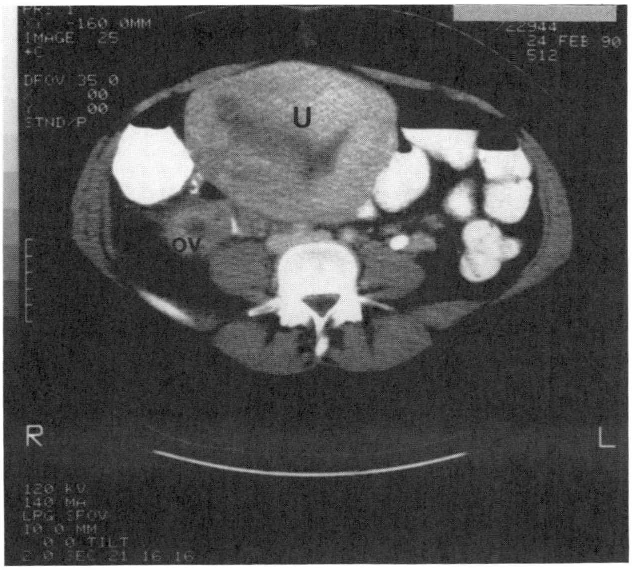

Figure 10-2 CT scan in a second patient with persistent postoperative fever shows similar abnormality in right ovarian vein (OV). U = enlarged uterus.

extended easily to provide access to vessels in the upper abdomen. The precise surgical approach must then be tailored to the intraoperative findings in each patient. In many instances, simple ligation of the affected vessel(s) is adequate to prevent further propagation of the thrombus and facilitate resolution of the patient's fever. If the thrombus extends into the inferior vena cava, ligation or plication of this vessel or insertion of an umbrella filter is indicated. If the ovarian vein thrombosis has extended to the origin of the renal veins, embolectomy may be necessary. Actual excision of the infected vessel and removal of the ipsilateral adnexa and uterus are indicated only in the presence of a well-defined abscess. Whenever any of these procedures is contemplated, the obstetrician must work in close consultation with an experienced vascular surgeon.

Prognosis

In the early 1900s the mortality from septic pelvic vein thrombophlebitis was alarmingly high, approaching 50 percent in some reports.[15] With the advent of modern antibiotics and anticoagulants and the improvement of supportive care for the critically ill patient, mortality now is uncommon. When deaths do occur, they usually result from uncontrolled sepsis, pulmonary embolism, or intraoperative cardiac arrest. This last event is a well-

Table 10-4 Antibiotic Therapy for Septic Pelvic Vein Thrombophlebitis

Drug	Intravenous Dose
Clindamycin +	900 mg q8h
penicillin +	5 million units q6h
gentamicin	1.5 mg/kg q8h
Clindamycin +	900 mg q8h
penicillin +	5 million units q6h
aztreonam	2 g q8h
Metronidazole +	500 mg q6h
penicillin +	5 million units q6h
gentamicin or	1.5 mg/kg q8h
aztreonam	2 g q8h
Imipenem-cilastatin	500 mg q6h

recognized, albeit rare, complication of vena cava ligation.

Long-term morbidity in affected patients also is uncommon unless surgical intervention has been necessary. In this circumstance, one possible complication is persistent pain and edema in the ipsilateral lower extremity.[5] In addition, several reports have described an increased frequency of obstetric complications in patients who have had ligation of the ovarian vessels and/or vena cava.[1,5,9] These complications have included spontaneous abortion, preterm delivery, and intrauterine fetal demise. However, these reports have not been properly controlled for other confounding variables, such as low socioeconomic status, consistency of prenatal care, prior obstetric history, and concurrent medical illnesses that may adversely affect subsequent pregnancy outcome.

There is no published information regarding recurrence risk for septic pelvic vein thrombophlebitis in a future pregnancy. Similarly, no studies specifically address the issue of use of oral contraceptives in patients who have sustained this complication. In the absence of definitive information, caution dictates that these agents not be used because of their recognized thrombogenic effects.

References

1. Allan TR, Mill GC, Wabrek AJ, Burchell RC. Postpartum and postabortal ovarian vein thrombophlebitis. Obstet Gynecol 1976; 47:525–528.
2. Brown CEL, Lowe TE, Cunningham FG, Weinreb JC. Puerperal pelvic vein thrombophlebitis: impact on diagnosis and treatment using x-ray computed tomography and magnetic resonance imaging. Obstet Gynecol 1986; 68:789–794.
3. Brown TK, Munsick RA. Puerperal ovarian vein thrombophlebitis: a syndrome. Am J Obstet Gynecol 1971; 109:263–273.
4. Collins CG. Suppurative pelvic thrombophlebitis. Am J Obstet Gynecol 1970; 108:681–687.
5. Collins JH, Cohen CJ. Pregnancy subsequent to ligation of the inferior vena cava and ovarian vessels. Am J Obstet Gynecol 1959; 77:760–769.
6. Darney PD, Wilson EA. Intravenous pyelography in the diagnosis and management of postpartum ovarian vein thrombophlebitis: a case report. Am J Obstet Gynecol 1977; 127:439–440.
7. Duff P. The pathophysiology and management of postcesarean endomyometritis. Obstet Gynecol 1986; 67:269–276.
8. Duff P. Antibiotics for pelvic infections. In Rayburn W, Zuspan FP, eds. Drug therapy in obstetrics and gynecology. Ed 3. St Louis: Mosby–Year Book Inc, 1992.
9. Duff P, Gibbs RS. Pelvic vein thrombophlebitis: diagnostic dilemma and therapeutic challenge. Obstet Gynecol Surv 1983; 38:365–373.
10. Dunn LJ, VanVoorhis LW: Enigmatic fever and pelvic thrombophlebitis. N Engl J Med 1967; 276:265–268.
11. Gibbs RS. Treatment of refractory postpartum fever. Clin Obstet Gynecol 1976; 19:83–95.
12. Hodgkinson CP. Physiology of the ovarian veins during pregnancy. Obstet Gynecol 1953; 1:26–35.
13. Josey WE, Staggers SR. Heparin therapy in septic pelvic vein thrombophlebitis: a study of 46 cases. Am J Obstet Gynecol 1974; 120:228–233.
14. Khurana BK, Rao J, Friedman SA, Cho KC. Computed tomographic features of puerperal ovarian vein thrombosis. Am J Obstet Gynecol 1988; 159:905–908.
15. Miller CF. Ligation or excision of the pelvic veins in the treatment of puerperal pyemia. Surg Gynecol Obstet 1917; 25:431–439.
16. Munsick RA, Gillanders LA. A review of the syndrome of puerperal ovarian vein thrombophlebitis. Obstet Gynecol Surv 1981; 36:57–66.
17. Rudoff JM, Astrauskas LJ, Rudoff JC, et al. Ultrasonographic diagnosis of septic pelvic thrombophlebitis. J Ultrasound Med 1988; 7:287–291.
18. Sharma GVRK, Cella G, Parisi AF, Sasahara AA: Thrombolytic therapy. N Engl J Med 1982; 306:1268–1226.

PART II

Mother and Fetus

CHAPTER 11

Viral Infections

Antonio V. Sison, M.D.
John L. Sever, M.D., Ph.D.

INTRODUCTION

The major breakthroughs in the discovery and characterization of several viruses that play a major role in perinatal infections have been reported in the last 50 years. Some important historical facts are shown in Table 11-1. For example, *Parvovirus* B19 was fortuitously discovered by Cossart and associates in 1975, and only in the last 10 years has its role in perinatal infections leading to disease been described. Similarly, the human immunodeficiency virus (HIV) has only recently been shown to be the causative agent for the acquired immunodeficiency syndrome (AIDS) in humans. Its relevance to perinatal medicine has been that more than 80 percent of infants with AIDS in this country have acquired the infection by maternal transmission of the virus.

The roles of antiviral chemotherapeutic agents and prophylactic agents such as vaccines have also only been recently recognized. Rubella vaccine was introduced in 1969 and has been solely responsible for the dramatic decrease by over 95 percent in the incidence of the congenital rubella syndrome in the United States since 1969. Vaccine against hepatitis B virus was introduced in 1981, and its prophylactic use in infants born to pregnant women with acute HBV infection or who are chronic hepatitis B surface antigen (HB_sAg) carriers has signif-

Table 11-1 Historical Facts on Perinatal Viral Infections

Virus	Year	Facts
Rubella	1941	Australian ophthalmologist, M. Gregg, first reports congenital defects in infant of mother who developed German measles in pregnancy[7] 1969: Rubella vaccine introduced
Varicella-zoster (VZV)	1947/1953	Laforet and Lynch first report congenital defects following maternal VZV infection[10] VZV isolated by Weller.[18a]
Herpes simplex (HSV)	1934/1935	Batignani and Hass report first case of neonatal HSV infection[28]
Cytomegalovirus	1956	Weller and Rowe and associates successfully isolate cytomegalovirus in tissue culture[14,18]
Hepatitis B virus	1965 1981	Blumberg and associates discover the Australia antigen[3] Hepatitis B vaccine introduced from pooled human sera; bioengineered vaccine later introduced
Parvovirus B19	1975 1984	Cossart and associates discover parvovirus while assaying sera for hepatitis virus[5] Brown and associates links parvovirus B19 infection to fetal hydrops[4]
Human immunodeficiency virus type 1 (HIV-1)	1983 1985	Barre-Sinoussi and associates isolate the virus from an AIDS patient[1] Mitsuya and associates discover nucleoside analogue, azidothymidine (AZT)[11]

Table 11-2 Viruses That Cross the Placenta

Virus	Reference Number
Parvovirus B19	4
Cytomegalovirus	16
Influenza	19
Rubella	6
Hepatitis B	17
Herpes simplex	20
Human immunodeficiency virus	12
Varicella-zoster	13
ECHO virus	15
Coxsackievirus B	9

icantly reduced the chronic carrier state in infants who received the vaccine. More recently, 3′-azido-2′,3′-dideoxythymidine (AZT) was shown by Mitsuya and coworkers in 1985 to be useful in treating HIV infection.[11] This nucleoside analogue competes with thymidine during DNA transcription and has been shown to effectively diminish the progression of symptomatic disease in AIDS.

It is beyond the scope of this text to describe all the viruses known to affect the fetus and the newborn. Other volumes of this series will discuss specific viruses and their clinical effects in detail. This chapter is limited to the viruses that have been commonly associated with fetal and neonatal infection. In general, mother-to-child transmission of viral disease leading to fetal infection generally occurs either through the placenta or through direct contact of the infant with an infected delivery tract. Those viruses that have been shown to cross the placenta are listed in Table 11-2. The presence of the viruses on this list has been documented by virus isolation from amniotic fluid or from the fetus/abortus material or by presence of virus-specific immunoglobulin M (IgM) in cord blood.

Other viruses that have been associated with perinatal infection leading to fetal or neonatal disease that are not covered in this chapter include enteroviruses (poliomyelitis virus, ECHO virus, group B Coxsackievirus), mumps (parotitis) virus, influenza viruses, smallpox virus, measles (rubeola) virus, and the viruses that causes western equine encephalomyelitis (WEE) and Venezuelan equine encephalomyelitis (VEE).

References

1. Barre-Sinoussi F, Chermann JC, Rey F, et al. Isolation of T lymphotropic retrovirus from a patient at risk for acquired immunodeficiency syndrome (AIDS). Science 1983; 220:868–871.
2. Batignani A. Conjunctivite da virus erpetico in neonato. Bull Ocul 1934; 13:1217–1221.
3. Blumberg BS, Alter HJ, Visnich S. A "new" antigen in leukemic sera. Lancet 1965; 191:541–546.
4. Brown T, Anand, A. Ritchie LD, et al. Intrauterine parvovirus infection associated with hydrops fetalis. Lancet 1984; 2:1033–1034.
5. Cossart YE, Field AM, Cant B, Widdows D. Parvovirus-like particles in human sera. Lancet 1975; 1:72–73.
6. Daffos F, Forestier F, Grangeot-Keros L, et al. Prenatal diagnosis of congenital rubella. Lancet 1984; 2:1–3.
7. Gregg NM. Congenital cataract following German measles in the mother. Trans Ophthalmol Soc Aust 1941; 3:35–41.
8. Hass M. Hepatoadrenal necrosis with intranuclear inclusion bodies: report of a case. Am J Pathol 1935; 11:127–142.
9. Kaplan MH, Klein SW, McPhee J, Harper RG. Group B coxsackievirus infections in infants younger than three months: a serious childhood illness. Rev Infect Dis 1983; 5:1019–1032.
10. Laforet EG, Lynch C. Multiple congenital defects following maternal varicella. N Engl J Med 1947; 236:534–537.
11. Mitsuya H, Wienhold KJ, Furman PA, et al. Proc Natl Acad Sci USA 1984; 82:7096–7100.
12. Mundy D, Schinazi R, Gerber A, et al. Human immunodeficiency virus isolated from amniotic fluid. Lancet 1987; 2:459–460.
13. Paryani SG, Arvin AM. Intrauterine infection with varicella-zoster virus after maternal varicella. N Engl J Med 1986; 314:1542–1546.
14. Rowe WP, Hartley JW, Waterman S, et al. Cytopathogenic agent resembling human salivary gland virus recovered from tissue culture of human adenoids. Proc Soc Exp Biol Med 1956; 92:418–424.
15. Skeels MR, Williams JJ, Ricker FM. Perinatal echovirus infection. N Engl J Med 1981; 305:1529. (letter).
16. Stagno S, Pass R, Reynolds DW, et al. Comparative study of diagnostic procedures for congenital cytomegalovirus infection. Pediatrics 1980; 65:251–257.
17. Stevens C, Beasley R, Tsui J, and Lee WC: Vertical transmission of hepatitis-B antigen in Taiwan, N Engl J Med 1975; 292:771–774.
18. Weller TH: Serial propagation of agents producing inclusion bodies derived from varicella and herpes zoster. Proc Soc Exp Biol Med 1953; 83:340–346.

18a. Weller TH, Macauley JC, Craig JM, and Wirth P. Isolation of intranuclear inclusion producing agents from infants with illnesses resembling cytomegalic inclusion disease. Proc Soc Exp Biol Med 1957; 94:4-12.

19. Yawn D, Pyeatte J, Joseph M, et al. Transplacental transfer of influenza virus. JAMA 1971; 216:1022–1023.
20. Zervoudakis I, Silverman F, Senterfit L et al. Herpes simplex in the amniotic fluid of an unaffected fetus. Obstet Gynecol 1980; 55[supp]:16S–17S.

RUBELLA VIRUS INFECTIONS

Although the clinical manifestations of rubella infections were well described in the mid-18th century, it was in 1941 that the Australian ophthalmologist McAlister Gregg reported the association between rubella infection during pregnancy and congenital defects in the offspring.[14] In that study, following an epidemic of rubella in Sydney, 68 of 78 infants with congenital cataracts (many of whom also had cardiac defects) were born to mothers who had rubella during their pregnancies. The full-blown congenital rubella syndrome was not described until after the worldwide rubella epidemic in 1962 to 1964.

The introduction of rubella vaccine has significantly reduced the incidence of congenital rubella infection in the United States. It is important, however, to recognize that rubella vaccine is not generally used in most countries of the world; therefore, in those areas rubella in the adult and congenital rubella continue to occur.

Epidemiology

Before the introduction and utilization of the rubella vaccine, approximately 85 percent of individuals had rubella by age 15 to 19 years and were immune. Almost 100 percent of individuals age 35 to 40 years had been infected and were immune. In the rubella pandemic of 1962 to 1964, 12.5 million cases of rubella infection were reported globally. There were 11,000 fetal deaths attributable to maternal rubella infection and 20,000 infants were born with congenital rubella syndrome (CRS) worldwide.[27]

Following the introduction of rubella vaccine in the United States in 1969, the total number of cases of CRS decreased 99 percent during the period 1969 to 1986.[2] Individuals over 15 years of age accounted for 56 percent of all cases of rubella infection, and by 1986 the total number of cases in this age group was reduced by 95 percent compared to 1969. In 1969, for example, 62 cases of CRS were reported to the National Congenital Rubella Syndrome Registry (NCRSR) of the Centers for Disease Control, resulting in an incidence rate of 1.72 per 100,000 live births. By 1984 and 1985, the number of reported cases of CRS totaled two for each year, significantly reducing the annual incidence rate to 0.05/100,000.[2] In 1986, 12 cases of CRS were reported, 8 of whom were from New York City. This unprecedented rise in CRS was probably due to the rubella outbreak in New York City in 1984 through 1985. Since that time, only 1 or 2 cases of CRS have been reported each year in this country.

Despite the routine use of rubella vaccine in childhood in the United States, approximately 10 percent of women of childbearing age are susceptible to infection with rubella. This is due to failure to immunize some children and to a low rate of vaccine failures. These susceptible women need to be identified and immunized.

In most developing countries rubella vaccine is available only to affluent patients, and the great majority of children are not immunized. In addition, in some industrialized countries only female children are immunized at puberty. As a result, rubella and CRS are still major problems in most of the world.

The attack rates after exposure to rubella depend largely on the population being studied. In a study of military recruits, more than 90 percent developed rubella infection after exposure, compared to only 50 to 90 percent among college students.[26,27] A true indication of attack rates after exposure to the general population has been difficult to assess, primarily because its mild clinical course produces underreporting of rubella infections.

Outbreaks of rubella infection in unvaccinated general populations peak during the spring months, and epidemics usually occur every 6 to 7 years. Rubella most commonly affects children 5 to 14 years of age.

Biology

Rubella is a 58-nm virus that belongs to the family Togaviridae and genus *Rubivirus*. The viral genome consists of RNA of 3×10^6 MW. The genome is enclosed in a viral envelope derived from the infected host cell membrane. The envelope has characteristic spherical projections made of glycoprotein. The viral genome encodes for three structural proteins called E_1, E_2, and protein C. The E_1 codes for the part of the protein comprising the spikelike projections, and protein C forms the viral nucleocapsid along the genomic RNA. Rubella has only one serologic type.

Rubella was first isolated in tissue culture in 1962 by two independent investigators.[25,34] One series of isolations was achieved by direct inoculation onto a monolayer of primary green monkey kidney (GMK) tissue culture. Because rubella virus does not produce a cytopathic effect in such cultures, the cell cultures were challenged with an enterovirus known to produce cytopathic effects. Presence of rubella virus inhibited the ability of this second virus to produce the cytopathic effect. The other isolations were achieved by inoculation of human amnion cell cultures with resulting cytopathic changes. Several different serial cell lines are now generally used for the culture of rubella. There are no animal models for the study of congenital rubella syndrome.

Routes of Transmission

Acquired Infection

The common mode of transmission is through respiratory droplets shed from infected individuals. The virus enters the nasopharynx of the host and invades the mucosal tissue. Virus may then spread locally to nearby lymph nodes (such as posterior auricular or suboccipital systems). Viremia begins after 7 days, continues 7 to 10 days, but ceases 1 to 2 days after the onset of the rash. The incubation period to onset of symptoms is 14 to 21 days. Peak viremia occurs at the onset of the rash. Patients are infectious by the respiratory route from 7 days prior to and up to 5 days after the appearance of the rash. Virus can be isolated from nasopharyngeal swabs during this phase. Acquired rubella is highly contagious, and about 25 to 33 percent of cases may be asymptomatic.[7,18]

Congenital Infection

Vertical transmission of rubella virus occurs transplacentally in association with maternal viremia (Table 11-3). Terry and colleagues[31] detected the presence of rubella antigen and RNA sequences by nucleic acid hybridization of chorionic villus samples from 11-week pregnancies that had been complicated by maternal infection with rubella in the first trimester. Other studies on abortus material have also shown the presence of rubella infection in these tissues.[28,32]

The CRS results from in utero infection of the fetus following primary infection of the pregnant woman during the first 20 weeks of gestation. However, fetal infection has been documented to occur following maternal rubella at virtually any time in pregnancy (Table 11-3). The frequency and severity of fetal damage is directly associated with the gestational age of the fetus. As a rule, the earlier the infection, the more frequent and severe the fetal damage.

Major defects are found in half the children when maternal infection occurs in the first month of gestation, 22 percent in the second month, and 10 percent in the third month.[30] Lower rates of fetal damage (about 6 percent) are seen with maternal infection in the fourth or fifth month of gestation.

If the mother has rubella at delivery, it is possible that a very small percentage of infants become infected during the delivery process through contact with infectious maternal fluids. Virus has been detected in cervical secretions, and therefore this route may also potentially transmit the infection from the mother to the infant. There is also a theoretical risk of mother-to-infant infection through infectious breast milk.[21]

Table 11-3 Timing of Maternal Rubella in Relation to Frequency of Fetal Infection

Time of Maternal Infection (Weeks in Gestation)	Fetal Infection (%)
Less than 11	90 (9/10)
11–12	67 (4/6)
13–14	67 (12/18)
15–16	47 (17/36)
17–18	39 (13/33)
19–22	34 (20/59)
23–26	25 (8/32)
27–30	35 (11/31)
31–36	60 (15/25)
Greater than 36	100 (8/8)

Adapted from Miller E, Cradock-Watson JE, and Pollock TM: Consequences of confirmed maternal rubella at successive stages of pregnancy, Lancet 2:781, 1982.

Fetal Infection Following Maternal Rubella Very Early in Gestation

The effects of rubella infection prior to pregnancy and in the first weeks of pregnancy have been investigated. Enders and associates[11] followed 61 pregnant women who had rubella from 5 weeks before to 6 weeks after their last menstrual period (LMP). Of the 38 pregnancies that carried to term, no clinical or serologic evidence of CRS was found in the pregnancies in which the rubella rash appeared before the LMP or within 11 days after the LMP. The earliest maternal infection that resulted in CRS was at 12 days after the LMP (about the time of implantation). In addition, the infant developed CRS in all cases in this study when the maternal rash appeared 3 to 6 weeks after the LMP.

Congenital Infection After Maternal Reinfection with Rubella

There have been rare reports of maternal-to-fetal transmission of rubella after reinfection of seropositive pregnant women.[4,6,8,9,12,22,29] In some cases, maternal reinfection with rubella resulted in CRS.[9,12] Reinfection with rubella has been reported after primary infection and following vaccination.[12] Reinfections in the pregnant woman are usually asymptomatic. Viremia is also possible but uncommon. Reinfections probably result from low levels of antibody in the host.

Clinical Manifestations

Mother

The most frequent clinical finding of acquired rubella is a fine macular rash starting on the face and extending 1 to 2 days later to the trunk and extremities. There may be prodromal symptoms 1 to 5 days before the onset of the rash, including malaise, fever, headaches, and conjunctivitis. Frequently there is posterior auricular, suboccipital, and posterior cervical lymphadenopathy. In more than one-third of adult patients, arthralgias are common. Women have a higher incidence of joint complications than men. The small distal joints of the fingers and the wrist are most frequently involved, although more proximal joints such as knees and elbows may be involved as well.[18] In some cases, arthralgias may be the only presenting symptom of rubella infection. Less frequent findings include tenosynovitis, myalgia, and peripheral neuritis.[18] The virus has been recovered from synovial fluid of patients with arthralgias.[16,18]

Infant

Table 11-4 summarizes the clinical findings associated with the CRS. Hearing loss is the most common clinical manifestation and can result from maternal infection at any time in the first 5 months of gestation. Cardiac defects are more commonly associated with maternal infection in the first trimester.[24] Overall, the most serious cardiac, ophthalmologic, and neurologic fetal damage results from maternal infection very early in pregnancy, usually in the first several months.

Most clinical manifestations of the CRS may be apparent at birth, but others may not be evident until later in life.[13] Late-onset findings occur in 10 to 20 percent of CRS cases, usually present in the second decade of life, and include diabetes mellitus, thyroid disorders, and ophthalmologic disorders such as glaucoma.

Table 11-4 Clinical Manifestations of Congenital Rubella Syndrome

General
- Intrauterine growth retardation
- Prematurity
- Abortion
- Stillbirth

Neurologic
- Meningoencephalitis
- Microcephaly
- Intracranial calcifications
- Psychomotor retardation
- Behavioral disorders
- Autism
- Chronic progressive panencephalitis
- Hypotonia
- Speech defects
- Hearing loss (most common symptom)

Ophthalmologic
- Cataracts
- Retinopathy
- Glaucoma
- Cloudy cornea
- Microphthalmia
- Subretinal neovascularization

Cardiac
- Patent ductus arteriosus
- Pulmonary artery stenosis
- Pulmonary artery hyperplasia
- Coarctation of the aorta
- Ventricular septal defect
- Atrial septal defect
- Myocarditis
- Myocardial necrosis

Dermatologic
- Thrombocytopenia purpura ("blueberry muffin" spots)
- Chronic rubelliform rash
- Dermatoglyphic abnormalities

Hepatic
- Jaundice
- Hepatosplenomegaly
- Hepatitis

Hematologic
- Anemia
- Hemolytic anemia

Miscellaneous
- Interstitial pneumonia
- Bone lesions (micrognathia, radiolucency of long bones)
- Immunologic abnormalities (hypogammaglobulinemia, thymic hypoplasia)
- Endocrinologic abnormalities (diabetes mellitus, thyroid disease, growth hormone deficiency)
- Genitourinary abnormalities (cryptorchism, polycystic kidney)

Adapted from Freij BJ, South MA and Sever JL: Maternal rubella and the congenital rubella syndrome, Clin Perinatol 15:247, 1988.

Diagnosis

Mother

The 3-day rash, lymphadenopathy, and mild constitutional symptoms are usually diagnostic of rubella, particularly during an epidemic. To confirm the diagnosis, maternal sera can be tested for rubella-specific IgM antibody. The most reliable method for testing IgM to rubella at this time is the ELISA method. This IgM test becomes positive approximately 1 week after the onset of the rash and remains positive for 1 to 2 months. Infection can also be diagnosed by demonstrating seroconversion with rubella-specific IgG antibody. However, this requires paired sera specimens with the first specimen obtained before or at the onset of the rash and the second specimen obtained 2 to 3 weeks later. Other methods for the detection of rubella-specific IgG or IgM antibody include radioimmunoassay (RIA), immunofluorescence (IFA), and latex agglutination (LA).

Immunity has been determined to be associated with rubella-specific IgG antibody levels of greater than 15,000 IU per l or an HAI titer of greater than or equal to 1:8.[7,17] Rubella-specific IgM may be detectable by the third or fourth week after exposure to the virus (or about 1 week after the onset of the rash), persists for 1 to 2 months, and is virtually undetectable by the eighth to ninth week.[25] In rare instances rubella-specific IgM has been reported to persist for years.[1,19]

Other methods for diagnosing rubella infection in the mother include the demonstration of the presence of viral antigen in throat swab specimens by immunofluorescence or by virus isolation in tissue culture.[3,15] Virus has also been isolated from blood, urine, amniotic fluid, and placenta of infected individuals.[7] The cell culture systems most commonly used include rabbit kidney (RK13), rabbit cornea (SIRC), and monkey kidney (Vero).[7] Virus has been isolated from synovial fluid of individuals who developed arthralgias.[18] Rubella has also been demon-

Table 11-5 Centers for Disease Control Classification for Congenital Rubella Syndrome Cases

I. CRS CONFIRMED—Defects present and one or more of the following:
   A. Rubella virus isolated
   B. Rubella-specific immunoglobulin G (IgG) present
   C. Infant's rubella IgG antibody titer persists above and beyond that expected from passive transfer of maternal antibody

II. CRS COMPATIBLE—Laboratory data insufficient for confirmation and any two complications listed in A or one from A and one from B:
   A. Cataracts and congenital glaucoma, congenital heart disease, loss of hearing, pigmentary retinopathy
   B. Purpura, splenomegaly, jaundice, microcephaly, mental retardation, meningoencephalitis, radiolucent bone disease

III. CRS POSSIBLE—Some compatible clinical findings that do not fulfill the critieria for a compatible case

IV. CONGENITAL RUBELLA INFECTION ONLY—No defects present but laboratory evidence of infection

V. STILLBIRTHS—Stillbirths that are thought to be secondary to maternal rubella infection.

VI. NOT CRS—One or more of any of the following inconsistent laboratory findings for a child without evidence of an immunodeficiency disease:
   A. Rubella antibody titer absent in a child less than 24 months
   B. Rubella antibody titer absent in mother
   C. Rubella antibody titer decline in an infant consistent with the normal decline of passively transferred maternal antibody after birth (The expected rate of decline of maternal antibodies is one twofold dilution/month)

Adapted from Epidemiologic notes and reports: rubella and congenital rubella—United States, 1984–1986.

strated in abortus material using tissue culture or nucleic acid hybridization techniques.[3,28,32]

Infant

Clinical diagnosis of CRS involves identifying the constellation of symptoms identified as CRS (see Table 11-4). Serology can confirm the diagnosis. Rubella-specific IgM antibody is present in the infected child at birth and remains detectable for 6 months. The ELISA test is most useful for this determination. Persistently elevated rubella-specific IgG antibody beyond 6 to 12 months of life also confirms the diagnosis.

Virus isolation by cell culture is also possible from the infant's respiratory secretions, blood, stool, cerebrospinal fluid, and urine.[7,13] Table 11-5 summarizes the clinical and serologic criteria established by the Centers for Disease Control for the diagnosis of CRS.[2]

The prenatal diagnosis of rubella has been reported in several studies.[5,10] Daffos and associates[5] measured rubella-specific IgM by cordocentesis in 18 pregnancies at 20 to 26 weeks gestation. All of the mothers had primary rubella infection before 18 weeks of gestation. The same infants were tested again for IgM antibody at birth. The fetal blood tests properly identified 12 of 13 infants who were later shown to be positive for rubella-specific IgM. One infant who tested negative for the rubella-specific IgM from the cordocentesis sample was found to have IgM antibody at birth.

Placenta

Histologic findings consistent with or suggestive of rubella infections complicating pregnancy include a lymphocytic deciduitis, necrotizing endarteritis of the fetal villous vessels, edematous villous stroma with increased Hofbauer cells, and fibrin deposition and neutrophilic infiltration of trophoblasts.[20,32] Eosinophilic viral inclusions have also been reported in these placentas.[32]

Management

Mother

Acquired rubella in adults is a mild, self-limited disease. Most patients have a 3-day rash, low-grade fever, and lymphadenopathy. Generally, only assurance and symptomatic treatment is necessary. About 20 percent of infected women develop transient arthralgias that usually respond to analgesics.

Infant

Infants with CRS shed virus from the nasopharynx and are potentially infectious for up to 1 year. They should therefore be isolated from pregnant women to reduce the risk of transmission of the virus. Management of CRS mainly involves treatment of the organs damaged from the infection. Both symptomatic infants with CRS and asymptomatic infected infants should be followed for the development of abnormalities after birth and for late-onset disease in the second decade of life.

Prevention

The rubella vaccine has been available since 1969. The strain of live attenuated rubella vaccine currently used in the United States is the RA27/3, grown in human diploid fibroblast cultures. Seroimmunity is achieved in more than 95 percent of individuals who receive the vaccine. Universal immunization against rubella infection has been the prime target in the United States. All children should be immunized at 15 months of age. Because some children do not respond to the vaccine or miss immunization, about 10 percent of women of childbearing age are susceptible. For this reason, all women of childbearing age should be tested for antibody to rubella, and those found susceptible should receive the vaccine when not pregnant. Mild, transient arthralgia occurs in some women who receive the vaccine. Rarely, other serious sequelae have been reported, including neurologic findings and a state of chronic rubella viremia.[33]

Accidental administration of rubella vaccine to a pregnant woman can result in fetal infection in some cases. To date, however, there have been no reports of fetal damage due to the vaccine virus. It is now estimated by the Centers for Disease Control that the risk of CRS in these cases, if present, is less than 2 percent. Because the vaccine virus crosses the placenta, however, it is recommended that pregnant women not be immunized and that women who are immunized be instructed not to become pregnant for 3 months.

Conclusions

1. With the use of rubella vaccine, congenital rubella syndrome and acquired rubella infections have been markedly reduced in the United States and most other industrialized countries. However, rubella vaccine is generally not used in most of the world, particularly in developing countries.
2. About 10 percent of women of childbearing age in the United States are susceptible to rubella and should be immunized when not pregnant.
3. Maternal rubella is usually mild and includes a 3-day macular rash, lymphadenopathy, and possibly arthralgia.
4. The frequency and severity of CRS is linked to the time of maternal infection. Infants of mothers infected in the first months of gestation have the greatest risk of major fetal damage.
5. Infants with CRS are usually infectious for 6 to 12 months and should be isolated. Management of CRS involves treatment of the organs damaged resulting from the infection. A small portion of infants with CRS are asymptomatic at birth. Late-onset symptoms of CRS appear in the second decade of life in about 10 percent of all cases of CRS.
6. The rubella vaccine results in antibody response and immunity in more than 95 percent of immunized individuals. Side effects from the vaccine are usually mild. Accidental immunization of pregnant women with rubella vaccine carries a theoretical risk of less than 2 percent for CRS. However, because the vaccine virus does cross the placenta in some cases, the vaccine should not be given to pregnant women, and women who receive the vaccine should be instructed not to become pregnant for 3 months.

References

1. Baubalis JV, Brown JC. Specific response of the immunoglobulins to rubella infection. Proc Soc Exp Biol Med 1968; 128:206–210.
2. Center for Disease Control. Rubella and congenital rubella—United States, 1984–1986. MMWR 1987; 36:664–675.
3. Cradock-Watson JE, Miller E, Ridehalgh MK, et al. Detection of rubella virus in fetal and placental tissue and in the throats of neonates after serologically confirmed rubella in pregnancy. Prenat Diag 1989; 9:91–96.
4. Cradock-Watson JE, Ridehalgh MK, Anderson MJ, Pattison JR. Rubella reinfection and the fetus. Lancet 1985; 1:1039.
5. Daffos F, Forestier F, Grangeot-Keros L, et al. Prenatal diagnosis of congenital rubella. Lancet 1984; 2:1–3.
6. Das BD, Lakhani P, Kurtz JB, et al. Congenital rubella after previous maternal immunity. Arch Dis Child 1990; 65:545–556.
7. Dascal A, Libman MD, Mendelson J, Cukor G. Laboratory tests for the diagnosis of viral disease in pregnancy. Clin Obstet Gynecol 1990; 33:218–231.
8. Eilard T, Strannegard O. Rubella reinfection in pregnancy followed by transmission to the fetus. J Infect Dis 1974; 129:594–596.
9. Enders G, Calm A, Schaub J. Rubella embryopathy after previous maternal rubella vaccination. Infection 1984; 12(2):96–98.
10. Enders G, Jonatha W: Prenatal diagnosis of intrauterine rubella. Infection 1987; 15:162–164.
11. Enders G, Nickerl-Pacher U, Miller E, and Cradock-Watson JE: Outcome of confirmed periconceptional maternal rubella. Lancet 1988; 1:1445–1447.
12. Forsgren M, Soren L. Subclinical rubella reinfection in vaccinated women with rubella-specific IgM response during pregnancy and transmission of virus to the fetus. Scand J Infect Dis 1985; 17:337–341.
13. Freij BJ, South MA, Sever JL. Maternal rubella and the congenital rubella syndrome. Clin Perinatol 1988; 15:247–257.
14. Gregg NM. Congenital cataract following German measles in the mother. Trans Ophthalmol Soc Aust 1941; 3:35–41.
15. Haire M, Hadden DS. Rapid diagnosis of rubella by direct immunofluorescent staining of desquamated cells in throat swabs. J Med Microbiol 1972; 5:231–235.
16. Heggie AD, Robbins FC. Natural rubella acquired after birth: clinical features and complications. Am J Dis Child 1969; 118:12–18.
17. Herrmann KL. Available rubella serologic tests. Rev Infect Dis 1985; 7:S108–S112.
18. Horstman DM. Rubella. Clin Obstet Gynecol 1982; 25:585–597.
19. Hossain A, Bakir TM. Rubella and cytomegalovirus (CMV) infections: laboratory aspects of investigation of antenatal, congenital, persistent and subclinical infections. J Trop Pediatr 1989; 35:225.
20. Kaplan C. The placenta and viral infections. Clin Obstet Gynecol 1990; 33:232–241.
21. Klein EB, Bryne T, Cooper LZ: Neonatal rubella in a breast-fed infant after postpartum maternal infection. J Pediatr 1980; 97:774–775.
22. Levine JB, Berkowitz CD, St Geme JW. Rubella virus reinfection during pregnancy leading to late-onset congenital rubella syndrome. J Pediatr 1982; 100:589–591.
23. Miller E, Cradock-Watson JE, Pollock TM. Consequences of confirmed maternal rubella at successive stages of pregnancy. Lancet 1982; 2:781–784.
24. Overall JC. Intrauterine virus infections and congenital heart disease. Am Heart J 1972; 84:823–833.

25. Parkman PD, Buescher EL, Artenstein MS. Recovery of rubella virus from army recruits. Proc Soc Exp Biol Med 1962; 111:225–230.
26. Pollard RB, Edwards EA. Epidemic survey of rubella in a military recruit population. Am J Epidemiol 1975; 101:431–437.
27. Preblud SR, Alford CA. Rubella. In: Remington, J, Klein J, eds. Infectious diseases of the fetus and newborn. Ed 3. Philadelphia, WB Saunders Co, 1990; 196–240.
28. Rawls WE, Desmyter J, Melnick JL. Serologic diagnosis and fetal involvement in maternal rubella. JAMA 1968; 203:627–631.
29. Saule H, Enders G, Zeller J. Congenital rubella infection after previous immunity of the mother. Eur J Pediatr 1988; 147:195–196.
30. Sever JL, Larsen JW, Grossman JH. Handbook of perinatal infections. Ed 2. Boston: Little, Brown Inc, 1989.
31. Terry GM, Ho-Terry L, Warren RC, et al. First trimester prenatal diagnosis of congenital rubella: a laboratory investigation. BMJ 1986; 292:930–933.
32. Thompson KS, Tobin JO. Isolation of rubella virus from abortion material. BMJ 1970; 2:264–266.
33. Tingle AJ, Chantler JK, Pot KH, et al. Postpartum rubella immunization: association with development of prolonged arthritis, neurological sequelae, and chronic rubella viremia. J Infect Dis 1985; 152:606–612.
34. Weller TH, Neva FA. Propagation in tissue culture of cytopathic agents from patients with rubella-like illness. Proc Soc Exp Biol Med 1962; 111:215–225.

HERPES SIMPLEX VIRUS INFECTIONS

The first cases of neonatal herpes virus infections were reported in 1934 and 1935 by Batignani and Hass, respectively,[8,19] but knowledge of herpes simplex virus infections in humans dates back to the ancient Greeks. Herpes simplex virus (HSV) infections in adults commonly present as oral lesions (gingivostomatitis) or genital lesions (herpes genitalis) in the acute stage of infections and may clinically recur. Perinatal transmission of HSV leading to neonatal herpes is commonly acquired from a pregnant woman with an infected vaginal tract at the time of delivery. The incidence of neonatal herpes in the United States is about 1 in 7,500 births.

Epidemiology

Maternal Infection Rates

Seroprevalence studies in adult populations have been difficult largely because of the lack of highly specific serologic assays for herpes simplex virus type 1 (HSV1) and type 2 (HSV2). Recently data on seroepidemiologic trends for HSV2 have been obtained with the development of enzyme immunoassays to detect type-specific antibodies to HSV2 glycoprotein G.[1,5,10] These studies suggest that seroprevalence of HSV2 infections is closely associated with race, maternal age, and socioeconomic status. Ades and associates[1] tested 3,533 pregnant women in London, England, antenatally for serologic evidence of HSV2 by ELISA for antibodies to HSV2 type-specific antigen. In this study, the seropositivity rate to HSV2 was 0 percent at age 16 compared to 40 percent by age 35 among black women. The incidence of primary HSV2 infection was 2.4 per 1,000 pregnancies among pregnant Asian women, 5 per 1,000 pregnancies among white women, and 20 per 1,000 pregnancies among black women.[1] In another study, only 10 to 20 percent of women of high socioeconomic status showed seropositivity to HSV2.[31]

Using a similar immunoassay to HSV2-glycoprotein G, Boucher and coworkers[10] identified 311 of 1,891 pregnant women (16.5 percent seroprevalence rate) in California who had serologic evidence of past infections with HSV2. Four of 1,580 seronegative women seroconverted during pregnancy, yielding an annualized rate of acquisition of HSV2 infection of 0.58.[10]

Neonatal Infection Rates

The incidence of neonatal HSV infection today is approximately 1 in 7,500 live births in the United States. Several studies suggest an increasing trend in the incidence of neonatal HSV, probably due to the increasing HSV2 rates in women.[24] The majority of neonatal HSV is acquired through contact with the virus in the vagina and cervix during delivery. Prophylactic cesarean section has therefore been shown to significantly reduce the risk of neonatal exposure to the virus at the time of delivery.[26] However, vertical transmission of HSV has been reported to occur transplacentally, and children and infants can be infected postnatally as well.[24]

High neonatal morbidity and mortality rates caused by neonatal HSV infection reflect the severe risk to the newborn. Close to 60 percent of infants born with HSV infection die from the infection, and more than half of surviving infants show permanent damage.

Biology

Herpes simplex virus is a member of the *Herpesvirus* group. It contains a double-stranded DNA surrounded by a 162-subunit nucleoprotein coat called the *capsid*, which is arranged in an icosahedral configuration. The capsid, in turn, is surrounded by an envelope composed of glycoprotein, lipids, and polyamines. In humans, there are two serotypes: HSV type 1 (HSV1) and HSV type 2 (HSV2). The former is responsible primarily for gingivostomatitis and pharyngitis in children and adults. The latter serotype (HSV2) is associated primarily with genital herpes. However, HSV1 has been identified in 15 to 30 percent of cases of genital herpes.

The viral genome encodes for about 70 polypeptides, which account for the virus's antigenic diversity. The genome is comprised of two major components, the L and S components. The viral genome of subtypes HSV1 and HSV2 exhibit close homology, and subsequently their glycoproteins have significant antigenic cross-reactivity. This explains the inherent difficulty in serologically differentiating the two serotypes of HSV.

An intact viral envelope is essential to the infectivity of HSV. Nonenveloped mutations of the virus have been shown not to be infectious.[24] After infection, the viral envelope fuses with the host cell membrane; the nucleocapsid is then released into the cytoplasm. By mechanisms not yet fully understood, the viral genome is then incorporated into the host cell nucleus. Morphologic changes in infected cells are usually evident within 48 hours of infection and include presence of eosinophilic intranuclear inclusion bodies and margination of nuclear chromatin. This process of margination gives the nucleus the typical "ground-glass" appearance of HSV-infected cells. Replication and viral assembly take place in the host cell nucleus.

HSV is neurotropic; that is, it has the ability to infect neural ganglia and use these cells as "privileged sites" in which the virus is protected from usual host cell immune mechanisms. Latent infections take place in these neural ganglia and can be reactivated. Reactivation of HSV2 is clinically manifested as recurrent genital ulcers.

Routes of Transmission

Horizontal Transmission

Primary HSV2 infection results from direct contact of the patient's mucous membranes or intact skin with infectious material, most commonly by sexual contact. HSV2 has been cultured from urine, cervix, nasopharynx, blood, and conjunctiva of infected individuals.[9,16] Fomites have been reported to be a potential source of infection.[28] Additionally, asymptomatic cervical shedding has been widely reported.[4,17,30,32] Prevalence of asymptomatic HSV shedding from the cervix at the time of labor has been reported to range from 0.09 to 0.96 percent. Simkovich and associates performed cervical cultures on 2,013 consecutive pregnant women in labor with no previous history of genital HSV and reported a rate of 0.2 percent of positive cultures.[30]

Table 11-6 Perinatal Transmission Rate Following HSV2 Infection

	Risk of Infection of Newborn
Primary HSV2 infection at vaginal delivery	50–60%
Recurrent HSV2 genital infection at vaginal delivery	5%
Primary HSV2 infection before delivery	5%

Asymptomatic viral shedding at term has been reported.[21] However, Nerurkar and colleagues tested a random group of 786 asymptomatic pregnant women in Miami, Florida, and Honolulu, Hawaii, and no cultures were positive for HSV. Conflicting rates of asymptomatic viral shedding probably reflect differences in the type of population studied. Jacob and coworkers, for example, cited a rate as high as 5 percent in pregnant women tested in the late third trimester.[21]

Unfortunately, viral shedding during pregnancy is a poor prognostic indicator of viral shedding at the time of delivery. Hence, testing pregnant women by virus isolation in the third trimester for HSV may not accurately identify the group of women who will be infected or shed virus at the time of delivery.

Vertical Transmission

Fetal infection with HSV following maternal infection can occur through three different mechanisms: (1) in utero transplacental infection leading to congenital HSV,[11,12,15,18,20,2-] (2) by an ascending infection from the cervix, or (3) more commonly, by intrapartum transmission through direct contact of the infant with infectious maternal genital lesions. In utero transmission accounts for about 5 to 10 percent of all cases of neonatal HSV infection.[5] The risk of intrapartum transmission associated with primary genital HSV is 40 to 50 percent.[33]

Recurrent HSV infections in pregnant women are also associated with perinatal transmission of HSV, but the rate of transmission is only about 5 percent. In addition, congenital HSV infections following recurrent HSV in the pregnant women are usually less severe, probably because of the protective role played by maternal HSV-specific antibody.

Table 11-6 summarizes the risks of transmission.

Clinical Manifestations

Mother

Primary infections with either HSV1 or HSV2 have an incubation period of 3 to 7 days, following which local symptoms appear. The most common symptoms with HSV1 are gingivostomatitis and pharyngitis[33]; less common symptoms include genital herpes, herpetic whitlow, keratitis, encephalitis, esophagitis, pneumonitis, and hepatitis. Rarely, HSV2 infections of the cervix present as a vaginal discharge not due to bacterial vaginosis or monilia.

Genital herpes is usually due to HSV2, and primary infection commonly presents as multiple vesicular lesions in the genital area, usually starting out as papules, which may ulcerate and become exquisitely painful. The ulcerations have an indurated erythematous base and resolve within 4 to 6 weeks without scarring.[24] The mean duration of viral shedding in primary infections is 8 to 17 days.[13] The lesions may be accompanied by constitutional symptoms such as malaise and fever. Extragenital lesions may occur as a result of autoinoculation.

Recurrences following a primary episode of HSV2 infection occur in 38 to 56 percent of individuals.[23] Reactivation is thought to follow stimulation of a latent virus infection in HSV-infected neural ganglia. Recurrences usually present with genital lesions similar to those of primary HSV infections. Compared to primary episodes of HSV, recurrences are usually associated with a shorter duration of viral shedding and of symptoms and are usually not accompanied by systemic illness.

Viral meningitis and encephalitis have been reported as sequelae of a primary HSV infection in adults, but fortunately these complications are extremely rare.

Fetus

Table 11-7 summarizes the risk factors for transmission of HSV during delivery. Spontaneous abortions have been reported to be increased in cases of antepartum HSV infection.[6,7,16,26] Nahmias and associates reported a 54 percent miscarriage rate in pregnant women who developed primary HSV infection before 20 weeks of gestation.[26] The same study reported a 35 percent prematurity rate for pregnant women who developed primary HSV before the second trimester. Other reports concur with this finding.[11,35] Of 196 infants studied from 1982 to 1987 with neonatal HSV infection, 24 percent were found to be premature.[35] Brown and colleagues reported an association between early HSV infection and intrauterine growth retardation.[11] Congenital malformations, such as chorioretinitis and hydranencephaly, following primary infection in the first 20 weeks of gestation have been reported.[7,15]

Infant

The clinical manifestations of HSV infection in the newborn range from mild vesicular lesions to a disseminated infection. Almost all neonatal HSV infections, regardless of the timing of infection, become symptomatic. Infants with in utero infection usually present at birth or within 24 to 48 hours of life with the symptoms listed in Table 11-8. Those infants who acquire the infection during delivery present with clinical findings within the first 1 to 2 weeks of life.

HSV infections acquired during delivery present as three distinct syndromes: (1) those involving mainly the skin, eyes, and mouth; (2) those with CNS symptoms, with or without skin, eye, and mouth involvement; and (3) disseminated infections where multiple organs are involved.

Infections of the skin, eyes, and mouth progress to CNS symptoms or disseminated HSV infection in 70 percent of untreated cases.[3,36] The overall mortality with disseminated HSV is 80 percent. With antiviral chemotherapeutic agents, this rate is reduced to 20 percent. The most common cause of neonatal death in disseminated HSV is pneumonitis or disseminated intravascular coagulopathy (DIC).

Table 11-7 Risk Factors for Increased Intrapartum Transmission of HSV

Maternal primary infection with HSV
Multiple lesions
Premature delivery
Premature rupture of membranes (PROM)
Placement of fetal scalp electrode (FSE)

Diagnosis

Mother

The clinical diagnosis of maternal primary infection requires a thorough history and physical examination to rule out other causes of ulcerative genital lesions. A Tzanck smear of freshly ulcerated vesicles is not pathognomonic but suggestive of HSV infection. In the presence of infection, the smear usually shows multinucleated giant cells in 40 to 50 percent of cases. Scraping samples may also be smeared onto glass slides and tested for HSV by indirect fluorescence or in situ hybridization techniques with a sensitivity of 60 to 90 percent.

Viral culture is the most accurate method for diagnosing HSV infection at this time. A swab of the lesion or ulcer is obtained and placed in a viral transport medium. Most cases of primary, recurrent, or asymptomatic HSV infection are virus culture positive. Virus has been isolated from the cervix, skin, feces, urine, throat, conjunctiva, nasopharynx, blood, and cerebrospinal fluid.

Serologic tests for HSV-specific IgM can be helpful in confirming the diagnosis of acute HSV infection. Because the antibody does not appear until 3 to 5 days after the appearance of genital lesions, it does not have clinical value for the rapid diagnosis of HSV in pregnant women at term. It also has no value for diagnosing recurrent infection. Antigens can be detected by immunofluorescence antibody (IFA) in exfoliated cells.

The new "shell vial" method of detection is now available in some laboratories. It involves inoculation of the sample onto tissue culture vials. The vials are then centrifuged, which increases viral attachment to the cells by distorting the tissue culture cell surfaces. Detection of HSV is then accomplished in 24 hours by ELISA or fluorescence.[25]

Table 11-8 Clinical Manifestations of Neonatal HSV Infections

Site	Early Symptoms*	Late Symptoms†
Skin	Vesicles Exanthem	Recurrent cutaneous lesions
Eye	Chorioretinitis Keratoconjunctivitis Microphthalmia Cataracts Retinal dysplasia	Chorioretinitis Blindness Cataracts Retinal detachment
Mouth	Ulcerations	
CNS	Microcephaly Cerebral atrophy Hydranencephaly Intracranial calcifications Encephalitis (bulging fontanelles, pyramidal tract signs, tremors, poor feeding, temperature instability)	Seizures Psychomotor retardation Learning disability Spasticity Microcephaly Porencephalic cysts Hydranencephaly
Miscellaneous	Hepatosplenomegaly Pneumonitis Purpura/petechiae Bone abnormalities Disseminated HSV (shock, bleeding diathesis, jaundice, respiratory distress, seizures, irritability, thrombocytopenia)	Hearing loss Dental anomalies Pneumonitis Disseminated intravascular coagulopathy

*Early symptoms refer to clinical manifestations within 24 to 48 hours of life usually seen with congenital (in utero) HSV infections or within 5 to 15 days of life as seen with infections acquired during or after delivery.
†Late symptoms refer to clinical findings that develop as sequelae from early clinical disease, whether or not treatment was instituted.

Infant

The clinical symptoms of neonatal HSV infections are often nonspecific. Only 50 percent of cases develop vesicular lesions. Almost 40 percent of infected infants who develop CNS symptoms do not have skin or eye lesions. Early diagnosis is essential for the infants because intervention with chemotherapeutic agents such as acyclovir must be initiated as early as possible.

Virus isolation may be accomplished from vesicle fluid, ulcerated lesions of the conjunctiva, nasopharynx, skin, and cerebrospinal fluid. HSV-specific IgM develops in infants infected at birth but usually does not appear for several days after the development of symptoms.

Management

Mother

Treatment of painful genital lesions is mainly symptomatic. Lesions usually heal spontaneously without scar formation. Individuals are infectious when lesions are present and should use a barrier type of contraception during sexual contact.

Acyclovir is a synthetic purine analogue whose mechanism of action involves inactivating HSV-specific thymidine kinase.[24] The infected host cell preferentially phosphorylates this analogue, which then acts as an inhibitor of HSV DNA polymerase. Acyclovir has been shown to reduce the severity of symptoms and shorten the duration of viral shedding in primary HSV infection.[14]

The use of acyclovir in pregnancy is currently not approved by the Food and Drug Administration (FDA) for HSV infections. However, its use has been reported in severe cases of maternal infection. A registry of pregnant women who have received acyclovir during pregnancy has been established to identify and monitor infants for any adverse effects.[2] There is at present no definitive evidence for any teratogenic effects of acyclovir in infants born to women who took acyclovir.

Infant

Infants born to pregnant women with active HSV infection should be carefully observed for development of neonatal HSV. Cultures should be obtained from the conjunctiva, skin, and pharynx at birth and repeated at 24 hours. Acyclovir has been successfully used in the treatment of local or CNS-related HSV infection in infants. Vidarabine, another nucleoside analogue, has also been equally effective in neonatal infections, primarily in disseminated HSV. Nahmias and associates have shown a 75 percent rate of progression from local neonatal HSV infection to CNS involvement in untreated

Table 11-9 Guidelines for the Management of Pregnant Women at Delivery with HSV Infections

Pregnant woman with *primary infection* at delivery (lesions present) or with clinically suspicious HSV genital lesions at delivery, regardless of clinical history of HSV infection:
- Culture genital lesions to confirm diagnosis
- Perform cesarean section.
- Culture infant at birth; repeat at 24 hours.
- Observe infant carefully for symptoms of neonatal HSV.
- If cultures are positive or if symptoms develop, treat with acyclovir or vidarabine.

Pregnant women with a history of past HSV infection but without lesions:
- Look carefully and thoroughly for presence of lesions.
- Attempt vaginal delivery unless obstetric indications for cesarean delivery are present.
- Observe infant carefully for symptoms of neonatal HSV.
- If symptoms develop, culture infant and then treat with acyclovir or vidarabine.

cases compared to only 15 percent of cases where vidarabine (15 mg per kilogram) was used.[26] With a higher dose (30 mg per kilograms vidarabine), none of the infants with neonatal HSV progressed to CNS involvement.

Prevention

Women who shed virus in the third trimester are not predictive of those who shed virus at delivery.[21,30] Hence, viral cultures near delivery have little value in identifying pregnant women at risk for transmitting HSV to their infants at delivery. In addition, asymptomatic rates of infection are high.

Arvin and coworkers[4] have shown that among 414 pregnant women with a history of recurrent HSV, 17 women had antepartum viral cultures that were positive for HSV. None of these pregnancies resulted in an infected infant at birth. In contrast, 1.4 percent of pregnant women who were virus culture negative during the antepartum period had infants with proven neonatal infection.

Prober and colleagues examined 6,904 deliveries without regard for the mother's history of HSV infection and found 0.2 percent (14 cases) of neonatal HSV infection, all of whom were from pregnancies whose mothers had no clinical evidence or history of HSV infection.[29] They concluded that a positive or negative clinical history was not predictive of neonatal risk for HSV infection.

To resolve these difficulties, Table 11-9 summarizes guidelines for the management of pregnant women with HSV infection. Any pregnant woman in labor who clinically shows active HSV genital lesions or who reports symptoms suggestive of reactivated disease in the absence of visible lesions should be delivered abdominally regardless of status of amniotic membrane (intact or ruptured). Viral cultures should be obtained from the maternal cervix as well as from the infant at birth. Cultures should be repeated in the infant at 24 hours and the child carefully observed for symptoms of neonatal HSV. If cultures are positive or if the infant develops symptoms, treatment with acyclovir or vidarabine should be initiated.

Pregnant women with a history of past HSV infection but without any visible lesions or symptoms should be managed expectantly. Vaginal delivery may be attempted unless obstetric indications for cesarean delivery are present. The child should be observed carefully for symptoms of HSV and, if symptoms develop, should be cultured and treated with acyclovir or vidarabine after viral cultures are obtained.

Conclusions

1. The majority of neonatal HSV infections occur by exposure of the child to infected lesions at the time of delivery. Other modes of transmission such as in utero (or transplacental) infection, postnatal infection by exposure to lesions on the mother, or contact with infected individuals in the first month of life may prevail.
2. Primary HSV infection is more severe and more likely to result in transmission to the child during vaginal delivery in contrast to recurrent HSV infection. Primary HSV carries a perinatal transmission rate of 40 to 50 percent, whereas recurrent infection results in neonatal infection in only 5 percent of cases.
3. The majority (80 percent) of primary genital infections are due to HSV2. Almost all recurrent infections are due to HSV2.
4. Almost all cases of neonatal HSV infection present with symptoms (either at birth or shortly thereafter). If untreated, localized infections with skin, eyes, and mouth involvement progress to CNS symptoms in 70 percent of cases. Fifteen percent of neonatal infections are localized (skin, eye, and mouth lesions only), another 15 percent are CNS-associated, and the remaining 70 percent are disseminated infections.
5. Disseminated neonatal HSV infection carries the worst prognosis. The mortality rate is about 80 percent.
6. Clinical history is extremely unreliable in predicting who will shed virus at the time of delivery and whether the infant will become infected.
7. The most common cause of death in disseminated HSV infection in infants is either pneumonitis or disseminated intravascular coagulopathy.
8. Acyclovir has very limited use in pregnancy, but reports to date have not shown any teratogenic effects. Acyclovir and vidarabine are used for infected newborns to reduce the morbidity and mortality from the disease.

References

1. Ades AE, Peckham CS, Dale GE, et al. Prevalence of antibodies to herpes simplex virus types 1 and 2 in pregnant women, and estimated rates of infection. J Epidemiol Community Health, 1989; 43:53–60.
2. Andrews EB, Tilson HH, Cordero JF, and Hurn BA: Acyclovir in pregnancy registry: an observational epidemiologic approach. Am J Med (suppl 2A) 1988; 85:123–128.
3. Arvin AM. Antiviral treatment of herpes simplex infection in neonates and pregnant women. J Am Acad Dermastol 1988; 18:200–203.
4. Arvin AM, Hensleigh PA, Prober CG, et al. Failure of antepartum cultures to predict the infant's risk of exposure to herpes simplex virus at delivery. N Engl J Med 1986; 315:796–800.
5. Baker DA. Herpesvirus. Clin Obstet Gynecol 1983; 26:165–172.
6. Baker DA: Herpes and pregnancy: new management. Clin Obstet Gynecol 1990; 33:253–257.
7. Baldwin S, Whitley RJ. Teratogen update: intrauterine herpes simplex virus infection. Teratology 1989; 39:1–10.
8. Batignani A. Conjunctivite de virus erpetico in neonato. Bull Ocul 1934; 13:1217–1221.
9. Binkin NJ, Kaplan JP, Cates W. Preventing neonatal herpes: the value of weekly viral cultures in pregnant women with recurrent genital herpes. JAMA 1984; 251:2816–2821.
10. Boucher FD, Yasukawa LL, Bronzan RN, et al. A prospective evaluation of primary genital herpes simplex virus type 2 infections acquired during pregnancy. Pediatr Infect Dis J 1990; 9:499–504.
11. Brown ZA, Vontver LA, Benedetti J, et al. Effects on infants of a first episode of genital herpes during pregnancy. N Engl J Med 1987; 317:1246–1251.
12. Christie JD, Rakusan TA, and Martinez MA: Hydrancephaly caused by congenital infection with herpes simplex virus. Pediatr Infect Dis 1986; 5:473–478.
13. Corey L, Adams HG, Brown ZA. Genital herpes simplex virus infections: clinical manifestations, course, and complications. Ann Intern Med 1983; 98:958–961.
14. Corey L, Fife KH, Benedetti JK, et al. Intravenous acyclovir for the treatment of primary genital herpes. Ann Intern Med 1983; 98:914–921.
15. Florman AL, Gershon AA, Blackett PR, Nahmias AJ. Intrauterine infection with herpes simplex virus: resultant congenital malformations. JAMA 1973; 225:129–132.
16. Freij BJ, Sever JL. Herpesvirus infections in pregnancy: risks to embryo, fetus, and neonate. Clin Perinatol 1988; 15:203–231.
17. Hankins GD, Cunningham FG, Luby JP, et al. Asymptomatic genital excretion of herpes simplex virus during early labor. Am J Obstet Gynecol 1984; 150:100–101.
18. Harris HH, Foucar E, Anderson RD, Ray TL. Intrauterine herpes simplex infection resembling mechanobullous disease in a newborn infants. J Am Acad Dermatol 1986; 15:1148–1155.
19. Hass M. Hepatoadrenal necrosis with intranuclear inclusion bodies: report of a case. Am J Pathol 1935; 11:127–142.
20. Hutto C, Arvi A, Jacobs R, et al. Intrauterine herpes simplex virus infections, J Pediatr 1987; 110:97–101.
21. Jacob AJ, Epstein J, Madden DL, Sever JL. Genital herpes infections in pregnant women near term. Obstet Gynecol 1984; 63:480–484.
22. Karesh JW, Kapus S, MacDonald M. Herpes simplex virus and congenital malformations. South Med J 1983; 76:1561–1563.
23. Kaufman RH, Adam E, Mirkovic RR, et al. Treatment of genital herpes simplexvirus infection with photodynamic inactivation. Am J Obstet Gynecol 1978; 132:861–865.
24. Landy HJ, Grossman JH. Herpes simplex virus. Obstet Gynecol Clin North Am 1989; 16:495–515.
25. Michalski F, Shaikh M, Sahraie F, et al. Enzyme-linked immunosorbent assay spin amplification technique for herpes simplex antigen detection. J Clin Microbiol 1986; 24:310–311.
26. Nahmias AJ, Josey WE, Naib Z, et al. Perinatal risk associated with maternal genital herpes simplex virus infection. Am J Obstet Gynecol 1971; 110:825–837.
27. Nerurkar LS, Jensen LP, McCalum P, Sever JL. Frequency of asymptomatic genital herpes in pregnant women at term. Obstet Gynecol Surv 1988; 43:132–134.
28. Nerurkar LS, West F, May M, et al. Survival of herpes simplex virus in water specimens collected from hot tubs in spa facilities and on plastic containers. JAMA 1983; 250:3081–3083.
29. Prober CG, Hensleigh PA, Boucher FD, et al. Use of routine viral cultures at delivery to identify neonates exposed to herpes simplex virus. N Engl J Med 1988; 318:887–891.
30. Simkovich JW, Commander MC, Soper DE. Asymptomatic shedding of herpesvirus during labor. Am J Obstet Gynecol 1988; 158:588–589.
31. Stavraky KM, Rawls WE, Chiavetta J, et al. Sexual and socioeconomic factors affecting the risk of past infections with herpes simplex type 2. Am J Epidemiol 1983; 118:109–121.
32. Tejani N, Klein SW, Kaplan M. Subclinical herpes simplex genitalia infections in the perinatal period. Am J Obstet Gynecol 1984; 63:480–484.
33. Whitley RJ. Neonatal herpes simplex virus infections. Clin Perinatol 1988; 15:903–919.
34. Whitley RJ. Herpes simplex virus infections. In: Remington J, Klein J, eds. Infectious diseases of the fetus and newborn. Ed 3. Philadelphia: WB Saunders Co 1990; 282–305.
35. Whitley RJ, Corey L, Arvin A, et al. Changing presentation of herpes simplex virus infection in neonates. J Infect Dis 1988; 158:109–116.
36. Whitley RJ, Nahmias AJ, Visintine AM, et al. The natural history of herpes simplex infection of mother and newborn. Pediatrics 1980; 66:489–494.

VARICELLA-ZOSTER VIRUS INFECTIONS

Varicella-zoster virus (VZV) infections in adults present either as a primary infection (chickenpox) or as a reactivation of latent infection of neural ganglia by the virus in the form of herpes zoster (shingles). VZV infections in neonates clinically present as (1) full-blown congenital varicella syndrome (CVS), (2) neonatal varicella, (3) disseminated varicella, or (4) neonatal zoster. Fortunately, congenital varicella is infrequent, neonatal varicella and zoster are usually mild diseases, and disseminated varicella can be prevented by the use of varicella-zoster immune globulin. These different clinical syndromes in pregnant women and infants are discussed in this section.

Epidemiology

Maternal Infection

Chickenpox is a very common childhood disease. Seroprevalence studies in adults in the United States and in Europe show that about 85 to 95 percent have serologic evidence of previous chickenpox.[11,27] The frequency of antibody increases with age; by 60 years of age, almost all persons have antibody to VZV.[35] The virus is extremely infectious; when an individual has chickenpox, more than 90 percent of susceptible household contacts become infected.[13] Almost all varicella infections are symptomatic, and almost all individuals who give a definite history of having had chickenpox have antibody to VZV. Even among individuals who do not have a history of chickenpox, about 70 to 90 percent have antibody to the virus indicating previous infection.[2,23,29] Because most adults have had chickenpox and are immune, only 1.8 percent of all cases of chickenpox are in individuals over 20 years of age in industrialized countries.

Because susceptibility for VZV infections in adults is small, the incidence of infection in pregnancy is low. The incidence of primary infection in pregnancy ranges from 1.3 to 7 cases per 10,000 pregnancies.[5,11]

Adults who have chickenpox are at increased risk for developing severe disease and significant sequelae when compared to children. In addition, some investigators report that pregnant women have a greater risk of developing complications than nonpregnant adults. Stagno and Whitley, for example, reported that among 29 pregnant women with chickenpox, 14 developed varicella pneumonia and 3 percent died from the infection.[31] In contrast, among 236 nonpregnant adults with chickenpox, only 11 percent developed pneumonia, and there were no reported deaths. Studies by Paryani and Arvin showed similar results.[26]

Among individuals who have had chickenpox, 10 to 20 percent eventually develop shingles.[32] The frequency and recurrences of shingles are directly associated with increasing age, with immunosuppressive disease states (such as malignancies or AIDS), and with the use of immunosuppressive drugs.[32]

Neonatal Infection

The first reported case of congenital varicella syndrome was described in 1947 by Laforet and Lynch.[21] This was an infant born at term to a mother who developed chickenpox at 8 weeks gestation. The infant showed evidence of cortical atrophy, cerebellar hypoplasia, cicatricial lesions of the skin, and muscular atrophy of the leg. Since then, additional investigators[1,25,30] have provided data associating maternal chickenpox with the congenital varicella syndrome (CVS). The rate of infants with CVS born to mothers with chickenpox in the first half of pregnancy has been reported to be 2.3 percent by Higa and coworkers,[20] 3.7 percent by Enders,[11] and 4.9 percent by Fox and Strangarity.[13] Chickenpox in the second half of pregnancy is rarely associated with CVS.

There are conflicting data on whether shingles during pregnancy can lead to CVS. Studies by Paryani[26] and Enders[11] concluded that shingles during pregnancy does not pose a significant risk for CVS. They argued that pre-existing maternal antibody to VZV may play a role in protecting the fetus from transplacental infection.[26] Other reports, however, cite cases of CVS in infants or mothers with shingles during pregnancy.[12,34]

Disseminated VZV infection in neonates is a severe, frequently fatal illness. Infants at risk for developing this complication are those born to mothers who develop chickenpox near term. The risk of fetal infection with maternal infection near term is 24 percent.[24]

Biology

Although there are related viruses in other species, the human is the only natural host for VZV. VZV is a member of the *Herpesvirus* group, along with herpes simplex virus, Epstein-Barr virus, and cytomegalovirus. Its viral and genetic makeup is almost identical to herpes simplex virus (HSV). VZV has a molecular weight of 150 to 200 with an icosahedral nucleocapsid of 162 capsomeres.[32] The nucleocapsid is surrounded by a protein envelope, within which is an amorphous layer called the *tegument*.[32] The genome is comprised of a double-stranded DNA that encodes for about 75 proteins.

Pathogenesis and Routes of Transmission

Horizontal Transmission

Varicella is usually transmitted by the respiratory route by droplets from the host's nasopharynx or from vesicular fluid and cells from fresh skin lesions. Fomites have not been shown to contribute to the transmission of VZV.[32] During the incubation period of 9 to 21 days (shorter in immunocompromised patients), VZV first replicates in the nasopharynx, followed by a period of viremia and infection of the reticuloendothelial system (e.g., the spleen). The viremic phase precedes the development of clinical symptoms by as much as 11 days but usually by about 5 days.[3] Patients usually complain of fever and malaise during the viremic phase. Infection of the reticuloendothelial system is followed by replication at this same site. The rash of chickenpox appears within a week of the onset of the viremia. Successive crops of vesicular lesions develop which eventually dry and crust over in a week.

VZV is neurotropic and becomes latent in dorsal root ganglia. Immunity to VZV, once established, is usually lifelong but exceptions have been reported in immunocompromised patients and rarely in normal individuals.[3,14,32]

Vertical Transmission

The transmission of VZV from an infected mother to the fetus has been well documented.[1,11,20,25,26,30] The spectrum of clinical disease in newborns as well as the severity of clinical presentation depends mostly on the timing of the maternal infection (Table 11-10): (1) maternal infection within the first 20 weeks of gestation results in CVS in 2 to 5 percent of cases; (2) maternal infection a few weeks before delivery can be transmitted in utero and result in chickenpox in the newborn; (3) maternal infection that occurs from 5 days before to 2 days after delivery can result in severe disseminated varicella infection; (4) maternal infection 2 days after delivery can result in chickenpox in the newborn. There is a slightly increased incidence of severe chickenpox in children infected in the newborn period compared to older children.

Clinical Manifestations

Acquired Infection with VZV (Child and Adult): Chickenpox

More than 93 percent of chickenpox cases in the United States and Europe occur in individuals younger than 20 years of age. There is a 14- to 21-day incubation period, sometimes associated with mild prodromal constitutional symptoms. The characteristic vesicular rash usually begins on the head and neck and extends to the trunk and extremities. Viremia precedes the rash by about 5 days and continues for about 2 days after the onset of the rash. Pruritus is a major complaint. Viral shedding usually begins 48 hours before the onset of the skin lesions and continues for several days. The fluid from the vesicles contains large amounts of virus during the active stage of the disease. The lesions begin to dry by day 6, at which point patients are no longer infectious.[32] Patients who are immunocompromised may have a more prolonged course.

Herpes Zoster

Zoster or shingles follows the reactivation of latent VZV in dorsal root ganglia. Usually this occurs many years after the episode of chickenpox. The lesions follow the dermatomal distribution of the dorsal root nerve in-

Table 11-10 Fetal Effects of Maternal VZV Infection in Relation to Gestation

Time of Maternal Disease	Fetal Effects
First 20 weeks of gestation	Congenital varicella syndrome (2–5% risk) Spontaneous abortion(?) Fetal demise(?) Prematurity(?) Growth retardation(?)
Third trimester 20 days prior to and until 5 days prior to delivery	Varicella in newborn (rare and mild disease)
5 days prior to and until 2 days after delivery	Severe disseminated VZV (30% risk) With VZIG suppression, some may develop zoster later
Postnatal First year after delivery	Chickenpox (increased risk for fatal disease compared to infants over 1 year with chickenpox)

volved. Reactivation of latent infection is increased in patients with decreased cellular immunity.[32,35]

Overall, 10 percent of adults experience zoster and 30 percent of patients with malignancies such as Hodgkin's disease have this disease. A prodromal phase consisting of extreme pain along dermatomal lines often accompanies reactivation. Most adults carry latent VZV in sensory ganglia of the facial and spinal nerves.

Recently several reports have shown an increased risk of developing zoster in patients with human immunodeficiency virus type 1 (HIV1) infection.[14,32] The decline of cellular immunity in HIV disease may explain the higher risk of zoster in such individuals.

Complications of Primary or Recurrent VZV Infection

The complications of varicella-zoster infection are listed in Table 11-11. It is evident that zoster infections can also lead to serious complications.

Varicella pneumonia is the most common serious, life-threatening complication of primary VZV infection.[15,32] The progression to pneumonia after primary infection is more common in adults than in children. Sixteen percent of adults progress to VZV pneumonia compared to only 1 percent in children and infants.[33] Patients usually develop pulmonary symptoms within 1 week after the onset of the cutaneous lesions, characterized by respiratory distress, dyspnea, and pleuritic chest pain. Chest x-rays usually show a nodular infiltrate with prominent peribronchial distribution.[33]

Varicella pneumonia in pregnancy when compared to pneumonia in nonpregnant women has been reported to be more common and have a more severe clinical course.[4,10,18,26] In 1965 Harris and Rhoades reported a 41 percent mortality in 17 cases of varicella pneumonia in pregnancy, with a corresponding fetal mortality of 65 percent.[18] A more recent study, however, reported a mortality rate of only 3 percent.[31] Paryani and Arvin reported a mortality rate among 43 pregnant women with varicella pneumonia of 2 percent.[26]

Varicella encephalitis is another complication. It usually has a worse prognosis in adults than in children. The mortality rate with VZV encephalitis is as high as 35 percent. Symptoms may include seizures, nystagmus, ataxia, and nuchal rigidity.[32]

Table 11-12 lists some important differences between adults and children.

Table 11-11 Complications of VZV Infection in Adults and Children

Primary infection (chickenpox)
Pneumonia
Encephalitis
Reye's syndrome
Aseptic meningitis
Transverse myelitis
Guillain-Barré syndrome
Bacterial superinfection
Ocular manifestations (lid ulcerations, conjunctivitis, uveitis)
Hepatitis
Recurrent infection (zoster)
Shingles-type pain (neuralgia)
Skin lesions in dermatome pattern
Pneumonitis
Esophagitis
Myocarditis
Herpes gangrenosum
Corneal scarring

Pregnancy-Associated Varicella: Effects on the Child

There are four distinct clinical manifestations of VZV infection in neonates born to mothers who experienced a VZV infection (primary or recurrent) in pregnancy: (1) congenital varicella syndrome (CVS), (2) disseminated VZV infection, (3) neonatal chickenpox, and (4) herpes zoster. These findings are discussed in this section.

Congenital Varicella Syndrome

The clinical manifestations of this syndrome are listed in Table 11-13. The most consistent findings include (1) cicatricial skin lesions (scarring) that follow a dermatomal pattern, (2) neurologic abnormalities including limb paresis and cortical atrophy, (3) ophthalmologic abnormalities such as chorioretinitis and anisocoria, and (4) skeletal deformities such as limb hypoplasia. Most commonly the hypoplastic limb is ipsilateral

Table 11-12 Differences Between Adult and Pediatric VZV Infections

Child	Adult
Over 98% of all cases of chickenpox in cases less than 20 yrs of age*	About 2% in adults more than 20 yrs of age*
Most common complication following primary VZV is bacterial superinfection of skin lesion	Most common complication following primary VZV is varicella pneumonia
Incidence of VZV pneumonia low (about 1%)	Incidence of VZV pneumonia significant (about 16%)
Neurologic sequelae such as encephalitis and Reye's syndrome in this age group	Rare neurologic sequelae
Mortality rate = 2/100,000 (high in infants less than 1 year = 8/100,000)	Mortality rate = 15 times rate in children

*In developed countries.

and distal to the observed skin lesion. Other anomalies such as duodenal stenosis, atresia of the colon, and genitourinary abnormalities are rare.[1]

CVS is usually associated with maternal infection in the first 20 weeks of gestation, but there are reports of CVS resulting from pregnancies where infection occurred after 20 weeks.[11,26,30] The risk for CVS following maternal infection in the first 20 weeks of gestation is about 2 to 5 percent.

Disseminated VZV Infection

Infants born to mothers who develop chickenpox within 5 days of delivery and up to 2 days after delivery carry a 30 percent risk of developing disseminated varicella in the newborn period. The clinical findings include disseminated skin lesions, pneumonia, and hepatic involvement. The fetus appears to be infected transplacentally. The infant is infected in utero but has no protection with passive maternal anti-VZV antibody and is at risk of developing serious clinical disease a few days after birth. The mean incubation period is about 11 days.[24]

The risk of disseminated VZV infection following maternal disease near delivery is about 25 to 30 percent.[24] The infection in the child, especially if maternal infection occurs within 5 days prior to delivery and 2 days after delivery, can be severe and carries a mortality rate of about 30 percent in untreated cases.

Varicella in the Newborn

Infants born to mothers who develop chickenpox 5 days to 20 days prior to delivery are at risk for developing neonatal varicella or chickenpox. The vesicular lesions usually develop within 3 to 4 days after delivery of the infant. The course of this disease is usually mild compared to disseminated neonatal VZV infection, presumably because of the protective role played by maternally transferred anti-VZV antibody. No deaths from neonatal varicella have been reported.

Zoster in the Newborn

Limited data are available associating maternal chickenpox with development of zoster in newborns and infants.[7,8,11,17] Paryani and Arvin report an infant exposed to VZV in utero in the second trimester who developed herpes zoster at 7 months of age.[26] The clinical course of neonatal zoster is usually mild with development of the zosteriform skin lesions following a dermatomal pattern. As in adult zoster, lesions are usually unilateral, involving the sixth to eighth cervical, third thoracic, and fourth lumbar dermatomes.[11] There is usually no evidence of systemic illness accompanying the lesions in neonatal zoster.

Other Fetal and Neonatal Effects of VZV Infection

Prematurity, Spontaneous Abortion, and Fetal Death

There are conflicting data regarding the association between in utero VZV infection and increased risk for prematurity, miscarriage, and fetal death. Alkalay and coworkers[1] reviewed all of the cases of CVS reported through 1987. Twenty-two cases satisfied their criteria for CVS, which included evidence of maternal VZV infection in pregnancy, presence of congenital skin lesions with a dermatomal distribution in the infant, and immunologic evidence of in utero infection with VZV.[1] Of the 22 cases, 33 percent were premature and 39 percent were small for gestational age. Enders also suggested that early first-trimester maternal VZV infection may result in spontaneous abortion or fetal death.[11]

An earlier cohort study of 190,000 pregnancies by Siegel,[30] however, identified 135 pregnancies complicated by VZV infection. The study showed no significant correlation between maternal VZV infection and spontaneous abortion, fetal death, low birth weight, or prematurity. There were also no statistically significant differences in these parameters between the 135 pregnancies with VZV infection and a matched cohort of pregnancies without VZV infection.

Diagnosis

Mother

Accurate diagnosis of maternal infection is crucial to the management of VZV infections. The exanthem of VZV is usually pathognomonic; in some cases, however, other causes of pruritic skin lesions need to be ruled out. The Tzanck test on cells from skin lesions may be helpful in the diagnosis, but only 50 to 60 percent of lesions tested are positive, and the Tzanck test may also be positive in lesions due to herpes simplex virus. VZV antigen from cells derived from the skin lesions can be detected by precipitation, fluorescence, and ELISA methods. Virus isolation of VZV is also possible in human fetal fibroblast cultures, but cytopathic effects in such tissue cultures may require 1 week or more to develop. VZV-specific IgM is helpful in diagnosing recent infections, but the test does not become positive for several days after the onset of the rash.

Infant

Both CVS and disseminated VZV infection are characterized by the clinical manifestations listed in Table 11-13. In addition, zoster can also be a clinical finding among infants born to mothers who acquired VZV infection during pregnancy. VZV cannot be cultured from infants who present with CVS as the infection occurred much earlier in gestation. However, VZV can be cultured from the lesions of infants with disseminated VZV infection or with neonatal varicella.

Management

Mother

Table 11-14 presents an algorithm for the management of pregnant women who are exposed to chickenpox or who develop chickenpox or zoster while pregnant. VZV infection from community outbreaks is highly contagious. Fortunately, seropositivity rates for VZV are also high (about 95 percent). The incidence of chickenpox in pregnancy in this country is about 1 to 5 cases per 10,000 pregnancies.

Table 11-13 Clinical Manifestations of the Congenital Varicella Syndrome

Dermatologic	Scarring
	Hyperpigmented skin lesions with dermatomal pattern
Neurologic	Cerebral cortical atrophy
	Microcephaly
	Encephalitis
	Seizures
	Mental retardation
	Limb paresis
	Intracranial calcifications
	Bulbar palsy
	Cerebellar hypoplasia
Ocular	Microphthalmia
	Optic atrophy
	Cataract
	Chorioretinitis
	Nystagmus
	Anisocoria
	Corneal opacity
Miscellaneous	Limb hypoplasia

Pregnant Women with History of VZV Exposure

Pregnant women exposed to chickenpox should be tested for VZV-specific IgG; seropositive patients are immune and can be reassured. If the patient is found to be seronegative by ELISA, administration of varicella-zoster immune globulin (VZIG) is recommended at a dose of 0.125 ml per kilogram intramuscularly.[9] Susceptible pregnant women exposed to VZV infection more than 96 hours prior to investigation may be offered VZIG, but its efficacy is doubtful.

Efficacy of VZIG

In Enders' study, of 25 susceptible pregnant women who were exposed to VZV infection and were given VZIG, 20 (80%) women did not develop VZV infection in pregnancy.[11] No cases of CVS was reported in this group. In contrast, of 18 susceptible pregnant women who were exposed to VZV infection and did not receive VZIG, 16 (89 percent) women developed VZV infection. The study concluded that administration of VZIG not only reduces the risk of VZV infection in pregnancy after exposure but also effectively reduces the risk of CVS. Similarly, Hanngren and colleagues reported 33

Table 11-14 Management of VZV Infections and Exposures in Pregnancy

Pregnant woman exposed to VZV with questionable or no history of previous VZV

Confirm serology
(VZV-specific IgG)

↓ IgG +

Patient immune

↓ IgG −

Patient not immune
VZIG* 0.125 mg/kg IM
within 96 hours of exposure**
Observe for chickenpox

Pregnant woman with chickenpox infection

Infection in first 20 weeks of gestation
- Counsel 2–5% risk of CVS or very low risk of neonatal zoster
- Counsel risk for spontaneous abortion, prematurity, fetal demise, low birth weight
- Observe for complications (e.g., varicella pneumonia)
- Consider acyclovir therapy for severe pneumonia in mother (5–18 mg/kg IV every 8 hours)

Infection 5 days to 20 days prior to delivery
- Counsel low risk of neonatal varicella (chickenpox)
- Observe infant for chickenpox
- VZIG not indicated

Infection 5 days before to 2 days after birth
- Administer VZIG (1.25–2 ml IM) to infant immediately
- Counsel 30% risk of disseminated VZV in infant
- Observe infant for disseminated VZV
- Acyclovir or vidarabine for severe disseminated VZV

Pregnant woman with herpes zoster

Counsel probably low risk, if any, of CVS or neonatal zoster
VZIG not indicated
Symptomatic treatment

* Varicella immunoglobulin.
** VZIG may not be effective after 96 hours from exposure.

of 41 infants born to women who were exposed to VZV infection in pregnancy and who received VZIG were either not infected at birth or showed mild symptoms of VZV infection.[16] Two cases were severe and there were no infant deaths.

Pregnant Women with Chickenpox

Pregnant women who develop chickenpox in the first trimester should be warned about the low risk of CVS (about 2 to 5 percent). They should also be counseled on the controversial risk of spontaneous abortion, prematurity, fetal demise, and low birth weight following the infection. Those who acquire chickenpox 5 to 20 days prior to delivery should be informed as to the risk of neonatal varicella and informed that the latter is commonly mild. Those who acquire chickenpox 5 days before to 2 days after delivery should be counseled on the 30 percent risk of disseminated VZV in the infant. Infants born to these mothers should receive VZIG at a dose of 1.25 to 2 ml intramuscularly soon after birth. The infant should be observed closely for symptoms of disseminated VZV.

Mothers who develop primary VZV postnatally are at risk in transmitting the virus to their infants as well. Management includes isolation of the mother from the infant till the skin lesions begin to crust. Others have recommended prophylactic administration of VZIG to the infants in these cases, although its efficacy is also doubtful.

Pregnant Women with Varicella Pneumonia

Although there are no well-established protocols for the use of acyclovir in pregnancy, several case reports cite the successful management of varicella pneumonia in pregnancy with acyclovir therapy along with respiratory support.[6,10,22] Reported dosages range from 5 to 8 mg per kilogram intravenously every 8 hours.[6] There are presently no data bearing on the safety of using acyclovir in pregnancy. However, of reported cases of VZV pneumonia in pregnancy treated with acyclovir, there are no reports of an adverse fetal outcome.

Pregnant Women with Zoster

Pregnant women who develop zoster in pregnancy should be counseled on the very small risk of CVS to their infants. Management of zoster in pregnancy mainly consists of symptomatic relief from the painful lesions. It is advisable to confirm the diagnosis by viral culture or immunofluorescence antibody (IFA) to differentiate a zosteriform herpes simplex from zoster. VZIG is not recommended in women with recurrent zoster.[11]

Infant

Infants born to mothers who develop chickenpox 5 days before to 2 days after delivery should receive VZIG immediately after birth or within 24 to 48 hours of onset of maternal chickenpox. The recommended dose is 1.25 to 2.0 ml given intramuscularly. Immune serum globulin (1.0 to 1.5 ml per kilogram) may be used if VZIG is not readily available, although its efficacy may not be comparable.[19]

Infants with CVS are usually not infectious and therefore do not require isolation. Treatment should be directed to the organ damage resulting from VZV infection. Unfortunately, some of the clinical manifestations of CVS are irreversible.

The mortality rate of untreated disseminated VZV infection in neonates is about 30 percent. The use of acyclovir (500 mg per square meter of body surface) or vidarabine (10 mg per kilogram per day) in severely affected infants with disseminated VZV has been reported.[28] Infants with disseminated VZV infection are highly contagious and therefore require isolation. Therapy for these infants involves symptomatic treatment as well.

Conclusions

1. Four distinct clinical manifestations of VZV infection have been identified in infants whose mothers developed primary or recurrent VZV infection during pregnancy: (a) Congenital varicella syndrome (or CVS) occurs in about 2 to 5 percent of infants born to pregnant women who have had chickenpox in the first 20 weeks of gestation. CVS developing from maternal infection in the second half of pregnancy is extremely rare but has been reported. Also very rarely, recurrent VZV infection in the form of zoster complicating pregnancy has been reported to result in CVS. CVS commonly involves multiple organs, but findings frequently include cicatricial skin lesions following dermatomal patterns, limb paresis, chorioretinitis, and limb hypoplasia. (b) Disseminated VZV infection in infants occurs when maternal infection with VZV takes place from 5 days before delivery up to 2 days following delivery. The risk of fetal infection is about 25 to 30 percent, and the infection carries a mortality rate of 30 percent in untreated cases. (c) Neonatal varicella occurs when maternal chickenpox develops 5 days to 20 days prior to delivery. The course of this disease is usually mild. (d) Zoster has been reported in infants who otherwise have had no clinical history of primary VZV infection. This is believed to have originated from in utero infection of the fetus following maternal chickenpox.[11,26]

2. VZV infections in pregnant women are very infrequent (1 to 5 per 10,000) in industrialized societies, but 25 percent of all deaths due to VZV infection in all age groups belong to this group of individuals. Some studies suggest that pregnant women with VZV also may be at greater risk for developing complications such as varicella pneumonia.

3. Passive immunization with VZIG of the mother exposed to VZV infection reduces the risk of developing full-blown VZV infection.

4. Administration of VZIG to newborns of mothers infected near term reduces the risk of disseminated infection.

5. Acyclovir and vidarabine have been successfully used in the management of varicella pneumonia in pregnancy. Their toxic and teratogenic potential is not clearly defined at this time.

References

1. Alkalay AL, Pomerance JJ, Rimoin DL. Fetal varicella syndrome. J Pediatr 1987; 111:320–323.
2. Arbeter AM, Baker L, Starr SE, et al. Combination measles, mumps, rubella, and varicella vaccine. Pediatrics 1986; 78:742–747.
3. Asano Y, Itakura N, Hiroishi Y, et al. Viremia is present in incubation period in nonimmunocompromised children with varicella. J Pediatr 1985; 106:69–71.
4. Batik O and Stevens N. Varicella in pregnancy, J Fam Pract 1989; 28:315–321.
5. Bolognese RJ, Aldinger R, Roberts N. Prenatal care in the prevention of infection. Clin Perinatol 1981; 8:605–606.
6. Brown ZA, Baker DA. Acyclovir therapy during pregnancy. Obstetr Gynecol 1989; 73:526–531.
7. Brunell PA, Kotchmar GS. Zoster in infancy: failure to maintain virus latency following intrauterine infection. J Pediatr 1981; 98:71–73.
8. Brunell PA, Miller LH, Lovejoy F. Zoster in children. Am J Dis Child, 1968; 115:432–437.
9. Centers for Disease Control. Varicella-zoster immune globulin for the prevention of chickenpox: recommendations of the immunization practices advisory committee. Ann Intern Med 1984; 100:859–865.
10. Eder SE, Apuzzio JJ, Weiss G. Varicella pneumonia during pregnancy. Am J Perinatol 1988; 5:16–18.
11. Enders G. Varicella-zoster virus infection in pregnancy. Prog Med Virol 1984; 29:166–196.
12. Eyal A, Friedman M, Peretz BA, Paldi E. Pregnancy complicated by herpes zoster: a report of two cases and literature review. J Reprod Med 1983; 28:600–603.
13. Fox GN, Strangarity JW. Varicella-zoster virus infections in pregnancy, Am Fam Physician 1989; 39:89–98.
14. Friedman-Kien AE, LaFleur FL, Gendler E, et al. Herpes zoster: a possible early clinical sign for development of acquired immunodeficiency syndrome in high-risk individuals. J Am Acad Dermatol 1986; 14:1023–1028.
15. Guess HA, Broughton DD, Metton LJ, Kurland LT. Population-based studies of varicella complications. Pediatrics 1986; 78:723–727.
16. Hanngren K, Grandien M, Grunstrom G. Effect of zoster immunoglobulin for varicella prophylaxis in the newborn. Scand J Infect Dis 1985; 17:343–347.
17. Hanshaw JB, Dudgeon JA, Marshall WC. Viral disease of the fetus and newborn. Ed. 2, Philadelphia: WB Saunders Co, 1985; 161–174.
18. Harris RE, Rhoades ER. Varicella pneumonia complicating pregnancy: a report of a case and review of the literature. Obstetr Gynecol 1965; 25:734–740.
19. Herrmann KL. Congenital and perinatal varicella. Clin Obstet Gynecol 1982; 25:605–622.
20. Higa K, Dan K, Manabe H. Varicella-zoster virus infections during pregnancy: hypothesis concerning the mechanism of congenital malformations. Obstetr Gynecol 1987; 69:214–222.
21. Laforet EG, Lynch C. Multiple congenital defects following maternal varicella. N Engl J Med 1947; 236:534–537.
22. Landsberger EJ, Hager WD, Grossman JH. Successful management of varicella pneumonia complicating pregnancy. J Reprod Med 1986; 31:311–314.
23. McGregor JA, Mark S, Crawford GP, Levin MJ. Varicella-zoster antibody testing in the care of pregnant women exposed to varicella. Am J Obstet Gynecol 1987; 157:281–284.
24. Meyers JD. Congenital varicella in term infants: risk considered. J Infect Dis 1974; 129:215–218.
25. Miller HC, Clifford SH, Smith CA, et al. Study of the relation of congenital malformations to maternal rubella and other infections: preliminary report. Pediatrics 1949; 3:259–270.
26. Paryani SG, Arvin AM. Intrauterine infection with varicella-zoster virus after maternal varicella. N Engl J Med 1986; 314:1542–1546.
27. Prober CG, Arvin, AM. Perinatal viral infections. Eur J Clin Microbiol, 1987; 6:245–261.
28. Rosenfeld JA. Chickenpox and pregnancy: what are the risks? Postgrad Med 1989; 85(8):297–300.
29. Shehab ZM, Brunell PA. Susceptibility of hospital personnel to varicella-zoster virus. J Infect Dis 1984; 150:786.
30. Siegel M. Congenital malformations following chickenpox, measles, mumps, and hepatitis. JAMA 1973; 226:1521–1524.
31. Stagno S, Whitley RJ. Herpesvirus infections of pregnancy, part II: herpes simplex virus and varicella-zoster virus infections. N Engl J Med 1985; 313:1327–1330.
32. Strauss SE, Ostrove JM, Inchauspe G, et al. Varicella-zoster virus infections: biology, natural history, treatment, and prevention. Ann Intern Med 1988; 108:221–237.
33. Triebwasser JH, Harris RE, Bryant RE, Rhoades E. Varicella pneumonia in adults: report of seven cases and a review of literature. Medicine 1967; 46:409–423.
34. Webster MH, Smith CS. Congenital abnormalities and maternal herpes zoster. BMJ 1977; 2:1193.
35. Weller TH. Varicella and herpes zoster: changing concepts of the natural history, control and importance of a not-so-benign virus. N Engl J Med 1983; 309:1362–1368, 1434–1440.

CYTOMEGALOVIRUS INFECTIONS

Cytomegalovirus (CMV) is the most common congenital infection in the United States. About 40,000 infants are born annually with CMV infection.[8,29,35] Approximately 10 percent of these infants (about 4,000) each year are damaged by the virus. In the world, approximately 1 percent of all newborns are infected with CMV. Most infants have an asymptomatic infection in the neonatal period. The infection in these infants becomes apparent later when these infants present with mental retardation and/or deafness. Of the infants that are severely infected, 20 percent die from the infection.[29] Both primary infection and reactivation of a latent CMV infection in pregnant women have been associated with congenital CMV, but only the former has been linked to significant fetal and neonatal damage. Women who are child-care workers carry an 8 to 12 percent risk of infection with cytomegalovirus and therefore constitute a high-risk population who should be counseled when pregnant.

Epidemiology

Maternal Infection

The frequency of CMV antibody among pregnant women varies with geographic location, socioeconomic status, and occupation. For example, in the United States, Yow and associates[36] tested 4,578 pregnant women in Texas of middle and upper socioeconomic status over a period of 5 years and found that 48 percent were seronegative. The seroconversion rate was 2.2 percent. In studies in Great Britain the rate of susceptible (seronegative) pregnant women ranged from 42 to 46 percent.[10,11,20] The seroconversion rate during pregnancy ranged from 0.7 to 3.7 percent.[2,10,27] However, in some tropical areas infection rates approach 100 percent in early childhood.

Several epidemiologic studies showed higher rates of congenital infection when the frequency of maternal antibody is highest.[4,17,18,27,29] Factors that may explain this finding are that (1) more maternal infections mean a higher likelihood of primary infection in pregnancy and thus a higher likelihood of perinatal infection, and (2) more maternal infections mean a higher rate of reactivation during pregnancy.

Several studies also indicate that the rate of congenital CMV infections is higher in women of low socioeconomic status than in women of middle or upper socioeconomic status; this was observed in mothers who had *reactivation* of a CMV infection but not in mothers who developed *primary* CMV infection during pregnancy.[8,29]

Congenital Infection

On the average, 0.4 to 2.3 percent of all births globally are complicated by congenital CMV infection.[8,36] Primary infection with CMV in pregnancy has been reported to have a 20 to 50 percent transmission rate.[2,12,20,31] Of these, approximately 1 to 2 percent result in overt congenital CMV disease presenting at birth. Pregnancies complicated by reactivation of a latent CMV infection result in congenital CMV infection in approximately 0.5 to 1 percent of cases.

Neonatally Acquired CMV Infection

There is a positive correlation between the frequency of maternal antibody and CMV infections acquired in the first year of life.[21] Forty-one of 123 infants (33 percent) born to seropositive mothers developed subclinical CMV infections within the first year of life, compared to only 5 of 123 (4 percent) of CMV-seronegative mothers.[21] Two of the latter five infants probably acquired the infection from transfusion with documented CMV-positive blood. In Finland, where the maternal seroprevalence rate is about 82 percent,[9] 32 percent of 128 infants developed CMV infections by the first year of life. It appears, then, that about one-third of infants born to seropositive mothers acquire the infection in the home during the first year of life.

Two other factors that correlate with the rate of acquired CMV infections are breast-feeding and the rate of maternal cervical shedding of CMV.[21,23] Among seropositive mothers, the odds ratio for infants acquiring CMV within 1 year in breast-fed infants over non-breast-fed infants is 2.3 (95 percent confidence interval).[21] Mothers who consistently shed virus in cervical secretions were also shown to more likely to have children with neonatally acquired CMV infections.[23]

Biology

Cytomegalovirus is a member of the *Herpesvirus* group. The virus has an icosahedral capsid of 162 capsomeres.[33] The genome contains double-stranded DNA of about 240 kilobases and encodes for about 25 to 35 structural proteins. The name *cytomegalic inclusion disease* is derived from the virus's ability to induce cellular cytomegalia or "swelling" of infected cells. The virus also has the ability to produce characteristic intranuclear and cytoplasmic inclusion bodies in infected cells.

Human fibroblasts are the most efficient tissue cultures for the propagation of the CMV virus.[25] In vitro studies of CMV infectivity demonstrated that the spread of infection is primarily through direct cell-to-cell infection.[33] At least three closely related antigenic types of CMV infect humans.[32]

Routes of Transmission

Horizontal transmission of CMV occurs primarily through infected respiratory secretions, infected urine, and sexual contact and less frequently through blood transfusions and tissue transplantations.[1,13,14,28,34] Nasopharyngeal secretions and urine are common sources of CMV among children in day-care centers.[19] Both semen and cervical secretions have been implicated in the horizontal spread of CMV as well.[13,29]

Maternal-to-fetal transmission of CMV appears to take place through several routes: (1) transplacentally by direct infection of fetal trophoblast; (2) via an ascending infection from the cervix, which may be infected; or (3) by direct fetal contact with infected maternal secretions (such as from the cervix or urine) during delivery. Postnatal infection occurs through contact of the infant with the mother or from infected breast milk. Asymptomatic cervical shedding of CMV in pregnant women can be substantial. In one study 7.6 percent of pregnant women in the third trimester were found to be asymptomatically shedding virus from the cervix compared to 2.6 percent of women in the first trimester.[29] Three to 9 percent of pregnant women in the third trimester were also found to be seropositive for CMV.[29] Overall, about 3 percent of all pregnant women shed CMV from the cervix near the time of delivery, and 1 percent of all newborns are infected at the time of birth. However, a high percentage of uninfected newborns (up to 33 percent) become infected shortly after birth.

Clinical Manifestations

Mother

Maternal infection with CMV is almost always asymptomatic. A few pregnant women, however, present with a heterophile-negative mononucleosis-type syndrome. These patients usually have fever, pharyngitis, generalized malaise, lymphadenopathy, and other nonspecific constitutional symptoms. There is usually no hepatosplenomegaly, although a mild hepatitis with slight elevation in liver enzymes may be seen. There is no clear evidence that pregnancy increases the risk of CMV infection in women.

Following primary infection, CMV usually become latent. Reactivation of a latent CMV infection often occurs in pregnant women but is almost always asymptomatic. Reactivated CMV has been associated with congenital CMV infections, although symptomatic neonatal disease usually results from a primary infection in the pregnant women.

Infant

About 1 percent of all newborns are congenitally infected with CMV. Most are asymptomatic at birth. Approximately 10 percent of infants with asymptomatic congenital CMV infections are later found to have hearing loss, mental retardation, or both. Less often, congenitally infected infants are symptomatic at birth and are diagnosed as having cytomegalic inclusion disease. This occurs in about 1 per 10,000 births in the United States. Table 11-15 summarizes both early and late findings in infants with severe congenital CMV. Almost all affected children reflect a primary infection in the mother.[18] Infections earlier in pregnancy are more likely to cause severe congenital CMV.[28] Acute infection is followed by viral shedding in the urine and nasopharynx that may persist for several years.

Table 11-15 Clinical Manifestations of Severe Congenital CMV Infection*

Early findings	Late findings
Thrombocytopenia	Mental retardation
Hepatosplenomegaly	Hearing loss
Purpura (petechial rash)	Learning disability
Jaundice	Neuromuscular defects
Hemolytic anemia	Psychomotor retardation
Hepatitis	
Cerebral calcifications	**Findings that may present as an early or late finding**
Seizures	Chorioretinitis
Cerebellar or cerebral atrophy	Optic atrophy
Microphthalmia	Dental defects
Intrauterine growth retardation	Spasticity
Interstitial pneumonia	Microencephaly
Pneumonitis	
Mononucleosis-like illness	
Cardiovascular lesions	
Gastrointestinal defects	

*All bold-faced findings are those most frequently recognized in severe congenital CMV infection.

Diagnosis

Mother

Most primary CMV infections in pregnant women are asymptomatic. The rare symptomatic patient has nonspecific clinical findings, such as a mononucleosis-like syndrome. For this reason, unless routine serial antibody titers are obtained, most primary infections are unrecognized. In the United States, one-third to two-thirds of all pregnant women have antibody to CMV, indicating that they have had a prior infection and thus carry latent virus. Patients with symptoms can be tested for IgM-specific antibody to confirm the diagnosis of an acute CMV infection, but only 80 percent of primary CMV infections demonstrate CMV-specific IgM antibody.[30] In addition, 20 percent of women with reactivation also show CMV-specific IgM. Seroconversion of pregnant women may be useful in the diagnosis of acute CMV, but this requires testing sera obtained before and during the acute phase for CMV IgG antibody.

Virus culture is the most specific diagnostic test for documenting maternal infections. However, culture of the virus does not differentiate a primary from a recurrent CMV infection. Cultures should be taken from the cervix, vagina, and urine.

Recent advances in molecular technology have enabled the detection of CMV DNA sequences through in situ hybridization[16,24,26] and polymerase chain reaction.[5,7,24] These applications of molecular biology research appear promising for the accurate diagnosis of CMV infections.

Routine testing for CMV in pregnant women is not recommended by the authors for the following reasons: (1) To establish a primary infection, serial antibody titrations would have to be made on all women beginning early in pregnancy to identify the 2 percent who have a primary infection. Less than 10 percent of this 2 percent would have an affected child and most of these would be mildly affected; (2) for recurrent infections, virus isolation would have to be used, and almost all of the infected children born to these cases are asymptomatic. The authors recommend that women with symptomatic disease be tested for IgM antibody and that virus isolation be obtained to confirm the diagnosis. Molecular techniques such as those described previously are being investigated for in utero diagnosis of CMV infection.

Infant

Almost all congenital CMV infections are asymptomatic. Clinical findings of the rare symptomatic infants are given in Table 11-15. Presence of CMV-specific IgM is helpful to confirm the diagnosis, but only 80 percent of congenitally affected infants demonstrate this antibody. Virus culture of the infant's urine and nasopharynx is the best method to confirm the diagnosis. Several reports describe the use of the polymerase chain reaction to detect CMV in the urine of infected infants.[7]

Prenatal diagnosis of CMV may be established by measurement of CMV-specific IgM antibody from cordocentesis samples. Hogge and associates reported a CMV-specific IgM antibody titer of 1:256 in a cordocentesis sample from a 36-week hydropic infant suspected of having CMV infection.[15] Virus has also been recovered from amniotic fluid.[6]

Treatment

Mother

Asymptomatic pregnant women need no specific therapy. Treatment of maternal symptoms, when present, is symptomatic. Use of antiviral drugs such as acyclovir in the treatment of symptomatic pregnant women has not been established.

Infant

There is presently no established protocol for the treatment of congenital CMV. Antiviral agents such as acyclovir and vidarabine have very limited use in severe congenital CMV and appear only to suppress the infection. Ganciclovir, an analogue of acyclovir, has been used in the management of CMV-induced chorioretinitis.[3] Ganciclovir works by interrupting viral DNA production, as well as in viral packaging.[3] Ganciclovir has been found to reduce viral shedding in symptomatic infants, but the suppression is effective only while the patient is under treatment. Foscarnet (phosphonoformic acid) has also been shown to have activity against CMV infections, specifically in reducing viral shedding. Infected symptomatic infants need to be placed in isolation while in the nursery.

Prevention

A live attenuated CMV vaccine (Towne strain) has been developed and used experimentally in renal transplant patients.[22,36] Plotkin and colleagues studied prospective renal transplant patients who were susceptible to CMV infection and received either a placebo vaccine or the Towne strain vaccine.[22] Only 6 percent of patients who received the vaccine developed acute CMV infection, compared to 35 percent of those who received placebo. However, currently there are no vaccines available for use in susceptible individuals or pregnant women.

The most important approach to prevent congenital CMV is to minimize infection among serosusceptible pregnant women. Approximately 2 percent of women in the United States develop a primary infection with CMV during pregnancy. Proper handwashing techniques and extra care in handling infected body fluids should be used to minimize exposure to CMV during pregnancy.

Conclusions

1. Cytomegalovirus is the most common congenital infection in the United States, and 40,000 infants are infected annually.
2. About 2 percent of pregnant women develop primary infection with CMV. Reactivation of latent infections in pregnant women results in another 1 percent of infected women (total of 3 percent). Approximately one-third of these infected women transmit the infection to their infants. This results in 1 percent of all newborns being infected at birth. About 10 percent of these infected infants later show some damage, mainly some degree of hearing loss and mental retardation. Severe congenital CMV apparent at birth occurs in about 1 of 10,000 births.
3. The great majority of primary infections with CMV in adults are asymptomatic. Both primary and latent CMV infections in pregnancy have been associated with congenital CMV infection. However, significant damage to the child rarely results from latent CMV infections in pregnancy.
4. Routine screening for antibody to CMV is not presently recommended by the authors.

References

1. Adler SP, Chandrika T, Lawrence L, Baggett J. Cytomegalovirus infections in neonates acquired by blood transfusions. Pediatr Infect Dis J 1983; 2:114–118.
2. Ahlfors K, Ivarsson SA, Johnson T, Svanberg L. Primary and secondary maternal cytomegalovirus infections and their relation to congenital infection: analysis of maternal sera. Acta Paediatr Scand 1982; 71:109–113.
3. Alford CA, Stagno S, Pass RF, Britt WJ. Congenital and perinatal cytomegalovirus infections. Rev Infect Dis 1990; 12:S745–S753.

4. Andersen HK, Brostrom K, Hansen KB and others. A prospective study on the incidence and significance of congenital cytomegalovirus infection. Acta Paediatr Scand 1979; 68:329–336.
5. Buffone GJ, Hine E, Demmler GJ. Detection of mRNA from the immediate early gene of human cytomegalovirus in infected cells by in vitro amplification. Mol Cell Probes 1990; 4:143–146.
6. Davis LE, Tweed GV, Chin RD, Miller GL. Intrauterine diagnosis of cytomegalovirus infection: viral recovery from amniocentesis fluid. Am J Obstetr Gynecol 1971; 109:1217–1219.
7. Demmler GJ, Buffone GJ, Schimbor CM, May RA. Detection of cytomegalovirus in urine from newborns by using polymerase chain reaction DNA amplification. J Infect Dis 1988; 158:1177–1184.
8. Freij BJ, Sever JL. Herpesvirus infections in pregnancy: risk to embryo, fetus, and neonate. Clin Perinatol 1988; 15:203–231.
9. Granstrom M, Leinikki P, Santavuori P, Pettay O. Perinatal cytomegalovirus infection in man. Arch Dis Child 1977; 52:354–359.
10. Grant S, Edmond E, Syme J. A prospective study of cytomegalovirus infections in pregnancy: laboratory evidence of congenital infection following maternal primary and reactivated infection. J Infect 1981; 3:24–29.
11. Griffiths P, Baboonian C, Ashby D. The demographic characteristics of pregnant women infected with cytomegalovirus. Int J Epidemiol, 1985; 14:447–452.
12. Griffiths PD, Baboonian C. A prospective study of primary cytomegalovirus infection during pregnancy: a final report. Br J Obstet Gynaecol 1984; 91:307–315.
13. Handsfield HH, Chandler SH, Caine VA, et al. Cytomegalovirus infection in sex partners: evidence for sexual transmission. J Infect Dis 1985; 151:344–348.
14. Ho M, Suwansirkul S, Dowling JN, et al. The transplanted kidney as a source of cytomegalovirus infection. N Engl J Med 1975; 293:1109–1112.
15. Hogge WA, Tweed GV, Chin TD, Harbert GM. Fetal evaluation by percutaneous blood sampling. Am J Obstet Gynecol 1988; 158:132–136.
16. Lohr JM, Oldstone MB. Detection of cytomegalovirus nucleic acid sequences in pancreas in type 2 diabetes. Lancet 1990; 336:644–648.
17. MacDonald H, Tobin JO. Congenital cytomegalovirus infection: a collaborative study on epidemiological, clinical and laboratory findings. Dev Med Child Neurol 1978; 20:471–82.
18. Montgomery J, Mason JR, Williamson AP, et al. Prospective study of congenital cytomegalovirus infection. South Med J 1980; 73:590–595.
19. Pass RF, Little EA, Stagno S, et al. Young children as a probable source of maternal and congenital cytomegalovirus infection. N Engl J Med 1987; 316:1366–1370.
20. Peckham CS, Chin KS, Coleman JC, et al. Cytomegalovirus infection in pregnancy: preliminary findings from a prospective study. Lancet 1983; 1:1352–1355.
21. Peckham CS, Johnson C, Ades A, et al. Early acquisition of cytomegalovirus infection. Arch Dis Child 1987; 62:780–785.
22. Plotkin SA, Friedman HM, Fleisher GR, et al. Towne-vaccine-induced prevention of cytomegalovirus disease after renal transplants. Lancet 1984; 1:528–530.
23. Reynolds DW, Stagno S, Hosty TS, et al. Maternal cytomegalovirus excretion and perinatal infection. N Engl J Med 1973; 289:1–5.
24. Shibata DS, Martin WJ, Appleman MD, et al. Detection of cytomegalovirus DNA in peripheral blood of patients infected with human immunodeficiency virus. J Infect Dis 1988; 158:1185–1192.
25. Smith MG. Propagation in tissue cultures of a cytopathogenic virus from human salivary gland virus (SGV) disease. Proc Soc Exp Biol Med 1956; 92:424–430.
26. Sorbello AF, Elmendorf SL, McSharry JJ, et al. Rapid detection of cytomegalovirus by fluorescent monoclonal antibody staining and *in situ* DNA hybridization in a dram vial cell culture system. J Clin Microbiol 1988; 26:1111–1114.
27. Stagno S, Pass RF, Dworsky ME, et al. Congenital cytomegalovirus infection: the importance of primary and recurrent maternal infection. N Engl J Med 1982; 306:945–949.
28. Stagno S, Pass RF, Cloud G, et al. Primary cytomegalovirus infection in pregnancy: incidence, transmission to fetus and clinical outcome. JAMA 1984; 256:1904–1908.
29. Stagno S, Pass RF, Dworsky ME, Alford CA. Maternal cytomegalovirus infection and perinatal transmission. Clin Obstet Gynecol 1982; 25:563–576.
30. Stagno S, Tinker MK, Elrod C, et al. Immunoglobulin M antibodies detected by enzyme-linked immunosorbent assay and radioimmunoassay in the diagnosis of cytomegalovirus infections in pregnant women and newborn infants. J Clin Microbiol 1985; 21:930–935.
31. Stern H, Tucker SM. Prospective study of cytomegalovirus infection in pregnancy. BMJ 1973; 2:268–270.
32. Volk WA. Essentials of medical microbiology. Ed 2, Philadelphia, JB Lippincott, 1982: 578–580.
33. Weller TH. The cytomegaloviruses: ubiquitous agents with protean clinical manifestations (part 1 of 2). N Engl J Med 1977; 285:203–214.
34. Yeager AS, Grumet FC, Hafleigh EB, et al. Prevention of transfusion-acquired cytomegalovirus infection in newborn infants. J Pediatr 1981; 98:281–287.
35. Yow MD. Congenital cytomegalovirus disease: a NOW problem. J Infect Dis 1989; 159:163–167.
36. Yow MD, Williamson DW, Leeds LJ, et al. Epidemiologic characteristics of cytomegalovirus infection in mothers and their infants. Am J Obstet Gynecol 1984; 158:1189–1195.

HEPATITIS B VIRUS INFECTIONS

Globally, it is estimated that approximately 200 million people are chronic carriers of hepatitis B virus (HBV). The annual incidence of HBV infections in this country is about 200,000 cases. Infants born to mothers who developed acute HBV infection near term or who are chronic HBV carriers are at significant risk for acquiring HBV infection at delivery and becoming chronic carriers of HBV themselves later on. Long-term sequelae from chronic HBV infection have included hepatocellular carcinoma and cirrhosis of the liver. Because of the worldwide prevalence of the disease and the significant risks of newborn hepatitis, cancer, and cirrhosis, interruption of the transmission of HBV from the infected mother to her child is a primary goal for obstetricians and pediatricians.

Epidemiology

Viral hepatitis infections, primarily HBV, are among the most prevalent infectious diseases in the world. In endemic areas such as Southeast Asia, sub-Saharan Africa, the Pacific islands, and Haiti, the prevalence of chronic carriers is as high as 15 percent. Among Alaskan Eskimos, the rate of chronic HBV carriers is 14 percent. In the continental United States the rate is about 0.5 percent.[4]

Approximately 16,500 infants are born each year in the United States to mothers who are either chronic HBV carriers or who have had acute HBV infection near delivery. These infants are at significant risk of acquiring HBV infection.[9]

In a prospective study of approximately 22,700 Taiwanese middle-aged men, chronic HBV carriers were 200-fold more at risk for developing hepatocellular carcinoma than noncarriers.[2,4] These male chronic carriers were also found to be significantly at risk for liver cirrhosis later on in life.

Biology

Hepatitis B virus is a member of the family *Hepadnaviridae*. The virus contains a partially double-stranded DNA of about 3,200 kilobases. HBV is highly species-specific, infecting only humans and a few nonhuman primates.[22] The intact virion or "Dane particle" consists of outer and inner shells. The outer shell, which measures about 42 nm, contains a serologically detectable coating called *hepatitis B surface antigen* (HB_sAg). This antigen, formerly called the *Australian antigen,* was discovered in 1965 by Blumberg and associates[7] in the serum of an Australian aborigine. The inner shell of the virus contains the *hepatitis B core antigen* (HB_cAg), the viral genome, and another antigen called *hepatitis B e antigen* (HB_eAg). Both HB_sAg and HB_eAg can be detected serologically, whereas HB_cAg cannot. In addition, HB_eAg is detected only in patients who are positive for the HB_sAg.

HBV has a special predilection for hepatocytes, although the virus has been reported to infect leukocytes and pancreatic cells.[22] There are usually no cytopathic effects seen following infection of the host cell by HBV.

There are four other types of hepatitis virus: hepatitis A (HAV), hepatitis D or delta virus, and two types of non-A, non-B hepatitis virus (hepatitis C and enterically transmitted non-A, non-B hepatitis). Both HAV and hepatitis D are RNA viruses. Hepatitis D has been found only in chronic carriers of HBV and is endemic in Italy and the Middle East. Non-A, non-B hepatitis is now recognized to be due to hepatitis C and, less frequently, to other non-A, non-B, and non-C hepatitis viruses that are presently not seriologically detectable. Laboratory tests are now available to detect antibody to hepatitis A, B, and C.

Natural Course of Antigen and Antibody Production to HBV Infection

The course of antigen and antibody production following infection with HBV is shown in Figure 11-1. An understanding of these changes is necessary for the diagnosis of acute and chronic HBV infection.

Following parenteral or sexual exposure to HBV, the incubation period is about 45 to 150 days, after which clinical symptoms may appear. Antigenemia with HB_sAg usually precedes the onset of clinical findings by 4 to 7 days. HB_eAg may also be detected about the time that HB_sAg appears in the patient's sera. This period of antigenemia is followed by a rise in HBV-specific anti-HB_c IgM and IgG antibody. Complete recovery from HBV is serologically manifested by the disappearance of HB_sAg and the appearance of HB_sAB. There may be a period during which the patient has lost detectable HB_sAg, and HB_sAB has not yet appeared. This period is the "window" when HBV infection cannot be detected by these methods. However, patients who have had acute

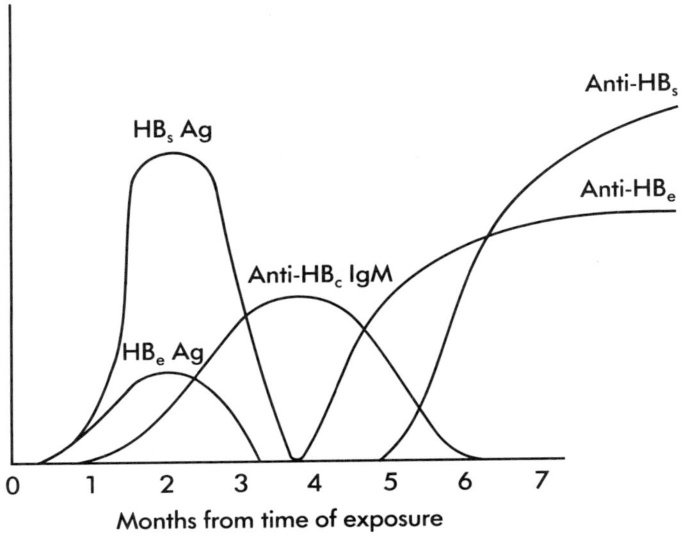

Figure 11-1 Serologic course and humoral response to acute HBV infection. HB_sAg, hepatitis B surface antigen; HB_eAg, hepatitis B e antigen; anti-HB_s, anti-hepatitis B surface antibody; antiHB_c, anti-hepatitis B core IgM antibody; anti-HB_e, anti-hepatitis B e antibody.

Table 11-16 Risk Factors for Hepatitis B Virus Infections

Geographic location (Southeast Asian, Pacific islander, Haitian, sub-Saharan African, Alaskan Eskimo)
Intravenous drug abuser
Male homosexual
History of liver disease
History of transfusion of blood or blood components
Individuals on dialysis or organ-transplant recipients
Individuals with multiple and repeated sexually transmitted diseases
Institutionalized and/or mentally handicappped individuals
Individuals exposed by household contact to persons with acute infection or to chronic carriers
Health care personnel

infection can be identified during this window by the presence of anti-HB_c IgM antibody.

The chronic carrier state occurs when there is persistent detectable HB_sAg for longer than 6 months. These individuals may or may not have persistent HB_eAg as well. There is production of HB_cAB but not HB_sAB. These individuals are a potential source of infection via both horizontal and vertical transmission and are at significant risk for long-term sequelae such as liver cirrhosis and hepatocellular carcinoma.[2]

Routes of Transmission

Mother

Horizontal transmission of HBV occurs through either parenteral exposure to infected materials or sexual contact. Infectious HBV particles have been identified in serum, saliva, and semen.[22] Individuals at increased risk for HBV infection are shown in Table 11-16. The secondary infection rate among spouses of chronic HBV carriers is 25 percent.[15] Accidental needle stick among health care personnel, tattooing, acupuncture, and dental surgery are all possible routes of transmission.

Infant

Mother-to-fetus transmission of HBV infection was first reported by Stokes and colleagues[33] in 1951. Since then, a significant body of literature has confirmed the role of vertical transmission in the spread of HBV infection.[1,6,24,25,32] In fact, globally, perinatal transmission probably represents the most prevalent route of transmission of HBV.

The majority of perinatal infections occur during the delivery process, when there is significant neonatal exposure to HBV either transplacentally or through contact with infectious secretions such as maternal blood. A minority of infants may be infected in utero.[39] Transplacental leakage of HB_eAg-positive maternal blood to the fetus has been reported.[17] Fetal swallowing at the time of delivery has been postulated as a possible route of infection.[16,28] The evidence for this is that more than 90 percent of gastric aspirates from infants born to mothers who are positive for both HB_sAg and HB_eAg were also positive for HB_sAg.[16]

Table 11-17 Risk of Perinatal Transmission of HBV Associated with Maternal HBV Status

Mother	Infection Rate in Infants
Acute infection at or near delivery	50–60%
Chronic infection	
HB_sAg+ only	12–25%
HB_sAg *and* HB_eAg+	70–90%

Assessment of Perinatal Risk

Table 11-17 summarizes the levels of risk for mothers transmitting HBV to their infants. Pregnant women who develop acute HBV infection near or at delivery carry a 50 to 60 percent risk of having an infected infant.[28] Pregnant women who are chronic carriers (persistent HB_sAg positive) have a transmission rate that is dependent on whether they are HB_eAg positive. Pregnant women who are positive for *both* antigens carry the highest risk for transmitting HBV (70 to 90 percent.)[5,21,29,31] Pregnant women who are HB_sAg positive but HB_eAg negative have a significantly reduced risk of perinatal transmission (10 to 25 percent).[5,20,21,28] *Clearly, presence of HB_eAg in a pregnant woman significantly increases the risk of her transmitting HBV to her infant.*

Of those infected infants born to pregnant women who carry both HB_sAg and HB_eAg, 80 to 90 percent become chronic HB_sAg carriers.[5,21,30,31,32]

Clinical Manifestations

Mother

Acute HBV infection in adults results in symptoms in 50 percent of cases. After an incubation period of 2 to 6 months, systemic symptoms may develop that include nausea, vomiting, malaise, myalgia, anorexia, right upper quadrant pain, and low-grade fever. The physical findings are not diagnostic. Patients may have clinical jaundice, hepatic tenderness, light-colored stools, and dark urine, but no other findings. Occasionally, a serum sickness-like illness develops that includes urticaria, arthralgia, and arthritis.[29] The clinical disease may last from 3 to 4 weeks but has been reported to persist as long as 6 months. Laboratory findings include mildly elevated hepatic enzymes. The serologic findings have been described earlier in this chapter.

After acute infection with HBV, 90 percent of cases undergo complete recovery with production of HB_sAB detectable in sera. Fewer than 10 percent of cases progress to a chronic carrier state in which there is persistent HB_sAg without production of HB_sAB. The carrier state may be lifelong. Fulminant hepatitis occurs in less than 1 percent of cases of acute infection and carries a 70 to 80 percent mortality.[22] Progression to fulminant hepatitis commonly presents as hepatic encephalopathy.

There is considerable evidence for the association between chronic HBV infection and hepatocellular carcinoma.[3,4,19,26,34] In several reports, 40 to 80 percent of patients who developed hepatocellular carcinoma were HB_sAg carriers.[3,34] The relative risk for developing hepatocellular carcinoma among HB_sAg-positive carriers in one study was 223 as compared to HB_sAg-negative controls.[4]

Infant

At birth, the great majority of HBV-infected children are asymptomatic.[23,28] The rare symptomatic infant may present with jaundice and mild elevation of liver transaminases. Of 200 infants found to have perinatal HBV infection documented by development of HB_sAg, only one infant had symptomatic hepatitis.[29]

Serious sequelae of perinatal infection include fulminant hepatitis B infection and chronic active hepatitis.[9,11] An equally significant sequela from long-term chronic HBV infection following perinatal acute infection is the increased risk of developing hepatocellular carcinoma and liver cirrhosis. Beasley and associates reported that the annual incidence of hepatocellular carcinoma in 22,700 Taiwanese males studied was 3.5 per 1,000 among HB_sAg carriers compared to 0.015 per 1,000 among HB_sAg-negative controls.[4] In the same study, 17 of 19 patients who died from liver cirrhosis were chronic HB_sAg carriers. Without a previous history of cirrhosis, patients who were chronic carriers were fivefold more at risk for death from cirrhosis than HB_sAg-negative patients.[4] Primary hepatocellular carcinoma has been reported in a 5-year-old child following HBV infection during delivery of the mother.[35]

There is no strong association between primary HBV infection in pregnancy with congenital malformations, stillbirth, miscarriage, and intrauterine growth retardation.[13,27] One study reported an increased prematurity rate among pregnancies complicated with acute HBV infection in the third trimester as compared to noninfected controls.[13]

Diagnosis

Mother

Clinical symptoms of HBV infection in pregnant women are not pathognomonic for hepatitis B virus infection. Therefore, a thorough study of viral and nonviral etiologies of hepatitis should be undertaken. Screening tests should include HB_sAg, HB_cAB, HB_sAB, and hepatitis A IgG and IgM. The diagnosis of HBV can be confirmed by serology.

Pregnant women with acute HBV infection first have HB_sAg. HB_cAB is detectable within days after HB_sAg appears. HB_sAB then becomes detectable 4 to 5 days after HB_sAg has disappeared.

In situ hybridization techniques for viral genome sequences have shown HBV genome sequences in hepatocellular carcinoma cells.[8,26]

Infant

Presence of HB_sAg in cord blood or fetal blood is usually diagnostic of fetal infection. A small proportion of infants are infected in utero and have HB_sAg in the cord blood. Infants who acquire HBV infection during delivery are HB_sAg negative at birth. Follow-up serology of these infants shows HB_sAg by 1 month of age.[29] Clinical symptomatology is often unreliable in infants because of the high asymptomatic rate of infection.

Management

Mother

Acute uncomplicated symptomatic infections with HBV are usually self-limited, and full recovery occurs in 3 to 4 months. Pregnant women who develop acute symptoms should be treated symptomatically. Patients should be observed for development of fulminant hepatitis, which usually presents with neurologic symptoms such as encephalopathy or with symptoms of severe liver damage such as a blood coagulopathy. Patients are usually infectious until HB_sAg disappears, and caution should be used in the handling and disposal of infected blood, needles, and body fluids.

Infant

Most children are asymptomatic and require no treatment. Symptomatic infants usually also have a self-limited course and should be managed with symptomatic therapy. No special isolation is required for infected infants except proper caution and disposal of blood, needles, and body fluids.

Prevention

The prevention of transmission of HBV from the mother to the infant requires the recognition of the infection in the mother through the use of routine testing for HB_sAg and the judicious use of hepatitis B immune globulin (HBIG) and hepatitis B vaccine (Heptavax, Recombivax, or Engerix-B) for the infant (Fig. 11-2).

Hepatitis B Immune Globulin

The recommended dose for HBIG is 0.5 ml given intramuscularly at birth to infants born to pregnant women who are either chronic carriers or develop acute HBV near term. Infants treated with three doses of HBIG at birth, 3 months, and 6 months had a substantially lower percentage of chronic carrier state (22.5 percent) as compared to infants who received placebo (91.4 percent chronic carrier state) or to infants who received only one dose of HBIG (50 percent chronic carrier state).[5,29]

Hepatitis B Vaccine

Heptavax (Merck Sharp & Dohme) was licensed in 1981. It was prepared from pooled sera of individuals with high titers of HB_sAg. The seroconversion rate of susceptible individuals after three doses was greater than 90 percent.[22] The usual dose is 10 mcg (1 ml) given intramuscularly and repeated at 1 month and 6 months. This material, however, is no longer being manufactured, and the limited supplies that remain have been reserved for individuals who have allergies to yeast. Recombivax (Merck Sharp & Dohme) was licensed in 1986 and is derived from *Saccharomyces cerevisiae* into which has been introduced the HBV gene sequence responsible for HB_sAg production.[22] The usual dose is 10 mcg (1 ml) for adults over 20 years given intramuscularly and repeated at 1 month and 6 months. The dose for newborns up to 10 years of age is 2.5 mcg (0.25 ml) given intramuscularly at the same schedule. Use of HBIG along with three doses of Recombivax prevented primary HBV infection in more than 90 percent at 6 months of age.

Engerix-B (Smith Kline & French) was recently introduced and is also a noninfectious recombinant DNA hepatitis B vaccine derived from *Saccharomyces cerevisiae*. The adult dose (11 years and older) is 20 mcg (1 ml) given intramuscularly and repeated at 1 month and 6 months. The dose for newborns and children up to 10 years is 10 mcg (0.5 ml) given intramuscularly at the same dosing schedule.

Recommendations for Prevention of HBV Transmission

Figure 11-2 summarizes the recommendations for preventing the transmission of HBV from the pregnant woman to her child.[9,14,18]

1. *Routine screening of all pregnant women.* The Centers for Disease Control (CDC) and the American College of Obstetricians and Gynecologists (ACOG) recommend universal screening of pregnant women for HB_sAg early in pregnancy. Several reports have shown the problem with risk-directed screening for HBV infection.[10,12,14,18] Cruz and associates showed that the prevalence of HB_sAg in pregnant women in Gainesville, Florida, was 0.54 percent.[10] In this study, 67 percent of pregnant women who tested positive for HB_sAg had no risk factors for HBV infection and would have been missed if screening were directed only at "at-risk" pregnancies. The difficulty in universal screening is the cost in areas where the incidence of HBV and the chronic carrier state is very low. The test may not be available, especially for women who have not had prenatal care.
2. *Protection of infants of HB_s Ag-positive women with HBIG and HBV vaccine.* Infants born to women who are shown to be chronic carriers of HBV or become infected when pregnant should receive HBIG within 12 hours of birth, followed by HBV vaccine immediately and repeated at 1 month and 6 months. Serologic tests for HB_sAg and HB_sAB should then be done at 10 to 15 months to assess the infant's immune response to the vaccine and the effectiveness of the program. Household

Screen *all* pregnant women for HB_sAg as early as possible (if no prenatal screening was done, obtain one at the time of admission for delivery)

↓ HB_sAg −

Retest later in pregnancy if clinical symptoms develop, or history of exposure to HBV, or high-risk behavior in pregnant women

↓ HB_sAg +

Administer HBIG immediately and 3 doses of HBV vaccine to the child

Figure 11-2 Recommendations for prevention of HBV transmission and management of HBV in pregnancy.

members of pregnant women who develop acute HBV infection should also be screened for HB_sAg and, if susceptible, should be offered the vaccine. Mothers who test positive for HB_sAg shortly after delivery or postnatally should have their infants screened for HB_sAg. Infants who are HB_sAg-negative should receive HBIG and HBV vaccine.

3. *Route of delivery*. There is at present no association between route of delivery and risk of perinatal HBV transmission. Hence, the decision to perform cesarean delivery should be made for obstetric reasons only.
4. *Isolation of infected individuals*. Mothers and infants with acute HBV infection do not require special isolation except for blood, needle, and body fluid precautions.

Non-HBV Viruses and Perinatal Transmission

Hepatitis A virus (HAV) is a 27-nm RNA virus that is transmitted horizontally primarily through the fecal-oral route. Clinical symptoms are generally similar to HBV infection. The diagnosis of HAV can be confirmed by presence of anti-HAV IgM or IgG. There is at present no evidence of fetal or perinatal infection following HAV infection in pregnant women. Infants born to mothers who have acute infection during delivery should receive 0.5 ml of immune serum globulin (ISG) at birth and at 1 month.

Non-A, non-B hepatitis virus is most commonly transmitted through transfusion of infected blood. This group of viruses have recently been classified further into hepatitis C and enterically transmitted non-A, non-B hepatitis viruses. An ELISA test for anti-hepatitis C virus (HCV) antibody is presently available.[37] The clinical course of HCV resembles that of HBV. The possibility of mother-to-fetus transmission of non-A, non-B hepatitis has been suggested but is not definitive.[36,38] Wejstal and Norkrans studied 14 pregnancies complicated by chronic non-A, non-B hepatitis and identified eight infants with elevated transaminases before 1 year of life, suggesting the possibility of mother-to-infant transmission of this virus.[38] Treatment of an exposed infant is debatable but may be reasonable as prophylaxis. The usual dose is 0.5 ml ISG at birth and at 1 month.

Hepatitis D or delta is an incomplete RNA virus that presents as a coinfection with HBV. Hepatitis D is endemic to Italy and some parts of the Middle East. In some estimates, the rate of hepatitis D infection is about 50 percent in chronic HB_sAg carriers. Mother-to-fetus transmission of hepatitis D has been reported.[40]

Conclusions

1. Hepatitis B virus can be transmitted from the infected mother to her child. Transmission can occur in utero (5 percent) or at the time of delivery (95 percent). Vertical transmission rates in infants born chronic carriers positive for HB_sAg alone range from 12 to 25 percent. Pregnant women who carry HB_sAg and HB_eAg have an 85 to 90 percent risk of transmitting HBV to their infants. Pregnant women with acute HBV near or at delivery have a 50 to 60 percent risk of transmission.
2. *All* pregnant women should be screened for HB_sAg during pregnancy.
3. Infants born to mothers who are HB_sAg positive should receive 0.5 ml of HBIG intramuscularly at birth, followed by HBV vaccine (Recombivax or Engerix-B) at the recommended doses at birth, 1 month, and 6 months. This regimen reduces chronic carrier state in infants by 80 to 90 percent.
4. Hepatitis D (delta) virus, non-A, non-B hepatitis virus, but not hepatitis A virus have been reported to be transmitted from mothers to their children.

References

1. Adams RH, Combes B. Viral hepatitis during pregnancy. JAMA 1965; 192:195–198.
2. Arevalo JA. Hepatitis B in pregnancy. West J Med 1989; 150:668–674.
3. Beasley RP. Hepatitis B virus as the etiologic agent in hepatocellular carcinoma: epidemiologic considerations. Hepatology 1982; 2(Suppl):21s.
4. Beasley RP, Hwang LY, Lin CC. Hepatocellular carcinoma and hepatitis B virus: a prospective study of 22,707 men in Taiwan. Lancet 1981; 2:1129–1133.
5. Beasley RP, Hwang LY, Lin CC, et al. Hepatitis B immune globulin (HBIG) efficacy in the interruption of perinatal transmission of hepatitis B virus carrier state: initial report of a randomised double-blind placebo-controlled trial. Lancet 1981; 2:388–393.
6. Beasley RP, Trepo C, Stevens CE, Szmuness W. The e antigen and vertical transmission of hepati-

tis B surface antigen. Am J Epidemiol 1977; 105:94–98.
7. Blumberg BS, Alter HJ, Visnich S. A "new" antigen in leukemia sera. JAMA 1965; 191:541–546.
8. Brechot C, Pourcel C, Louise A, et al. Presence of integrated hepatitis B virus DNA sequences in cellular DNA of human hepatocellular carcinoma. Nature 1980; 286:533–535.
9. Centers for Disease Control. Prevention of perinatal transmission of hepatitis B virus: prenatal screening of all pregnant women for hepatitis B surface antigen. MMWR 1988; 37:341–351.
10. Cruz AC, Frentzen BH, Behnke M. Hepatitis B: a case for prenatal screening of all patients. Am J Obstet Gynecol 1987; 156:1180–1187.
11. Delaplane D, Yogev R, Crussi F, Shulman ST: Fatal hepatitis B in early infancy: the importance of identifying HB_sAg-positive pregnant women and providing immunoprophylaxis to their newborns. Pediatrics 1983; 72:176–180.
12. Greenspoon JS, Martin J, Greenspoon RL, McNamara BT. Necessity for routine obstetric screening for hepatitis B virus surface antigen. J Reprod Med 1989; 34:655–658.
13. Hieber JP, Dalton D, Shorey J, Combes B. Hepatitis and pregnancy, J Pediatr 1977; 91:545–549.
14. Immunization Practices Advisory Committee. Postexposure prophylaxis of hepatitis B. MMWR 1984; 33:285–290.
15. Judson FN. Epidemiology of sexually transmitted hepatitis B infections in heterosexuals: a review. Sex Transm Dis 1981; 8:336–343.
16. Lee AK, Ip HM, Wong VC. Mechanisms of maternal-fetal transmission of hepatitis B virus. J Infect Dis 1978; 138:668–671.
17. Lin H, Lee T, Chen D. Transplacental leakage of HB_eAg-positive maternal blood as the most likely route in causing intrauterine infection with hepatitis B virus. J Pediatr 1987; 111:877–881.
18. MMWR. Prevention of perinatal transmission of hepatitis B virus: prenatal screening of all pregnant women for hepatitis B surface antigen. JAMA 1988; 260:165–170.
19. Ohbayashi A, Okochi K, Mayumi M. Familial clustering of asymptomatic carriers of Australia antigens and patients with chronic liver disease or primary liver cancer. Gastroenterology 1972; 62:618–625.
20. Ohto H, Lin H, Kawan T, et al. Intrauterine transmission of hepatitis B virus is closely related to placental leakage. J Med Virol 1987; 21:1–6.
21. Okada K, Kamiyama I, Inomata M, et al. e Antigen and anti-e in the serum of asymptomatic carrier mothers as indicators if positive and negative transmission of hepatitis B virus to their infants. N Engl J Med 1976; 294:746–749.
22. Pastorek JG. Hepatitis B. Obstet Gynecol Clin North Am 1989; 16:645–657.
23. Pickering LK. Management of the infant of a mother with viral hepatitis. Pediatr Rev 1988; 9:315–320.
24. Schweitzer IL, Dunn AE, Peters RL, Spears RL. Viral hepatitis B in neonates and infants. Am J Med 1973; 55:762–771.
25. Schweitzer IL, Spears RL. Hepatitis-associated (Australian antigen) in mother and infant. N Engl J Med 1970; 283:570–572.
26. Shafritz DA, Shouval D, Sherman HI, et al. Integration of hepatitis B virus DNA into the genome of liver cells in chronic liver disease and hepatocellular carcinoma. N Engl J Med 1981; 305:1067–1073.
27. Siegel M. Congenital malformations following chickenpox, measles, mumps and hepatitis: results of a cohort study. JAMA 1973; 226:1521–1524.
28. Snydman DR: Hepatitis in pregnancy. N Engl J Med 1985; 313:1398–1401.
29. Stevens CE. Viral hepatitis in pregnancy: the obstetrician's role. Clin Obstet Gynecol 1982; 25:577–585.
30. Stevens CE, Beasley RP, Tsui J, Lee W-C. Vertical transmission of hepatitis B antigen in Taiwan. N Engl J Med 1975; 292:771–774.
31. Stevens CE, Neurath RA, Beasley RP, Szmuness W. HB_eAg and anti-HB_e detection by radioimmunoassay: correlation with vertical transmission of hepatitis B virus in Taiwan. J Med Virol 1979; 3:237–241.
32. Stevens CE, Toy PT, Tong MJ, et al. Perinatal hepatitis B virus transmission in the United States. JAMA 1985; 253:1740–1745.
33. Stokes J, Wolman IJ, Blanchard MC, Farquhar JD. Viral hepatitis in the newborn: clinical features, epidemiology, and pathology. Am J Dis Child 1951; 82:213–216.
34. Szmuness W. Hepatocellular carcinoma and the hepatitis B virus: evidence for a causal association. Prog Med Virol 1978; 24:40–69.
35. Tong MJ, Govindarajan S. Primary hepatocellular carcinoma following perinatal transmission of hepatitis B. West J Med 1988; 148:205–208.
36. Tong MJ, Thursby M, Rakela J, et al. Studies on the maternal-infant transmission of viruses which cause acute hepatitis. Gastroenterology 1981; 80:999–1004.
37. Wejstal R, Hermodsson S, Iwarson S, Norkrans G. Mother to infant transmission of hepatitis C virus infection. J Med Virol 1990; 30:178–180.
38. Wejstal R, Norkrans G. Chronic non-A, non-B hepatitis in pregnancy: outcome and possible transmission to the offspring. Scand J Infect Dis 1989; 21:485–490.
39. Wong VC, Lee AK, Ip HM. Transmission of hepatitis B antigens from symptom free carrier mothers to the fetus and the infant. Br J Obstet Gynaecol 1980; 87:958–965.
40. Zannetti AR, Ferroni P, Magliano E, et al. Perinatal transmission of the hepatitis B virus and of the HBV-associated delta agent from mothers to offspring in northern Italy. J Med Virol 1982; 9:139–148.

PARVOVIRUS B19 INFECTIONS

Epidemiology
Biology
Pathogenesis and Routes of Transmission
Clinical Manifestations
  Erythema Infectiosum or Fifth Disease
  Arthralgias
  Hemolytic Anemia
  Parvovirus B19 Infection During Pregnancy
  Fetal Hydrops and Congenital Anomalies
Diagnosis
  Mother
  Fetus and Infant
Management
  Mother
  Fetus

Parvovirus B19 was discovered fortuitously by Cossart and associates[26] in 1975 in England while they were screening for hepatitis B in blood donors. They detected 9 units of blood that had false-positive results for the hepatitis B surface antigen by counterimmunoelectrophoresis (CIE) but that had negative results with the passive hemagglutination test. Electron microscopy revealed 23-nm particles, which were recognized as parvovirus. These particles differed from the 27-nm particles of hepatitis B surface antigen.

Parvovirus B19 infections in humans have several clinical manifestations, including the classic "fifth disease" of childhood and pregnancy-related findings, which are discussed in this section.

Epidemiology

The major clinical presentations of *Parvovirus* B19 in humans are given in Table 11-18. Erythema infectiosum (EI) is a common exanthem of childhood. EI, also called *fifth disease,* was the fifth of the classic exanthema of childhood following rubeola, scarlet fever, rubella, and Filatov-Dukes disease.[27] EI is most common in childhood, and prevalence of antibody markedly differs between children and adults. For children younger than 5 years, seroprevalence ranges from 2 to 10 percent, whereas for adults over 20 years it is 40 to 60 percent.[5,52,53] EI peaks in late winter to early spring but may persist until the beginning of summer.[55] Because the incidence of the disease is highest among children, outbreaks of EI are most common in places with high concentrations of children: schools, day-care centers, and households with several young family members.

During outbreaks, the infection rate for seronegative susceptibles is approximately 50 percent but ranges from 50 to 90 percent.[3,8,27,43,55,57,65] Infection rates among susceptible individuals were reported to have no association with age.[38] However, the place of exposure to parvovirus B19 may affect infection rates. Shmoys and Kaplan have reported a rate of 20 to 30 percent in school outbreaks,[57] which is significantly lower than most other quoted rates for household exposures (about 50 percent).

Biology

Parvovirus B19 is a member of the family Parvoviridae. It can only infect humans. Other members of the family are known to affect various animal species.[4,22,60] The virus contains a single-stranded DNA of about 5.5 kilobases. It can be seen on electron microscopy as intranuclear particles about 20 to 24 nm in size. The viral genome is surrounded by an icosahedral protein coat and the gene locus codes for two capsid proteins and nonstructural proteins.[40]

Pathogenesis and Routes of Transmission

The primary site of *Parvovirus* B19 infections is within erythroid precursor cells.[4] In vitro studies involving bone marrow explant cultures have shown that *Parvovirus* B19 replicates in erythroid precursor cell lines.[41,42] DNA replication occurs in the cell nucleus only during the S phase. Rapid multiplication eventually leads to cell lysis and release of viral progeny. Reticulocytopenia is typically observed in infected patients, usually within 7 days after infection. Among patients with no known hemolytic disorders, a slight fall in hemoglobin may be manifest during this period. Patients who suffer from hemolytic disorders, such as sickle cell disease or hereditary spherocytosis, or whose immune status may be compromised, such as bone marrow transplant patients, may experience a more dramatic (or even fatal) drop in hemoglobin. This marked anemia is called *transient aplastic crisis* (TAC).

Table 11-18 Clinical Manifestations of *Parvovirus* B19 in Humans

Dermatologic
Erythema infectiosum (EI) or fifth disease
Macular rash in adults
Hematologic
Mild anemia
Transient aplastic crises (TAC)
Chronic anemia
Rheumatologic
Arthralgia in adults
Pregnancy-associated
Spontaneous abortion
Nonimmune hydrops fetalis
Stillbirth
Myocarditis (?)
Congenital malformations

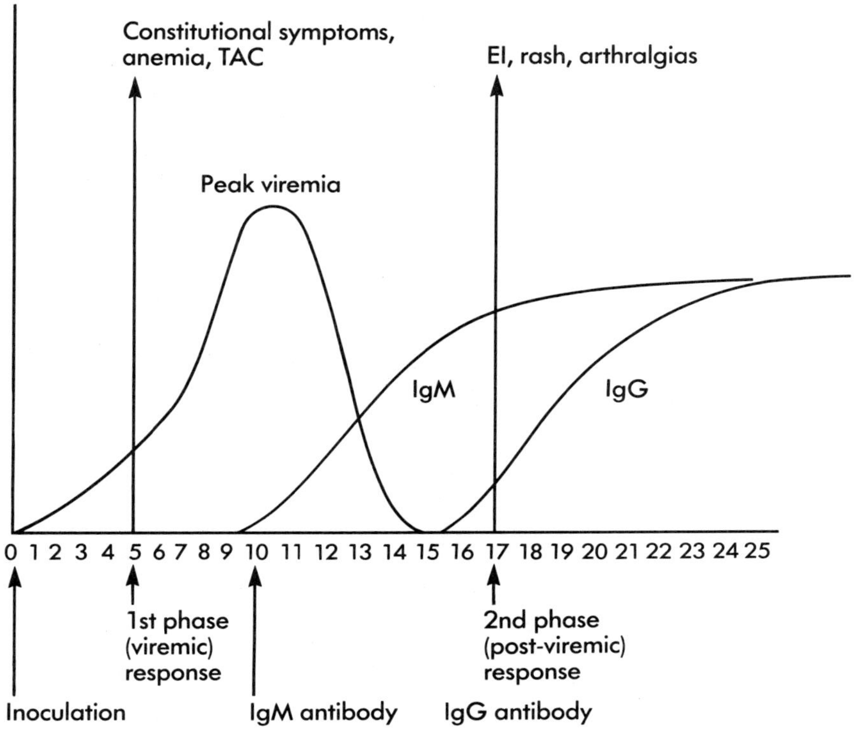

Figure 11-3 Clinical manifestations and antibody response to artificial inoculation with *Parvovirus* B19 virus in serosusceptible individuals. (Data from Anderson et al. 1985.[7])

Viral replication takes place by first synthesizing complementary DNA to form a monomer duplex DNA, followed by another replication back on itself to form dimer duplex DNA.[4] This process of replication requires cellular function expressed only during the S phase of the infected cell's DNA synthesis.[57]

Entry of the virus into an erythroid cell line occurs via cell surface receptor. Viral replication, leading to cell lysis, has been shown to be stimulated by erythropoietin in vitro.[61]

The most common route of horizontal transmission is through respiratory secretions. In addition, sexual transmission via infected semen,[55] transmission from infected blood products such as clotting factors,[61] and vertical transmission transplacentally[57] have been reported.

The pathophysiology of the disease and development of clinical symptoms produced by *Parvovirus* B19 have been delineated by Anderson and coworkers.[7] Healthy adult volunteers were artificially inoculated intranasally with *Parvovirus* B19 from an asymptomatic blood donor. Figure 11-3 summarizes the findings from that report. The study involved seven healthy volunteers, two of whom had IgG antibody to *Parvovirus* B19. The remaining five were seronegative. The volunteers were inoculated with 0.5 ml of diluted plasma from a seropositive individual with dilutions varying from 10^{-1} to 10^{-4}. The volunteers were then monitored for development of symptoms and for presence of virus in urine, serum, nasal washes, and stool suspensions, visualizing viral DNA by dot-blot hybridization with P^{32}-labeled DNA probes.

In this study, clinical symptoms were divided into two separate phases, as shown in Figure 11-3. The first phase, or the viremic phase, was characterized by development of constitutional symptoms such as fever, malaise, myalgias, headache, chills, and mild pruritus that occurred within 5 to 7 days after inoculation and were related to the viremia, which peaked on day 8. Maximum titers of 10^{11} genome copies per milliliter of blood were detected during peak viremia. The symptoms were secondary to production of immune complexes in the blood stream. During the viremic phase, nasal washes and gargle specimens showed the presence of virus. Virus shedding occurred via the respiratory secretions, and the highest viral load was observed during the first symptomatic phase of the illness, prior to the onset of rash. The viremic phase lasted 5 to 7 days and *Parvovirus*-specific IgM antibody was detectable in patient's sera by day 10. Interestingly, the smallest inoculum size (plasma dilution of 10^{-4}) did *not* result in a detectable viremia or in detectable *Parvovirus*-specific IgM antibody; no virus shedding was noted in this patient. As expected, volunteers who had had previous infection (those who were IgG positive) showed no evidence of clinical symptoms.

The second phase, or postviremic phase, began on day 15 to 17 and was characterized by pruritus and the rash of EI, followed 1 to 2 days later by arthralgia.

Table 11-19 Rash of Erythema Infectiosum: Adults and Children

	Adults	Children
Incidence of rash	Low frequency	High frequency
Type of rash	Macular	Classic "slapped cheeks" with reticular, lacelike pattern
Location of rash	Usually trunk and extremities	Face, extending to trunk and extremities

Viremia usually terminated by the time the rash developed. This information is significant in that children who present with the rash of EI probably need not be placed in isolation because viral shedding has usually ceased by that time.

In the same study, hematologic examinations showed a consistent fall in hemoglobin of about 1.2 to 1.8 percent per day among the infected individuals. Mild neutropenia and thrombocytopenia were also detected within 2 weeks after inoculation.

In conclusion, the Anderson group's study showed that (1) infection of seronegative individuals can occur via the intranasal route; (2) development of symptoms and the corresponding immune response require a minimum threshold of viral load (plasma dilution less than 10^{-4}); (3) constitutional symptoms occur during the viremic phase, when patients are usually shedding virus via the nasopharynx; (4) the rash and arthralgia associated with *Parvovirus* B19 infection occurs in the postviremic phase, when patients no longer have virus in the nasopharynx and both IgM and IgG antibodies specific to *Parvovirus* B19 are usually detectable; and (5) mild hematologic changes are usually seen during the second week of infection.

Clinical Manifestations

Erythema Infectiosum or Fifth Disease

Erythema infectiosum (EI) is one of the most common exanthema of childhood. The rash is usually described as a reticulate, lacelike, and macular rash, usually erupting initially on the face but then extending to the trunk and extremities. On the face, the rash is usually confluent and erythematous, giving the patient's face the appearance of slapped cheeks. The rash can also be pustular.[9] EI in adults usually presents as a macular rash on the trunk and extremities. The rash is pruritic and may be recurrent. The recurrences may be brought on by external stimuli such as changes in temperature or stress. The exanthem usually lasts about 1 to 3 weeks in both children and adults.

The onset of the rash of EI usually signals the beginning of the postviremic phase. Hence, patients are usually *not* infectious at this time. Viremia is absent, and nasal swab examinations for presence of *Parvovirus* are usually negative. EI in children is also usually preceded by constitutional symptoms that include headaches, pharyngitis, fever, coryza, diarrhea, nausea, cough, and conjunctivitis.[27] There appear to be no significant sequelae following the infection.[9,12,27,63] Seroprevalence rates for infants under 5 years range from 2 to 15 percent, for children between 5 and 19 from 15 to 60 percent, and for adults over 20 years well over 60 percent. Minor differences in clinical presentation of the disease between children and adults are shown in Table 11-19. Arthralgias are more common in EI for adults than for children.

Arthralgias

Arthralgia may be the only clinical manifestation of a *Parvovirus* B19 infection.[47,59] Its incidence is over 60 percent for adults compared to only 3 percent for children from 3 to 9 years.[1] The joints involved are usually the wrists, hands, knees, and ankles. The arthralgia is polyarticular and symmetric. Synovitis is unusual. Arthralgia usually appears within 2 to 7 days after the onset of the rash of EI, when patients are usually past their viremic phase. The symptoms are associated with the development of immune complexes. The symptoms usually resolve after several weeks but have been reported to last up to several years.[57] There is a slight predilection of this clinical symptom for women.

Hemolytic Anemia

Primary infection with *Parvovirus* B19 in normal volunteers has been shown to result in reticulocytopenia followed by mild anemia.[7] *Parvovirus* infections in patients with hemolytic disorders may be life-threatening.[4] Transient aplastic crises (TAC) may develop in patients with hereditary spherocytosis,[32] sickle cell disease,[56] and chronic hemolytic anemia.[46,50,61] Immunocompromised (e.g., bone marrow transplant patients, patients with leukemia, or patients on chemotherapeutic agents that affect bone marrow red cell precursors) patients who are infected may also be at significant risk of aplastic crisis.[36,62]

TAC occurs at the time the patient is viremic. Hence, patients with this clinical manifestation are usually infectious. Examination of the bone marrow at this time reveals a hypoplastic erythroid series.[57] The disruption in erythropoiesis usually lasts from 7 to 10 days, and some patients require hospitalization. Isolation precautions should be practiced because such patients are infectious.

A syndrome of chronic hemolytic anemia has also been reported in immunodeficient patients in which the decrease in hemoglobin and the reticulocytopenia is less acute.[36,62] Such patients develop *Parvovirus*-specific IgM antibody, but IgG antibody may be absent or persistently low for many years.[36]

Thrombocytopenia and neutropenia have also been

Table 11-20 Reported Fetal Loss Rates After Acute Parvovirus B19 Infection

Reference	Fetal Loss Rate (%)	Number of Women
Mortimer, et al.[39]	37.5	3 of 8 IgM+ pregnant women miscarried
Anand, et al.[2]	33	2 of 6 IgM+ women had stillbirth
Schwarz, et al.[54]	26	10 of 42 IgM+ pregnant women with hydropic stillbirths
Woernle, et al.[66]	25	1 of 4 IgM+ pregnant women with stillbirth at 24 weeks
U.K. study[45]	9.2	30 of 186 IgM+ pregnant women with stillbirth or miscarried; 8 of 14 abortus B19 DNA+
Rodis, et al.[49]	5	2 of 39 IgM+ pregnant women miscarried
MMWR[38]	4	2 of 95 IgM+ pregnant women miscarried

described in *Parvovirus* infections in normal seronegative susceptible individuals who have no hemoglobinopathies. Platelet counts may sometimes fall to 40 to 70 percent of preinfection values.[7]

Parvovirus B19 Infection During Pregnancy

Parvovirus infections in hamsters, pigs, cattle, and other species have been known to cause fetal death in early gestation.[16] Late infections cause cerebellar hypoplasia in cats and viral myocarditis in dogs and geese.[58] The first report that *Parvovirus* B19 can produce intrauterine infections and that these infections can lead to fetal damage appeared in 1984.[18,35] Since that time, fetal effects that have been associated with in utero *Parvovirus* B19 infections include spontaneous abortion, intrauterine fetal death, nonimmune hydrops fetalis, and congenital malformations.

Since the initial paper of Knott and colleagues[35] associating intrauterine *Parvovirus* infection with fetal death, more than a hundred cases of B19 infections in pregnancy have been reported.[11,15,17,28,29,37,39,64,66,67] Intrauterine infections have been reported in all trimesters of pregnancy.

The association between B19 infection and increased rates of abortion and stillbirth is controversial (Table 11-20). A review of studies of fetal loss possibly associated with maternal *Parvovirus* infection during pregnancy points to a fetal loss rate of 38 percent.[2,39,48,49,54,66] The most recent data, however, were provided by Rodis and colleagues,[49] who, during an outbreak of fifth disease in Connecticut in 1988, identified 39 pregnant women who had serologic evidence of recent *Parvovirus* B19 infection. Two of the 39 women had miscarriages, yielding a fetal loss rate of 5 percent. However, in neither case of miscarriage was *Parvovirus* DNA detected or hydropic changes evident. The only histologic evidence that could suggest an in utero infection in the abortus samples was evidence of severe erythroblastosis in one placenta. No age-matched controls were obtained for this study. It would not be unreasonable to assume that a control group would have had a similar rate of fetal loss. In fact, the authors mentioned that one of the two miscarriages was probably in the process of miscarriage when the woman was exposed to a child with EI.[49]

Kinney and coworkers[33] studied specimens that had been obtained from 96 women with stillbirths and another 96 women with spontaneous abortions randomly sampled from a pool of about 54,000 pregnant women who were part of the large Collaborative Perinatal Study at the National Institutes of Health (NIH). Age-matched controls were tested as well. None of the 96 women with stillbirths and only one of the 96 women with spontaneous abortions showed evidence of IgM antibody to *Parvovirus* B19. Additionally, the same study examined 1,035 deliveries in the Atlanta area during an EI outbreak in the winter of 1985. Thirty women were identified whose pregnancies resulted in stillbirths. Twenty of the 30 were enrolled in the study; none showed presence of IgM antibodies to *Parvovirus* B19. The investigators concluded that B19 infection was *not* a major cause of stillbirths and is probably not a major cause of spontaneous abortions in the general population.

In another study, Woernle and colleagues[66] examined the pregnancy outcomes of 31 pregnant women during an outbreak of EI in Mississippi in the winter of 1984. Four of the 31 women were IgM positive, indicating a recent infection during pregnancy. One of the four gave birth to a stillborn hydropic infant whose tissues were positive for B19 DNA by nucleic acid hybridization assay. They concluded that in utero infections with *Parvovirus* may be associated with stillbirths, but the extent of association is probably very small.

A Centers for Disease Control (CDC) study[38] that identified 95 pregnant women with *Parvovirus*-specific IgM antibody showed that 2 of 49 pregnancies followed to term resulted in fetal loss, yielding a fetal loss rate of only 4 percent.

Clearly, investigations reported to date have found a wide range of fetal loss rates associated with *Parvovirus* infections during pregnancy. Future research into this question will need to provide data on age-matched controls, study women early in pregnancy, and use hybridization techniques to establish the presence of infection in fetal tissue.

Fetal Hydrops and Congenital Anomalies

Hydrops fetalis has been reported with maternal B19 infection and appears to be due primarily to fetal anemia and resulting cardiac failure induced by the anemia.

Teratogenic effects of *Parvovirus* B19 have been reported in animals.[16,58] The role of B19 in human embryogenesis is controversial. Hartwig and associates reported an incomplete embryo of 9 weeks gestation born to an IgM positive mother.[30] One eye of the embryo showed evidence of microphthalmia, aphakia, and dysplasia of the sclera, anterior segment, and retina. There was also eosinophilic degeneration of skeletal and smooth muscle. From this study, the Hartwig group concluded that *Parvovirus* B19 may have teratogenic effects in the developing human embryo.

To assess the frequency of this association, Kinney and colleagues[33] conducted a prospective, case-control study of infants born in Cleveland during an EI outbreak in 1984. Of the 47 infants with congenital anomalies who were identified, none had B19-specific IgM antibody at birth. Fifty-five percent of the infants showed IgG-specific antibody, and the controls had the same frequency (57 percent). The Kinney group concluded that no strong evidence associates in utero *Parvovirus* B19 infections with congenital malformations. The incidence of congenital anomalies after maternal infection is probably no higher than the rate observed in the general population. Other studies[19,39] corroborate this finding.

From these data there is no strong correlation to date between intrauterine *Parvovirus* B19 infections and congenital anomalies. Future investigations of the teratogenic potential of *Parvovirus* B19 must include virologic studies to document the presence of the virus in the fetal tissues.

Diagnosis

Mother

Diagnosis of *Parvovirus* B19 infection in children and adults includes recognition of the clinical manifestations listed in Table 11-18. Diagnosis based on clinical findings alone can be unreliable. Serologic assays for B19 antibody are now available. The presence of B19 IgM indicates recent infection, and IgG antibody indicates past infection and immunity.

Table 11-21 summarizes laboratory methods for the detection of B19 infections. Approximately 50 percent of adults have B19-specific IgG antibody, compared to only 5 to 10 percent of preschool children.[49] Serum *Parvovirus*-specific IgM is a relatively sensitive and specific indicator of recent (acute) infection.[6,13] The specificity and sensitivity is 100% and 89%, respectively.[4] Unfortunately, these assays are available in only a few laboratories because of the lack of B19 antigen required for the assays. Recently, Kaligaya and associates have developed a cloned source of B19 antigen using a genetically engineered Chinese hamster ovary cell line.[31]

IgM antibodies usually appear within days after infection and may persist for 3 to 4 months.[49] The IgG antibody, by contrast, persists for years. Detection of viral antigens in maternal serum and cordocentesis samples has been suggested for diagnosing acute material or fetal infection, but no specific assay has been reported.[27,49]

Table 11-21 Methods in Diagnosing *Parvovirus* B19 Infections

Serology
- Maternal B19-specific IgG (indicates past infection/immunity)
- Maternal B19-specific IgM (indicates recent infection)
- Cordocentesis for B19-specific IgM

Presence of virus
- DNA in amniotic fluid or fetal tissue
    - Southern blot hybridization
    - In situ hybridization
    - Polymerase chain reaction
- Virus particles
    - Electron microscopy

Cytopathic effects
- Gross examination of tissue (fetus, placenta)
- Histology of erythroid cells

Markers of infection
- Maternal serum alpha-fetoprotein (MSAFP)
- Ultrasound (fetal hydrops)

Fetus and Infant

Gross and histologic examinations of blood and fetal tissues have been used for the diagnosis of *Parvovirus* infection.[2,36] Typically, giant pronormoblasts in Wright-Giemsa-stained bone marrow preparations are seen by light microscopy. Large normoblasts with marginated chromatin and eosinophilic nuclear inclusions in hematoxylin-and-eosin-stained tissues are also suggestive of B19 infection.[2] Electron microscopic evaluation of blood and fetal tissue has also proved helpful in the diagnosis of parvovirus infections.[21,24,34] By electron microscope (EM), the virus may be identified as 25-nm *Parvovirus*-like particles in paracrystalline arrays.

Gross examination of fetuses infected with *Parvovirus* B19 usually reveals a markedly hydropic stillborn with multiorgan involvement. Hepatomegaly, cardiomegaly, pulmonary hypoplasia secondary to long-term pleural effusions, and ascites are common findings.[57] The placenta is usually enlarged. Histologic examination of fetal tissues reveals extensive iron deposition in the liver and erythroblasts saturating fetal and placental capillaries.

The culture of B19 is limited but has been shown to be successful in bone marrow cultures with erythropoietin.[41]

DNA hybridization techniques have been the most promising to date in the accurate diagnosis of *Parvovirus* infections. There are several reports of Southern blot hybridization in detecting intrauterine *Parvovirus* infections.[2,10,15,28,36,64] In situ hybridization techniques have also been successfully utilized in detecting B19 infection.[23,44] Finally, the technique of polymerase chain re-

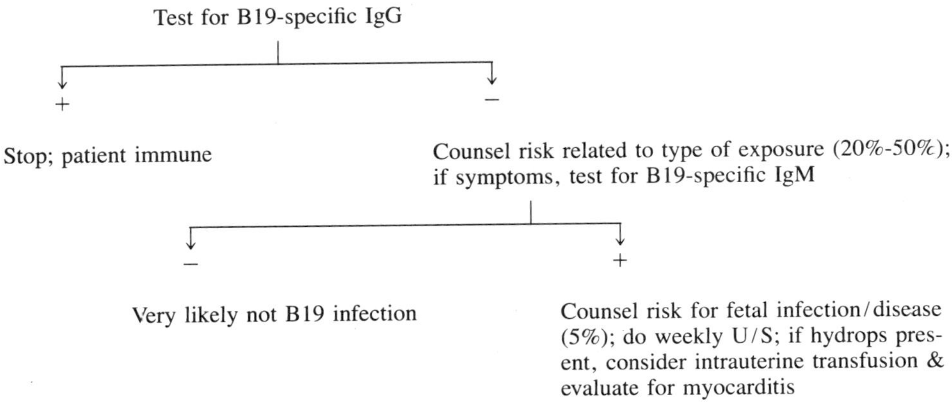

Figure 11-4 Management of pregnant women exposed to *Parvovirus* B19.

Table 11-22 Indications for Suspecting and Testing for *Parvovirus* B19 Infection

Unexplained pregnancy loss or fetal demise
Nonimmune hydrops
High-risk pregnant women
Exposure to outbreak of EI in school, day-care center, or household contact
Health care personnel taking care of patients with TAC secondary to *Parvovirus* infection
Unexplained rubellalike rash in pregnancy or nonspecific arthralgia

action (PCR) has recently shown significant promise in the detection of *Parvovirus* infections.[12,23,51]

Management

Mother

The management of pregnant women who may have been exposed to *Parvovirus* has been controversial. Table 11-22 lists the circumstances in which B19 infections should be evaluated. Figure 11-4 is the authors' recommended protocol. Individuals at high risk for exposure to the virus should be tested for IgG B19-specific antibody. Pregnant women who are IgG positive are immune and can be reassured and informed of their status. Pregnant mothers who show evidence of recent infection (i.e., IgM positive) should undergo sonographic evaluation to rule out hydrops fetalis. If the ultrasound is normal, it should be repeated every 1 to 2 weeks for 6 to 8 weeks, and maternal serum alpha-fetoprotein (MSAFP) should be drawn. If possible, sonographic evidence of fetal hydrops, depending on the severity, should be followed by cordocentesis and fetal blood tested by dot-blot hybridization or serology for presence of infection. A full workup of nonimmune hydrops fetalis should also be initiated at this time. A few studies have shown the efficacy of following MSAFP to detect fetal hydrops.[14,20]

Finally, women who show no antibodies to *Parvovirus* (IgG or IgM) at the time of exposure are susceptible to infection. Their risk of becoming infected for the remainder of their pregnancies should be minimized. They should also be counseled about the risks of infection after exposure and the risks of fetal effects.

Fetus

Management of severely anemic fetuses diagnosed by cordocentesis in documented B19 infections with intrauterine transfusions has been reported but has not received widespread acceptance.[54] The use of immune globulin in affected fetuses is also investigational at this point.

Conclusions

1. *Parvovirus* B19 infections in children usually present as erythema infectiosum with rash, whereas adults usually have arthralgias with or without the rash. Individuals with hemoglobinopathies may have serious consequences following *Parvovirus* B19 infection due to the red cell hypoplasia that develops.

2. Infection with *Parvovirus* B19 can be classified into two distinct phases: an early viremic phase when patients may have constitutional symptoms and shed virus from the nasopharynx, and a postviremic phase when patients no longer shed virus but clinically present with EI or arthralgia.

3. The rate of susceptibility of pregnant women is about 50 percent. Infection rates after exposure range from 20 percent (from household contact) to about 50 percent (from outbreaks of EI in school children and day-care centers). The risk of fetal death by spontaneous abortion before 20 weeks or intrauterine fetal death after 20 weeks range is about 5 percent.

4. There is no clear association between maternal B19 infection and congenital malformations.

5. Diagnosis of *Parvovirus* B19 infections largely depends on clinical findings, but serologic assays can be used to confirm the diagnosis. DNA hybridization techniques (dot-blot, in situ hybridization, and polymerase chain reaction) show the most promise in the definitive diagnosis of B19 infections.

References

1. Ager EA, Chin TD, Poland JD: Epidemic erythema infectiosum. N Engl J Med 1966; 275:1326–1331.
2. Anand A, Gray ES, Brown T. Human parvovirus infection in pregnancy and hydrops fetalis. N Engl J Med 1987; 316:183–186.
3. Anderson LJ. Role of parvovirus B19 in human disease. Pediatr Infect Dis J 1987; 6:711–718.
4. Anderson LJ. Human parvoviruses. J Infect Dis 1990; 161:603–608.
5. Anderson MJ, Cohen BJ. Human parvovirus B19 infections in United Kingdom 1984–86. Lancet 1987; 1:738 (letter).
6. Anderson MJ, Davis LR, Jones SE, et al. The development and use of an antibody capture radioimmunoassay for specific IgM to a human parvovirus-like agent. Journal of Hygiene 1982; 88:309–324.
7. Anderson MJ, Higgins PG, Davis LR, et al. Experimental parvoviral infection in humans. J Infect Dis 1985; 152:257–265.
8. Anderson LJ, Hurwitz ES. Human parvovirus B19 and pregnancy. Clin Perinatol 1988; 15(2); 273–286.
9. Anderson MJ, Jones SE, Fosher-Hoch SP, et al. Human parvovirus, the cause of erythema infectiosum (fifth disease). Lancet 1983; 1:1378.
10. Anderson MJ, Jones SE, Minson AC. Diagnosis of human parvovirus infection by dot-blot hybridization using cloned viral DNA. J Med Virol 1985; 15:163–172.
11. Anderson MJ, Khousam MN, Maxwell DJ. Human parvovirus B19 and hydrops fetalis. Lancet 1988; 1:535 (letter).
12. Anderson MJ, Pattison JR. The human parvovirus: brief review. Arch Virol 1984; 82:137–148.
13. Anderson LJ, Tsou C, Parker RA, et al. Detection of antibodies and antigens of human parvovirus B19 by enzyme-linked immunoadsorbent assay. J Clin Microbiol 1986; 24:522–526 (letter).
14. Bernstein IM, Capeless EL. Elevated maternal serum alpha-fetoprotein and hydrops fetalis in association with fetal parvovirus B19 infection. Obstet Gynecol 1989; 74:456-457.
15. Bond PR, Caul EO, Usher J, et al. Intrauterine infection with human parvovirus. Lancet 1986; 1:448–449.
16. Brown KE. What threat is human parvovirus B19 to the fetus? A review. Br J Obstetr Gynaecol 1989; 96:764–767.
17. Brown T, Anand A, Ritchie LD, et al. Intrauterine parvovirus infection associated with hydrops fetalis. Lancet 1984; 2:1033–1034.
18. Brown T, Ritchie LD. Infection with parvovirus during pregnancy. BMJ 1985; 290:559–560.
19. Canadian Pediatric Society (Infectious Disease and Immunization Committee). Erythema infectiosum and parvovirus B19 infection in pregnancy. Can Med Assoc J 1988; 139:633–634.
20. Carrington D, Gilmore DH, Whittle MJ, et al. Maternal serum alpha-fetoprotein: a marker of fetal aplastic crises during intrauterine human parvovirus infection. Lancet 1987; 1:433–435.
21. Caul EO, Usher MJ, Burton PA. Intrauterine infection with human parvovirus B19: a light and electron microscopic study. J Med Virol 1988; 24:55–66.
22. Chorba T, Coccia P, Holman HC, et al. The role of parvovirus B19 in aplastic crises and erythema infectiosum (fifth disease). J Infect Dis 1986; 154:383–394.
23. Clewley JP. Detection of human parvovirus using a molecularly cloned probe. J Med Virol 1985; 15:173–181.
24. Clewley JP, Cohen BJ, Field AM. Detection of parvovirus B19 DNA, antigen and particles in the human fetus. J Med Virol 1987; 23:367–376.
25. Committee on Infectious Disease (American Academy of Pediatrics). Parvovirus, erythema infectiosum, and pregnancy. Pediatrics 1990; 85:131–133.
26. Cossart YE, Field AM, Cant B, Widdows D. Parvovirus-like particles in human sera. Lancet 1975; 1:72–73.
27. Feder HM, Anderson I. Fifth disease: a brief review of infections in childhood, in adulthood, and in pregnancy, Arch Intern Med 1989; 149:2176–2178.
28. Gray ES, Anand A, Brown T. Parvovirus infections in pregnancy. Lancet 1986; 1:208.
29. Hall S. Infection with parvovirus during pregnancy. BMJ 1985; 290:713–714.
30. Hartwig NG, Vermeij-Keers CM, Van Elsacker–Niele A, Fleuren GJ. Embryonic malformations in a case of intrauterine parvovirus B19 infection. Teratology 1989; 39:295–302.
31. Kaligaya S, Shimada T, Fujita S, Young NS. A genetically engineered cell line that produces empty capsids of B19 (human) parvovirus. Proc Natl Acad Sci U S A 1989; 86:7601–7605.
32. Kelleher JF, Luban NL, Mortimer PP, Kamimura T. Human serum "parvovirus": a specific cause of aplastic crises in children with hereditary spherocytosis. J Pediatr 1983; 102:720–722.
33. Kinney JS, Anderson LJ, Farrar J, et al. Risk of adverse outcome of pregnancy after human parvovirus B19 infection. J Infect Dis 1988; 157:663–667.
34. Knisely AS, O'Shea PA, McMillan P, et al. Electron microscopic identification of parvovirus virions in fatal hydrops fetalis. Pediatr Pathol 1988; 8:163–170.
35. Knott PD, Weply GA, Anderson MJ. Serologically proved intrauterine infection with parvovirus. BMJ 1984; 289:1660.
36. Kurtzman GJ, Ozawa K, Cohen B, et al. Chronic bone marrow failure due to persistent parvovirus B19 infection. N Engl J Med 1987; 317:287–294.
37. Lafrere JJ, Dumez Y, Courouce AM, Deschene G. Intrauterine infection with human parvovirus.

Lancet 1986; 1:448–449.
38. Massachusetts Medical Society. Risks associated with human parvovirus B19 infection. MMWR 1989; 38(6):81-8.93–97.
39. Mortimer PP, Cohen BJ, Buckley MM. Human parvoviruses and the fetus. Lancet 1985; 2:1012 (letter).
40. Ozawa K, Ayub J, Kaligaya S. The gene encoding the nonstructural protein of B19 (human) parvovirus may be lethal in transfected cells. J Virol 1987; 61:2395–2406.
41. Ozawa K, Kurtzman G, Young N. Replication of the B19 parvovirus in human bone marrow cell cultures. Science 1986; 233:883–886.
42. Ozawa K, Kurtzman G, Young N. Productive infection by B19 parvovirus of human erythroid bone marrow cells in vitro. Blood 1987; 70:384–391.
43. Plummer FA, Hammond GW, Forward K, et al. An erythema-infectiosum-like illness caused by human parvovirus infection. N Engl J Med 1985; 313:74–79.
44. Porter HJ, Khong TY, Evands MF, et al. Parvovirus as a cause of hydrops fetalis: detection by *in situ* DNA hybridization. J Clin Pathol 1988; 41:381–383.
45. Public Health Laboratory Service Working Party of Fifth Disease. Study of human parvovirus B19 infection in pregnancy. Commun Dis Rep 1987; 87:3–6.
46. Rao KR, Patel AR, Anderson MJ, et al. Infection with parvovirus-like virus and aplastic crises in hemolytic anemia. Ann Intern Med 1983; 98:930–932.
47. Reid DM, Reid TMS, Brown T, et al. Human parvovirus-associated arthritis: a clinical and laboratory description. Lancet 1985; 1:422–425.
48. Rodis JF, Hovick TJ, Quinn DL, et al. Human parvovirus infection in pregnancy. Obstet Gynecol 1988; 72:733–738.
49. Rodis JF, Quinn DL, Gary GW, et al. Management and outcomes of pregnancies complicated by human B19 parvovirus infection: a prospective study. Am J Obstet Gynecol 1990; 163:1168–1171.
50. Saarinen UA, Chorba TL, Tattersall P, et al. Human parvovirus B19-induced epidemic red cell aplasia in patients with hereditary hemolytic anemia. Blood 1986; 67:1411–1417.
51. Salimans MM, Holsappel S, van de Rijke FM, et al. Rapid detection of human parvovirus B19 DNA by dot-hybridization and the polymerase chain reaction. J Virol Methods 1989; 23:19–28.
52. Samra JS, Obhrai MS, Constantine G. Parvovirus infection in pregnancy, Obstet Gynecol 1989; 73:832–834.
53. Schwarz TF, Rogendorf M, Deinhardt F. Human parvovirus B19 infections in United Kingdom 1984–86. Lancet 1987; 1:739 (letter).
54. Schwarz TF, Rogendorf M, Hottentrager B, et al. Human parvovirus B19 infection in pregnancy. Lancet 1988; 2:566–567.
55. Semble EL, Agudelo CA, Pegram PS. Human parvovirus B19 arthropathy in two adults after contact with childhood erythema infectiosum. Am J Med 1987; 83:560–562.
56. Serjeant GR, Topley JM, Mason K, et al. Outbreak of aplastic crises in sickle cell anemia associated with parvovirus-like agent. Lancet 1981; 2:595–597.
57. Shmoys S, Kaplan C. Parvovirus and pregnancy. Clin Obstet Gynecol 1990; 33:268–275.
58. Siegl G. Biology and pathogenicity of autonomous parvoviruses. In Berns KI, ed. The Parvoviruses, New York: Plenum Press, 1984.
59. Simpson RW, McGinty L, Simon L, et al. Association of parvovirus with rheumatoid arthritis of humans. Science 1984; 223:1425–1428.
60. Summers J, Jones SE, Anderson MJ. Characterization of the genome of the agents of erythrocyte aplasia permits its classification as a human parvovirus. J Gen Virol 1983; 64:2527–2532.
61. Thurn J. Human parvovirus B19: historical and clinical review. Rev Infect Dis 1988; 10:1005–1011.
62. VanHorn DK, Mortimer PP, Young N, Hanson GR. Human parvovirus-associated red cell aplasia in the absence of underlying hemolytic anemia. Am J Pediatr Hematol Oncol 1986; 8:235–239.
63. Wadlington WB. Erythema infectiosum. JAMA 1965; 192:58–60.
64. Weiland HT, Vemey-Keers C, Salimans MM, et al. Parvovirus B19 associated with fetal abnormality. Lancet 1987; 1:682–683.
65. White G, Woold AD, Mortimer PP. Human parvovirus arthropathy. Lancet 1985; 1:1419–1421.
66. Woernle CH, Anderson LJ, Tattersall P, Davison JM. Human parvovirus B19 infection during pregnancy. J Infect Dis 1987; 156:17.
67. Wright EP, Dyson AJ, Alaily A. Infection with parvovirus during pregnancy. BMJ 1985; 290:241.

CHAPTER 12

Acquired Immunodeficiency Syndrome

Howard L. Minkoff, M.D.

The growing threat that human immunodeficiency virus (HIV) poses to reproductive health has become increasingly apparent. By 1990 acquired immunodeficiency syndrome (AIDS) was the fifth leading cause of death of reproductive-age women in the United States and ranked first as a cause of death among minority women in certain large urban areas.[11] Public health officials estimate that during the decade of the 1990s 3 million women will die of AIDS worldwide. AIDS is also increasing as a cause of infant mortality in the United States, ranking as the number one cause of infant mortality in many inner city areas. AIDS, however, is no longer confined to the nation's urban areas. In 1989 the number of AIDS cases increased 5 percent in the nation's cities but 37 percent in the nation's rural areas.

Obstetricians and gynecologists have become increasingly involved in this epidemic. They provide reproductive health care to tens of thousands of HIV-infected women, they are involved in government-recommended HIV testing programs, and perhaps most importantly they provide care to hundreds of thousands of women "at risk." Physicians' interactions with sexually active women, particularly those with "casual" partners or multiple partners, provide a unique opportunity to educate patients about risks and ways to reduce them. In so doing they have an opportunity not only to reduce the incidence of HIV but also to reduce, from 13 million, the number of sexually transmitted diseases (STDs) diagnosed annually in the United States.

This chapter offers a primer on HIV disease in women and in so doing covers a range of issues, including the basics of HIV disease (pathophysiology, epidemiology) and clinical aspects relevant to gynecologists and obstetricians. It is hoped that this information will enable them to provide care to women infected or at risk.

Virology and Pathology

HIV is a retrovirus, an RNA virus, from which DNA can be reverse transcribed. It consists of an outer envelope, whose chief function is binding to target cells; core proteins; and polymerase, which allows the transcription of the RNA into DNA so that it can be incorporated into host cells. Tests used to identify people infected with HIV are dependent upon the recognition of antibodies to the different portions of the HIV virus. HIV-I is one of five human T-cell lymphotropic viruses (HTLVs) that have been identified to date. HTLV-I causes T-cell leukemia and tropical spastic paraparesis; HTLV-II causes hairy cell leukemia; HTLV-III is another name for HIV-I; HTLV-IV is HIV 2, an AIDS virus found predominantly in western Africa; and HTLV-V causes cutaneous T-cell lymphoma and leukemia.[53] Other than HIV-I (HTLV-III), these viruses are rarely found in the United States, although HTLV-I is being reported with increasing frequency among intravenous drug users.

A portion of the envelope of the HIV virion, called qp120, contains the segment that binds with cells containing the CD4 antigen. Cells with a high density of CD4 on their surface include monocytes, macrophages, lymphocytes, neural cells, and, according to some recent evidence, trophoblastic cells.[35] After the virus enters the cell, its RNA is transcribed into DNA, in a reaction mediated by reverse transcriptase, and then incorporated into the host genome. The virus then remains dormant for a varying duration of time, with the approximate median time till symptoms being a decade.[20] The reasons why activation occurs or why its timing is so variable have not been clearly elucidated. When the virus is activated, it leads to a reduction in the number of CD4 lymphocytes. These "helper cells" normally perform the critical function of coordinating a variety of host immune activities. As their numbers diminish, the infected host becomes susceptible to a wide variety of opportunistic infections.

Epidemiology

An appreciation of the potential impact of HIV infection on the professional lives of obstetricians and gynecologists is best provided through an understanding of the epidemiology of the virus in reproductive-age women. Although there are currently almost 10 men with AIDS for each woman, there is evidence that heterosexual transmission of HIV is already increasing the relative frequency of infection among women. The percentage of AIDS patients who are female increased 40 percent in 2 years from 7 to 10 percent. Cases among males increased only 18 percent in the same time frame.

Thirty percent of women with AIDS contracted it heterosexually. A large percentage of these women are sexual partners of intravenous drug–using (IVDU) men, who seem to be particularly efficient heterosexual transmitters of HIV. The demography of infected women therefore reflects that of communities where intravenous drug use is relatively common. It is not surprising that the overwhelming majority of infected women are indigent, minority, inner city inhabitants. The prevalence of HIV infection among pregnant women in New York City, for example, is 1.3 percent, with even higher rates reported from the Bronx (1.9 percent), Newark (4.3 percent), Miami (4.2 percent), and Brooklyn (2 percent).[30] Reported prevalence among women attending sexually transmitted disease (STD) clinics is even higher (e.g., Connecticut, 4.8 percent; Baltimore, 1.6 percent; New York City, 3.1 percent).[46] Because there is evidence that heterosexual spread can be bidirectional, as is seen in central Africa, HIV can potentially spread to a wider community, as have all other STDs.

Alkaloidal cocaine ("crack") may also be playing a role in the heterosexual spread of HIV. Women using crack have been reported to have more sexual partners than others. This behavior may explain, in part, the high incidence of sexually transmitted diseases such as syphilis reported among crack-using women. In one study parturients with cocaine derivatives in their urine were approximately six times more likely to have syphilis and HIV infections than were women with negative urine toxicologies.[37]

Because more than 75 percent of children with AIDS acquire it perinatally, most of them are also members of minority groups. It has been projected that in 1991 there was a cumulative total of 10,000 to 20,000 cases of pediatric HIV disease in the United States. That number is particularly alarming because nationally there are a total of 40,000 infant deaths per year, fewer than 10 fatal cases of congenital rubella, and approximately 400 fatal cases of congenital herpes. As testing programs for HIV are instituted on a broader scale during pregnancy, physicians must be prepared to deal with many women who will be identified as infected.

Current Standards of Care

Testing

As knowledge about AIDS has increased and as therapeutic interventions have become available, testing programs in the United States have evolved. Initially, selectively offering the HIV test was the standard. Women appearing for care would be questioned about risks (drug use, etc.) and would be offered HIV testing only if risks were acknowledged. This approach failed because most risks were stigmatizing and many infected women refused to acknowledge them.[30] Subsequently recommendations were made to offer HIV tests routinely, and increased numbers of women, many not acknowledging risks, accepted testing under those conditions. When zidovudine (ZDV) treatment was shown to improve substantially the outcome for asymptomatic individuals and became the standard of care, testing policy shifted from "offering" to recommending. Currently it is recommended that all sexually active women be given an opportunity to have an HIV test, and those in high-risk groups, including all those in communities with a high seroprevalence, be advised to have an HIV test.

The mechanics of testing have not changed in the last several years. All testing should be consented to and preceded by counseling. Counseling regarding testing should include information on the meaning of the test, advantages and disadvantages of testing, and institutional policies regarding the charting of results. If the results indicate infection, it is important to remember that care of seropositive pregnant women begins with the transmittal of test results.[26] The initial post-test discussion should cover the meaning of the patient's positive HIV antibody test result, a brief review of HIV infection and how it is transmitted (and how it is *not* transmitted), a discussion of "safer sex" and "safer needle use" if appropriate, and the implications of HIV infection during pregnancy.

If abortion is still an option, it should be discussed. The woman's choice, whether or not to abort, should be supported. Several studies of seropositive women's pregnancy decisions have shown that they generally do not choose to abort and that decisions about abortion are independent of serostatus[52] (although those who are not drug users may be more influenced in reproductive choice by serostatus than drug users).[56] Childbearing and rearing may be of greater importance to women than a 25 to 50 percent risk of perinatal transmission.

The clinician's "duty to warn" patients' partners is another concern. Ideally the patient should be convinced to relay the information to her partner. If not, clinicians must consider working with local health departments to notify a patient's sexual contacts. The balance between confidentiality and the duty to warn is delicate and warrants thoughtful consideration.[1]

It is important to stress the continued availability of the clinician to discuss issues of HIV infection. Referrals should be made at the initial counseling session for appropriate medical evaluation and follow-up. If a woman has other children who might have been perinatally infected (older siblings born after 1975), these children should be evaluated by a pediatrician who is familiar with HIV infection. Women should be told where their partners can be tested for HIV. The need or desire for psychosocial or psychiatric referrals should also be assessed at this time.

Counseling should also provide women with relevant information on HIV infections in pregnancy, including data on transmission, immune effects, and the effect of HIV disease on pregnancy outcome, as outlined in this chapter.

Transmission of HIV

Vertical transmission of HIV was first suggested in 1983 by Rubenstein and associates, who reported on seven children with AIDS, the mothers of 5 of whom belonged to risk groups for AIDS.[48] In a review of all pediatric AIDS cases reported as of 1984, Thomas and coworkers supported the concept of perinatal transmission, showing that 30 of 35 babies appeared to have acquired the infection from a parent who was from a risk group.[56a]

Early in the epidemic it had been suggested that all babies born to HIV-positive mothers be delivered by cesarean section in order to avoid the possibility of peripartum transmission of the virus during passage through an infected birth canal.[10] Although this recommendation was supported by reports of isolation of HIV or its antibody from cervical-vaginal secretions[2,59,64] and cervical tissue itself,[44] the frequency of viral isolation and quantity of virus isolated have been low. There is, at present, no direct evidence that HIV is acquired by the infant during its passage through the birth canal. Additionally there is clear evidence that cesarean section does not prevent infection in all children.[12,38,47,51] A 1987 report on 34 babies with symptomatic HIV disease noted that 10 of the infants were delivered by cesarean section, suggesting that operative delivery would not be protective.[41]

The timing of perinatal transmission has been difficult to determine. Lapointe and associates described a 28-week-old fetus that was delivered from a terminally ill AIDS patient by cesarean section and in whom viral antigen was detected in the thymus.[31] Peutherer and colleagues isolated HIV virus from two of six pregnancies that were terminated in the middle trimester.[42a] HIV has been directly isolated from the placenta at 34 weeks[40] and the amniotic fluid[10,40] and fetuses as early as 15 weeks gestation.[31,45] The possibility of contamination during the delivery process, however, cannot be ruled out in many of these cases.

The efficiency of vertical transmission is also unclear. The passive transfer of maternal antibody to the fetus and its persistence in the neonate's circulation for 18 months mean that in the absence of symptoms and more specific tests it may be impossible to determine if the child is infected before it is 18 months old. New research on specific immunologic markers, such as IgA, may reduce time till diagnosis. Based on studies with sufficient follow-up to assure accurate diagnosis, it appears that the risk of prenatal transmission of infection is between 20 percent and 35 percent. The largest studies to date are those from the European collaborative group[42] and the Italian Multicenter Study.[57] In the former study 271 children born to HIV-infected mothers in eight European centers are being followed. Of 100 children followed for more than 15 months, 19 had persistent antibody and 5 were antibody negative but presumed to be infected because of virus isolation or antigen detection. The estimated vertical transmission rate was therefore 24 percent. In the Italian study 486 children born to HIV-positive mothers were studied. Of 89 over 15 months of age, 29 (32.8 percent) were considered to be infected. Data from Third World countries have been in concert with these results.[22,49]

At present there is no doubt that the transplacental route is the major route of infection among infants, accounting for between 75 and 80 percent of all pediatric AIDS cases.[113] Approximately 14 percent of HIV-infected infants acquired their infection through blood transfusions.[60,62]

Although there have been isolated reports of the horizontal spread of infection to siblings by bites through intact skin[29] and the reuse of needles for administration of medications,[18] there is no substantive evidence that even close household contact can lead to transmission of the infection to other family members.

Immune Effects

HIV has a predilection for cells with the CD4 antigen on the surface, such as lymphocytes (helper cells), macrophages, neural cells, and some placental cells.[35] As a result of infection, a reduction in the T4 population occurs, along with a decrease in proliferation of T4 cells, impairment of lymphokine production, and defective cytotoxic activity by natural killer cells. B-cell abnormalities have also been observed, including poor antibody response to new antigens and inappropriate polyclonal activation with resultant elevated levels of serum immunoglobulins, circulating immune complexes, and various autoimmune phenomena.[7] These multiple defects in immune response render the host susceptible to an array of opportunistic infections seen in patients with AIDS.

Pregnancy may also influence immune function. The obstetric literature supports the belief that a pregnant woman is more susceptible to various viral, bacterial, and fungal infections and is more likely to die from these infections than her nonpregnant counterpart. In an epidemic of Asian influenza, for example, 50 percent of women who died were pregnant, although pregnant women comprised only 7 percent of women in the reproductive age group.[17]

Because the host response to most of the infectious disorders discussed is cell mediated, it is thought that pregnancy may be associated with a decrease in cell-mediated immunity. The demonstrated ability of pregnant women to mount a satisfactory response to intradermal skin antigens and their ability to reject skin grafts suggests, however, that only selective functions of cell-mediated immunity are depressed during pregnancy.

It is not entirely clear in what manner T-cell function is compromised in pregnancy. Sridama and associates showed that there was a significant decrease in the relative and absolute number of helper T lymphocytes (CD4) throughout pregnancy and that normalization of these cells occurred during the third and fifth month postpartum.[55] Bailey and coworkers also observed a decrease in T helper cells in pregnancy but thought patients had adequate T helper cell function as determined by in vitro immunoglobulin synthesis assay.[13] A small but significant reduction in whole circulating lymphocytes and T helper subsets was reported by Vanderberken and colleagues, but no change in T suppressor and cytotoxic cells (CD8) was found.[58] In contrast, a progressive increase in the total number of T cells during the first two trimesters of pregnancy was reported by Fiddes and associates, and a decrease only noted in the third trimester.[15]

Although evidence is conflicting, most investigators

agree that there is a decrease in cell-mediated immunity during pregnancy that is probably mediated through an altered ratio of T helper cell to T suppressor cell. Other factors contributing to the immunosuppression of pregnancy may be increased levels of total steroids and other pregnancy-specific plasma proteins and hormones like HCG, alpha-fetal protein, and pregnancy-associated alpha 2-glycoprotein.[63]

Because pregnancy as well as HIV may be associated with a significant depression of cell-mediated immunity, pregnancy could theoretically have an adverse effect on the natural history of HIV disease by enhancing immunoincompetence. Recently several controlled studies have prospectively followed HIV-positive mothers. Schaeffer and associates followed 32 HIV-positive women and 40 HIV-negative women during pregnancy for 6 months following delivery and did not observe any clinical progression of illness during pregnancy among seropositive women.[50] The authors felt that pregnancy had only a minor effect on the course of HIV disease. Bigger and colleagues showed that the direction of immunologic changes seen in HIV-positive mothers was the same as that in HIV-negative control pregnancies except that drops in CD4 counts were 10 to 20 percent greater among seropositive women.[6]

Other investigators have failed to show any evidence of progression of disease during pregnancy.[41] In a follow-up of 88 postpartum patients, MacCallum was unable to demonstrate any adverse effect of pregnancy on the course of HIV disease.[33] Similarly, Berrebi and coworkers followed 23 pregnant patients for 2 years following delivery and their matched seropositive nonpregnant controls and could not find any statistical difference between the two groups in the number of opportunistic infections.[4] Most recently Bledsoe reported on a matched group of approximately 50 infected pregnant women and 50 infected nonpregnant women. Follow-up for 12 to 18 months revealed no difference between the groups in the rate of clinical progression or immunologic deterioration.[5]

At present a significant influence of pregnancy on the course of HIV disease has not been documented. More prospective, long-term studies are needed before the impact of pregnancy will be clearly delineated.

Care of the Asymptomatic Patient

The HIV-infected asymptomatic individual should be under the care of a physician versed in the management of HIV disease. Recent advances allow clinicians to be proactive in maintaining the health of asymptomatic individuals. Patients should receive influenza and pneumonia vaccines. They should be screened for tuberculosis and have baseline toxoplasmosis titers. Advice should also be offered on life-style changes such as elimination of illicit drug use and alcohol, proper nutrition, rest, and avoidance of infections (reduced sexual exposure). Most interventions are currently linked to CD4 counts, which should be obtained regularly. Given variations due to laboratory techniques and day-to-day changes in an individual's counts, it is wise to repeat an unusually low count before acting on it. If the count drops below 500 per cubic millimeter antiretroviral therapy is warranted. When the count drops below 200 per cubic millimeter, prophylaxis for *Pneumocystis carinii* pneumonia (PCP) should commence.[43] Therapeutic agents utilized in the management of HIV-infected individuals are used either to prevent and treat specific opportunistic infections or to attack the virus directly. The agent currently in wide clinical use for the latter purpose is zidovudine (ZDV). ZDV interferes with reverse transcriptase and thereby prevents incorporation of the viral genome into the host DNA. Its clinical efficacy has been well documented in several large prospective studies. Among patients with initial CD4 counts under 500 per cubic millimeter, those receiving ZDV had a significantly slower rate of T-cell depletion and a slower progression to clinical illness.[16] A dose of 500 mg per day has been shown to have an efficacy equal to the originally recommended dose of 1500 mg. Among the problems associated with the use of ZDV have been anemia, lethargy, and muscle aches, as well as eventual breakthrough and resistance. Newer antiviral agents such as dideoxyinosine (DDI) have also been shown to have efficacy and may be used in patients who develop either intolerance or resistance to ZDV.

HIV and the Gynecologist

Standards for testing sexually active, nonpregnant women are the same as for those who are pregnant. All women should be given the opportunity to have an HIV test, and those engaged in high-risk behaviors or residing in high-prevalence communities should be advised to take the test. The pretest and post-test counseling are the same as those previously described.

Beyond testing, the gynecologist has obligations to two groups: those at risk and those infected. His or her chief obligation to women at risk is to inform them of their risk status and to help them institute measures to minimize their risks. This process begins with the sexual history. Taking an adequate sexual history should be a routine component of care. Surveys have shown that patients are receptive to inquiries about sexual health but that most clinicians do not ask. At a time when 13 million Americans acquire STDs annually, the importance of sexual health to general health is readily apparent.

The preventive message is the safer sex message. Absolutely safe sex is mutual monogamy with an uninfected partner. Although it would be beneficial to counsel patients to know their potential sexual partners for "longer" times before engaging in sexual activity, it should be recognized that casual contacts will still occur, and certainly learning a partner's serostatus is an elusive goal. Therefore, sexual contacts should involve condoms. Although clearly not foolproof, several avenues of investigation, both in vivo and in vitro, have demonstrated a protective effect with condoms. The role of antiviral agents such as nonoxynol-9 is less certain. Although these agents inactivate virus, they also can potentially cause inflammatory reactions that could enhance viral acquisition.

Recently a great deal of interest has focused on the unique ways in which HIV disease may affect women. Although a large amount of research remains to be performed before as much is known about women as is currently known about men, there are already clearly delineated areas of concern specific to women. Included in these are contraception, gynecologic infections, and gynecologic malignancies.

Contraceptive issues of relevance to infected women include the potential for various methods to affect a women's infectivity and to affect her immune status. Oral contraceptives (OCs) could theoretically influence the course of HIV disease. Both estrogen and progesterone have immune effects.[28] In vivo animal studies show that estrogens increase mortality from *Toxoplasma* infection, decrease the delayed skin reaction to tuberculin, and decrease rejection of skin and corneal transplants.[28,32,61] These effects indicate that estrogen inhibits cell-mediated immune responses. Estrogens also facilitate the development of antibodies and retard their decline, probably as a result of their functional inhibition of T-suppressor cells. Estrogen receptors have been detected on human T-cells, but only supraphysiologic concentrations of estrogen alter T-cell activity in vitro.

Progesterone at physiologic concentrations increases the activity of T-suppressor lymphocytes in vitro and inhibits the transformation of T-lymphocytes by mitogens.[23] This direct effect of progesterone on T-suppressor cells is one of the mechanisms preventing fetal rejection during pregnancy. The greatly increased progesterone levels obtained during pregnancy also produce a decreased response to rubella virus, a decrease in the response of T-lymphocytes to phytohemagglutinin (PHA), a decreased reactivity to intradermal purified protein derivative, and a lessened rejection of skin grafts. Several studies have found up to a 50 percent decrease in the T-lymphocyte response to PHA in women who are long-term users of OCs.[27,54] This alteration has never been directly linked to a clinical outcome in women who use OCs, but it is possible that the mechanisms involved are responsible for the reported decreased incidence of rheumatoid arthritis in OC users. Although no viral disease has yet been associated with the use of OCs, this observed decrease in cell-mediated immunity raises the suspicion that the use of OCs might increase an infected woman's response to HIV infection. There are no extant empiric data, however, to suggest harm to infected women from the use of hormonal contraception. At the current time, therefore, guidelines for the use of oral contraceptives should not be modified on the basis of serostatus. Concerns about disease transmission favor the use of alternative methods, particularly among discordant couples.

Intrauterine devices have the theoretical ability to enhance viral transmission from infected women. They can increase the amount of menstrual flow and may cause microabrasions on the head of the penis. Preliminary data suggestive of frequent abscesses among HIV-infected women with pelvic inflammatory disease (PID) would suggest caution before recommending a device that itself can be associated with PID.

Barrier methods would appear to have the least potential for either harmful effects on the infected women or viral transmission to uninfected sexual contacts.

Vaginal moniliasis has been reported to be a presenting symptom among a large minority of HIV-infected women. These infections may be recurrent and refractory to standard, topical therapies. Oral ketoconazole may be beneficial in cases of refractory moniliasis. When this agent is used, however, caution must be exercised in monitoring liver function tests.[36]

PID affects 1 million women annually, and recent reports suggest that among women in HIV-endemic communities those with PID are disproportionately infected with HIV. Information on the course of PID among HIV-infected women is quite preliminary. In one study HIV-seropositive women with PID were more likely than their seronegative counterparts with PID to be admitted with a low white blood cell count.[25] The authors also reported a trend toward more abscesses among seropositive women as well as toward more surgical intervention. These latter findings were not statistically significant, however.

Recent evidence is consistent with an HIV-mediated effect on cervical human papilloma virus (HPV) disease. These data are preliminary and mostly observational and should be interpreted with caution. Thus, although many studies have now shown that HIV-infected individuals are more likely to have HPV changes on pap smears, control groups were not matched for important covariables such as smoking and number of sexual partners.[9] Advanced cervical cancer has also been reported to be more fulminant in the setting of HIV disease.[34] Some data suggest that the accuracy of pap smears in predicting histologic and colposcopic abnormalities may be compromised in HIV-infected individuals. All these studies together raise concerns about the course of HPV in HIV-infected women. Although further study is clearly needed, in the interim clinicians caring for HIV-infected women should be assiduous in regularly assessing the cervix.

Obstetrical Management

The first obligation of the obstetric care provider is to assure that the patient has received adequate counseling to empower informed reproductive choice. Once the patient has made her choice, the provider should be supportive and make efforts either to provide the necessary service or to make an appropriate referral. If the patient opts to continue the pregnancy, as most women have to date, the clinician must be prepared to link the patient with support networks in the hospital and the community at large.

The guiding principle in providing care to the HIV-infected individual is not to modify the standard of care on the basis of gender or pregnancy status unless there are compelling reasons to do so. Thus, CD4 counts should be monitored and antiretroviral and prophylactic therapies should be considered when immune status warrants. The substantive risk to the mother, and hence to the pregnancy, from withholding indicated medications because of concerns about their unknown effects on the fetus must be recognized. Pursuant to that understanding, the mother's primacy in deciding about therapeutic interventions should be honored.

In addition to guiding pharmacologic interventions, CD4 counts provide the clinician with a reliable prediction of the potential for complications during pregnancy and hence allow the obstetrician to tailor care to the patient's needs. If the CD4 count is consistently over 500 per cubic millimeter, then it is probable that the pregnancy will proceed unremarkably, and consultations with infectious disease experts and the institution of drug therapies can safely be postponed until the postpartum period. Conversely, if CD4 levels drop below that mark, then the obstetrician should be prepared for possible complications. At the least, consultation with an expert in the care of HIV disease and close follow-up are warranted.

Under all circumstances the clinician should thoroughly assess the patient's clinical and immunologic status at the time of her first prenatal visit. Physical assessment should include an evaluation of lymph nodes, the oral cavity (for thrush or leukoplakia), and general body habitus (wasting, etc.). A careful evaluation for the presence of coincident infections should be undertaken. That assessment should include appropriate tests for chlamydia, gonorrhea, syphilis, and toxoplasmosis. A Mantoux test for tuberculosis should be performed. If the patient is in need of vaccination for hepatitis B, pneumonia, or influenza, it should be administered. Patients and clinicians should be aware of HIV-related symptoms (weight loss, diarrhea, night sweats, etc.) and investigate them expeditiously, particularly if they involve the respiratory system. Finally, if CD4 counts drop to levels consistent with an emergent risk for opportunistic infections, then consideration should be given to the institution of antiviral agents and PCP prophylaxis. Discussions about the risks and benefits of these agents, particularly in the setting of pregnancy, should cover all the material outlined in the section on care of the asymptomatic HIV-infected individual. In pregnancy, however, additional considerations regarding the risks and benefits of antiviral agents are warranted. The risks of withholding therapy in the setting of markedly depleted CD4 cells include the development of opportunistic infections during pregnancy. Progression to clinical illness has been reported among a substantial proportion of women who had documented low CD4 counts (less than 300 per cubic millimeter) during pregnancy.[39] The risks that the agents themselves pose to the fetus are not as clearly delineated. It is known that ZDV can cross the placenta and produce roughly equivalent fetal blood levels. Animal studies and small numbers of reports on human fetal exposure have not, however, documented a teratogenic risk. In mice and rats, lifetime exposure to doses several multiples of human doses have resulted in nonmetastasizing vaginal tumors at the end of the animals' natural lives.[21] The unique manner in which these animals excrete the drug and the occurrence of contamination of the vaginal vault during urinary excretion makes extrapolation of risk from the animal data very tenuous.

Management in the intrapartum period should not be substantively altered by serostatus. The mode of delivery should be based on obstetric indications only. HIV infections are indications neither to perform cesarean sections more aggressively nor to avoid them more assiduously. There are no data extant to prove that operative delivery modifies the perinatal transmission of the virus, although there are no appropriately designed studies that document the converse. Whether cesarean birth before the onset of labor or rupture of membranes can influence perinatal transmission remains to be investigated. In the interim, obstetric circumstance should guide clinical decisions regarding mode of delivery.

Monitoring of the fetus should be noninvasive if at all possible. Although only a minority of neonates are infected with HIV, all are potentially exposed to vaginal secretions contaminated with virus. Thus it would seem prudent to maintain the integrity of the fetal scalp by avoiding the use of scalp clips and scalp pHs when clinical circumstances allow.

The postpartum course of seropositive women has not been shown to be substantively different from that of other women. If a woman is known to have markedly depressed CD4 counts, however, it would be best to institute perioperative antibiotic prophylaxis if delivery is by cesarean section. Universal blood and body secretion precautions should be extended to the child at birth, but bonding between the mother and child should be encouraged.

Breast feeding, however, is not advisable in countries where safe alternatives to breast milk are readily accessible. Several cases of infection via breast milk have been documented. These cases generally involved women who were seronegative during their pregnancies but who received HIV-contaminated blood in the immediate postpartum period. They subsequently breast-fed children who seroconverted. Breast feeding might be particularly dangerous around the time of seroconversion when a coincident peak in p24 antigen has been reported. In large cohort studies of HIV-infected mothers, few authors have found a substantial difference in the ultimate infection rate between breast-fed and bottle-fed infants.

Finally, the obstetrician is responsible for assuring appropriate follow-up for those patients who have been diagnosed as having an HIV infection during their pregnancy. Many protocols are already available for infected mothers and children that can materially improve their prognosis. Access to those protocols are dependent on appropriate and timely referral.

Strategies for Preventing Fetal Damage from HIV

Despite public health efforts to prevent infection in women, it is estimated that close to 6,000 HIV-infected women gave birth in 1990. In the absence of intervention strategies, close to 2,000 infected children emerged from that cohort. Several avenues of investigation are now being pursued that are designed to reduce the perinatal transmission of HIV. A multicenter, NIH-funded study of zidovudine in pregnancy and in the early neonatal period began in 1991. Zidovudine is an inhibitor of reverse transcriptase, the enzyme that allows HIV to be reverse transcribed into DNA, permitting the virus to be integrated into the host genome. By administering zidovudine in pregnancy and early in the neonatal period, it is hoped that the free viral load will be reduced and the ability of the virus to integrate into fetal cells will also be diminished. Clearly this strategy will fail for fetuses who are infected before therapy begins.

A second approach is to administer soluble CD4 bound to gamma globulin. The CD4 antigen is the receptor for HIV. It is found on lymphocytes, monocytes, Hofbauer cells, trophoblastic cells, and vascular cells in the placenta.[35] It is possible that viral attachment to any of the latter three cell types could be the mechanism by which the fetus becomes infected. Soluble CD4 could act as a false receptor for HIV, causing the virus to bind to the soluble antigen rather than to native, cell-bound antigen. Binding the CD4 to IgG would help to overcome the otherwise extremely short half-life of CD4. Phase-one trials of CD4 in pregnancy are currently ongoing.

A third avenue of research is based on studies of immunoblot patterns of HIV-infected mothers who give birth. Geodert and colleagues reported that the children of mothers who had high-affinity antibody to the gp-120 segment of the envelope of HIV were significantly more likely to serorevert (i.e., be uninfected) than children of mothers who lacked high-affinity antibody to that segment. The gp-120 segment is the portion of the virus that binds to the CD4 antigen. Subsequent research has shown that the particular portion of gp-120 that is most crucial is the principal neutralizing domain.[14] Antibody to the segment may in fact be protective for the child. Attempts to produce monoclonally an antibody to various portions of the envelope of HIV or to immunize a mother passively or actively might therefore be reasonable approaches to the prevention of perinatal transmission.

Beyond reducing the incidence of HIV among reproductive-age women and interfering with vertical transmission, fetal damage can be reduced by preventing opportunistic infections among pregnant women. Opportunistic infections can be lethal; even if not, they may result in the preterm birth of an asphyxiated infant. Experience with HIV-infected, nonpregnant individuals suggests that preventive strategies can be successfully implemented.

Infection Control

One major concern of clinicians is nosocomial acquisition of HIV. Recommendations for risk-reduction techniques are based on a standard approach designed to prevent direct skin contact with potentially infected secretions.[19] In endemic areas caution must be exercised when handling secretions of all patients, not only those known to be infected. Focusing only on those patients known to be infected creates a two-tier infection control system that puts the clinician at risk from patients infected but not yet identified, who are therefore not appropriately managed. Studies from emergency room settings in endemic communities have shown a high prevalence of infection in reproductive-age individuals and have also shown that patient history (drug use, etc.) does not efficiently identify the infected. Moreover, even seronegative patients can pose a risk of transmitting CMV or hepatitis or other retroviruses (HTLV-I, II, IV, or V).

Specific control measures include the use of gowns and gloves (both latex and vinyl appear to effective) during deliveries, the use of gloves while handling the neonate as long as any maternal secretions remain, and frequent handwashing.[8] The added protection afforded by goggles, the use of which has been advocated, is purely speculative. Recent reports of infections of health care providers after skin contact with infected blood, however, justify maximum caution. Oral suction should be replaced with devices attached to wall suction. Wall suction should be kept below 140 mmHg to avoid harm to the fetus.

Caution is also important in the operating room. Tearing of gloves can be common (10 to 20 percent) and is sometimes associated with skin punctures. Double-gloving can reduce skin exposure from 15 to 5 percent of cases. By being aware of the presence of sharp instruments and by not leaving them on the field, surgeons can help to reduce their risks.

In all medical settings, needles should never be resheathed, bent, or broken before discarding. Impenetrable needle-disposal containers should be conveniently placed on all wards. By using all of these precautions, risk of HIV infection can be minimized. Finally, although HIV-infected individuals are often co-infected with CMV, hepatitis B, and the like, no increase in these infections has been documented among health care workers caring for AIDS patients.

There is some evidence from animal models that ZDV may reduce the chance that inoculation with a retrovirus will result in infection. Consequently, trials of ZDV for health care workers sustaining serious injury with HIV-contaminated secretions have been instituted. Clinicians' hesitation about being placed in placebo groups has hampered completion of the studies. All institutions should have a needle stick policy in place that allows rapid access (within hours) to ZDV for injured health workers who, after being fully informed, choose a trial of zidovudine.

Conclusion

In the history of the AIDS epidemic, the decade of the 1990s will be remembered as the decade of women. Millions are currently infected and millions will die before the turn of the century. The predominant mode of spread will no longer be homosexual activity but rather intravenous drug use and heterosexual behavior. The medical needs of infected women will no longer be confined to AIDS clinics but will spill into the offices of all providers who see women. HIV infections will disproportionately be seen among women with abnormal pap smears, pelvic inflammatory disease, and recurrent candidiasis. Obstetricians and gynecologists will be counseling and caring for infected women and advising their at-risk patients about preventive behaviors. In a decade in which HIV will assume new prominence as a cause of morbidity among women, obstetricians and gynecologists will be asked, once again, to assume their traditional roles as primary advocates for women. An understanding of the standards of care for HIV disease, as well as concern and compassion, will empower that role.

References

1. ACOG Committee: Statement 85, HIV infection: physicians' responsibilities, Washington DC, 1990.
2. Archibald DW, Witt DJ, Craven DE, et al. Antibodies to HIV in cervical secretions from women at risk for AIDS. J Infect Dis 1987; 156:240–241 (letter).
3. Bailey K, Herrod HG, Younger R, Shaver D. Functional aspects of T-lymphocytes subsets in pregnancy. Obstet Gynecol 1985; 66:211–215.
4. Berrebi A, Puel J, Grandjean H, et al. The influence of pregnancy on the evolution of HIV infection. Paper presented at the fourth international conference on AIDS. Stockholm, 1988. Abstract 4041.

5. Bledsoe K. The effect of pregnancy on HIV infection. Proceedings of the sixth international AIDS meeting. San Francisco, 1990.
6. Bigger RJ, Pahwa S, Landesman S, Goedert JJ. Helper and suppressor lymphocyte changes in HIV-infected mothers and their infants. Paper presented at the fourth international conference on AIDS, Stockholm, 1988. Abstract 4031.
7. Bowen DL, Lane HC, Fauci AS. Immunopathogenesis of the acquired immunodeficiency syndrome. Ann Intern Med 1985; 103:704–709.
8. Centers for Disease Control. Summary: recommendations for preventing transmission of infection with HTLV-III/LAV in the work place. MMWR 1985; 34:681–699.
9. Centers for Disease Control. Risk for cervical disease in HIV-infected women in New York City. MMWR 1990; 39:846–850.
10. Chiodo F, Ricchi E, Costigliola P, et al. Vertical transmission of HTLV-III. Lancet 1986; 1(8483):739.
11. Chu SY, Buehler JW, Berkelman RL. Impact of the human immunodeficiency virus epidemic on mortality in women of reproductive age, United States. JAMA 1990; 264:225–229.
12. Cowen MJ, Hellmar G, Chudwin D, et al. Maternal transmission of acquired immune deficiency syndrome. Pediatrics 1984; 73(3):382–386.
13. Desposito F, McSherry GD, Oleske JM. Blood products acquired HIV infection in children. Pediatr Ann 1988; 17(5):341–345.
14. Devash Y, Calvelli TA, Wood DG, et al. Vertical transmission of human immunodeficiency virus is correlated with the absence of high-affinity/avidity maternal antibodies to the gp120 principal neutralizing domain. Proc Natl Acad Sci USA 1990; 87:3445–3449.
15. Fiddes TM, O'Reilly DB, Cetrulo CL, et al. Phenotypic and functional evaluation of suppressor cells in normal pregnancy and in chronic aborters. Cell Immunol 1986; 97:407–418.
16. Fischl MA, Richman DD, Grieco MH, et al. The efficacy of aziodothymidine (AZT) in treatment of patients with AIDS and AIDS related complex: a double blind, placebo controlled trial. N Engl J Med 1987; 317:185–191.
17. Freeman DW, Barno A. Deaths from influenza epidemic associated with pregnancy. Am J Obstet Gynecol 1969; 78:1172.
18. Friedland GH, Saltzman BR, Rogers MF, et al. Lack of transmission of HTLV-III/LAV infection to household contacts of patients with AIDS or ARC with oral candidiasis. N Engl J Med 1986; 314(6):3444–3449.
19. Gerberding JL. Recommended infection-control policies for patients with human immunodeficiency virus infection. N Engl J Med 1986; 315:1562–1564.
20. Goedert JJ, Kessler CM, Aledort LM, et al. A prospective study of human immunodeficiency virus type 1 infection and the development of AIDS in subjects with hemophilia. N Engl J Med 1989; 321:1141–1148.
21. Goedert JJ, Mendez H, Drummond JE, et al. Maternal infant transmission of HIV Type 1: Association with prematurity or low anti-gp120. Lancet 1989; 2:1351–1353.
22. Halsey NA, Boulos R, Holt E, et al Transmission of HIV-1 infections from mothers to infants in Haiti. JAMA 1990; 264:2088–2092.
23. Hill JA, Barbieri RL, Anderson DJ. Immunosuppressive effects of danazol in vitro. Fertil Steril 1987; 48(3):414–418.
24. Hill WC, Bolton V, Carlson JR. Isolation of acquired immunodeficiency syndrome virus from the placenta. Am J Obstet Gynecol 1987. 157:10–11.
25. Hoegsberg B, Minkoff HL, Abullafia O, et al. Sexually transmitted diseases and human immunodeficiency virus infection among women with P.I.D. Am J Obstet Gynecol 1990; 163:1135–1138.
26. Holman S, Sunderland A, Berthard M, et al. Prenatal HIV counseling and testing. Clin Obstet Gynecol 1989; 445–455
27. Kasakura S. A factor in maternal plasma during pregnancy that suppresses the reactivity of mixed leukocyte cultures. J Immunol 1971; 107(5):1296–1301.
28. Kittas C, Henry L: Effect of sex hormones on the response of mice to infection with *Toxoplasma gondii* British Journal of Experimental Pathology 1980; 61:590.
29. Koenig RE, Gautier T, Levy JA. Unusual intrafamilial transmission of HIV. Lancet 1986; 2(8507):337.
30. Landesman S, Minkoff H, Holman S, et al. Serosurvey of HIV infections in parturients JAMA 1987; 258:2701–2703.
31. Lapointe N, Michaud J, Pekovik D, et al. Transplacental transmission of HTLV-III virus. N Engl J Med 1985; 312:1325.
32. Lurie MB, Harris TN, Abranson S, and Allison JM. Constitutional factors in resistance to infection II: The effect of estrogen on tuberculin skin sensitivity and on the allergy of the internal tissues. Am Rev Tuberculosis 59:186, 1949.
33. MacCallum LR, France AJ, Jones ME and others. The effects of pregnancy on the progression of HIV disease. Paper presented at the fourth international conference on AIDS. Stockholm, 1988. Abstract 4032.
34. Maiman M, Fruchter R, Serur E, et al. Human immunodeficiency virus infection and cervical neoplasia. Gynecol Oncol 1990; 38:377–382.
35. Maury W, Potts BJ, Rabson AB. HIV-1 infection of the first-trimester and term human placental tissue: a possible mode of maternal-fetal transmission. J Infect Dis 1989; 160:583–588.
36. Minkoff HL. Care of pregnant women infected with human immunodeficiency virus. JAMA 1987; 258:2714–2717.
37. Minkoff H, McCalla S, Delke I, et al. Cocaine and sexually transmitted diseases including HIV. Paper presented at the fifth international AIDS conference. Montreal, 1989.
38. Minkoff H, Nanda D, Menez R, Fikrig S. Pregnancies resulting in infants with acquired immunodeficiency syndrome or AIDS related complex. Obstet Gynecol 1987; 69:285–287.
39. Minkoff HL, Willoughby A, Mendez H, et al.

Serious infections among women with advanced HIV infection. Am J Obstet Gynecol 1990; 162:30–34.
40. Mundey DC, Schinzai RF, Gerber AR, et al. HIV isolated from amniotic fluid. Lancet 1987; 2:459–460.
41. Nanda D, Minkoff H. HIV in pregnancy: transmission and immune effects. Clin Obstet Gynecol 1989; 456–466
42. Peckham CS, Sentuna YD, Ades AE, et al. Mother to child transmission of HIV infection. Lancet 1988; 2:1039–1043.
42a. Peutherer JF, Rebus S, Pu D, et al. Fourth international conference on AIDS, 1988, Stockholm, Abstract #7235.
43. Phair J, Munoz A, Detels R, et al. The risk of pneumocystis carinii pneumonia among men infected with human immunodeficiency virus type I. N Engl J Med 1990; 322:161–165.
44. Pomerantz RJ, De la Monte SM, Dongan SP, et al. HIV infection of the uterine cervix. Ann Intern Med 1988; 108:321–327.
45. Qazi QH, Sheikh TM, Fikrig S. Lack of evidence for craniofacial dysmorphism in perinatal HIV infection. J Pediatr 1988; 112:7–11.
46. Quinn TC, Glasser D, Cannon RO, et al. Human immunodeficiency virus infection among patients attending clinics for sexually transmitted diseases. N Engl J Med 1988; 318:197–203.
47. Romano N, De-Crescenzo L, Lupo G, et al. Main routes of transmission of HIV infection in a family in Palermo, Italy. Am J Epidemiol 1988; 128:254–260.
48. Rubenstein A, Sicklic M, Gupta A, et al. AIDS with reversed T4 to T8 ratios in infants born to promiscuous and drug addicted mothers. JAMA 1983; 249:2350–2356.
49. Ryder RW, Nsa W, Hassia SE, et al. Prenatal transmission of the human immunodeficiency virus type 1 to infants of seropositive women in Zaire. N Engl J Med 1989; 320:1837–1842.
50. Schaefer A, Grosch-Woerner, Friedman I, et al. The effect of pregnancy on the natural course of HIV disease. Paper presented at the fourth international conference on AIDS, Stockholm, 1988. Abstract 4039.
51. Scott GB, Burke BE, Letterman JG, et al. Acquired immune deficiency syndrome in infants. N Engl J Med 1984; 310:76–81.
52. Selwyn PA, Carter CJ, Schoenbaum EE, et al. Knowledge of HIV antibody status and decisions to continue or terminate pregnancy among intravenous drug users. JAMA 1989; 261:1289–1294.
53. Sever JL. HIV: Biology and immunology. Clin Obstet Gynecol 1989; 32:423–428.
54. Siiteri PK, Stites DP. Immunologic and endocrine interrelationships in pregnancy. Biol Reprod 1982; 26:1–14.
55. Sridama V, Pacini F, Yang SL, et al. Decreased level of helper T cells: a possible cause of immunodeficiency in pregnancy. N Engl J Med 1982; 307:352–356.
56. Sunderland A, Moroso GN, Holman S, et al. Influence of HIV infection on pregnancy decisions. Paper presented at the fifth international conference on AIDS, Montreal, 1989.
56a. Thomas P, Jaffe N, Spira TJ, et al. Unexplained immune deficiency in children: a surveillance report. JAMA 1984; 292:639.
57. Tovo PA, de Martino M, Caramia G, et al. Epidemiology, clinical features and prognostic factors of pediatric HIV infection. Lancet 1988; 2:1043–1045.
58. Vanderberken Y, Vheghe MP, Velespesse G, et al. Clin Exp Immunol 1982; 48:1118–1120.
59. Vogt MW, Witt DJ, Craven DE. Isolation of HTLV-III/LAV from cervical secretions of women at risk for AIDS. Lancet 1986; 1:525–527.
60. Wahn V, Kramer HH, Brusten HT, et al. Horizontal transmission of HIV infection between two siblings. Lancet 1986; 2:694(letter).
61. Waltman ST, Burde RM, Berrios J. Prevention of corneal homograft rejection by estrogens. Transplantation 1971; 11(2):194–196.
62. Ward JW, Holmberg SD, Allen JR, et al. Transmission of HIV by blood transfusion screened as negative for HIV antibody. N Engl J Med 1988; 318(8):473–478.
63. Weinberg ED. Pregnancy associated depression of cell mediated immunity. Review of infectious diseases. 1984, 6(6)814–831.
64. Wofsy CB, Cohen JB, Haven LB, et al. Isolation of AIDS associated retrovirus from vaginal and cervical secretions from women with antibody for the virus. Lancet 1986; 1:527–529.

CHAPTER 13

Toxoplasmosis

Jacques Couvreur M.D.
Philippe Thulliez M.D.
Fernand Daffos M.D.

Toxoplasma gondii was discovered in 1908 in Tunis by Nicolle and Manceaux[98] in the spleen and liver of *Ctenodactylus gondii,* a North African rodent, and isolated the same year from a rabbit by Splendore in Brazil.[124] The important milestones that led to our consideration that this agent is an important, ubiquitous parasite in animal and human pathology were the discovery of "parasitic cysts" in the retina of a child who died with hydrocephaly, microphthalmia, and coloboma by Janku in Czechoslovakia in 1923;[75] the identification of this organism as *Toxoplasma* by Levaditi in Paris in 1923;[87] the discovery of an encephalitozoic infantile granulomatous encephalitis and the establishment of its prenatal transmission by Wolf and associates in 1937–1939;[138-140] the identification of this encephalitozoon as *Toxoplasma* by Sabin and Olitsky in the United States[115] and its etiologic role in an acquired fatal disease in an adult by Pinkerton and Weinman in 1940;[101] and the development of a valuable serologic technique, the dye test, by Sabin and Feldman in 1948.[114] Finally in 1969 *Toxoplasma gondii* was identified as a coccidian and its definitive host the cat by Frenkel and colleagues[58] and concomitantly by two other groups.[73,137]

The Organism and Its Life Cycle

Toxoplasma gondii is an intracellular protozoan parasite that can infect humans and any other warm-blooded animal. This coccidian exists in three forms: the oocyst, the resistant form; the tachyzoite, the proliferative form; and the bradyzoite, a quiescent intracystic tissue stage. The life cycle of *T. gondii* is divided into two parts: a sexual cycle, confined to the intestine of felids; and an asexual cycle that occurs in the extraintestinal tissues of felids and all other hosts.

Nonimmune cats become infected by the ingestion of meat harboring tissue cysts. In the intestine, the sexual cycle results in the production of oocysts, which are shed in the feces for 1 to 3 weeks and rarely thereafter. The proportion of cats excreting oocysts at any moment is usually not more than 2 percent in most countries, but a cat may excrete millions of oocysts in a single day.[45] When sporulation is complete, 1 to 5 days after they are excreted, the oocysts become infective and remain viable in soil for a year or more, depending upon climatic conditions.

On ingestion by intermediate hosts, organisms invade

the intestinal epithelium and associated lymph nodes as tachyzoites; then they spread through the circulation and tissues. Tachyzoites are crescent shaped, 2 to 4 μm by 4 to 8 μm; they actively penetrate host cells and multiply in parasitophorous vacuoles that do not fuse with lysosomes and are thus not destroyed. Host cell rupture can be followed by parasitization of contiguous cells. This process continues until the host develops immunity: extracellular parasites are eliminated, intracellular multiplication slows, and tissue cysts containing bradyzoites are formed within the host cell. Tissue cysts have a diameter of 20 to 200 μm, contain hundreds of organisms, and are usually subspherical or conform to the shape of the host cell. Although they may exist in virtually every organ, the brain and skeletal and heart muscles appear to be the most common sites where they persist as viable parasites throughout the life of the host.[105] Tissue cysts provoke little or no inflammatory response as long as the cyst wall is not disrupted. When an intermediate host, such as a bird or rodent, is the prey of a cat, the cycle is repeated.

Human infection is incidental and a dead end in the life cycle. It may occur via the oral route by ingestion of oocysts or tissue cysts and via the transplacental route by transmission of tachyzoites when a previously uninfected woman acquires the infection during pregnancy.

Transmission

There are two major routes of transmission: oral through ingestion of oocysts and tissue cysts in acquired toxoplasmosis and congenital by transplacental spread of tachyzoites.

Oral Transmission

Oocysts

Thousands of oocysts may be shed in a single stool of an infected cat. In freshly passed cat feces, they are unsporulated and thus not infective; they become infectious in 1 to 4 days. They can persist in a moist environment for months. Studies have demonstrated that deposits of infected cat feces remained infectious to mice for a year in Costa Rica and in Kansas.[61] Rain, earthworms, dung beetles, and cockroaches may be instrumental in spreading the oocysts in the environment.[57] These characteristics explain why infections are common in tropical countries, and in children who frequently play on the ground around houses where cats are present.[61,125] The transmission of *Toxoplasma* oocysts is similar to that of eggs of *Ascaris* or *toxocara*. Adult transmission can occur through soil contamination of improperly washed vegetables, strawberries, and the like. Dust borne outbreaks have occurred.

Cysts

Undercooked or raw meat is the most common route of transmission in adults. It is reported that 10 to 70 percent of mutton, 25 percent of pork, and 10 percent of beef samples may contain *Toxoplasma* cysts.[14,74,141] Cysts remain viable for 4 days at 4°C in refrigerators and after cooking for 20 minutes at 45°C. The wall of the cyst is digested by peptic and tryptic digestive juices in the gastrointestinal tract but the endozoites can survive 3 hours in the juices, which allows them to invade the mucosa of the digestive tract and to spread. The meat-to-human route of transmission of *Toxoplasma* was demonstrated by Desmonts and Couvreur in a group of children fed with raw or undercooked meat.[41] It is obvious that prevalence of toxoplasmosis is much higher in countries where the practice of eating raw or undercooked meat is common.

Transplacental Transmission

Transplacental infection has been documented in animals. In sheeps and goats as in humans, it occurs following an infection acquired during pregnancy.[12] In mice and goats, transmission in successive pregnancies has been observed.[46]

Other Means of Transmission

Transmission of *Toxoplasma* by blood transfusion has never been proven but may occur. Parasitemia has been observed in apparently normal animals, sometimes for months following inoculation of avirulent strains of *Toxoplasma*. It has been demonstrated in acute latent infections,[77] and recurrent parasitemia may occur in chronic toxoplasmosis in human beings. *Toxoplasma* was isolated from the blood of a woman 14 months after the delivery of a newborn with severe, fatal congenital toxoplasmosis.[95] *Toxoplasma* invades and remains viable in leukocytes. The organisms can survive in whole citrated blood stored at 4°C for up to 50 days. Venereal or salivary transmission has never been demonstrated. Toxoplasmosis presenting mainly as encephalitis has been reported in cardiac, kidney, bone marrow, and liver transplant recipients.[90] The heart transplant population seems particularly at risk,[89] with development of toxoplasmosis in 5 to 15 percent of recipients.

Transmission of *Toxoplasma* from mother to infant by milk has been observed in one case.[129] It seems exceptional but has been documented in animal experiments.[46] Oral transmission by goat milk has been observed in humans.[116]

Epidemiology

Toxoplasma is ubiquitous in nature. It is encountered wherever cats are present. The organism is found in herbivorous, omnivorous, and carnivorous animals and in some birds.

Toxoplasmosis is probably one of the most common infections of humans. There is no difference in prevalence between the sexes. Serologic investigations reveal considerable geographic differences in prevalence rates. Colder regions have fewer human infections than warmer areas. In the tropics and subtropics, the highest incidence of infection is during childhood, with contaminated soil being the major source of infection.[60,61] In developed countries where the meat-to-human route is the prevalent way of transmission, seroconversion occurs later in life and seropositivity increases with age. The prevalence of antibodies to *T. gondii* in various countries is summa-

Table 13-1 Prevalence of Antibodies to *Toxoplasma gondii* in Some Countries Throughout the World

Country (Senior Author, Year, Reference)	Percent Positive
Algeria (Schneider, 1979[119])	52
Brazil (Ferraroni, 1982[54])	74
Costa Rica (Frenkel, 1981[60])	61
England (Ruoss, 1972[113])*	22
El Salvador (Remington, 1970[108])	75
France (Desmonts, 1974[36]*)	87
Hong Kong (Ko, 1980[79])	10
Iran (Ghorbani, 1981[66])	13
Jordan (Abdel-Hafez, 1986[1]*)	26
Malaysia (Saleha, 1984[117])	4.5-27
Norway (Stray-Petersen, 1980[126]*)	13
Somalia (Zardi, 1980[142])	53
Tahiti (Wallace, 1976[131])	71
Taiwan (Wallace, 1976[132])	4
United States (Feldman, 1965[53])	8-20
United States (Sever, 1988[121]*)	38
United States (Remington, 1988[107]*)	27
Zaire (Wery-Paskoff, 1970[133])	40

*Studies limited to pregnant women or women of childbearing age.

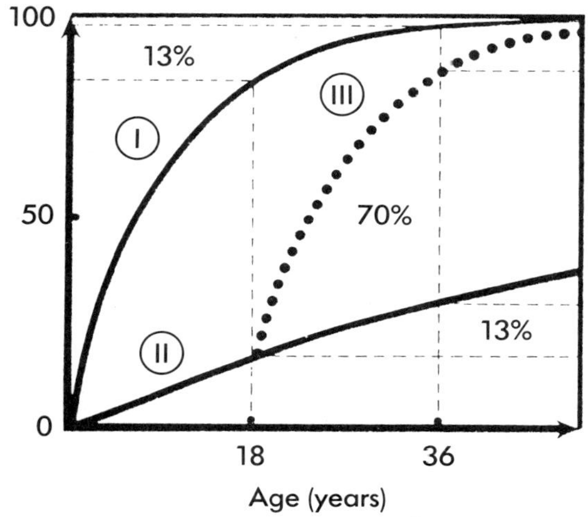

Figure 13-1 Toxoplasmosis incidence rates between 18 and 36 years of age. Curve I: theoretical antibody prevalence for a yearly rate of 10 percent acquisitions. Curve II: prevalence for a rate of 1 percent acquisitions. Curve III: prevalence for a rate increasing from 1 to 10 percent at age 18. (From Desmonts G, Couvreur J. 1975.[39])

rized in Table 13-1. Variations in the nature of the serologic techniques used in different surveys must be taken into account. However, there are striking differences in prevalence rates between geographic areas: Paris (France), 87 percent, or Amazonia (Brazil), 74 percent versus Taiwan, 4 percent, or Navajo Indians (United States), 0. These differences are related to the presence of cats and eating habits. Wherever meat is eaten raw or undercooked, toxoplasmosis is widespread. Conversely, the prevalence is low in communities where people eat well-cooked or deep-frozen meat.

The risk of acquired toxoplasmosis in pregnant women depends on three factors: (1) the prevalence in the community, (2) the number of contacts with a source of infection, and (3) the number of pregnant women in the community who have not developed antibody as a result of a prior infection. In a community with a high prevalence rate, only a few women are at risk during their childbearing years. If the prevalence is low, a large proportion of women are at risk because they have not been immunized by a prior infection. This explains why the number of infections during pregnancy and consequently the incidence of congenital toxoplasmosis may be similar to communities where epidemiologic conditions are quite different (Fig. 13-1).

It must be emphasized that the risk of acquired infection is markedly increased for women migrating from a community with a low prevalence of toxoplasmosis to a country with high prevalence.[37] The authors have observed that Vietnamese women coming from areas where the prevalence is probably below 5 percent to France, where it is above 80 percent are at high risk if they change their eating habits.

The prevalence of congenital infection in a community is directly related to the rate of acquired infection in pregnant women. Several facts are worth considering: about 40 percent of maternal acute infections are transmitted to the fetus;[36] the majority of congenital infections are subclinical; the prevalence can vary over years; and it is influenced by preventive measures. In Paris compulsory routine screening for seroconversion in pregnant women started in 1978, and subsequent preventive measures reduced the prevalence of congenital toxoplasmosis. There was a decrease from more than 3 to fewer than 1 per 1,000 live births.[83] In Alabama it varied from 0.6 to 2 per 1,000.[3]

Clinical Patterns

Acute Infection in the Pregnant Woman

Following an incubation period of 10 to 17 days, the most common clinical manifestation is lymphadenopathy, particularly involving the suboccipital and supraclavicular regions. Nodes are moderately enlarged and can be tender for a few days. There may be fatigue, headache, and myalgia, yet fever is rare. Other signs of infection, such as sore throat or splenomegaly, are not

Table 13-2 Clinical Findings in 210 Infants with Congenital Toxoplasmosis*

Clinical Findings	Number Examined	Number Positive	(%)
Prematurity			
Birth weight below 2,500 g	210	8	(3.8)
Birth weight of 2,500-3,000 g		5	(2.4)
Intrauterine growth retardation		13	(6.2)
Jaundice	201	20	(10)
Hepatosplenomegaly	210	9	(4.2)
Thrombocytopenic purpura	210	3	(1.4)
Abnormal blood count (anemia, eosinophilia)	102	9	(8.8)
Microcephaly	210	11	(5.2)
Hydrocephalus	210	8	(3.8)
Hypotonia	210	2	(1)
Convulsions	210	8	(3.8)
Psychomotor retardation	210	11	(5.2)
Intracranial calcifications (x-ray)	210	24	(11.4)
Abnormal transfontanellar sonography	49	5	(10)
Abnormal tomodensitometry of the brain	13	11	(84)
Abnormal electroencephalographic pattern	191	16	(8.3)
Abnormal cerebrospinal fluid	163	56	(34.2)
Microphthalmia	210	6	(2.9)
Strabismus	210	11	(5.2)
Chorioretinitis			
Unilateral	210	34	(16.1)
Bilateral		12	(5.7)
Subclinical pattern	210	116	(55.2)

*Infants were 0 to 11 months of age with congenital toxoplasmosis diagnosed through prospective studies of women with acquired *Toxoplasma* infection during pregnancy.
Adapted from Couvreur et al. 1984.[28]

present. Blood studies can reveal atypical lymphocytes as in infectious mononucleosis.

Several facts must be emphasized: the possible long persistence in the nodes (3 to 6 months), the absence of any tendency to suppurate, and the lack of correlation between the relatively benign clinical syndrome and the risk and severity of fetopathy.[36] In fact, signs of the acute infection are most of the time unrecognized.

Congenital Infection

Following the initial observations by Wolf and Cowen,[138] the signs and symptoms of congenital toxoplasmosis have been well documented.[3,22,47,51,127] Four entities were originally considered as the main features of the disease: chorioretinitis, hydrocephaly or microcephaly, cerebral calcifications, and neurologic injury.

However, prospective studies of infected infants born to women with acute infection diagnosed during pregnancy revealed that the most common form of congenital toxoplasmosis is subclinical.[36] Consequently, analytic inventory of the signs and clinical syndromes is considered separately. Table 13-2 summarizes clinical findings in 210 infants.

Inventory of the Clinical Signs

Ocular Involvement. Focal chorioretinitis is the most frequent sign of congenital toxoplasmosis: 76 percent in patent cases.[36] This complication has been extensively studied by ophthalmologists.[69] Usual presenting

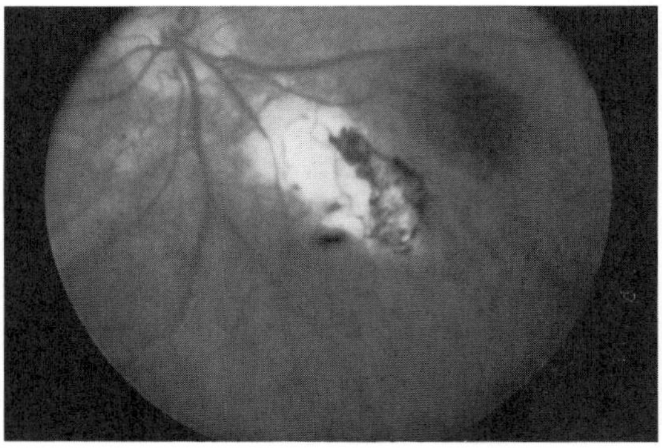

Figure 13-2 Chorioretinitis scar in a 7-year-old girl. (From Desmonts G, Couvreur J. 1985.[40])

symptoms are strabismus and nystagmus (in bilateral cases) and less often microphthalmia, small cornea, or cataract. Lesions can be found more or less fortuitously, years after birth.

Active lesions appear on fundoscopic examination as a white or yellowish focus. There is edema of the retina. Vitreous inflammatory exudate can impede visualization of the ocular fundus.

Older lesions appear as glial scars with a punched-out pattern (Fig. 13-2); areas of destruction of the retina, choroid, and sclera are visible. Around the depigmented areas, there are pigment deposits. The lesion can be solitary or associated with other smaller lesions of various ages. The surrounding retina and vasculature are normal.

Chorioretinitis in congenital toxoplasmosis has a predilection for the macular area, is bilateral in severe cases, and has a tendency to relapse.

Chorioretinitis can be associated with inflammatory involvement of the anterior uvea, iris, and ciliary bodies, with subsequent posterior synechiae and a risk of cataract. Functional disability can be severe. One study found that ocular toxoplasmosis was responsible for 5 percent of blindness in children.[50]

Hydrocephalus. This is almost always related to obstruction of the aqueduct of Sylvius. It has been encountered in 20 to 22 percent of patients with congenital toxoplasmosis.[36,51] Our personal experience of 21 cases with a follow-up of 6 months to 15 years[26] indicates that there are three types of presentation: detection in utero by sonography in fetuses at risk (2 cases)(Fig. 13-3), recognition in patients with known congenital toxoplasmosis (17 cases), and presenting sign of the disease (2 cases). Toxoplasmic hydrocephalus developed within 4 months following birth in 71 percent of the patients. There was spontaneous stabilization in 9.5 percent, and hydrocephalus occurred as late as at 14 and 17 years of age in two cases.

Hydrocephalus was associated with chorioretinitis in 78 percent, signs of neurologic injury in 43 percent, and IQ below 100 in 57 percent of the patients. Local antibody synthesis can be a sign of activity. Shunting was necessary in 90 percent of the patients. Transfontanellar sonography can detect ventricular dilation in 23 percent of patients with hyperproteinorachia and ocular involvement.[97] Computed tomography is mandatory to detect the site of the obstruction, to evaluate the degree of cerebral atrophy, and to look for granulomatous lesions.[103]

Microcephaly. Microcephaly, when present, reflects severe brain damage but is not specific to this disease.[107]

Neurologic Signs. The clinical spectrum of neurologic signs is protean, ranging from massive to subtle. Computed tomography allows a detailed study of the neuroanatomic lesions that include porencephaly encephalomalacia, and hydraencephaly.

Calcifications. Calcifications (Fig. 13-4) are of two types: small nodular deposits of 1 to 3 mm or more in diameter, scattered in the white matter, often in a subependymal location; and curvilinear streaks in the periventricular areas or basal ganglia. In cytomegalic inclusion disease, calcification, in contrast, is often periventricular.

Convulsions. Convulsions are the presenting sign in about 50 percent of clinical cases.[52]

Mental Retardation. Congenital toxoplasmosis with neurologic injury often leads to mental retardation. Numerous retrospective studies have been made to delineate the role of congenital toxoplasmosis in mentally retarded children. The results ranged from no significant data to 4 to 20 percent of cases in which *Toxoplasma* was implicated. Prospective controlled studies are mandatory for accurate evaluation of a causative relationship. Preliminary data obtained by Alford and coworkers[2] show that congenital toxoplasmosis in a subclinical form can cause intellectual impairment.

Cerebrospinal Fluid Abnormalities. Among the CSF abnormalities, a high protein content is the most frequent. It ranges from slight to massive amounts (up to 800 mg per milliliter) with a xanthochromic color. The number of cells, mostly lymphocytes, is normal or moderately elevated. Cerebrospinal fluid study is mandatory in cases of congenital toxoplasmosis for several reasons:

1. It is the most frequent abnormality encountered in infected infants (34 percent) and may be the only finding in subclinical cases.[28]
2. A high protein content is of poor prognostic significance.
3. *Toxoplasma* can be isolated from CSF for the first few weeks.[38]

Other Visceral Manifestations. These manifestations are less frequent. Jaundice is related to liver damage or hemolysis. Toxoplasmosis occurred in 2.2 percent of a series of 225 patients with neonatal jaundice.[22] It is generally associated with hepatosplenomegaly. Liver calcifications are exceptional. The nephrotic syndrome associated with the presence of *Toxoplasma* in glomeruli has been observed in severe cases.[21] Subclinical interstitial pneumonia has been documented by histologic studies.[20] Although *Toxoplasma* is frequently isolated from the myocardium in fatal cases, interstitial myocarditis is not associated with symptoms.

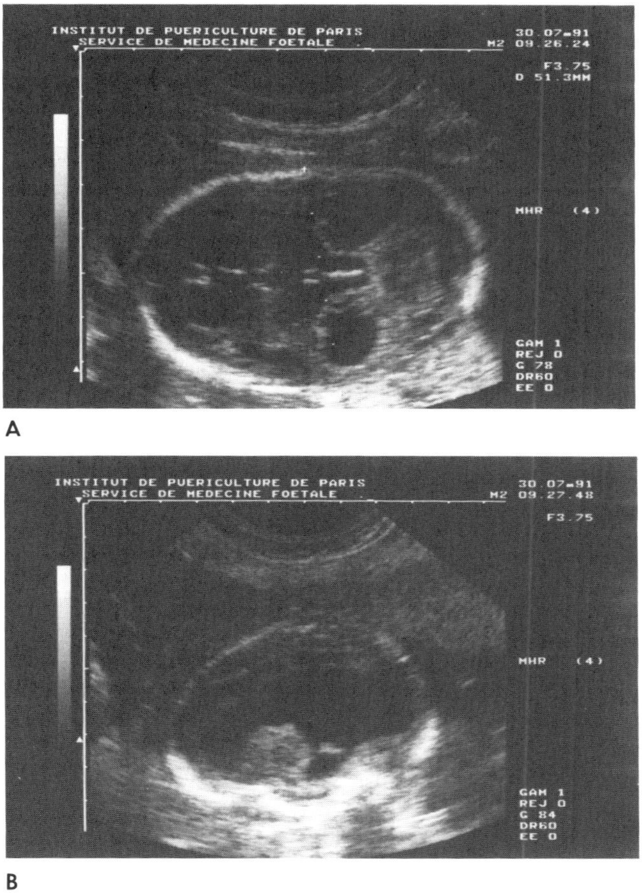

Figure 13-3 A, Hydrocephalus diagnosed through sonography in a 22-week-old fetus. **B,** Fetopathy proved in utero by a fetal blood examination.

Purpura, petechiae, and ecchymosis reflect the thrombocytopenia occurring in severe systemic disease. Erythroblastosis and hydrops fetalis are rarely observed.[10,17]

Prematurity. Prematurity and intrauterine growth retardation are more frequent in infected infants than in the general community.[28]

Toxoplasmosis in Twins. Toxoplasmosis in twins has an identical pattern when they are monozygotic. Wide discrepancies between the infants are the rule in dizygotic twins[24,123] and often there is no infection in one of the twins.[24] These facts are important with respect to the pathophysiology of maternal-fetal infection (see Pathophysiology section).

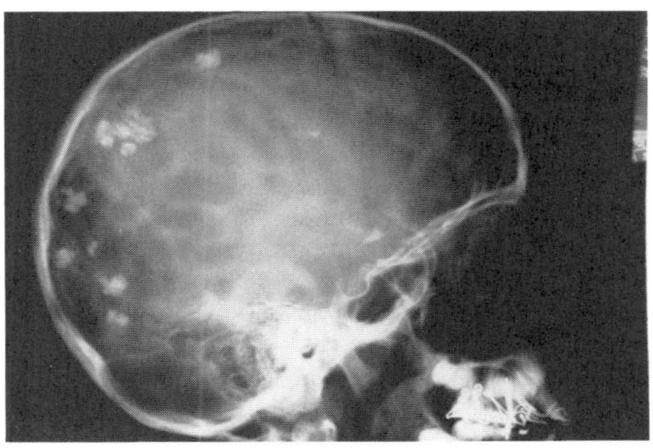

Figure 13-4 Huge cerebral calcifications discovered fortuitously in an 11-year-old girl. Chorioretinitis and minimal brain dysfunction are present.

Syndromes

Although wide variations are encountered, most cases are of one of the following four forms:

Neonatal Patent Disease. Neonatal patent disease is generally severe with signs of systemic, multivisceral involvement: prematurity, jaundice, hepatosplenomegaly, purpura, bulging of the fontanelle and neurologic signs, chorioretinitis, high protein CSF content, and ventricular dilation. Severe sequelae including death are common. However, some infants with no signs of encephalitis can recover despite systemic disease when they are treated early. Sometimes infection is not clinically recognizable in the neonatal period, but severe central nervous system involvement (hydrocephaly, encephalitis, evolutive eye lesions) occurs after several weeks or months.

Sequelae with Signs of Cerebral Damage. This clinical pattern includes chorioretinal scars and often cerebral calcifications. Convulsions, developmental retardation, and neurologic signs are the presenting manifestations.

Mild Sequelar Disease. This clinical pattern includes patients with mild chorioretinitis or with a few cerebral calcifications but without clinical evidence of cerebral damage. The intellectual and neurologic development is normal.

Subclinical or Inapparent Infection. The most common form of congenital toxoplasmosis is this pattern. Its incidence was demonstrated by prospective studies of maternal infection.[36] The diagnosis relies on laboratory data: infected placenta, signs of antibody synthesis, and persistence of antibodies. The label *subclinical* applies to a patient who has had a thorough yet negative physical examination that includes a fundoscopic examination, transfontanellar sonography, and CSF study.

Secondary Progress

The fact that congenital toxoplasmosis can progress further in weeks, months, or many years following birth is of importance.

Secondary chorioretinitis has been described,[2] in particular in patients with subclinical disease. Prospective studies confirm these data. In Holland, Koppe and associates[80] followed 12 children from birth and found that 66 percent developed chorioretinitis before 15 years of age. In the United States Wilson and colleagues[135] found that among 13 infants with subclinical infection in the neonatal period, 11 (85 percent) developed eye involvement between 1 month and 9.3 years of age. In Paris, in a group of 48 infants with congenital toxoplasmosis discovered through a routine screening program at 10 months of age, 10 percent had chorioretinitis at the time of the diagnosis, 16 percent at 2 years of age, and 18 percent at 4 years of age.[83] Among 172 patients (of whom 119 had subclinical infection) followed for 2 to 11 years, 14 (8.1 percent) developed new ocular lesions between 4 months and 7.5 years, despite the fact that all patients had been treated.[23]

A prospective clinical study revealed an increased rate of deafness, microcephaly, and low IQ values at a 7-year follow-up.[119] Clinical onset of hydrocephaly can be very late:[111] among 21 cases with a mean follow-up of 6.1 years, 2 became active and required surgery at 13 and 17 years of age, respectively.[26]

Evidence of a secondary period of activity is also supported by biological data. A secondary rise of antibodies is frequent during the second year and sometimes occurs many years later. There may be local synthesis of antibodies, as for instance in the eye and subarachnoid space. Examination of more than 2,000 samples of aqueous humor of the eye in patients with chorioretinitis (most of them with congenital infection) revealed that the aqueous humor/serum ratio was greater than 2 in 34 percent between 4 and 9 years of age, 32 percent between 10 and 14, 40 percent between 15 and 19, and 33 percent between 20 and 24 years of age.[35] Significant local synthesis of antibodies in cerebrospinal fluid (CSF:serum ratio approximately 4) was observed in 19 of 46 patients 2 to 27 years of age (41 percent). This proportion rose to 61.5 percent in patients with recent clinical activity, that is, chorioretinitis or convulsions.[27] Sequential determinations in 13 patients with hydrocephaly revealed a CSF:serum ratio greater than 4 in 11 of them. In five patients, the value correlated well with progress of the disease and may correlate with an increase in intracranial pressure.[27]

Prognosis

In order to evaluate potential risk factors that might indicate that the congenital disease would progress, 85 patients with fetopathy were studied prospectively. They were divided in two groups: 30 who developed secondary chorioretinitis and 55 who never developed ocular lesions following birth. Patients were significantly more prone to have short- or long-term flare-ups of chorioretinitis if the maternal infection occurred before week 26 of pregnancy and if their initial check-up revealed cerebral calcifications, neurologic changes, bilateral chorioditis, and local synthesis of antibodies in the CSF. The mean specific IgG titer at birth was elevated in those with chorioretinitis and was twice that observed in those who did not develop ocular lesions.[31]

Laboratory Diagnosis

Serologic methods are the main tools for the diagnosis of *Toxoplasma* infection. In the fetus and the newborn, the diagnosis can also be established by isolation of organisms.

Serologic Methods

In some tests entire organisms are used as antigens; they mainly demonstrate antibodies directed against the antigens of the parasite membrane.[40] These are the Sabin-Feldman dye test (DT), the immunofluorescent antibody (IFA) test, the agglutination test, and the IgM-immunosorbent agglutination assay (ISAgA).

Other methods use an antigenic extract from lysed parasites, including the CF test, the indirect hemagglutination (IHA) test, the latex agglutination test, and the ELISA. The antigenic extract contains many antigens that originate from both the membrane and the cytoplasm of the parasite.[40] After infection, the detection of IgG antibodies is delayed with lysed parasites in comparison with methods using intact organisms. However improved ELISA with membrane antigens are now being introduced.

The DT is a standard reference test. In this test live parasites exposed to antibody-containing serum die after formation of antigen-antibody complexes on the surface of the organism. The DT primarily measures IgG that usually appears 1 to 2 weeks after initiation of infection. Peak titers are reached in 6 to 8 weeks and then persist with gradually declining titers for years. The titer does not correlate with the severity of illness. The DT is used in relatively few laboratories because it employs live organisms.

Immunofluorescent Antibody Test

The IFA may be used to measure IgG or IgM antibodies. Slide preparations of fixed *Toxoplasma* are incubated with serial dilutions of the patient's serum. A specific reaction between the organismic antigenic sites and the antibodies is detected by using a fluorescein-tagged antiserum prepared against serum gamma globulins. In general, the qualitative agreement between results in DT and IFA tests is excellent, but false-positive results occur in some sera that contain antinuclear antibodies, and reliable quantitative titers may be difficult to obtain.

The IFA test has been adopted for the demonstration of specific IgM antibodies and has contributed to the diagnosis of acquired and congenital infection. However, the IgM-IFA test has two main drawbacks: the occurrence of false-positive results in sera that contain rheumatoid factor and a false-negative reactivity that is due to an inhibitory effect of high titers of IgG antibodies. Thus a recent acute infection may be missed. Moreover, the sensitivity of this method is insufficient to detect a specific IgM antibody response in the fetus or the newborn. Thus the IgM-IFA test should not be used to investigate congenital infection.

Indirect Hemagglutination Test

In the IHA test, red blood cells tagged with *Toxoplasma* antigen agglutinate when serum containing specific antibodies is added. Titers may lag several weeks or more behind those of the DT. The IHA test is not recommended for the diagnosis of congenital infection or for screening pregnant women because the test may be negative early in the infection. However, it is useful as an additional test in the diagnosis of acute acquired infection when the DT titer has already stabilized and a rising IHA titer can be demonstrated.

Agglutination Test

The agglutination test employs whole formalin-preserved parasites. The test is very sensitive to IgM antibodies, and "natural" IgM antibodies frequently cause nonspecific agglutination of the parasites in the serum of individuals who are negative when tested by the DT. This problem is avoided by including 2 mercapto-ethanol as a diluent to suppress the agglutination due to IgM antibodies. Several different antigen suspensions are available. High-sensitivity agglutination antigen (HS) is used to demonstrate the presence of IgG antibodies in screening pregnant women and in the diagnosis of infection in both mother and child. This method is accurate, simple to perform, and easy to read.[44]

If acetone or methanol is used instead of formalin as a fixative, an antigen preparation (AC) is obtained that contains stage-specific antigens that are recognized by IgG antibodies formed against *Toxoplasma* tachyzoites early in infection. The differential agglutination test (HS/AC test), which compares the titers obtained with both antigens, is useful for differentiating between infections acquired recently and those acquired is the more distant past.[33] In those adults who have both IgM and high IgG titers, a negative AC test signifies that the infection has been acquired at least 6 months before.

The same HS antigen is used in an antibody-trapping immunoassay (ISAgA) for detection of *Toxoplasma* IgM antibodies. It does not require use of an enzyme conjugate; it is simple to perform and is read in the same manner as the agglutination test.[44] The test is more sensitive and more specific than the IgM-IFA test and has been used effectively for diagnosis of infection in the fetus and the newborn.[43] Because of its high sensitivity, the ISAgA detects IgM antibodies earlier than other tests in recently acquired infections and also detects IgM antibodies for a longer period after infection.

Enzyme-Linked Immunosorbent Assay

The ELISA is an objective test that is widely used. Its efficacy in detecting an early IgG antibody response to *Toxoplasma* depends on the way the antigen is prepared. Antibody-trapping ELISAs, like double-sandwich ELISA, have been developed for detection of specific IgM. They are more sensitive and specific than the IgM-IFA test but may demonstrate as IgM-ISAgA the IgM antibodies for a year or longer.

More recently *Toxoplasma*-specific IgA antibody detection by ELISA or the ISAgA test has been considered as an additional diagnostic marker in congenitally infected newborns and in pregnant women with newly acquired infection. These promising results require further evaluation.

Enzyme-Linked Immunofiltration Assay

The enzyme-linked immunofiltration assay makes use of a micropore membrane and permits simultaneous study of antibody specificity by immunoprecipitation and characterization of G, M, A, or E antibody isotypes by immunofiltration with enzyme-labeled antibodies.[102] This method appears very useful for the diagnosis of congenital infection.

Detection and Isolation of *Toxoplasma Gondii*

A histologic examination is rarely performed when lymphadenopathy occurs in a pregnant woman. The histopathologic changes in *Toxoplasma* lymphadenitis would enable one to make a presumptive diagnosis of acute acquired toxoplasmosis, but the organisms themselves are rarely demonstrable.[107]

Isolation of *Toxoplasma gondii* provides unequivocal proof of congenital infection. The organisms can be isolated from cord blood sampled at birth or in utero under ultrasound guidance, from peripheral blood of the newborn, from the amniotic fluid, and from the placenta. Isolation procedures involve the inoculation of mice or the inoculation of tissue culture preparations.

Mouse Inoculation

The sediment from 10 to 30 ml of amniotic fluid, whole blood clot, or the cellular phase of heparinized blood is injected intraperitoneally or subcutaneously into mice.

For placental tissue, trypsin digestion is used;[107] this method makes it possible to isolate both tachyzoite and cyst forms. Approximately 100 g of placenta (without fixative) is first minced with scissors and passed through a meat grinder; it is then placed in trypsin solution (0.25% trypsin in buffered saline, pH 7.2) and incubated with constant agitation for 1 hour at 37°C. The suspension is passed through several layers of gauze to remove the large particles, and then the sediment is washed in saline to remove trypsin. The digested material is resuspended in saline, and 0.5 to 1 ml is inoculated into mice by the intraperitoneal or subcutaneous route.

Approximately 5 to 10 days after intraperitoneal injection of mice, the peritoneal fluid can be examined either fresh or in stained smears for the presence of intracellular and extracellular tachyzoites. Mice that die before 6 weeks are examined for the presence of the organism. With rare exceptions, isolates from congenitally infected infants are relatively avirulent for mice, and a period of 3 to 6 weeks is usually required for definitive demonstration of the parasite. Surviving mice are bled for serologic testing 3 and 6 weeks after inoculation. If antibodies are present, proof of infection must be obtained by examining wet preparations or stained smears of brain tissue for demonstration of cysts.

Tissue Culture

Because the main drawback of mouse inoculation is a 3- to 6-week delay before a result is definitive, inoculation into cell culture combined with immunoreagents offers the opportunity for more rapid detection of *Toxoplasma* in fetal samples.[34]

Amniotic fluid sediment is inoculated into a human embryonic fibroblast culture (cell line MRC5). After 4 days of incubation, parasites are identified in monolayers by an indirect immunofluorescence assay.

The buffy coat layer of fetal blood samples may be examined in the same way. Some studies have found tissue culture to be at least as sensitive as mouse inoculation, but in our experience on amniotic fluid samples, tissue culture is less sensitive (53 percent versus 73 percent, n = 53).

Because results are obtained within a few days, tissue culture isolation should be used in addition to mouse inoculation when early diagnosis is critical for the management of the patient, that is prenatal diagnosis of a congenital infection.

Demonstration of Specific Nucleic Acid Sequences

As in many other infectious diseases, the polymerase chain reaction (PCR) has been applied to detect *Toxoplasma gondii* DNA and has recently been evaluated in comparison with other diagnostic methods.[67] It correctly identified the presence of *Toxoplasma* in 8 of 10 samples of amniotic fluid from proven cases of congenital infection; no false-positive result was observed among 38 specimens from uninfected fetuses. Therefore, application of the PCR may be expected to change the diagnostic repertoire drastically in the near future. Nevertheless, further studies are required to assess the sensitivity and the specificity of PCR for the purpose of prenatal diagnosis.

Postmortem Examination

Organisms are regularly detected on wet preparations of brain tissue from infected fetuses after induced abortion. Fluorescent antibody and peroxidase-antiperoxidase techniques are applicable to unfixed or formalin-fixed paraffin-embedded tissue sections. Isolation of parasites is easiest from the brain and skeletal muscle of infants who die months or years after birth, although isolates have been obtained from virtually every organ and tissue.[107]

Diagnosis in the Pregnant Woman

Because the majority of cases of acute acquired *Toxoplasma* infection are asymptomatic, the diagnosis relies mainly on the results of serologic tests.

A positive titer indicates only that a toxoplasmic infection has occurred. Because IgG and IgM titers may remain elevated for a year or more, one cannot determine from a single high titer whether the infection is acute or chronic. A diagnosis of acute acquired infection is established by the demonstration of a rising titer in serial specimens: either conversion from a negative to a positive titer or a rise from a low to a higher IgG titer with demonstrable IgM. However, a stable high titer may have been reached if the time the first serum was obtained was delayed.

Ideally, every woman of reproductive age should know her *Toxoplasma* serologic status before conception. If the patient has specific IgG antibodies, she is protected and there is no fetal risk unless she is immunocompromised. Women with negative serologic tests are at risk of acquiring a primary infection during pregnancy, and education regarding preventive measures should be provided. Additionally, serologic testing should be repeated during pregnancy until delivery to detect those women who acquire primary infection so that they can be identified and their offspring appropriately managed. IgM antibodies are usually the first to appear, but IgG antibodies, as measured in the dye test, also appear early: sera in which only IgM antibodies are detectable are uncommon. A rise in IgM antibody titer is infrequently observed, suggesting that it does not last longer than 1 or 2 weeks before reaching its peak. In contrast, the rise in IgG antibody titer is initially very slow.

In the absence of positive preconception serology, serologic testing is recommended early in the first trimester. A positive IgG titer in the absence of IgM as measured by a suitable test (DS-ELISA or ISAgA) is consistent with a latent (chronic) infection acquired months or years earlier. It can be confirmed by finding a similar titer on a second specimen obtained 3 weeks later and run in parallel with the first one.

The presence of IgM antibodies suggests but does not prove an acute or recent infection because specific IgM may occasionally persist for months or years. Examination of paired sera, taken 3 weeks apart, is necessary. A significant rise in IgG titer confirms an acute infection. To assess the risk of transmission of the organism to the fetus, it is necessary to relate the date of acquisition of the infection to the date of conception. In this regard, knowledge of the relation of variations in titer depending on the serologic method employed is helpful.[40,107] IgG antibodies detected in the DT and IFA tests reach their peak within 2 months, whereas those measured in IHA test and some ELISAs may reach their maximum in 4 months. In the aggultination test, the rise in IgG antibody titer may parallel the DT pattern, or it may rise slowly. Specific treatment given early may suppress the rise in titer. If the IgG antibody titer is stable and the patient has not been treated in the interim, infection was acquired at least 2 months before the first serum was obtained.

Commonly, the asymptomatic woman is evaluated late in pregnancy. If her IgG and IgM antibodies titers are high and no significant rise in IgG titers in any test can be demonstrated, it is impossible to determine when her infection was acquired with respect to the time of conception. If, in this instance, the AC agglutination test is negative, the infection was most probably acquired prior to conception.[33]

Diagnosis in the Newborn Infant

Congenital infection is demonstrated by isolation of parasites from the placenta or from the newborn, by the demonstration of a specific humoral response in the infant, or by both. Isolation of parasites should be attempted whenever possible because the antibody response of a congenitally infected baby may be weak or delayed.

At delivery, unfixed placental tissue should be stored at 4°C until it can be injected into mice. The correlation between isolation of *Toxoplasma* from placental tissue and infection of the neonate is excellent. Cases in which placental isolation is obtained and the infant is not infected are very unusual.[107] Nevertheless, the frequency of isolation depends on whether the woman has been treated; organisms are isolated less often if spiramycin or pyrimethamine and sulphonamides have been administered during pregnancy (see Pathophysiology section).

Toxoplasma may also be isolated from cord or peripheral blood of the newborn. In a study of 69 infants with congenital infection, Desmonts isolated organisms from blood in 43 percent of cases, but no infant had detectable parasitemia after 4 weeks of age.[107]

The demonstration of specific IgM antibodies in the serum of a newborn is diagnostic of congenital infection. A positive result on a cord blood sample should be confirmed on a serum specimen obtained later to rule out the possibility of a placental leak. Specific IgM antibody is absent in the sera of 75 percent of neonates with a congenital infection when the IgM-IFA test is used, whereas false-negative result is obtained in only 30 percent with the ISAgA method. It is noteworthy that the proportion of infants showing IgM antibody is the same whether the illness is clinically manifest or subclinical. IgM antibodies may persist for months or disappear.

In the absence of demonstration of *Toxoplasma* or IgM antibodies, follow-up serologic testing of infants with a suspected infection is the only means of making a diagnosis. Maternally transmitted IgG antibodies may persist for 6 to 12 months, depending on the original titer. Thus the presence of IgG antibody at this age does not necessarily prove that the infant is infected. Synthesis of *Toxoplasma* IgG antibody may be demonstrable by comparing the "immune load" (ratio of specific serum antibody titer to the level of serum IgG) of a recent sample with that of earlier samples.[40] In the absence of infection, the immune load decreases because the infant produces IgG that does not contain specific *Toxoplasma* antibodies. In the presence of infection, the infant produces specific antibodies, and thus the immune load remains the same or increases. A definitive serologic diagnosis may be delayed for several months in treated children in whom development of a specific antibody response may sometimes be very slow.

Prenatal Diagnosis

When the diagnosis of postconceptionally acquired *Toxoplasma* infection is established in a pregnant woman, spiramycin treatment should be given, and procedures to detect fetal infection such as ultrasound examination, cordocentesis, and amniocentesis attempted.[43]

Ultrasonography

Repeated examinations are performed throughout pregnancy, with special emphasis on the size of the lateral ventricles, thickness of the placenta, fetal ascites, liver enlargement, and intracranial calcifications.

Cordocentesis and Amniocentesis

From 20 weeks of gestation, 1.5 to 4 ml of fetal blood are taken by direct puncture with a needle guided by ultrasound. At the same time and by the same procedure, 15 to 20 ml of amniotic fluid are obtained for inoculation into mice and into tissue cultures.[34]

Laboratory Diagnosis

Nonspecific tests on fetal blood include white blood cell, platelet and eosinophil counts, and measurement of total IgM and gamma-glutamyl transferase.[32] Gamma interferon production by the fetus can also be investigated.[104] None of these tests is 100 percent reliable. When the results of the various tests are grouped together, however, they have a remarkably high predictive value and a high degree of specificity. When the parents wish to continue the pregnancy, the presence of abnormal signs justifies commencing treatment with pyrimethamine plus sulfonamides without waiting for the final results of cultures.[32]

Definitive diagnosis of *Toxoplasma* fetal infection relies on isolation of the parasite from fetal blood or amniotic fluid and on serologic examination of fetal serum for evidence of synthesis of specific IgM antibodies.

A positive result in IgM must be taken into account only when contamination of the fetal blood sample by maternal blood is ruled out by several tests: hematologic indexes, Betke-Kleihauer staining procedure and beta-human chorionic gonadotropin. In a retrospective study on 105 infected fetuses, anti-*Toxoplasma* IgM was detected in only 29.5 percent of cases, despite the high sensitivity of the method used (ISAgA). None of the samples taken before week 22 was positive. The frequency of positive results significantly increased with the gestational age at time of sampling: 10 percent in fetuses from 20 to 24 weeks, 29.5 percent from 25 to 29 weeks, and 63 percent from 30 to 34 weeks. These results probably reflect the growth of the immune response of the fetus with advancing gestation age. In the majority of cases (55 of 105), *Toxoplasma* was isolated from both fetal blood and amniotic fluid. In 40 percent of cases, only one of the two samples was positive. If only amniotic fluid samples had been studied, infection of 29 (27.6 percent) fetuses would not have been demonstrated.

From the comparative study of inoculation of 53 amniotic fluid samples into mice and tissue culture, it appeared that tissue culture was significantly less sensitive (53 percent positive) than mouse inoculation (73.5 percent). However, when cell culture results were considered together with IgM detection in fetal serum, a diagnosis with certainty was obtained in 70 percent of cases within 4 days. These results emphasize the need to perform multiple diagnostic techniques to allow for an early and reliable prenatal diagnosis.

Prenatal Management

Overall results obtained by our group were recently reported.[32,70] Prenatal diagnosis identified 80 cases of fetal infection among 1,270 pregnant women infected during pregnancy. In nine other cases, all the tests were negative, but the infants showed congenital infection at birth or during the first months of life. Either the tests lacked sensitivity or else the fetuses were not infected at the time of cordocentesis and amniocentesis. In the very near future, the polymerase chain reaction technique might provide definitive information in such cases,[67] but it is noteworthy that parasite transmission from the placenta to the fetus may occur several weeks after the maternal infection.

Among the 80 pregnancies with a positive prenatal diagnosis, 34 were terminated. In 27 cases, the decision was based on obvious lesions detected by ultrasound; they were already present at the time of prenatal diagnosis in 18 cases and developed later in 9 fetuses. In some cases, ventricular dilatation developed within 10 days. Seven pregnancies with early maternal infection and a positive prenatal diagnosis performed before 24 weeks were also terminated because of the high risk to the fetus, although no lesions were detectable by ultrasonography; all seven fetuses showed severe brain damage at postmortem. These findings may justify a recommendation for termination of pregnancy when maternal infection occurs before 10 weeks and if the prenatal studies demonstrate that the fetus is infected. In our series, 2.7 percent of the pregnant women elected termination; this percentage was much lower than that when no effort at prenatal diagnosis was undertaken for in the past most physicians would decide to terminate the pregnancy solely on the basis of the statistical risk.

Follow-up of Infants

Fifty-two pregnancies were allowed to continue, resulting in the birth of 55 infants (three twin pregnancies). Treatment with pyrimethamine and sulfonamides was continued in the infants (see the Treatment section).

At birth, 44 infants (80 percent) had a subclinical infection (no signs of either ophthalmologic or cerebral abnormalities). Seven infants had intracranial calcifications with normal ophthalmoscopic and neurologic status, and three infants had a peripheral chorioretinitis scar with no other lesion (benign form, 18 percent). One twin pregnancy was allowed to continue despite known major cerebral lesions in one fetus because the other had no lesions on ultrasonograms. The critically ill twin died at birth.

The 54 infants were followed for periods of 6 months to 4 years. One infant developed bilateral chorioretinitis and ventricular dilatation necessitating a ventriculoperitoneal shunt at 1 month of life. This infant did not receive treatment during pregnancy (negative prenatal diagnosis). In five infants, peripheral chorioretinitis was demonstrated on ophthalmoscopy by a scar between 5 and 17 months of life; none of the five infants had visual impairment, and the lesions remained stable. On the whole, 53 infants had normal development and normal neurologic status. These results are promising, but these infants must be examined regularly throughout their entire childhood because complications such as chorioretinitis might appear later.

Pathology

Placenta

The major findings are chronic inflammatory reactions in the decidua capsularis and focal reactions in the villi. There are intravillous and perivillous infiltrates with lymphocytes and other mononucleate cells.[11,118] Parasites are rarely visualized. Inoculation into mice is the best way to perform parasitologic diagnosis. However, tissue cysts have been seen in the connective tissue of the amniotic and chorionic membrane and in the decidua. The discovery of tachyzoites widely dispersed in the chorionic plate, decidua, and amnion, and in placental villi and the umbilical cord in some cases, is considered as a proof of hematogenous dissemination.

Autopsy

According to the clinical pattern, either generalized lesions or central nervous system lesions predominate. There may be severe multivisceral involvement with pneumonia, hepatitis, myocarditis, and active encephalomyelitis with mononuclear reaction and tachyzoites at the periphery of the lesions[56,57] or, at the other extreme, only signs of encephalitis with microglial nodules, infectious necrosis, and small, scattered infarcts.

Central Nervous System

Extensive necrosis of the brain parenchyma due to vascular involvement is the main feature. The necrotic areas can progress to form cystic cavities containing homogeneous eosinophilic material. Areas of calcification are found either as broad bands or as diffusely scattered foci. The extent of calcification appears related to the duration of the infection and to the severity of the necrotic reaction.[13] Both tachyzoites and cysts are seen in and adjacent to the necrotic foci, near or in the glial nodules in perivascular regions, and in noninflammatory areas of cerebral tissue.[105] Periventricular and periaqueductal vasculitis with necrosis may be extensive. Ependymitis can lead to the obstruction of the aqueduct of Sylvios with ensuing obstructive hydrocephaly. The protein content of the ventricular fluid can be very high, and significant amounts of *Toxoplasma* antigens can be found. There is a more or less severe cellular reaction of the leptomeninges.

Lungs. There is an interstitial lymphocytic and mononuclear inflammatory infiltrate that also affects the walls of small vessels. Parasites are occasionally identified within the endothelial cells of the alveolar septa.[20]

Heart. *Toxoplasma gondii* has a great affinity for heart muscle and occurs as cysts in the myocardial fibers either without inflammatory reaction or with focal areas of infiltration that may be necrotic.

Liver. Usually no inflammatory reaction or parasites are seen in the liver. Erythropoiesis is observed in cases mimicking erythroblastosis. Calcifications and hepatic cirrhosis are infrequent.

Spleen. There is no necrosis or signs of direct destruction by the parasite.

Kidneys. Focal glomerulitis with areas of necrosis occurs. These lesions can extend into adjacent tubules and in severe cases to the collecting tubules in the medulla. Tachyzoites can be identified in these lesions. Lesions of immune complex nephritis or alterations of the basement membrane and glomerular deposits of IgM may be the basis of the nephrotic syndrome that is rarely observed.[21]

Eye. The principal lesions involve the retina and choroid.[69] The sequence of events is as follows: first inflammation of the retina with exudation into the vitreous producing opacity; next inflammation of the choroid; finally a healing process with proliferation of the pigment bordering the inflammatory foci. Secondary lesions include iridocyclitis and cataract. Large lesions with marked necrosis can result in central atrophy of the retina and of the choroid. Microphthalmia may result because of arrest of the development of the eye or secondary atrophy. The inflammatory process involves the choroid under the retinal lesions, and the retina and choroid can be bound together by connective tissue. Tachyzoites reach the inner layer of the retina through the capillaries and can be found in inflammatory foci or as cysts.

Miscellaneous. *Toxoplasma* are frequently observed in skeletal muscle fibers, often without inflammatory reactions.[105] Foci of necrosis have been identified in the thymus, adrenals, pancreas, thyroid, pituitary, testes, and ovaries.

Pathophysiology

Experimental data and observations on infections in domestic animals suggest that the sequence of events leading to congenital toxoplasmosis is acute maternal infection during pregnancy followed by parasitemia, infection of the placenta with multiplication of the parasites in placental tissue, and finally spread of the organisms in the fetal circulation.

Beyond this simple scenario, several facts require attention and must be explained:

1. Congenital toxoplasmosis is an extremely protean disease: it can be fatal in utero, a neonatal systemic disease with necrotizing encephalitis, a hydrocephaly that becomes apparent several months after birth, or an isolated chorioretinitis discovered at school age. In the majority of cases, it can remain subclinical.
2. Another surprising fact is the extreme diversity of the immunologic response. Prospective studies reveal that some fetuses have evidence of acute and complete prenatal synthesis of both IgG and IgM antibodies that was protracted for months but that others have practically no humoral response. The postnatal decrease of the IgG titer reflects the decay of passively transmitted maternal antibodies, but they may be detected for as long as 15 to 24 months.
3. Another striking feature is the lack of a close correlation between the fetal immunologic response and the presence or absence of clinical lesions. Although clinical infection in newborns is often associated with evidence of fetal synthesis of antibodies, it is not uncommon to see no immunologic response in newborns with severe lesions.
4. The tendency for late reactivation needs emphasis. Flare-ups of chorioretinitis can occur in children or adolescents close to an old scar or in a previously normal retina.

Date of Maternal Infection

As far as the frequency of fetal transmission is concerned, prospective studies performed between 1966 and 1974 in Paris[36] revealed that fetopathy occurs in 14 percent, 29 percent, and 59 percent of babies born to mothers with acquired infection during the first, second, and third trimesters, respectively. Experience accumulated over 20 years in our laboratory has confirmed these findings: the later maternal infection is acquired, the more frequently parasites are transmitted to the fetus.[107] Transmission is rare (about 1 percent) when maternal infection occurs during the first 4 weeks, but reaches 90 percent if acquired during the last weeks.

As to the clinical pattern, four possibilities can be considered: fatal disease (fetal wastage, neonatal death), severe disease with neurologic signs, mild disease without signs of neurologic involvement, and subclinical infection. The respective frequency of these clinical patterns and the proportion of uninfected babies according to the time of maternal infection as observed in the Paris studies is summarized in Table 13-3. It appears that if transmission is rare from infections during the first trimester, the fethopathy at this period is severe with 12 percent death or patent toxoplasmosis. Conversely, subclinical disease is the most frequent presentation following maternal infection during the third trimester, with 53 percent subclinically infected babies, 6 percent with mild infection, and no fatal disease. The data for the second trimester are intermediate.

Table 13-3 Effect of Trimester During Which Maternal Infection Was Acquired on Clinical Pattern of Congenital Toxoplasmosis*

Outcome in Offspring	Trimester During Which Maternal Infection Acquired					
	1		2		3	
	N	(%)	N	(%)	N	(%)
Congenital toxoplasmosis						
Subclinical	3	(18)	49	(67)	68	(89)
Mild	1	(6)	13	(18)	8	(11)
Severe	7	(41)	6	(8)	0	(0)
Stillbirth or perinatal death	6	(35)	5	(7)	0	(0)
Total	17	(100)	73	(100)	76	(100)

*Among 166 infants who either died or had proven infection.
Adapted from Desmonts G, Couvreur J. 1975.[39]

Determination of the date of maternal infection in a series of patients with severe congenital toxoplasmosis revealed that the majority of the mothers had been infected between the tenth and twenty-fourth weeks.[107] The twenty-sixth week seems to mark a turn in fetal risk. The evidence indicates that the earlier the maternal infection, the more severe the disease. This is confirmed by pathologic examination of fetuses whose mothers underwent termination. As a rule fetuses infected before the twenty-sixth week had brain involvement and necrotic foci. Conversely, the period from week 26 to week 40 is low risk. Again, there are exceptions to this rule as illustrated by the following case:

This woman was delivered at 40 weeks of a boy. She had been seronegative with the last negative test 25 days before delivery. One week before delivery she developed cervical lymphadenopathy with a low-grade fever. On the first day of life, this 2,920-g baby presented with jaundice and slight hepatosplenomegaly plus hypoprothrombinemia. Fundi and sonography of the brain were normal. On day 2, IgM ISAgA were detected both in the baby and in the mother. Both showed IgG specific antibody rises, and the dye test titer reached 6,400 UI on day 39 in the baby. Between day 25 and day 38, the baby developed chorioretinitis. Six weeks of treatment with pyrimethamine, sulfadiazine, and prednisone resulted in stabilization of the lesion. His subsequent development was normal.

Placental Infection

It appears that placenta involvement is influenced by the administration of spiramycin to the mother during pregnancy. There was a 50 percent positive isolation in untreated women and only 19 percent when women had received spiramycin. During a period of 11 years after routine screening of pregnant women became compulsory in France, some 9,000 placentas were studied by Desmonts.[107] The placenta was infected in 1 percent of those who seroconverted during the first weeks of pregnancy and in 90 percent for those converting during the ninth month. No placental isolations were obtained when maternal infection occurred before conception.

Delay Between Placental Infection and Fetal Contamination

Placental infection is a potential source of infection for the fetus long after maternal parasitemia has subsided.[107] Although the organism can be transmitted almost immediately following placental infection, this transmission can be delayed for weeks or possibly even months.[128] Studies of toxoplasmosis in twins revealed that the clinical pattern is similar in both of the twins when the pregnancy is monochorial, whereas discrepancies are the rule when the pregnancy is dichorial. In the latter situation it is possible that only one fetus may be infected.[24] This observation suggests that in dichorial pregnancies transmission of the parasite does not occur at the same time in both placentas and that it may not be transmitted at all to one of them. Moreover, separate parasitologic investigation of the fetus and of the placenta after termination of pregnancy has revealed that the placenta may be infected and not the fetus.[107]

Short-Term and Long-Term Relapses

The patient with congenital toxoplasmosis remains under a lifelong antigenic stimulus, as witnessed by the antibody pattern. That congenital toxoplasmosis can progress postnatally for a lengthy period is well documented by clinical, ophthalmologic, and biologic data. The mechanisms of late reactivity are not clear. Persistent parasitemia, which has been documented only during the first week of life,[38] is transitory and cannot account for late flare-ups. Recurrent parasitemia has been demonstrated in animals and seldom observed in humans. It could disseminate trophozoites in tissues, particularly in regions where immunologic mechanisms are weak, as, for instance, in the retina and nervous system.[90]

Persistence of Trophozoites

The persistence of trophozoites in cells is a hypothesis posed by Frenkel.[56] Destruction of the cells could lead to release of the organisms and to parasitism of contiguous cells.

Table 13-4 Congenital Toxoplasmosis in Mothers with Chronic Toxoplasmosis Before Pregnancy

Cases (Mother's Age in Years)	I (17)	II (22)	III (23)	IV (34)
Type of infection	Chronic	Chronic	Chronic	Chronic
Delay between positive serologic diagnosis and conception in years	5	3	11	Undetermined
Associated disease	Systemic lupus erythematosus	Hodgkin's disease	Pancytopenia	Systemic lupus erythematosus
Iatrogenic factors impeding immunity				
Before conception	Steroid therapy	Splenectomy Radiation Chemotherapy	Splenectomy Steroid therapy	Steroid therapy
During pregnancy	Steroid therapy		Steroid therapy	Steroid therapy
Abnormalities of T-cell subsets		+	+	
Clinical pattern of fetopathy	Subclinical Secondary systemic disease Death on day 81	Subclinical	Isolated retinochoroiditis	Twin I Severe fetopathy Death on day 9 Twin II Subclinical infection

Cyst Rupture

This mechanism appears to be the most likely source of continued antigenic stimuli. Cysts are surrounded by a membrane that inhibits the action of humoral antibody and possibly of cellular mediated immunity. However, the existence on histologic examination of large cysts and of adjacent smaller cysts in mice has been interpreted as a proof of cyst rupture.[85,130] The demonstration of antigen close to the cysts by immunofluorescent methods favors the hypothesis of leaks of antigen from the cyst.[72,89,90] Such leaks might induce an inflammatory process that in turn might release lymphokines and catabolic enzymes, with consequent disruption of the cyst wall. Traumatic rupture has also been suggested.

On rupture of cysts, viable bradyzoites are released into the surrounding tissues. Two theories may explain the subsequent tissue injury. There may be multiplication of trophozoites, cell colonization, and necrosis, which induce a minimal inflammatory process because cyst rupture often occurs in retinal and brain tissue where there are low antibody levels.[100] However, Frenkel and others believe that it is a hypersensitivity phenomenon.[56,99]

Chronic Maternal Infection

Data obtained in prospective studies have established that a woman with chronic or latent toxoplasmosis acquired before conception does not transmit the infection to a fetus and provide the basis for preventive measures proven effective in Austria and France.[39,107] However, any rule has exceptions, which in this instance concern women with depressed immunity. Four such cases have been observed in our laboratory.[42] Because this series seems unique, these cases are summarized in Table 13-4. They have several features in common. The infection had been demonstrated in the mothers 3, 5, and 11 years prior to pregnancy in three cases and had occurred an undetermined number of years before the gestation in the fourth case. All had an illness known to be associated with abnormalities of cell-mediated immunity that was confirmed in two cases by inversion of the CD4:CD8 ratio. All had had therapy known to alter immunity (see Table 13-4). In three cases a very high IgG *Toxoplasma* titer had persisted for years. Only one of the five infants born to these four women had a severe fetopathy.

Congenital toxoplasmosis following chronic maternal infection is extremely rare and represents fewer than 1 percent of congenital cases.[42] However, more such cases may be expected in the future as the number of immunodeficient fertile women increases because of progress in the treatment of malignant diseases, organ transplantation, or the increased incidence of the acquired immunodeficiency syndrome (AIDS). Two cases of congenital toxoplasmosis in infants of mothers with AIDS have been reported, but it is not known if the maternal infection was chronic.[16,120] All pregnant women undergoing splenectomy who are receiving steroid therapy or who have abnormalities of T-cell subsets should undergo serial *Toxoplasma* serologic investigations. Any increase in specific antibodies should suggest the possibility of a recurrent parasitemia.[96]

Chronic Toxoplasmosis and Abortion

Whether chronic toxoplasmosis is a cause of abortion has been a matter of debate. It has been claimed that

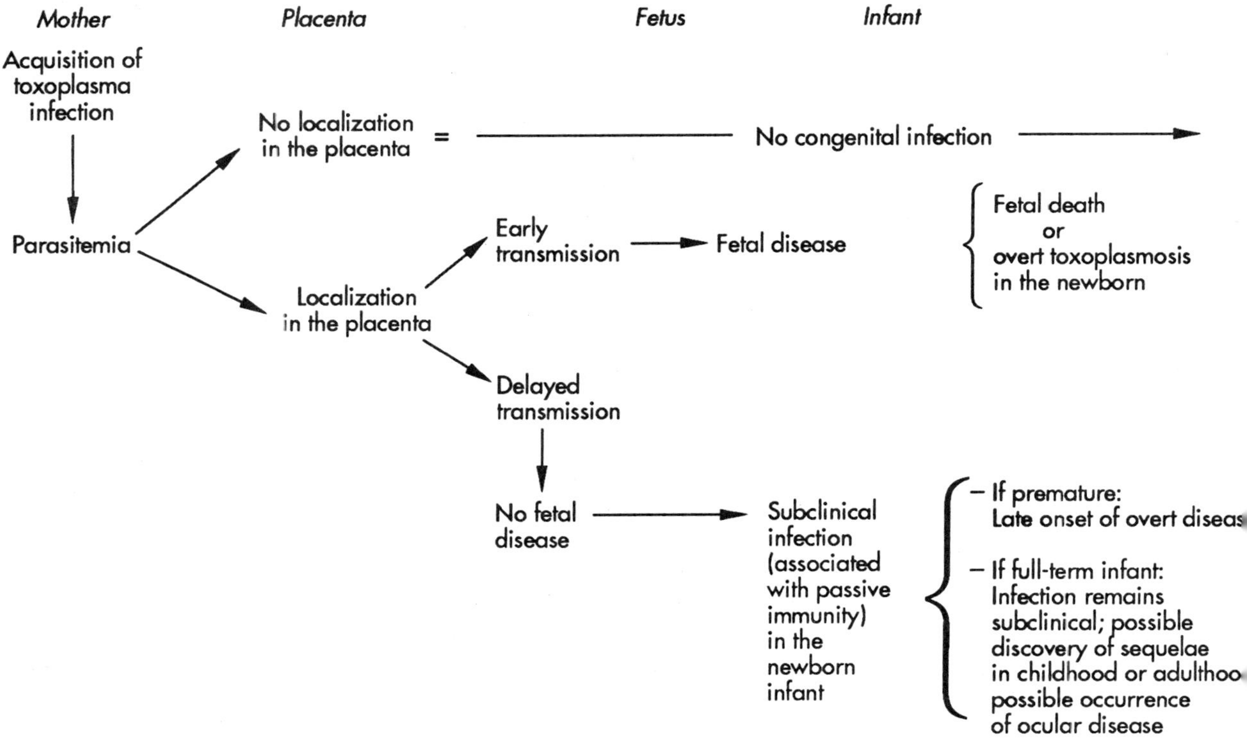

Figure 13-5 Pathogenesis of congenital infection with *Toxoplasma*. (From Desmonts G, Couvreur J. 1985.[40])

Toxoplasma can be identified in embryos or fetal brains, placenta or amniotic fluid, and menstrual fluid from one third of women with histories of repeated abortions, premature births, or stillbirths of unknown etiology.[86] These isolations are open to criticism[106] and have not been confirmed. However, *toxoplasma* has been isolated from uterine muscle,[109] indicating that *Toxoplasma* cysts may stay viable for years. The parasite has been also isolated from endometrial tissue and decidual or fetal tissue in a few women with positive dye tests who experienced a spontaneous abortion.[76,94,110] A unique case is an exception to Feldman's statement that "congenital toxoplasmosis does not occur in siblings of an affected child."[52] A woman gave birth by cesarean section to an infant who died at 24 hours of age with acute *Toxoplasma* infection. Five months later she was pregnant again; spontaneous abortion occurred at the sixth month, and microscopic examination revealed *Toxoplasma* in the fetus and the placenta.[62] However, the evidence was based on histologic grounds, a matter of controversy because histologic examination of tissues for *Toxoplasma* may be misleading. Other parasitologic studies of this matter have been unsuccessful.[75,113] It can be concluded that chronic *Toxoplasma* infection rarely causes abortion and fetal wastage.[78,107]

Summary: Patterns of Fetopathy

The interval between placental infection and fetal transmission determines the pattern of the fetopathy[37] (Fig. 13-5). If the interval between maternal infection and fetal transmission is very short, the fetopathy is severe. Conversely, a long interval allows the fetus to receive passively transmitted specific IgG maternal antibodies. The protective effect of these antibodies is limited because immunity against *Toxplasma* is mainly cell mediated. Antibodies impede extracellular dissemination but might favor intracellular multiplication and cyst formation. However, recognition of toxoplasmic antigen by fetal cells may be retarded, and the development of humoral and cellular immunity by the fetus may be impeded. A specific tolerance is induced.[7,8,37,122] This tolerance depends on an equilibrium between the titer of specific IgG and the degree of antigenic stimulation. Consequently, tolerance is transitory and ceases with the disappearance of passively transmitted IgG. Hence the clinical patterns of fetal damage vary between two extremes. If transmission occurs early in the pregnancy, the fetus is immature and the damage will be severe. With late transmission, there are minimal or absent clinical consequences after birth. One-fourth of such infants have no signs of antibody synthesis. However, subclin-

Table 13-5 Drug Dosages

Drugs	Presentation	Route	Doses	Observations
Pyrimethamine	Tablets: 50 mg	Oral	1 mg/kg/day	Half-life being 4.5 days, it can be given in loading doses every 2 or 3 days
Sulfadiazine	Tablets: 500 mg	Oral	50-80 mg/kg/day	Daily in 2 or 3 divided doses
Pyrimethamine plus Sulfadoxine	Tablets (Fansidar) Pyrimethamine: 25 mg plus Sulfadoxine: 500 mg	Oral	1 tablet per 20 kg every 10 days	Half-life of sulfadoxine: 8 days The interval between doses must never be less than 7 days Discontinue in case of rash Administration before 12 months of age not recommended.
Spiramycin	Tablets: 500 mg Syrup: 125 mg/5 ml	Oral	80-100 mg/kg/day (maximum: 3,000 mg/day in adults)	In 2 to 3 daily divided doses
Folinic acid	Vial: 5 mg, 50 mg Brewer's yeast	Oral or intramuscular Oral	Infants: 5 mg every 4 to 7 days Children: 50 mg every 15 days	Prevention of side effects related to pyrimethamine
Steroids	Prednisone tablets: 1, 5, 20 mg	Oral	Infants: 1 mg to 1.5 mg/kg/day	Used in cases with inflammatory reaction (eye, cerebrospinal fluid) (see text)

ical, low-grade, protracted infection is present. After 6 to 12 months, with the disappearance of maternal antibodies, there is generally active antibody synthesis as the host recognizes as foreigners parasites that multiplied during the tolerance phase. Then latent infection can progress into disease.

Treatment

Drugs

Table 13-5 lists drugs used in the treatment of toxoplasmosis, and their dosages.

Antitoxoplasmic Agents

Pyrimethamine. Pyrimethamine is a substituted phenylpyrimidine cleared by hepatic metabolism. It is a folic acid antagonist. Its plasma half-life in adults is approximately 100 hours, although individuals differ, as suggested by a range of 35 to 175 hours in patients submitted to malaria prophylaxis.[18] There is no positive correlation between dose and serum concentrations, a fact that may require monitoring when a serum assay is available. Penetration of pyrimethamine into the cerebrospinal fluid was shown to range from 10 to 25 percent in patients with meningeal leukemia[65] and in AIDS patients with encephalitis. It can be concentrated in brain tissue. Teratogenic effects have been demonstrated in animals, and thus it should not be administered during the first 14 weeks of pregnancy.[82] Pyrimethamine should always be administered in combination with sulfonamides.

Sulfonamides. The sulfonamides are well absorbed by the oral route and widely distributed in the body with good penetration into the cerebrospinal fluid. The most widely used—sulfadiazine—has a serum half-life of 10 to 12 hours.

Sulfapyrazine, sulfamerazine, and sulfadimidine are equally effective. All other sulfa drugs tested were found to be inferior.[49] Cotrimazole is not recommended.

Pyrimethamine-Sulfonamides Combination. It has been demonstrated that pyrimethamine and sulfonamides have a synergistic action against *Toxoplasma* about six times that which would be expected if their effects were merely additive.[48] The pharmacologic explanation is the sequential blocking of the metabolic pathways in the synthesis of folic acid: sulfonamides inhibit dihydrofolic acid synthetase, whereas pyrimethamine inhibits dihydrofolic reductase. Activity of the combination against trophozoites has been demonstrated in vitro and in vivo.[19]

If pyrimethamine is used alone because of side effects with sulfonamides, studies and experience with AIDS suggest that a higher dosage may achieve an anti-*Toxoplasma* effect.[93]

Pyrimethamine-Sulfadoxine Combination (Fansidar). This combination is very active in murine toxoplasmosis and seems to have effects similar to pyrimethamine-sulfadiazine. It has been used in congenital toxoplasmosis, but it can produce severe cutaneous side effects in adults[95] and should not be used in infants under 1 year of age.

Spiramycin. Spiramycin is a macrolide antibiotic that has been shown to be effective in experimental toxoplasmosis in animals[12,71] and to protect congenitally infected mice.[63,64] A reduced risk of congenital toxoplasmosis was observed in infants of women with toxoplasmosis acquired during pregnancy treated with spiramycin.[36] It is concentrated in placental tissue; on a regimen of 2 g per day, the spiramycin concentration in the placenta is 2.75 mg per kilogram and with a dosage of 3 g per day, it is more than twofold increased.[36,37] A study of 20 pregnant infected women revealed that between weeks 20 and 24 the mean fetal concentration was 47 percent maternal values. At birth, the placental concentration was four times the average blood concentration in mothers and 6.5 times the cord blood values.[55] Spiramycin is inactivated in the body; it is safe and causes gastrointestinal side effects only at high doses.

Other Drugs and Future Prospects. Clindamycin has an activity similar to that of spiramycin but cannot be used for long-term treatment because of digestive side effects.

Roxithromycin is active against acute murine toxoplasmosis. It produces a higher serum level and a longer half-life than spiramycin,[15] but data on human *Toxoplasma* infections are lacking.

Azithromycin is very active in preventing death and encephalitis in mice; it has not been tried in humans.[6]

Two folic acid antagonists, piritrexim[5] and trimetrexate,[4] both inhibitors of dihydrofolate reductase also gave good results against murine toxoplasmosis. Both showed synergistic activity with sulfonamides.

Arprinocid, a purine analogue, also protects mice.[88]

It has been demonstrated that interferon gamma is effective in vitro against *Toxoplasma* by stimulating macrophage activity.[92] The combination roxithromycin and recombinant interferon gamma has a synergistic effect against murine toxoplasmic encephalitis.[68]

Adjuvant Therapy

Folinic Acid. Bone marrow suppression can occur because of folic acid antagonism by pyrimethamine and sulfadiazine. Weekly blood counts should be performed to detect granulocytopenia, thrombocytopenia, and megaloblastic anemia. These side effects can be corrected or prevented by folinic acid or by brewer's yeast.[59] Folic acid should not be used because of its antagonistic activity on the effect of pyrimethamine on *Toxoplasma*.

Corticosteroids (Prednisone or Methylprednisone). Steroids are indicated when there is an inflammatory process reflected by a high level of CSF protein or a progressive chorioretinitis. They must be continued on full dosage until the process has subsided, when the dosage should be progressively reduced.

Management of Pregnant Women with Acute Infection

Spiramycin

Spiramycin is administered in a daily dose of 3 g and continued until delivery. Fetal infection was significantly reduced with this regimen: 61 percent of infants infected in untreated women and 23 percent in treated women.[36] Among infected patients, placental inoculation resulting in isolation of *Toxoplasma* was positive in 90 percent of untreated women and 75 percent of treated women.[25] However, if parasitic infection of the placenta and fetal infection are reduced in the treated groups, the proportion of severe cases in infected infants is not modified.[36] Thus it appears that whereas spiramycin during pregnancy has a preventive effect against maternal-fetal transmission, it does not alter the clinical pattern of overt congenital toxoplasmosis.

Pyrimethamine-Sulfadiazine Combination: In Utero Treatment of Congenital Toxoplasmosis

Earlier reports recorded the efficacy of this combination to prevent fetal infection. Kraübig, who treated infected women after 14 weeks of gestation, obtained a 70 percent reduction of fetopathy.[81,82] Aspockh and associates successfully used spiramycin before the twentieth week and pyrimethamine plus sulfonamides after the twentieth week with success.[9]

We have recorded our experience with the in utero treatment of proven fetopathies.[30,70] In 52 cases that were diagnosed from fetal blood, amniotic fluid, or both, the mothers received one or several courses of pyrimethamine plus sulfadiazine alternating with spiramycin.[30] This series was compared with a second group of 51 cases of congenital toxoplasmosis diagnosed after birth, whose mothers had received spiramycin alone. These two groups were identical as far as the date of maternal infection, and they were treated the same way after birth.

Parasitologic examination of the placenta was positive in 42 percent of the first group versus 83 percent of the second group, and the newborns had IgM-ISAgA in 17.4 percent versus 68 percent in the first and second groups respectively. There was also a significant reduction of the mean specific IgG immune load in the first group: 86 IU per milligram versus 137 IU per milligram at birth and 70 IU per milligram versus 135 IU per milligram at 4 to 6 months of age. The babies of the first group had a lower CSF protein level, and more had a subclinical pattern of the disease. In cases with clinical signs, however, the pattern and the sequelae were not altered significantly. The relatively long period between maternal infection and onset of treatment (7 weeks) might explain this relative clinical failure.

It can be concluded that the pyrimethamine-sulfadiazine combination is active against progressive fetopathy. The treatment should be given as soon as fetopathy is proved. The use of this drug combination in seroconverters lacking a prenatal diagnosis of fetopathy is controversial because the pharmacologic and teratogenic effects of these drugs have not been sufficiently documented.

Termination

Abortion should be considered only if maternal infection has definitely occurred between conception and the twenty-fourth week, that is, if there is significant risk of neurologic injury. The important basis for a decision is the degree of risk of fetopathy; it is almost negligible (1 percent) for a maternal infection in the first 4 weeks but rises thereafter.

It must be pointed out that *indiscriminate* termination because of early maternal infection leads to a considerable wastage of normal fetuses, that is, near 80 percent. Prenatal diagnosis prevents such a wastage by allowing *elective* abortion.

Postnatal Treatment

Drugs

Pyrimethamine Plus Sulfadiazine. Pyrimethamine plus sulfadiazine is the best treatment. It has been recommended that three to four 21-day courses[29] be given during the first year. Experience indicates that the longer the treatment is given, the better the results. Controlled studies are now ongoing with 6- and 12-month regimens.[91] Folinic acid is given routinely. The dosage may be doubled if signs of bone marrow depression occur. It may be necessary to discontinue the treatment if the white cell count is below 1,000 per milliliter. If granulocytopenia recurs, it is recommended to start again with pyrimethamine alone and then to add sulfadiazine to see which drug is responsible. If sulfadiazine is not tolerated, pyrimethamine alone for several months must be tried because the experience with AIDS demonstrates some efficacy.

Spiramycin. Spiramycin is administered between the pyrimethamine plus sulfadiazine courses. It is well tolerated, but its activity in congenital toxoplasmosis has not been established.

Indications

Every case of congenital toxoplasmosis, even those that are subclinical, must be treated. Our current recommendations are as follows:

1. Overt congenital toxoplasmosis. The course of treatment is for 1 year, the first 6 months with pyrimethamine plus sulfadiazine. During the following 6 months, 1 month of pyrimethamine plus sulfadiazine is alternated with 1 month of spiramycin. No treatment is usually given after 12 months of age except when there is evidence of activity of the infection, such as a flare-up of chorioretinitis.
2. Overt congenital toxoplasmosis with evidence of inflammatory process (chorioretinitis, high level of CSF protein, generalized infection, jaundice). As for overt congenital toxoplasmosis with the addition of corticosteroids.
3. Subclinical toxoplasma infection. Alternate pyrimethamine plus sulfadiazine for 6 weeks, with spiramycin for 6 weeks, and so on to complete a treatment course of 1 year.
4. Healthy newborn in whom serologic testing has not provided definitive results but maternal infection was proved to have been acquired during pregnancy. One course of pyrimethamine plus sulfadiazine for 1 month. The necessity for continued therapy and the drug regimen depend thereafter on multiple factors: date of maternal infection, antibody titers, immune load, and clinical findings. It must be kept in mind that passively transferred maternal antibodies can persist to 10 months of age, that an infected baby can have a negative parasitologic examination of the placenta, and that initially there may be a decrease of specific IgG titer.
5. Healthy newborn, born to a mother with high dye test titer; date of maternal infection undetermined. Spiramycin for 1 month. Then, follow #4. Continue clinical and serologic follow-up until there is complete disappearance of antibodies.

In our personal experience, 5 patients among 350 followed for more than 2 years became seronegative, a fact that raises the hitherto unsolved question, Does congenital toxoplasmosis undergo self-cure?

Prevention

The prevention of congenital toxoplasmosis is based on the prevention of maternal infection, a threefold program: detection of seronegative women, prevention of infection during pregnancy in these women, and detection of seroconverters.

Screening for Seronegative Women

Ideally, women should be tested just before pregnancy or at least before 12 weeks' gestation with a serologic test equal in sensivity, specificity, and reproductibility to the dye test.[107] The practical implementation of such a program depends on its cost and the epidemiology of toxoplasmosis in the community.[112]

Prevention of Infection in Seronegative Pregnant Women

Practical recommendations have been given by Wilson and Remington as follows:[134]

1. Cook meat to well done, smoke it, or cure it in brine.
2. Avoid touching mucous membranes of mouth and eyes while handling raw meat.
3. Wash hands thoroughly after handling raw meat.
4. Wash kitchen surfaces that come into contact with raw meat.
5. Wash fruits and vegetables before consumption.
6. Prevent access of flies, cockroaches, and the like to fruits and vegetables.

7. Avoid contact with materials that are potentially contaminated with cat feces, such as cat litter boxes, or wear gloves when handling such materials or when gardening.
8. Disinfect cat litter box for 5 minutes with boiling water, or line the litter box with the bag the litter come in; then the box does not come in contact with the used litter, and mess is prevented, not boiled away.

Detection of Seroconverters

Seronegative pregnant women should be tested at 22 to 26 weeks and then every 4 to 8 weeks, depending on the risk of acute toxoplasmosis in the community. Any conversion or significant rise of antibodies should be adequately confirmed by sending paired sera to a reference laboratory before decisions are made for the management of the pregnancy. Inappropriate laboratory techniques, misleading interpretation of test results, and lack of experience have proved often to be more harmful to the fetus than *Toxoplasma* itself.

Special Considerations

In counseling concerning the risk of conception following a recent acute infection, a delay of 6 months can be recommended. Pregnancy in immunodeficient mothers with chronic infection should be monitored to detect rises in antibody titer or a parasitemia by repeated examinations.

References

1. Abdel-Hafez SK, Sabeed I, Ismail NS. Serodiagnosis of *Toxoplasma gondii* in habitually aborting women and other adults from North Jordan. Folia Parasitol (Praha) 1986; 33:7–13.
2. Alford CA, Foft JW, Blankenship WJ. Subclinical central nervous system of neonates: a prospective study of infants born with increased levels of IgM. J Pediatr 1959; 75:1167–1178.
3. Alford CA, Stagno S, Reynolds DW. Congenital toxoplasmosis: clinical and therapeutic considerations with special reference to subclinical disease. Bull N Y Acad Med 1974; 50:160–181.
4. Allegra CJ, Kovacs JA, Drake JC, Chabner BA. Potent in vitro antitoxoplasma activity of the lipid soluble antifolate trimetrexate. J Clin Invest 1987; 79:478–482.
5. Araujo FG, Guptil DR, Remington JS. In vitro activity of piritrexin against *Toxoplasma gondii.* J Infect Dis 1987; 156:828–830.
6. Araujo FG, Guptil DR, Remington JS. Azythromycin, a macrolide antibiotic with potent activity against *Toxoplasma gondii*. Antimicrob Agents Chemother 1988; 32:755–757.
7. Araujo FG, Remington JS. Immune response to intracellular parasites: suppression by antibody. Proc Soc Exp Biol Med 1872; 139:254–258.
8. Araugo FG, Remington JS. Induction of tolerance to an intracellular protozoan *(Toxoplasma gondii)* by passively administered antibody. J Immunol 1974; 113:1424–1428.
9. Aspockh H, Flamm H, Picher O. Die toxoplasmse. Uberwachung wahrend der Schwangershaft. IO jahre Erfahrungen in Ostrerreich. Mitt Oestgerreichen Gesamte Tropenmedicine und Parasitologrer 1986; 8:105–113.
10. Bain AD, Bowe JH, Flint WP, et al. Congenital toxoplasmosis simulating hoemolytic disease in the newborn. Journal of Obstetrics and Gynaecology of British Commonwealth 1956; 63:826–832.
11. Benirshke K, Driscoll SG. The pathology of the human placenta. New York: Springer Verlag, 1967.
12. Beverley JKA, Freeman AP, Henry L, et al. Prevention of pathological changes in experimental congenital toxoplasmosis infection. Lyon Medical 1973; 17:491–496.
13. Callahan WP, Russell WO, Smith MG. Human toxoplasmosis. A clinicopathologic study with presentation of five cases and review of the literature. Medicine (Baltimore) 1946; 25:343–397.
14. Catar G, Bergendi L, Holkova R. Isolation of *Toxoplasma gondii* from swine and cattle. J Parasitol 1969; 55:952–955.
15. Chang HR, Pechere JCF. Activity of roxithromycin against *Toxoplasma gondii* in murine models. J Antimicrob Chemother 1987; 20B:69–74.
16. Cohen-Addad NE, Joshi VV, Sharer LG, et al. Congenital acquired immunodeficiency syndrome and congenital toxoplasmosis; pathologic support for a chronology of events. J Perinatol 1988; 8:328–331.
17. Conquy P, Niel G, Couvreur J, et al. Anasarque foeto-placentaire et toxoplasmose gravidique. J Gynecol Obstet Biol Reprod (Paris) 1982; 11:717–722.
18. Cook IF, Cochrane JP, Edstein MD. Race-linked differences in serum concentrations of dapsone, monoacetyldapsone and pyrimethamine during malaria prophylaxis. Trans R Soc Trop Med Hyg 1986; 80:897–901.
19. Cook MK, Jacobs L. In vitro investigations on the action of pyrimethamine against *Toxoplasma gondii*. J Parasitol 1958; 44:280–288.
20. Couvreur J. Le poumon et la toxoplasmose. Revue Française des Maladies Respiratorie 1975; 3:525–532.
21. Couvreur J, Alison F, Boccon-Gibod L, et al. Rein et toxoplasmose. Ann Pediatr (Paris) 1984; 31:847–852.
22. Couvreur J, Desmonts G. Congenital and maternal toxoplasmosis. A review of 300 congenital cases. Dev Med Child Neurol 1962; 4:519–530.
23. Couvreur J, Desmonts G, Aron-Rosa D. Le pronostic oculaire de la toxoplasmose congenitale: role du traitement. Ann Pediatr (Paris) 1984; 31:855–858.
24. Couvreur J, Desmonts G, Girre JY. Congenital toxoplasmosis in twins. A series of fourteen pairs of twins: absence of infection in two pairs. J Pediatr 1976; 89:235–240.
25. Couvreur J, Desmonts G, Thulliez P. Prophylaxis of congenital toxoplasmosis. Effects of spiramycin on placental infection. J Antimicrob Chemother 1988; 22B:193–200.
26. Couvreur J, Desmonts G, Thulliez P, et al. Sur 23 cas d'hydrocephalie de la toxoplasmose congenitale. Paper presented at the nineteenth Inter-

national Congress of Pediatrics, Paris, 1989, 110.
27. Couvreur J, Desmonts G, Tournier G, Collin F. La production locale accrue d'immunoglobulines specifiques G dans le liquide cephalo-rachidien au cours de la toxoplasmose congenitale. Ann Pediatr (Paris) 1984; 31:829–835.
28. Couvreur J, Desmonts G, Tournier G, Szusterkac M. Etude d'une serie homogène de 210 cas de toxoplasmose congenitale chez des nourrissons de O à 11 mois et dépistés de façon prospective. Ann Pediatr (Paris) 1984; 31:819.
29. Couvreur J, Nottin N, Desmonts G. La toxoplasmose congenitale traitée. Résultats cliniques et biologiques. Ann Pediatr (Paris) 1980; 27:647–652.
30. Couvreur J, Thulliez P, Daffos F, et al. Foetopathie toxoplasmique: traitement "in utero" par l'association pyrymethamine-sulfamides. Arch Fr Pediatr 1991; 48:397–403.
31. Couvreur J, Thulliez P, Flamenbaum F. Essai de determination facteurs de risque oculaire à moyen ou long terme chez le nouveau né atteint de toxoplasmose congenitale. Paper presented at the Nineteenth International Congress of Pediatrics, Paris, 1989, 111.
32. Daffos F, Forestier F, Capella-Pavlovsky M, et al. Prenatal management of 746 pregnancies at risk for congenital toxoplasmosis. N Engl J Med 1988; 318:271–275.
33. Dannemann BR, Vaughan WC, Thulliez P, Remington JS. Differential agglutination test for diagnosis of recently acquired infection with *Toxoplasma gondii*. J Clin Microbiol 1990; 28:1928–1933.
34. Derouin F, Thulliez P, Candolfi E, et al. Early prenatal diagnosis of congenital toxoplasmosis using amniotic fluid samples and tissue culture. Eur J Clin Microbiol Infect Dis 1988; 7:423–425.
35. Desmonts G. Toxoplasmose oculaire. Etude epidemiologique (Bilan de 2030 examens d'humeur aqueuse). Arch Ophthalmol (Paris) 1973; 33:87–102.
36. Desmonts G, Couvreur J. Congenital toxoplasmosis: a prospective study of 378 pregnancies. N Engl J Med 1974; 290:1110–1116.
37. Desmonts G, Couvreur J. Toxoplasmosis in pregnancy and its transmission to the fetus. Bull N Y Acad Med 1974; 50:146–159.
38. Desmonts G, Couvreur J. L'isolement du parasite dans la toxoplasmos congenitale. Intéret pratique et théorique. Arch Fr Pediatr 1974; 31:157–166.
39. Desmonts G, Couvreur J. Toxoplasmosis: epidemiolgic and serologic aspects of perinatal infection. In: Krugman S, Gershon AA, eds. Infections of the fetus and the newborn infant. Vol 3. Progress in clinical and biological research. New York: Alan Liss, 1975:115–132.
40. Desmonts G, Couvreur J. Toxoplasmosis. In: Conn RB, ed. Current diagnosis. Vol 7. Philadelphia: WB Saunders, 1985:274–287.
41. Desmonts G, Couvreur J, Alison F, et al. Etude epidemiologique sur la toxoplasmose: De l'influence de la cuisson des viandes de boucherie sur la frequence de l'infection humaine. Revue Francaise Etudes Cliniques Biologiques 1965; 10:952–958.
42. Desmonts G, Couvreur J, Thulliez P. Toxoplasmose congenitale. Cinq cas de transmission à l'enfant d'une infection maternelle antérieure à la grossesse. Presse Med 1990; 19:1445–1449.
43. Desmonts G, Daffos F, Forestier F, et al. Prenatal diagnosis of congenital toxoplasmosis. Lancet 1985; 1:500–504.
44. Desmonts G, Thulliez P. The *Toxoplasma* agglutination antigen as a tool for routine screening and diagnosis of *Toxoplasma* infection in the mother and infant. In: Development of biologic standard diagnostics and vaccines for parasitic diseases. Vol 62. Basel: S Karger, 1985:31–35.
45. Dubey JP, Beattie CP. Toxoplasmosis of animals and man. Boca Raton, Fla: CRC Press, 1988; 1–220.
46. Eichenwald H. Experimental toxoplasmosis. Transmission of the infection in utero and through the milk of lactating female mice. Am J Dis Child 1948; 76:307–315.
47. Eichenwald HA. A study of congenital toxoplasmosis. In: Siim JC, ed. Human toxoplasmosis. Copenhagen: Munksgaard, 1960:41–49.
48. Eyles DE, Coleman N. Synergistic effect of sulfadiazine and Daraprim against experimental toxoplasmosis in the mouse. Antibiot Chemother 1953; 3:483–490.
49. Eyles DE, Coleman N. The effect of sulfadimetine, sulfisoxazole and sulfapyrazine against mouse toxoplasmosis. Antibiot Chemother 1955; 5:525–528.
50. Fair JR. Congenital toxoplasmosis. III. Ocular signs of the disease in state schools for the blind. Am J Ophthalmol 1959; 48:165–172.
51. Feldman HA. Congenital toxoplasmosis. A study of one hundred and three cases. Amer J Dis Child 1953; 86:487–489.
52. Feldman HA. Toxoplasmosis. Pediatrics 1958; 22:559–574.
53. Feldman HA, Miller LT. Serological study of toxoplasmosis prevalence. American Journal of Hygiene 1956; 64:320–325.
54. Ferraroni JJ, Lacaz CZ. Prevalenca de anticorpos contra os agentes causadores da hepatite, malaria, sifilis e toxoplasose em cinco populacoes humanas distintas da amazonie brasileira. Rev Inst Med Trop (Sao Paolo) 1982; 24:155–161.
55. Forestier F, Daffos F, Rainaut M, et al. Suivi therapeutique foeto-maternel de la spiramycine en cours de grossesse. Arch Fr Pediatr 1987; 44:539–544
56. Frenkel JK. Pathology and pathogenesis of congenital toxoplasmosis. Bull N Y Acad Med 1974; 50:182–191.
57. Frenkel JK. Toxoplasmosis. In: Strickland GT, ed. Hunter's tropical medicine. Ed 6. Philadelphia: WB Saunders, 1984:593–605.
58. Frenkel JK, Dubey JP, Miller NL. *Toxoplasma gondii* in cats: fecal stages identified as coccidian oocysts. Science 1970; 167:893–896.
59. Frenkel JK, Hitchings GH. Relative reversal by

vitamins (p-aminobenzoic, folic and folinic acids) of the effects of sulfadiazine and pyrimethamine on toxoplasma, mouse and man. Antibiot Chemother 1957; 7:630–638.
60. Frenkel JK, Ruiz A. Endemicity of toxoplasmosis in Costa Rica. Amer J Epidemiol 1981; 113:254–269.
61. Frenkel JK, Ruiz A, Chinchilla M. Soil survival of *Toxoplasma* oocysts in Kansas and Costa Rica. Amer J Trop Med Hyg 1975; 24:439–443.
62. Garcia AGP. Congenital toxoplasmosis in two successive sibs. Arch Dis Child 1968; 43:705–709.
63. Garin JP, Eyles DF. Le traitement de la toxoplasmose de la souris par la spiramyucine. Presse Med 1958; 66:254–260.
64. Garin JP, Pellerat J, Maillard M, et al. Bases théoriques de la prevention de la toxoplasmose congenitale chez la femme enceinte. Presse Med 1968; 76:22–26.
65. Geils GF, Scott CW, Baugh CM, Butterworth CE. Tratment of menigeal leukemia with pyrimethamine. Blood 1971; 38:131–137.
66. Ghorbani M, Edrissian GH, Afshar A. Serological survey of human toxoplasmosis in mountainous regions of the north-west and south-west parts of Iran (1976-77). Trans R Soc Trop Med Hyg 1981; 75:38–41.
67. Grover CM, Thulliez P, Remington JS, Boothroyd JC. Rapid prenatal diagnosis of toxoplasma infection by using polymerase chain reaction and amniotic fluid. J Clin Microbiol 1990; 28:2297–2301.
68. Hofflin JM, Remington JS. In vivo synergism of roxithromycin (RU 965) and interferon against *Toxoplasma gondii*. Antimicrob Agents Chemother 1987; 31:346–348.
69. Hogan MJ, Kimura SJ, O'Connor GR. Ocular toxoplasmosis. Arch Ophthalmol 1964; 72:592–600.
70. Hohlfeld P, Daffos F, Thulliez P, et al. Fetal toxoplasmosis: outcome of pregnancy and infant follow-up after in utero treatment. J Pediatr 1989; 115:765–769.
71. Hudson DG, Yoshira GM, Kirby WM. Spiramycin: clinical and laboratory studies. Arch Intern Med 1956; 97:57–61.
72. Huldt G. Studies on experimental toxoplasmosis. Ann N Y Acad Sci 1971; 177:146–155.
73. Hutchison WM, Dunache JF, Work K. The fecal transmission of *Toxoplasma gondii*. APMIS 1968; 74:462–464.
74. Jacobs L, Remington JS, Melton M. A survey of meat samples from swine, cattle and sheep for the presence of encysted *Toxoplasma*. J Parasitol 1960; 46:11–21.
75. Janků J. Pathogenesa a pathologická anatomie tak nazuaného vrozeného kolobomu zluté skvrny v oku normálne velikém a mikrophthalmickém s nálezem parazitu v sítnici. Text in Czech. Quoted by Remington and Desmonts.[106] Cas Lek. Cesk 1923 62:1021–1027.
76. Janssen P, Piekarski G, Korte W. Zum Problem des Abortes bei latentes *Toxoplasma*. Infection der Frau. Klin Wochenschr 1970; 48:25–30.
77. Kayhoe DE, Jacobs L, McCullough NB. Acquired toxoplasmosis. Observations on two parasitologically proved cases treated with pyrimethamine and triple sulfonamides. N Engl J Med 1957; 257:1247.
78. Kimball AC, Kean BH, Fuchs T. Toxoplasmosis: risk variations in New York obstetric patients. Amer J Obstet Gynecol 1974; 119:208–214.
79. Ko RC, Wong FWT, Todd D. Prevalence of *Toxoplasma gondii* antibodies in the Chinese population of Hong Kong. Trans R Soc Trop Med Hyg 1980; 74:351–354.
80. Koppe JG, Loewer-Siegler DH, De Roever-Bonnet H. Results of 20 year follow up congenital toxoplasmosis. Lancet 1986; 1:254–256.
81. Kraübig H. Erste praktische Erfahrungen mit des Prophylaxe der Konnatalen Toxoplasmose. Med Klin 1963; 58:1361–1364.
82. Kraübig H. Praventive behandlung der Konnatalen toxoplasmose. In: Kirchof H, Kraübig H, eds. Toxoplasmose: praktische frogen und ergebnisse. Stuttgart: Georg Thiem Verlag, 1965:104–122.
83. Labadie MD, Hazemann JJ. Apport es bilans de santé de l'enfant pour l'étude épidemiologique de la toxoplasmose congénitale. Ann Pediatr (Paris) 1984; 31:823–828.
84. Labadie MD, Rossignol CL. Depistage de la toxoplasmose. Approche epidemiologique. Paper presented at the Nineteenth International Congress of Pediatrics, Paris, 1989, 249.
85. Lainson R. Observations on the development and nature of pseudocysts of *Toxoplasma gondii*. Trans R Soc Trop Med Hyg 1958; 52:396–407.
86. Langer H. Repeated congenital infection with *Toxoplasma gondii*. Obstet Gynecol 1963; 21:318–329.
87. Levaditi C. Au sujet de certaines protozooses hereditaires humaines à localisatios oculaires et nerveuses. C R Soc Biol (Paris) 1928; 98:297–299.
88. Luft BJ. Potent in vivo activity of arprinosid, a purine analogue, against murine toxoplasmosis. J Infect Dis 1986; 154:692–695.
89. Luft BJ, Naot Y, Araugo FG, et al. Primary and reactivated *Toxoplasma* infection in patients with cardiac transplants: clinical spectrum and problems in diagnosis in a defined population. Ann Intern Med 1983; 99:27.
90. Luft BJ, Remington JS. Toxoplasmic encephalitis. J Infect Dis 1988; 157:1–6.
91. MacLeod R. Personal communication 1991.
92. McCabe RE, Luft BJ, Remington JS. Effect of murine interferon gamma on murine toxoplasmosis. J Infect Dis 1984; 150:961–962.
93. McCabe RE, Oster S. Current recommendations and future prospects in the treatment of toxoplasmosis. Drugs 1989; 38:973–987.
94. Meylan J. Toxoplasmosis as a cause of repeated abortion. In: Hentsch D, ed. Toxoplasmosis. Bern: Hans Huber 1971:151–157.
95. Miller KD, Lobel HD, Satriale RF, et al. Severe cutaneous reactions among American travellers using pyrimethamine-sulfadoxine (Fansidar) for malaria prophylaxis. Am J Trop Med Hyg 1986; 35:451–458.

96. Miller MJ, Aronson WJ, Remington JS. Late parasitemia in asymptomatic acquired toxoplasmosis. Ann Intern Med 1969; 71:139–145.
97. Neuenschwander MD, Cordier MD, Couvreur J. Toxoplasmose congenitale: apport de l'echomotomographie transfontanellaire et de la tomodensitometrie. Ann Pediatr (Paris) 1984; 31:837–839.
98. Nicolle C, Manceaux L. Sur un protozoaire nouveau du *gondii: Toxoplasma*. Arch Inst Pasteur Tunis 1909; 2:97–103.
99. O'Connor GR. The influence of hypersensitivity on the pathogenesis of ocular toxoplasmosis. Trans Am Ophthalmol Soc 1970; 68:501–547.
100. O'Connor GR. Factors related to the initiation and recurrence of uveitis. XL Edward Jackson Memorial Lecture. Am J Opthamol 1983; 96:577–599.
101. Pinkerton H, Weihman D. *Toxoplasma* infection in man. Arch Pathol 1940; 30:374–392.
102. Pinon JM, Thoannes H, Gruson N. An enzyme linked immunofiltration assay used to compare infant and maternal antibody profiles in toxoplasmosis. J Immunol Methods 1985; 77:15–23.
103. Puri S. Positive brain scan in toxoplasmosis. J Nucl Med 1974; 15:641–643.
104. Raymond J, Poissonnier MH, Thulliez P, et al. Presence of gamma interferon in human acute and congenital toxoplasmosis. J Clin Microbiol 1990; 28:1434–1437.
105. Remington JS, Cavanaugh EN. Isolation of the encysted form of *Toxoplasma gondii* from human skeletal muscle and brain. N Engl J Med 1965; 273:1308–1310.
106. Remington JS, Desmonts G. Toxoplasmosis. In: Remington JS, Klein JO, eds. Infectious disease of the fetus and newborn infant. Ed 2. Philadelphia: WB Saunders, 1983:143–263.
107. Remington JS, Desmonts G. Toxoplasmosis. In: Remington JS, Klein JO, eds. Infectious diseases of the fetus and newborn infant. Ed 3. Philadelphia: WB Saunders, 1990:89–195.
108. Remington JS, Efron B, Cavanaugh EN. Studies on toxoplamosis in El Salvador; prevalence and incidence of toxoplasmosis as measured by the Sabin-Feldman dye-test. Trans R Soc Trop Med Hyg 1970; 64:252–267.
109. Remington JS, Melton M, Jacobs L. Chronic *Toxoplasma* infection in the uterus. J Lab Clin Med 1960; 56:879–883.
110. Remington JS, Newell JW, Cavanaugh E. Spontaneous abortion and chronic toxoplasmosis. Report of a case with isolation of the parasite. Obstet Gynecol 1964; 24:25–31.
111. Ribierre M, Couvreur J, Canetti J. Les hydrocephalies par stenose de l'aqueduc de Sylvius dans la toxoplasmose congenitale. Arch Fr Pediatr 1970; 27:501–510.
112. Roux C, Desmonts G, Mulliez N. Toxoplasmose et grossesse. Bilan de deux ans de prophylaxie de la toxoplasmose congenitale à la maternité de l'Hopital Saint Antoine (1973-1974). J Gynecol Obstet Biol Reprod (Paris) 1976; 5:249–264.
113. Ruoss CF, Bourne GL. Toxoplasmosis in pregnancy. Journal of Obstetrics and Gynecology of the British Commonwealth 1972; 79:1115–1118.
114. Sabin AB, Feldman HA. Dyes as micochemical indicators of a new immunity phenomenon affecting a protozoon parasite *(Toxoplasma)*. Science 1948; 108:660–663.
115. Sabin AB, Olitsky P. *Toxoplasma* and obligate intracellular parasitism. Science 1937; 85:336–337.
116. Sacks JJ, Roberto RR, Brooks NF. Toxoplasmosis infection associated with raw goat milk. JAMA 1982; 248:1728–1732.
117. Saleha AA. Observations on some epidemiological aspects of toxoplasmosis in Malaysia. International Journal of Zoonology 1984; 11:75–83.
118. Sarrut S. Renseignements fournis par l'étude histologique du placenta dans la toxoplasmose congénitale. Ann Pediatr (Paris) 1967; 14:2429–2435.
119. Schneider R, Tabet-Derraz O, Dedet JP. Etude du serodiagnostic de la toxoplasmose par immunofluorescence à l'Institut Pasteur d'Algérie. Arch Inst Pasteur Alger 1979; 52:95–104.
120. Scott GB, Fischl MA, Klimas N, et al. Mothers of infants with the acquired immunodeficiency syndrome. JAMA 1985; 253:363–366.
121. Sever JL, Ellenberg JH, Ley AC. Toxoplasmosis: maternal and pediatric findings in 23,000 pregnancies. Pediatrics 1988; 82:181–192.
122. Shimada K, O'Connor GR. Cyst formation by *Toxoplasma gondii* (RH strain) in vitro. The role of immunologic mechanisms. Arch Ophthalmol 1974; 92:496–501.
123. Sibalic D, Djurkovic-Djakoviv O, Nikolic R. Congenital toxoplasmosis in twins. Folia Parasitol (Praha) 1986; 33:1–6.
124. Splendore A. Un nuovo parasita dei conigli. Revista Societad Sciencias (Sao Paulo) 1908; 3:109–112.
125. Stagno S, Dykes AC, Amos CS, et al. An outbreak of toxoplasmosis linked to cats. Pediatrics 1980; 65:706–712.
126. Stray-Petersen B. A prospective study of acquired toxoplasmosis among 8043 pregnant women in the Oslo area. Am J Obstet Gynecol 1980; 13:399–406.
127. Thalammer O. Die angeborene Toxoplasomse. In Kirchhoff H, Kraübig H, eds. Toxoplasmose. Praktrische fragen und ergelnisse. Stuttgart: Georg Thieme Verlag, 1966:151–173.
128. Thalammer O. Prenatal incubation period. In: Thalammer O, ed. Prenatal infections. Stuttgart: Georg Thieme Verlag, 1971:70–71.
129. Thulliez P. Unpublished data.
130. Van der Waiij D. Formation, growth and multiplication of *Toxoplasma gondii* cysts in mouse brains. Trop Geogr Med 1959; 11:345–360.
131. Wallace GD. The prevalence of toxoplasmosis in Pacific islands and the influence of ethnic groups. Am J Trop Med Hyg 1976; 25:48–53.
132. Wallace GD, Laigret J, Kaeuffer H. A comparison of the prevalence of *Toxoplasma* antibody in Tahitians and Chinese living in Tahiti. Southeast Asian J Trop Med Public Health 1974; 5:350–352.
133. Wery-Paskoff J. 1970. Quoted by Zardi, Adorisio, Harare, and Nuti.
134. Wilson CB, Remington JS. What can be done to prevent congenital toxoplasmosis? Am J Obstet Gynecol 1980; 138:357–363.

135. Wilson CB, Remington JS, Stagno S, Reynolds DW. Development of adverse sequelae in children born with subclinical *Toxoplasma* infection. Pediatrics 1980; 66:767–774.
136. Wilson CB, Tsai V, Remington JS. Failure to trigger the oxidative metabolic burst by normal macrophages: possible mechanism for survival of intracellular pathogens. J Exp Med 1980; 151:328–356.
137. Witte HM, Pierkarsi G. Die Oocysten Ausscheidung bei experimentall infizierten Katzen in Abhängigkeit von Toxoplasma-Stamm. Zentralblatt Parasitenkunde 1970; 33:358–360.
138. Wolf A, Cowen D. Granulomatous encephalomyelitis due to an encephalitozoon (encephalitozoic encephalomyelitis). A new protozoan disease in man. Bulletin of the Neurological Institute New York 1937; 6:306–371.
139. Wolf A, Cowen D, Paige BH. Toxoplasmic encephalitis. III. A new case of granulomatous encephalomyelitis due to a protozoan. Am J Pathol 1939; 15:657–694.
140. Wolf A, Cowen D, Paige H. Human toxoplasmosis. Occurence in infants as an encephalomyelitis. Verification by transmission to animals. Science 1939; 89:226–227.
141. Work K. Isolation of *Toxoplasma gondii* from the flesh of sheep, swine and cattle. APMIS 1967; 71:296–306.
142. Zardi O, Adorisio E, Harare O, Nuti M. Serological survey of toxoplasmosis in Somalia. Trans R Soc Trop Med Hyg 1980; 74:577–581.

CHAPTER 14

Perinatal Chlamydial Infections

Cheryl K. Walker, M.D.
Richard L. Sweet, M.D.

Of the three distinct chlamydial species that are known to cause human disease, *C. trachomatis, C. psittaci,* and *C. pneumoniae,* only *C. trachomatis* is known to be transmitted sexually.[18] It is one of the most common sexually transmitted diseases (STDs) in the United States and has an estimated annual prevalence of over 4 million cases.[7] Its annual cost is projected in excess of $1.5 billion, and women account for 79 percent of these expenditures.[61]

Chlamydial cervicitis is notorious for its indolent course in women, with up to 70 percent of women being asymptomatic or harboring subclinical symptoms. Thus, women with lower genital tract chlamydial infection are identified commonly either through screening programs or after the infection's complications become manifest. Untreated chlamydial cervicitis may lead to pelvic inflammatory disease (PID) and sequelae, such as infertility, ectopic pregnancy, and chronic pelvic pain in nonpregnant women; during pregnancy it may be responsible for a number of adverse perinatal outcomes.

Epidemiology

Surveys estimate that up to 40 percent of sexually active women in the United States have antibodies to *C. trachomatis.*[42a] The prevalence varies according to the population studied. The rate for asymptomatic women attending family planning clinics ranges from 5.5 to 22.5 percent and rises to 34 to 63 percent in women with mucopurulent cervicitis (MPC).[26,30] Antenatal screening programs have recovered *C. trachomatis* from cervical swabs in 2 to 37 percent.[3,10,15,20,21,25,33,45,56] It is estimated that approximately 5 percent of pregnant women in the United States have chlamydial infection of the cervix.

Risk markers for chlamydial infection are similar to those for other STDs. For pregnant women, they include age under 20, unmarried status, multiple sexual partners, a new sexual partner in the last 3 months, poverty, urban dwelling, inadequate antenatal care, symptoms of MPC or sterile pyuria, and presence or history of other STDs.[4,9,46] Up to 60 percent of women with lower genital tract gonococcal infection harbor *C. trachomatis* concomitantly.[49,60] Finally, the greatest hazard is sexual contact with an infected partner.[4,14,38,55]

The Organism

Two of the species in the genus *Chlamydia* are characterized in Table 14-1. *Chlamydia psittaci* is a common pathogen in birds and lower mammals and is occasionally associated with human infections. A recently described *C. psittaci* strain, TWAR, has been demonstrated to be a human pathogen that is an increasingly recognized cause of acute respiratory tract disease.[19] *Chlamydia trachomatis* is predominantly a human pathogen. Whereas *C. trachomatis* is sensitive to sulfonamides and has iodine-staining inclusions, *C. psittaci* is resistant to sulfonamides and does not contain iodine-staining inclusions.

Chlamydia trachomatis can be differentiated on a serologic basis into 15 serotypes (Table 14-1). These serotypes are associated with three major groups of human infections. Serotypes L_1, L_2, and L_3 are the causative agents for lymphogranuloma venereum. Serotypes A, B, Ba, and C are associated with endemic blinding trachoma. The D, E, F, G, H, I, J, and K serotypes are orogenital and sexually transmitted strains that are responsible for inclusion conjunctivitis, newborn pneu-

Table 14-1 Chlamydia: Taxonomy and Association with Human Disease

Chlamydia psittaci		**Chlamydia trachomatis**	
Resistant to sulfonamides		Sensitive to sulfonamides	
Inclusions do not stain with iodine		Inclusions stain with iodine	
Common pathogen in man and lower animals		Predominantly human pathogen	
Serotypes	**Disease**	**Serotypes**	**Disease**
Many	Psittacosis	A, B, Ba, C	Endemic blinding trachoma
TWAR	Acute respiratory infections	D, E, F, G, H, I, J, K	Inclusion conjunctivitis Urethritis Cervicitis Pelvic inflammatory disease Epididymitis Newborn pneumonia
		L_1, L_2, L_3	Lymphogranuloma venereum

monia, urethritis, cervicitis, salpingitis, acute urethral syndrome, and perinatal infections.

Pathology

Chlamydiae are gram-negative obligate intracellular organisms that are classified as bacteria because they possess both DNA and RNA. Because of their restricted metabolic capacity, they require columnar or pseudostratified columnar cells for survival. Elementary bodies (EB), which are capable of extracellular survival for limited periods, are the infective form of the organism. They gain access to host cells through special surface receptors and the process of endocytosis. Once inside the cell, the bacterium undergoes reorganization into a reticulate body (RB). Larger and richer in RNA, RBs are metabolically active and multiply to create the characteristic intracellular inclusions. In turn, the reticulate body re-forms into EBs, which mechanically disrupt the host cell with resultant expulsion of EBs into the environment. This growth cycle requires approximately 48 hours.

Clinical Manifestations

The spectrum of disease in women includes lower genital tract infection such as cervicitis, urethritis, bartholinitis, proctitis, and lymphogranuloma venereum (LGV). Infection may extend to the upper genital tract and cause endomyometritis, salpingitis, peritonitis, and perihepatitis. Extragenital sites such as the pharynx and conjunctivae are also sometimes infected.

The incubation period for genital chlamydial infections ranges from 6 to 21 days. Following this, the infection may become symptomatic. As mentioned previously, the majority of women lack symptoms. A number of presentations have been described in pregnancy.

Endocervicitis

Infection of the endocervix is the most common chlamydial infection in women. When present, symptoms usually include an abnormal vaginal discharge, which typically is nonpruritic, not foul smelling, and yellow or green in color. The clinical syndrome is called mucopurulent cervicitis (MPC) and hinges on three findings: endocervical friability, erythema, or edema; yellow or green endocervical discharge, which may appear yellow when viewed on a white cotton-tipped swab (positive swab test); and more than 10 polymorphonuclear leukocytes per high-power field of a Gram-stained endocervical swab sample.

Acute Urethral Syndrome

Alternatively known as *sterile pyuria,* acute urethral syndrome is characterized by urinary frequency and dysuria that may last 2 weeks in the setting of pyuria in the absence of bacteriuria. *Chlamydia trachomatis* is the etiologic agent in 25 percent of women with this syndrome. *Chlamydia trachomatis* is more frequently recovered from the endocervix than from the urethra of women with this syndrome.[51]

Upper Genital Tract Infection

In women undergoing elective abortion, those with chlamydial cervicitis have a 35 percent chance of developing postabortal endomyometritis.[5,35,39,40,62] Thus, prior to instrumentation, antibiotic prophylaxis is recommended for women with known or suspected infection.

Although an association between chlamydia infection and postpartum endomyometritis has been suspected for more than 50 years,[58] it has not been proven. Wagner and associates described a characteristic syndrome of

Table 14-2 Experience with Antigen-Detection Methods for *Chlamydia trachomatis* in Women

	Sensitivity	Specificity	Positive Predictive Value	Negative Predictive Value
Direct Immunofluorescence				
High-prevalence population	89 (89–98)	98 (89–99)	90 (68–97)	98 (98–100)
Intermediate-prevalence population	79 (61–96)	98 (94–99)	79 (65–93)	98 (94–99)
Enzyme Immunoassay				
High-prevalence population	90 (70–98)	97 (86–98)	84 (61–94)	98 (97–99)
Intermediate-prevalence population	89 (82–96)	97 (93–98)	73 (45–80)	98 (98–99)

Modified from Stamm 1988.[48]

late-onset endomyometritis following vaginal delivery with mild symptoms of abdominal pain and uterine tenderness that were associated with antenatal presence of *C. trachomatis*.[59] Although several studies have reported a link,[13,28,58,59] others have not.[24,27,57]

In the nonpregnant woman, there is a tendency for ascending spread of lower genital tract chlamydial infection. Pelvic inflammatory disease (PID) is rare in pregnancy, although numerous case reports exist in the literature.[1,16,29,31,32,34,47] The diagnosis is confounded by the physiology of pregnancy, which under normal circumstances includes gastrointestinal disturbances and an elevation of the peripheral white blood cell count. Because the incidence of fetal wastage approaches 50 percent in women with gestational PID, broad-spectrum antibiotics must be administered whenever this infection is suspected.[6]

Diagnosis

A variety of techniques are used to confirm a clinical diagnosis of chlamydial infection. They include cytology, serology, culture, antigen detection, and identification with a DNA probe. The use of Papanicolaou smears to detect inclusion bodies has not been evaluated in comparison with culture.[41] Serologic tests are helpful in assessing previous exposure but have limited use in diagnosing active infection. Although promising, DNA hybridization technology is still investigational. Culture and antigen-detection systems, however, are widely used and remain the techniques that are clinically useful.

Care in the collection and proper handling of specimens is essential in order to ensure the reliability of cultures and antigen detection. Because *C. trachomatis* is an obligate intracellular organism, specimens must include infected cells. Debris should be minimized by carefully cleaning the cervix of extraneous mucus and secretions. The use of metal-shafted swabs is advocated because the presence of wood diminishes the number of inclusion-forming units in stored specimens. Use of the cytologic brush rather than the conventional swab appears to enhance both specimen collection and culture sensitivity.[37]

The optimal test for *C. trachomatis* infection is culture.[50] Unfortunately, the technique is long, tedious, expensive, and not universally available. It may take up to 7 days to obtain culture results. Isolation of this intracellular organism requires the collection of epithelial cells from the infected site, the use of refrigerated transport medium containing antibiotics to restrict overgrowth of other bacteria, and inoculation within 24 hours to a susceptible tissue culture cell line, such as the McCoy cell. Specimens may be frozen at $-70°C$ if timely inoculation is not possible. The sensitivity of this technique is proportional to laboratory experience. The use of fluorescein-labeled monoclonal antibodies for identification of inclusions, the use of microtiter plates rather than coverslip vials, and performance of a second passage are all recent innovations in culture techniques that have been shown to improve results.[52,63]

Two antigen-detection tests recently have become available for *C. trachomatis* infection. They are less expensive and cumbersome than culture, widely available, and provide a rapid result. The first utilizes fluorescent monoclonal antibody staining of chlamydial elementary bodies (MicroTrak, Syva Co., Palo Alto, CA), and the other detects antigen eluted from swabs and measured by an ELISA (Chlamydiazyme, Abbott Laboratories, North Chicago, IL). Both tests compare favorably with culture. When used in high-prevalence populations (15 to 26 percent), both tests have sensitivity, specificity, and positive predictive value assessments of over 90 percent (Table 14-2). Sensitivity and positive predictive value appear to decrease for both tests as the prevalence of infection decreases. In areas of medium prevalence (9 to 1[illegible] percent), the ELISA has better sensitivity, but both methods have positive predictive values less than 80 percent.[48] Neither test has been evaluated in low-prevalence populations, although it has been noted that use of a confirmatory blocking assay to validate positive ELISAs increases the specificity dramatically, making it a more useful test in low-risk women.[36] As with cultures, use of the cytobrush to obtain the specimen has been shown to enhance the predictive value of antigen-detection methods.[37]

Table 14-3 Pregnancy Outcome in IgM-Positive versus IgM-Negative Chlamydia-Infected Women

	Chlamydia Infected Women		
	IgM POSITIVE	IgM NEGATIVE	**Chlamydia Negative**
Harrison et al.[24]			
Number of patients	17	53	793
Low birth weight	4 (24%)	1 (2%)	52 (6.6%)
Mean gestational age (weeks)	37.9	39.6	39.3
PROM	7 (41%)	4 (8%)	74 (9%)
Sweet et al.[54]			
Number of patients	67	99	
PROM	13 (19.4%)	8 (8%)	
Preterm delivery (less than 37 weeks)	13 (19.4%)	8 (8%)	

Maternal and Fetal Risks

Maternal *C. trachomatis* infection has been implicated in the development of spontaneous abortion, fetal death, premature ruptured membranes (PROM), preterm delivery (PTD), and intrauterine growth retardation, although existing evidence is inconclusive. Concern was raised with the report by Martin and coworkers associating maternal chlamydial infection with spontaneous abortion, low birth weight, preterm delivery, and increased perinatal mortality.[33] Subsequent, larger prospective studies failed to confirm an association between maternal chlamydial infection and an increase in perinatal morbidity or mortality.[21,23,24] Two investigations have identified a subpopulation of infected women subject to adverse perinatal outcome; both found an association between maternal IgM seropositivity and PROM and PTD (Table 14-3).[24,54] Harrison and coworkers noted that in the subgroup of chlamydia culture–positive women with IgM antibody against *C. trachomatis*, there was a significantly increased risk for PROM, low birth weight, and shorter gestational age.[24] In the study by Sweet and associates, chlamydia-infected women with antichlamydial IgM were at significantly increased risk of PROM and preterm delivery.[54] Comparing women with chlamydial infection with uninfected controls, Gravett and coworkers detected an increase in preterm labor (36 percent versus 12 percent O.R. 4.3), preterm PROM (23 percent versus 11 percent O.R. 2.4), and low birth weight (less than 2,500 g) (32 percent versus 15 percent O.R. 2.7) in the former group.[17] Recently two retrospective studies on the effect of treatment for *C. trachomatis* during pregnancy have investigated the association between chlamydia cervical infection and adverse pregnancy outcome.[11,42] Cohen and coworkers studied three groups: chlamydia-infected women treated during pregnancy, chlamydia-infected women who did not receive treatment, and uninfected women. The untreated infected women had higher incidences of PROM and preterm delivery than the other groups, whereas the treated infected women and uninfected women were not significantly different.[11] Similarly, Ryan and associates demonstrated in a high-prevalence population (21 percent infected with chlamydia) that their untreated group had a significantly increased incidence of PROM and low birth weight and a decreased neonatal survival when compared to the culture-positive group receiving treatment (Table 14-4).[42] Logistic regression analysis revealed a significant decrease in PROM for the treated versus untreated group with chlamydia infection (O.R. 0.56; 95 percent C.I. 0.37–0.85). Because these studies were retrospective in nature, they suggest that treatment of chlamydia infection during pregnancy may reduce the incidence of adverse pregnancy outcomes. However, prospective and randomized studies that control for known risk factors of preterm delivery will be required to confirm this finding.

The risk for vertical transmission of *C. trachomatis* from pregnant women with cervical chlamydia infection to their neonates is well documented. Vertical transmission rates in untreated infected women approach 70 percent.[43,53] Symptoms of inclusion conjunctivitis develop within 2 weeks of birth in approximately 20 to 50 percent of exposed infants (Table 14-5). Another 10 to 20 percent develop chlamydial pneumonia in the first 4 months of life. Hammerschlag and coworkers reported that neonatal ocular prophylaxis with either erythromycin or tetracycline opthalmic ointment was ineffective in preventing chlamydial conjunctivitis.[22] Whereas the incidence of chlamydial conjunctivitis among infants born to chlamydia-infected mothers was 20 percent in the silver nitrate group, it was 14 percent and 11 percent in the erythromycin and tetracycline groups, respectively (*P* not significant). Thus, maternal screening and treatment is the most effective means of reducing chlamydial infection in infants.

Treatment

The agents most commonly used to treat chlamydial infection in adults, tetracycline and doxycycline, are contraindicated in pregnancy, as are the quinolones. Because erythromycin estolate may cause maternal hepatotoxicity, it is also not safe for use during pregnancy. The Centers for Disease Control recommends the use of erythromycin base, 500 mg orally four times daily for 7 days.[8] For women in whom tolerance is problematic,

Table 14-4 Pregnancy Outcome in Women Infected with Chlamydia: Effect of Treatment

Outcome	Chlamydia Positive				Chlamydia Negative (%) (n = 9,111)
	UNTREATED (%) (N = 1110)	P	TREATED (%) (N = 1323)	P	
PROM	58 (5.2)	<0.001	39 (2.9)	NS	243 (2.7)
Birth weight less than 2,500 g	218 (19.6)	<0.0001	145 (11)	NS	1,068 (11.7)
Newborn survival	1083 (97.6)	<0.001	1315 (99.4)	<0.01	8,973 (98.5)

Data from Ryan et al.[42]

Table 14-5 *Chlamydia trachomatis* Infection among Infants Born to Untreated Chlamydial Infected Mothers

Study	Conjunctivitis	Pneumonia
Alexander et al.[2]	9/18 (50%)	NS*
Frommell et al.[15]	7/18 (39%)	2/18 (11%)
Heggie et al.[25]	20/95 (21%)	3/95 (3%)
Hammerschlag et al.[21]	12/36 (33%)	3/36 (8%)
Schachter et al.[44]	16/89 (18%)	16/89 (18%)

**NS*, not stated.

one or two dosages of erythromycin ethylsuccinate is advocated, 800 mg four times daily for 7 days or 400 mg four times daily for 14 days. If gastrointestinal complications preclude the use of any of the erythromycins, amoxicillin, 500 mg three times daily for 7 days, has been shown in limited trials to reduce vertical transmission.[12] With tetracycline or doxycycline treatment for chlamydial infection, a test of cure is not recommended. However, with erythromycin, amoxicillin, or other antimicrobials, a test of cure should be obtained at a minimum of 3 weeks following completion of treatment.

Screening

The association of *C. trachomatis* with vertical transmission and a possible adverse perinatal outcome underscores the need for screening women at the first prenatal visit and, for those at high risk for contracting chlamydia, again during the third trimester.[8] Women with a positive test should be treated and retested in 3 to 4 weeks to ensure treatment efficacy. Partner screening and treatment as well as education about safe sexual practices are essential components of any treatment program. Finally, given that multiple sexually transmitted infections are often coexistent, women diagnosed with chlamydial infection should be tested for other STDs.

References

1. Acosta AA, Mabray CR, Kaurman RH. Intrauterine pregnancy and coexistent pelvic inflammatory disease. Obstet Gynecol 1971; 37:282.
2. Alexander ER, Chandler J, Pheifer TA, et al. Prospective study of perinatal *Chlamydia trachomatis* infection. In: Hobson D, Holmes KK, eds. Nongonococcal urethritis and related infections. Washington, DC: American Society Microbiology, 1977; 148–152.
3. Alexander ER, Harrison R. Role of *Chlamydia trachomatis* in perinatal infection. Rev Infect Dis 1983; 5:713–719.
4. Arya OP, Mallinson H, Goddard AD. Epidemiological and clinical correlates of chlamydial infection of the cervix. British Journal of Venereal Disease 1981; 57:118–124.
5. Barbacci MB, Spence MR, Kappus EW, et al. Postabortal endometritis and isolation of *Chlamydia trachomatis*. Obstet Gynecol 1986; 68:686–690.
6. Blanchard AC, Pastorek JG II, Weeks T. Pelvic inflammatory disease during pregnancy. South Med J 1987; 30:1363.
7. Centers for Disease Control. *Chlamydia trachomatis* infections: policy guidelines for prevention and control. MMWR 1985; 34:53S–74S.
8. Centers for Disease Control. 1989 Sexually transmitted diseases treatment guidelines. MMWR 1989; 38:28S–29S.
9. Chacko MR, Louchik JC. *Chlamydia trachomatis* infection in sexually active adolescents: prevalence and risk factors. Pediatrics 1984; 73:836.
10. Chandler JW Alexander ER, Pheiffer TA, et al. Ophthalmia neonatorum associated with maternal chlamydial infections. Transactions American Acadamy Ophthalmology Otolaryngology 1977; 83:302–308.
11. Cohen I, Veille JC, Calkins BM: Improved pregnancy outcome following successful treatment of chlamydial infection. JAMA 1990; 263:3160–3163.
12. Crombleholme WR, Schachter J, Grossman M, et al. Amoxicillin therapy for *Chlamydia trachomatis* in pregnancy. Obstet Gynecol 1990; 75:752–756.

13. Cytryn A, Sen P, Haingsub R, et al. Severe pelvic infection from *Chlamydia trachomatis* after cesarean section. JAMA 1982; 247:1732–1734.
14. Dunlap EMC, Jones BR, Darougar S. Chlamydia and non-specific urethritis. Br Med J 1972; 2:577.
15. Frommel GT, Rothenberg R, Wang S-P. Chlamydial infection of mothers and their infants. J Pediatr 1979; 95:28–32.
16. Fuselier P, Alam A. Pregnancy complicated by pelvic abscess. J Reprod Med 1978; 21:257.
17. Gravett MG, Nelson P, DeRouen T, et al. Independent associations of bacterial vaginosis *Chlamydia trachomatis* infection with adverse pregnancy outcome. JAMA 1986; 256:1899–1903.
18. Grayston JT, Kuo CC, Campbell LA, Wang SP. *Chlamydia pneumoniae* sp. nov. for *Chlamydia* sp. strain TWAR. Int J Syst Bacteriol 1989; 39:88.
19. Grayston JT, Kuo CC, Wang SP, Altman J. A new *Chlamydia psittaci* strain, TWAR, isolated in acute respiratory tract infections. N Engl J Med 1986; 315: 161–168.
20. Grossman M, Schachter J, Sweet R, et al. Prospective studies of chlamydia in newborns. In Mardh P-A, Holmes KK, Oriel JD, et al, eds. Chlamydial infections. Fernstrom Foundations Series, vol 2, Amsterdam. Elsevier, 1982; 213–216.
21. Hammerschlag MR, Anderka M, Semine DZ, et al. Prospective study of maternal and infantile infection with *Chlamydia trachomatis*. Pediatrics 1979; 64:142–148.
22. Hammerschlag MR, Cummings C, Roblin PM, et al. Efficacy of neonatal ocular prophylaxis for the prevention of chlamydial and gonococcal conjunctivitis. N Engl J Med 1989; 32:772–775.
23. Hardy PH, Hardy JB, Nell EE, et al. Prevalence of sexually transmitted disease agents in pregnant inner-city adolescents and pregnancy outcome. Lancet 1984; 2:333.
24. Harrison HR, Alexander ER, Weinstein L, et al. Cervical *Chlamydia trachomatis* and mycoplasmal infections in pregnancy: Epidemiology and outcomes. JAMA 1984; 250:1721–1727.
25. Heggie AD, Lumicao CG, Stuart LA, Gyues MT. *Chlamydia trachomatis* infection in mothers and infants: a prospective study. Am J Dis Child 1981; 135:507–511m.
26. Hobson D, Johnson FWA, Rees E, et al. Simplified method for diagnosis of genital and ocular infections with *Chlamydia*. Lancet 1974; 2:555–556.
27. Hoyme UB, Kiviat N, Eschenbach DA. Microbiology and treatment of late postpartum endometritis. Obstet Gynecol 1986; 68:226.
28. Ismail MA, Chandler AE, Beem MO, Moawad AH. Chlamydial colonization of the cervix in pregnant adolescents. J Reprod Med 1985; 30:549–553.
29. Jafari K, Vilovic-Kos J, Webster A, et al. Tubo-ovarian abscess in pregnancy. Acta Obstet Gynecol Scand 1977; 56:1.
30. Kuo C-C, Wang S-P, Wentworth BB, et al. Primary isolation of TRIC organisms in HeLa 229 cells treated with DEAE-dextran. J Infect Dis 1972; 125:665–668.
31. Lancet M, Cohen A. Acute prurulent salpingitis in late pregnancy. Obstet Gynecol 1957; 14:426.
32. Lennon GG. Acute salpingitis during pregnancy. Journal of Obstetrics and Gynaecology of the British Commonwealth 1949; 56:1035.
33. Martin DH, Koutsky L, Eschenbach DA, et al. Prematurity and perinatal mortality in pregnancies complicated by maternal *Chlamydia trachomatis* infections. JAMA 1982; 247:1585–1588.
34. McCord M, Simmons CM. Acute prurulent salpingitis during pregnancy. Am J Obstet Gynecol 1953; 65:1136.
35. Moller BR, Ahorns S, Laurin J, Mardh P-A. Pelvic infection after elective abortion associated with *Chlamydia trachomatis*. Obstet Gynecol 1982; 59:210–213.
36. Moncada J, Schachter J, Bolan G, et al. Confirmatory assay increases specificity of the chlamydiazyme test for *Chlamydia trachomatis* infection of the cervix. J Clin Microbiol 1990; 28:1770–1773.
37. Moncada J, Schachter J, Shipp M, et al. Cytobrush in collection of cervical specimens for detection of *Chlamydia trachomatis*. J Clin Microbiol 1989; 27:1863–1866.
38. Oriel JD, Reeve P, Powis P, et al. Chlamydial infection: isolation of *Chlamydia* from patients with non-specific genital infection. British Journal of Venereal Disease 1972; 48:419–436.
39. Osser S, Persson K. Postabortal pelvic infection associated with *Chlamydia trachomatis* and the influence of humoral immunity. Am J Obstet Gynecol 1984; 150:699.
40. Quigstad E, Skaug K, Jerve F, et al. Pelvic inflammatory disease associated with *Chlamydia trachomatis* infection after therapeutic abortion. British Journal of Venereal Disease 1983; 59:189.
41. Robson HG, Shah PP, Lalonde RG, et al. Comparison of rosaramicin and erythromycin stearate for treatment of cervical infections with *Chlamydia trachomatis*. Sex Transm Dis 1983; 4:747.
42. Ryan GM, Abdella TN, McNeeley SG, et al. *Chlamydia trachomatis* infection in pregnancy and effect of treatment on outcome. Am J Obstet Gynecol 1990; 162:34–39.

42a. Schachter J. Chlamydial infections. N Engl J Med 1978; 298:428.

43. Schachter J, Grossman M. Chlamydial infections. Annu Rev Med 1981; 32:45–61.
44. Schachter J, Grossman M, Sweet RL, et al. Prospective study of perinatal transmission of *Chlamydia trachomatis*. JAMA 1986; 255:3374–3377.
45. Schachter J, Holt J, Goodner E, et al. Prospective study of chlamydial infection in neonates. Lancet 1979; 2:377–380.
46. Schachter J, Stoner E, Moncoda J. Screening for chlamydial infections in women attending family planning clinics: evaluations of presumptive indicators for therapy. West J Med 1983; 138:375–379.
47. Scott TM, Hay D. Acute salpingitis and surgery. Journal of Obstetrics and Gynaecology of the British Commonwealth 1954; 61:788.

48. Stamm WE. Diagnosis of *Chlamydia trachomatis* genitourinary tract infections. Ann Intern Med 1988; 108:710–717.
49. Stamm WE, Guinan ME, Johnson C, et al. Effect of treatment regimens for *Neisseria gonorrhoeae* on simultaneous infection with *Chlamydia trachomatis*. N Engl J Med 1984; 311:1–6.
50. Stamm WE, Mardh P-A. Chlamydia trachomatis. In: Sexually transmitted diseases, Holmes KK, Mardh P-A, Sparling PF, et al, eds. McGraw Hill: New York. 1990:917–926.
51. Stamm WE, Wagner KF, Ansel R, et al. Causes of the acute urethral syndrome in women. N Engl J Med 1980; 303:956–958.
52. Stephen RS, et al. Sensitivity of immunofluorescence with monoclonal antibodies for detection of *Chlamydia trachomatis* inclusions in cell culture, J Clin Microbiol 1982; 16:4.
53. Sweet RL, Gibbs RS. Chlamydial infections. In: Infectious diseases of the female genital tract. Baltimore: Williams & Wilkins. 1990:45–74.
54. Sweet RL, Landers DV, Walker C, Schachter J. *Chlamydia trachomatis* infection and pregnancy outcome. Am J Obstet Gynecol 1987; 156:824–833.
55. Tait IA, Rees E, Hobson D, et al. Chlamydial infection of the cervix in contacts of men with nongonococcal urethritis. British Journal of Venereal Disease 1980; 56:37–45.
56. Thompson S, Lopez B, Wong KH, et al. The relationship of low birthweight and infant mortality to vaginal microorganisms. Paper presented at the third international meeting on sexually transmitted diseases. Antwerp, October 2–3, 1980.
57. Thompson S, Lopez B, Wong KG, et al. A prospective study of chlamydial and mycoplasmal infections during pregnancy. In Mardh P-A, Holmes KK, Oriel JD, and others, editors. Chlamydial infections. Fernstrom Foundation Series, vol 2, Amsterdam, 1982, Elsevier.
58. Thygeson P, Mengert WF. The virus of inclusion conjunctivitis: further observations. Arch Ophthalmol 1936; 15:377–410.
59. Wager GP, Martin DH, Koutsky L, et al. Puerperal infectious morbidity: relationship to route of delivery and to antepartum *Chlamydia trachomatis* infection. Am J Obstet Gynecol 1980; 138:1028–1033.
60. Washington AE. Update on treatment recommendations for gonococcal infections. Rev Infect Dis 1982; 4(suppl):S758–S771.
61. Washington AE, Johnson RE, Sanders LL. *Chlamydia trachomatis* infections in the United States: what are they costing us? JAMA 1987; 257:2070–2072.
62. Westergard L, Philipson T, Scheibel J. Significance of cervical *Chlamydia trachomatis* infection postabortal pelvic inflammatory disease. Obstet Gynecol 1982; 60:322.
63. Yoder BL, et al. Microtest procedures for isolation of *Chlamydia trachomatis*. J Clin Microbiol 1981; 13:1036.

CHAPTER 15

Genital Mycoplasmas

Marinella Cardello Cummings, M.S.
William M. McCormack, M.D.

In 1937 Dienes and Edsall were first to report the isolation of a mycoplasma, most likely *Mycoplasma hominis,* from a human who had a Bartholin's gland abscess.[6]

To date, 12 mycoplasmal species—*M. buccale, M. faucium, M. fermentans, M. genitalium, M. hominis, M. lipophilum, M. pneumoniae, M. orale, M. salivarium, Ureaplasma urealyticum, M. primatum,* and *Acholeplasma laidlawii*—have been isolated from the mucous membranes of the genital and upper respiratory tract in humans.

Three of the human mycoplasma species—*M. hominis, U. urealyticum,* and *M. genitalium*—have been shown to be genital pathogens and are discussed in this chapter.

Characteristics

Mycoplasmas have no cell wall and are thus resistant to antibiotics that affect the cell wall, such as penicillins and cephalosporins. Mycoplasmas differ from viruses in that they contain both RNA and DNA. They resemble chlamydiae, rickettsiae, and viruses in filterability through a 450-nm filter, but they differ in being able to grow on artificial media.[4] Although cell wall–deficient bacterial variants (L forms, spheroplasts, protoplasts) form colonies that are similar in appearance to those of mycoplasmas and share some other properties with the mycoplasmas, they are unrelated.

On a solid medium most mycoplasmas form very small colonies, 50 to 600 μm in diameter, which can be seen only with a hand lens or under the low-power objective of a microscope. The classic "fried egg" appearance of the usual colony is due to an opaque, granular central zone of growth down into the agar and a flat, translucent peripheral zone of growth on the surface.[4] Not all mycoplasmas produce "fried egg" colonies, and variations in colonial morphology are frequently dependent on the constituents of the medium, as well as atmosphere and inoculum size. Ureaplasmas were originally called *tiny* or *T-strains* because they form small (15 to 30 μm) colonies that lack the peripheral area of surface growth.[4] The ability of the genus *Ureaplasma* to hydrolyze urea sets it apart from the genus *Mycoplasma.*

By reason of their limited biosynthetic abilities, these organisms are highly fastidious and require complex enriched culture media for growth. Such media usually contain a peptone, animal serum as a source of cholesterol or related sterol, preformed nucleic acid precursors supplied by yeast extract, and metabolites, such as glucose, arginine, or urea.[21] Most mycoplasmas are facultatively anaerobic, but growth of some organisms is enhanced by incubation in air with 5 percent CO_2. The optimum incubation temperature is 37°C.

Differences in metabolic activity provide a useful means of identification of genital mycoplasmas. The specific metabolites, arginine and urea, along with a phenol red indicator, are added to separate tubes of liquid mycoplasma medium that has been adjusted to pH 6.0 for ureaplasma and pH 7.0 for *M. hominis.* These tubes are then inoculated with the sample. The *M. hominis* organisms convert arginine to ornithine, whereas ureaplasmas utilize urea. Both of these reactions are associated with a rise in pH. From tubes showing a change in color of the pH indicator, an aliquot is subcultured onto an appropriate agar for definitive identification. Colonies of *M. hominis* usually have a classic "fried egg" appearance. When crowded, the colonies appear smaller and have less peripheral growth. There is a zone of inhibition around a disc impregnated with specific antiserum. There are two colony types of *U. urealyticum:* small, even colonies looking like bits of dust, and large, uneven, textured colonies with dark black centers and very little peripheral growth. The addition of manganous sulfate to ureaplasma agar causes the colonies to appear quite dark, golden brown to chestnut, with a well-defined periphery. There is a zone of inhibition around an erythromycin disc.

Mycoplasma hominis produces nonhemolytic pinpoint colonies on blood agar, but the organisms cannot be visualized in Gram-stained smears of these colonies. It will also grow in routine blood culture media without changing the appearance of the medium. Blind subculture on to agar media is needed to identify the organisms.[49] Ureaplasmas and *M. genitalium* do not grow in ordinary microbiologic media.

Mycoplasma genitalium has been isolated in Sp4 medium.[46] It is a glucose fermenter that is more fastidious than *M. hominis* or *U. urealyticum* and does not grow in conventional mycoplasma media. These organisms require other supplements, such as CMRL 1066 tissue culture supplement with glutamine, yeastolate, and fetal bovine serum. Modification of Sp4 medium with polymyxin B and amphotericin prevents contamination. The Sp4 medium can also be used to isolate *M. hominis*.

Epidemiology

The genital mycoplasmas *M. hominis* and *U. urealyticum* are common inhabitants of the genitourinary mucous membranes of humans. Infants presumably become colonized with genital mycoplasmas during passage through the birth canal. Infants delivered by cesarean section are colonized less often than those delivered vaginally.[22] Ureaplasmas have been isolated from the genitalia of up to one-third of infant girls and *M. hominis* from a smaller proportion.[22] Mycoplasmas are recovered less frequently from infant boys.[9] Mycoplasmas, mainly ureaplasmas, have been isolated from the nose and throat of about 15 percent of infants of both sexes.[22]

Neonatal colonization tends not to persist. These organisms are seldom recovered from prepubertal boys.[25] Five to 22 percent of prepubertal girls are colonized with *U. urealyticum*, and 8 to 17 percent with *M. hominis*.[13,14,25] Following puberty, colonization is closely associated with sexual experience.[29] Colonization increases with increasing sexual experience more rapidly in women than in men, which suggests that it is easier to transmit the organisms from men to women than from women to men. Colonization rates with both *M. hominis* and *U. urealyticum* are higher among clinic populations than among the patients of private obstetricians and gynecologists.[30] Women who use nonbarrier methods of contraception are more likely to be colonized than women who use other methods or no method of contraception.[30] Thus, these organisms can be isolated from a significant proportion of normal sexually experienced men and women. The role of *M. hominis* and *U. urealyticum* in human disease must be viewed against this background.

Clinical Manifestations

Role of Genital Mycoplasmas in Disease of the Genital Tract in Women

Vaginitis

Mycoplasma hominis and *U. urealyticum* are both commonly isolated from women who have bacterial vaginosis; these organisms appear to be part of the abnormal polymicrobial flora of this condition.[42] Bacterial vaginosis (BV, formerly nonspecific vaginitis) is thought to be a flora shift from normal vaginal flora, dominated by lactobacilli, to a polymicrobic flora, which includes *Gardnerella vaginalis*, *Mobiluncus* species, and various anaerobic bacteria, as well as mycoplasmas and ureaplasmas. The change in flora is associated with a malodorous homogeneous vaginal discharge. Women who have BV are more likely to be colonized with *M. hominis* than women without BV.[37,45] In a study by Pheifer and associates, treatment with metronidazole was associated with the elimination of *M. hominis* from many patients.[38] Clinical response to therapy was unrelated to elimination of *M. hominis*.

Pelvic Inflammatory Disease

Although most cases of pelvic inflammatory disease (PID) are caused by *Chlamydia trachomatis* and/or *Neisseria gonorrhoeae*, *M. hominis* organisms have been isolated from upper genital tract specimens from some patients with PID and are probably important pathogens in some women who have this condition. Mardh and Westrom isolated *M. hominis* from the fallopian tubes of 4 of 50 women with salpingitis.[27] The organisms were not isolated from women without salpingitis. Serologic studies have shown a response to *M. hominis* in about 30 percent of patients who have PID.[35,50] Antibodies to *M. hominis* were found three times more often in women with tubal infertility than in other infertile women.[34] *Mycoplasma hominis* is part of the abnormal microbial flora of bacterial vaginosis, and the isolation of and serologic response to *M. hominis* may reflect the role of bacterial vaginosis organisms in PID.

Ureaplasma urealyticum has been isolated from the fallopian tubes in occasional cases of PID.[28] Attempts at producing salpingitis in grivet monkeys using *U. urealyticum* have failed.[28]

Mycoplasma genitalium is a pathogen of the urogenital tract of higher primates and probably plays a role in human genital tract infection.[47] These organisms have been implicated in PID. In one study, 38 percent of women with PID had no antibody to *M. hominis* or *C. trachomatis* but had a fourfold or greater rise in *M. genitalium* antibody titer.[33] However, the specificity of serologic tests for this agent remains uncertain.[50] *Mycoplasma genitalium* organisms have been shown to produce severe endosalpingitis in monkeys.[47] The recent introduction of a DNA probe for *M. genitalium* may increase our knowledge of the role of this organism in PID.[50]

Bartholin's Abscess

Although *M. hominis* was first isolated from a Bartholin's gland abscess, it does not appear that genital mycoplasmas are an important cause of this infection. In a study by Lee and colleagues, *M. hominis* was isolated from one and *U. urealyticum* from none of 34 abscesses.[26]

Fever Following Abortion

Mycoplasma hominis appears to cause some cases of fever following abortion. Harwick and associates reported isolation of *M. hominis* from the blood of 4 of 51 women who had febrile abortions but not from 53 women who had afebrile abortions.[18]

Postpartum Fever

Mycoplasma hominis organisms cause postpartum fever, presumably by causing endometritis. Lamey and colleagues isolated *M. hominis* from the bloodstream of 9 of 125 febrile postpartum women, compared with none of 60 afebrile postpartum patients.[24] Wallace and coworkers isolated *M. hominis* from the blood of 10 to 15 percent of women with postpartum fever.[49] Platt and associates evaluated 535 women who had been delivered vaginally and found that 23 of them had unexplained postpartum fever.[39] The only agent associated with it was *M. hominis*. Knowledge of *M. hominis* antibody status identified not only patients with a high incidence of postpartum fever but also the majority of all febrile patients. Fifty-seven percent (16 of 28) of all fevers and 70 percent (16 of 23) of fevers not explained by examination and bacterial cultures occurred in patients with low antibody titers. The evidence that *M. hominis* infection was the cause of fever and not a linked variable is that preexisting mycoplasmacidal antibody titers greater than 1:8 were strongly protective against postpartum fever. Although antibody titer rise was associated with fever, this association resided entirely within the subgroup that had low initial titers.

Disorders of Reproduction

Mycoplasma hominis and *U. urealyticum* organisms have been associated with disorders of reproduction such as infertility, habitual abortion, and low birth weight, but the role of the organisms in these conditions is unclear.

Involuntary Infertility

Harrison and coworkers treated couples who had primary infertility of unknown cause with doxycycline or placebo.[17] The 28-day course of the antibiotic eradicated both *M. hominis* and *U. urealyticum*, but the rate of conception was no higher in those treated with the drug than in those given placebo. Other studies reviewed by Glatt and associates also failed to show an association between administration of tetracycline to ureaplasma-colonized couples and conception.[12]

Habitual Spontaneous Abortion and Stillbirth

Most investigators[15,16,36] have found no relation between lower genital tract colonization with ureaplasmas and fetal loss. However, *U. urealyticum* organisms have been isolated more frequently from stillborns and spontaneous abortuses than from induced abortuses or full-term infants.[41] Although there is an association between infection of the products of conception by ureaplasmas and fetal loss, the association is difficult to evaluate because the comparability of the various groups of women remains unsure and because the role of other organisms often was not assessed. The role of antimicrobial agents in preventing spontaneous abortion remains unsettled because either antibiotic treatment trials have been uncontrolled or the number of persons studied has been too few.[12]

Chorioamnionitis

Several investigators[11,19,20,43] have reported a significant association between chorioamnionitis and mycoplasmal infection. Gibbs and colleagues[11] found *M. hominis* more often in amniotic fluid of patients with clinical evidence of intrauterine infection in late pregnancy than in amniotic fluid of asymptomatic patients. Hillier and coworkers[20] found that there was an association not only between *M. hominis* and chorioamnionitis but also between bacterial vaginosis and chorioamnionitis. It may be that the isolation of *M. hominis* is an indication of bacterial vaginosis and that the complex abnormal flora of bacterial vaginosis—and not *M. hominis* alone—is causally related to chorioamnionitis.

Low Birth Weight

Although Minkoff and associates found no evidence that *U. urealyticum* was associated with low birth weight, ureaplasma-colonized pregnant women were more likely to have preterm labor.[32] A prospective study was conducted in which specimens were taken from 484 prenatal patients at the time of the first prenatal visit and culture results tabulated in terms of birth weight. There was an association between the presence of *U. urealyticum* and low birth weight.[1] Embree and associates studied placentas and found that isolation of *U. urealyticum* was associated with prematurity and low birth weight.[7] McCormack and colleagues[30] demonstrated that among pregnant women who were colonized with *U. urealyticum*, erythromycin treatment in the third trimester, when compared with placebo treatment, was associated with a significantly higher infant birth weight. Erythromycin was ineffective in eradicating *U. urealyticum* from the vagina.

A recently published multicenter study involving much larger populations of pregnant women showed no association between ureaplasmal colonization and adverse pregnancy outcome.[2] In this population, erythromycin treatment of ureaplasma-colonized pregnant women was not associated with birth weight or gestational age.[8]

Neonatal Infections

Waites and coworkers studied meningitis in 100 predominantly preterm infants.[48] They found that *M. hominis* and *U. urealyticum* were the most common microorganisms isolated from the cerebrospinal fluid of these neonates. *Ureaplasma urealyticum* was isolated more often than *M. hominis*. Garland and Murton also described neonatal meningitis caused by *U. urealyticum*.[10] It has also been associated with lower respiratory tract infection and chronic pulmonary disease in infants with very low birth weight.[3]

Treatment and Prevention

Mycoplasmas are not sensitive to inhibitors of cell wall synthesis. Polyenes have variable effects, depending on the sterol content of the mycoplasmal cell membrane. The organisms are not susceptible to sulfonamides and trimethoprim because they do not synthesize folic acid. Protein synthesis in mycoplasmas is prokaryotic in nature, so that antibiotics such as chloramphenicol and tetracyclines inhibit protein synthesis and growth.[44] *Mycoplasma hominis* organisms are susceptible to lincomycin and clindamycin, moderately susceptible to chloramphenicol, and resistant to erythromycin and rifampin;

aminoglycosides have limited activity.[23] Tetracycline is the antibiotic that is most frequently used to treat infections caused by *M. hominis,* but with the emergence of tetracycline-resistant *M. hominis* strains[5,23,40] other agents should be considered. Clindamycin is the most reasonable alternative agent. Ureaplasmas are usually susceptible to tetracyclines and to erythromycin.

Because cultures for these organisms are not generally available, clinicians should recognize the syndromes that have been associated with genital mycoplasmas and prescribe antimicrobial agents known to be active. *Mycoplasma hominis* causes some cases of PID. Initial treatment for PID should include antibiotics active against *N. gonorrhoeae, C. trachomatis, M. hominis,* and anaerobes. The Centers for Disease Control currently recommends either cefoxitin and doxycycline or clindamycin and gentamicin. Treatment of fever following vaginal delivery or abortion with tetracyclines or clindamycin may also be warranted. Present data do not support treatment aimed at ureaplasmas in the management of infertility. Similarly, there is no convincing evidence that *U. urealyticum* should be sought or treated in pregnant women.

There are to date no immunizing preparations available for the genital mycoplasmas. Use of barrier methods of contraception retards colonization with mycoplasmas, but the organisms are so widespread that a significant number of sexually experienced adults will eventually become colonized.

References

1. Braun P, Lee Y-H, Klein JO, et al. Birthweight and genital mycoplasmas in pregnancy. N Engl J Med 1971; 284:167.
2. Carey JC, Blackwelder WC, Nugent RP, et al. Vaginal infection and prematurity study group: antepartum cultures for *Ureaplasma urealyticum* are not useful in predicting pregnancy outcome. Am J Obstet Gynecol 1991; 164:728–733.
3. Cassell GH, Waites KB, Crouse DT, et al. Association of *Ureaplasma urealyticum* infection of the lower respiratory tract with chronic lung disease and death in very low birth weight infants. Lancet 1988; 2:240–245.
4. Chanock RM, Tully JG. Mycoplasmas. In: Davis BD, Dulbecco R, Eisen HN, Ginsberg HS, eds. Microbiology. Ed 3. New York: Harper & Row, 1980:789–795.
5. Cummings MC, McCormack WM. Increase in resistance of *Mycoplasma hominis* to tetracyclines. Antimicrob Agents Chemother 1990; 34:2297–2299.
6. Dienes L, Edsall G. Observations on the L-organism of Klieneberger. Proc Soc Exp Biol Med 1937; 36:740–744.
7. Embree JE, Krause VW, Embil JA, MacDonald S. Placental infection with *Mycoplasma hominis* and *Ureaplasma urealyticum:* clinical correlation. Obstet Gynecol 1980; 56:475–481.
8. Eschenbach DA, Nugent RP, Rao AV, et al. Vaginal infections and prematurity study group: a randomized placebo-controlled trial of erythromycin for the treatment of *Ureaplasma urealyticum* to prevent premature delivery. Am J Obstet Gynecol 1991; 164:734–742.
9. Foy HM, Kenny GE, Levinsohn EM. Acquisition of mycoplasmata and T-strains during infancy. J Infect Dis 1970; 121:579–587.
10. Garland SM, Murton LJ. Neonatal meningitis caused by *Ureaplasma urealyticum.* Pediatr Infect Dis 1987; 6:868–870.
11. Gibbs RS, Blanco JD, St Clair PJ, Castaneda YS. *Mycoplasma hominis* and intrauterine infection in late pregnancy. Sex Transm Dis 1983; 10:303–306.
12. Glatt AE, McCormack WM, Taylor-Robinson D. Genital mycoplasmas. In: Holmes KK, Mardh P-A, Sparling PF, Wiesner PJ, eds. Sexually transmitted diseases. Ed 2. New York: McGraw Hill, 1990:279–293.
13. Hammerschlag MR, Alpert S, Rosner I, et al. Microbiology of the vagina in children: normal and potentially pathogenic organisms. Pediatrics 1978; 62:57–62.
14. Hammerschlag MR, Doraiswamy B, Cox P, et al. Colonization of sexually abused children with genital mycoplasmas. Sex Transm Dis 1987; 14:23–25.
15. Harrison HR. Prospective studies of *Mycoplasma hominis* in pregnancy. Sex Transm Dis 1983; 10:311–317.
16. Harrison HR. Cervical colonization with *Ureaplasma urealyticum* and pregnancy outcome: prospective studies. Pediatr Infect Dis J 1986; 5:S266–269.
17. Harrison RF, deLouvois J, Blades M, Hurley R. Doxycycline treatment and human infertility. Lancet 1975; 1:605–607.
18. Harwick HJ, Purcell RH, Iuppa JB, Fekety FR. *Mycoplasma hominis* and abortion. J Infect Dis 1970; 121:260–268.
19. Hillier SL, Krohn MJ, Kiviat N, et al. The association of *Ureaplasma urealyticum* with preterm birth, chorioamnionitis, postpartum fever, intrapartum fever and bacterial vaginosis. Pediatr Infect Dis J 1986; 5:S349.
20. Hillier SL, Martius J, Krohn M, et al. Case control study of chorioamnionic infection and chorioamnionitis in prematurity. N Engl J Med 1988; 319:972–978.
21. Kenny GE: Mycoplasmas. In: Lennette EH, Balows A, Hausler WJ, Shadomy HJ, eds. Manual of clinical microbiology. Ed 4. Washington, DC: American Society for Microbiology, 1985:407–411.
22. Klein JO, Buckland D, Finland M. Colonization of newborn infants by mycoplasmas. N Engl J Med 1969; 280:1025–1030.
23. Koutsky LA, Stamm WE, Brunham RC, et al. Persistence of *Mycoplasma hominis* after therapy: importance of tetracycline resistance and co-existing vaginal flora. Sex Transm Dis 1983; 10:374–381.
24. Lamey JR, Eschenbach DA, Mitchell SH, et al. Isolation of mycoplasmas and bacteria from the blood of postpartum women. Am J Obstet Gynecol 1982; 143:104–112.
25. Lee Y-H, McCormack WM, Marcy SM, Klein

JO. The genital mycoplasmas: their role in disorders of reproduction and in pediatric infections. Pediatr Clin North Am 1974; 21:457–466.

26. Lee Y-H, Rankin JS, Alpert S, et al. Microbiological investigation of Bartholin's gland abscesses and cysts. Am J Obstet Gynecol 1977; 129:150–153.
27. Mardh P-A, Westrom L. Tubal and cervical cultures in acute salpingitis with special reference to *Mycoplasma hominis* and T-strain mycoplasmas. British Journal of Venereal Disease 1970; 46:179–186.
28. Mardh P-A, Westrom L. T-mycoplasmas in the genital tract of the female. Acta Pathologica Microbiologica Scandinavia 1970; 78:367–374.
29. McCormack WM, Almeida PC, Bailey PE, et al. Sexual activity and vaginal colonization with genital mycoplasmas. JAMA 1972; 221:1375–1377.
30. McCormack WM, Rosner B, Lee Y-H. Colonization with genital mycoplasmas in women. Am J Epidemiol 1973; 97:240–245.
31. McCormack WM, Rosner B, Lee Y-H, et al. Effect on birth weight of erythromycin treatment of pregnant women. Obstet Gynecol 1987; 69:202–207.
32. Minkoff H, Grunebaum AN, Schwarz RH, et al. Risk factors for prematurity and premature rupture of the membranes: a prospective study of the vaginal flora in pregnancy. Am J Obstet Gynecol 1984; 150:965–972.
33. Moller BR, Taylor-Robinson D, Furr PM. Serological evidence implicating *Mycoplasma genitalium* in pelvic inflammatory disease. Lancet 1984; 1:1102–1103.
34. Moller BR, Taylor-Robinson D, Furr PM, et al. Serological evidence that chlamydiae and mycoplasmas are involved in infertility in women. J Reprod Fertil 1985; 73:237–240.
35. Moore DE, Cates W. Sexually transmitted diseases and infertility. In: Holmes KK, Mardh P-A, Sparling PF, Wiesner PJ, eds. Sexually transmitted diseases. Ed 2. New York: McGraw Hill, 1990:763–769.
36. Munday PE, Porter R, Falder PF, et al. Spontaneous abortion: an infectious etiology. Br J Obstet Gynaecol 1984; 91:1177–1180.
37. Paavonen J, Miettinen A, Stevens PA, et al. *Mycoplasma hominis* in nonspecific vaginitis. Sex Transm Dis 1983; 10:271–275.
38. Pheifer TA, Forsyth PS, Durfee MA, et al. Nonspecific vaginitis: role of *Haemophilus vaginalis* and treatment with metronidazole. N Engl J Med 1978; 298:1429–1434.
39. Platt R, Lin J-S, Warren JW, et al. Infection with *Mycoplasma hominis* in postpartum fever. Lancet 1980; 2:1217–1221.
40. Roberts MC, Koutsky LA, Holmes KK, et al. Tetracycline-resistant *Mycoplasma hominis* strains contain streptococcal tetM sequences. Antimicrob Agents Chemother 1985; 28:141–143.
41. Robertson JA, Honore LH, Stemke GW. Serotypes of *Ureaplasma urealyticum* in spontaneous abortion. Pediatr Infect Dis J 1986; 5:S270–272.
42. Shafer MA, Sweet RL, Ohm-Smith MJ, et al. Microbiology of the lower genital tract in postmenarchal adolescent girls: differences by sexual activity, contraception, and presence of nonspecific vaginitis. J Pediatr 1985; 107:974–981.
43. Shurin PA, Alpert S, Rosner B, et al. Chorioamnionitis and colonization of the newborn infant with genital mycoplasmas. N Engl J Med 1975; 293:5–8.
44. Stanbridge EJ, Reff ME. The molecular biology of mycoplasmas. In: Barile MF, Razin S, eds. The mycoplasmas. Vol 1. Cell Biology. New York: Academic Press, 1979: 157–185.
45. Taylor-Robinson D, McCormack WM. Mycoplasmas in human genitourinary infections. In: Tully JG, Whitcomb RF, eds. The mycoplasmas. Vol 3. New York: Academic Press, 1979:307–366.
46. Tully JG, Taylor-Robinson D, Cole RM, Rose DL. A newly discovered mycoplasma in the human urogenital tract. Lancet 1981; 1:1288–1291.
47. Tully JG, Taylor-Robinson D, Rose DL, et al. Urogenital challenge of primate species with *Mycoplasma genitalium* and characteristics of infection induced in chimpanzees. J Infect Dis 1986; 153:1046–1054.
48. Waites KB, Rudd PT, Crouse DT, et al. Chronic *Ureaplasma urealyticum* and *Mycoplasma hominis* infections of central nervous system in preterm infants. Lancet 1988; 2:17–21.
49. Wallace RJ, Alpert S, Browne K, et al. Isolation of *Mycoplasma hominis* from blood cultures in patients with postpartum fever. Obstet Gynecol 1978; 51:181–185.
50. Westrom L, Mardh P-A. Acute pelvic inflammatory disease (PID). In: Holmes KK, Mardh P-A, Sparling PF, Wiesner PJ, eds. Sexually transmitted disease. Ed 2. New York: McGraw Hill, 1990:593–613.

CHAPTER 16

Listeriosis

David Charles, M.D.

Listeriosis is a relatively infrequent infection, and not until 1986 did it become a reportable disease in the United States.

During the past decade listerial infections appear to have increased in incidence, and their clinical and demographic characteristics have also changed. Until the past few years, except for some microbiologists, immunologists, and pediatricians, very few people were interested in *Listeria monocytogenes*, which is the pathogen responsible for listerial infections. As recently as 1966 Gray and Killinger[28] referred to this bacterium as a "Cinderella among the pathogenic bacteria" because of failure to recognize the human pathogenicity of the organism, despite the fact that it was recognized to have an adverse effect on pregnancy ranging from stillbirth to perinatal infections.

Now that the news media in various parts of the globe have reported epidemiologic aspects of listerial infections, more especially their relationship to food contamination, the pathogen has suddenly become the object of great public concern. There is now an apparent effort among clinical laboratories to become more diligent in attempting to find this organism.

Historical Introduction

According to Gray and Killinger[28] in the 1890s Hayeme in France and Henle in Germany noted the presence of gram-positive bacilli in necropsy material from patients who in retrospect almost certainly had listeriosis. In the ensuing years the organism was isolated and named by a number of investigators. Hulphers in 1911 identified a gram-positive bacillus from microabscesses in the livers of rabbits, to which he gave the name *Bacillus hepatis*.[35] In 1921, Dumont and Cotoni[17] reported that the bacterium was present in spinal fluid cultures of a patient with meningitis, and Cotoni[11] subsequently identified it as *Listeria monocytogenes*. Murray and associates[56] recovered the bacterium from livers of rabbits and guinea pigs during a laboratory epidemic that was characterized by a septicemic illness associated with areas of hepatic necrosis and a marked monocytosis in the peripheral blood. In view of the monocytosis associated with the infection, they called the organism *Bacterium Monocytogenes*.

A year later Pirie[64] reported an epizootic among gerbils in the Tiger River region of South Africa. The organism that was isolated was identical to that noted in the epizootic recorded by Murray and associates.[56] The bacterium was initially known as the Tiger River Bacillus, but because of the constant finding of focal hepatic necrosis in the animals examined Pirie[65] proposed the name *Listerella hepatolyticus*. The appellation *Listerella* was in honor of Joseph Lister, the father of antisepsis. Although Lister was from his inborn scientific curiosity interested in physiology and in microbes, he derived great insight into the microbic world from his father, Joseph Jackson Lister, who was a microscopist and a wine merchant. It was the father who devised the achromatic lens that created the modern microscope. We

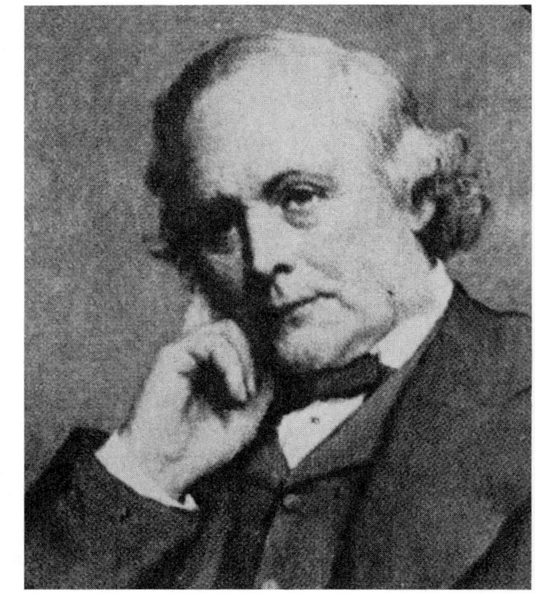

Figure 16-1 Joseph Lister: 1827–1912.

would therefore consider it correct to think that the present-day genus *Listeria* honors both father and son (Fig. 16-1).

Gill[25] is considered to be the first individual to isolate *Listeria monocytogenes* from farm animals. He studied a form of ovine meningoencephalitis which he named *circling disease,* a term still used by sheep farmers. From the brain of such animals he isolated a bacillus that proved to be *L. monocytogenes*. Since that time, the organism has been isolated from most domestic and feral animals.

In 1929 Nyfeldt[59] reported the isolation of this bacterium from the cerebrospinal fluid of a youth with infectious mononucleosis. Although we now recognize that mononucleosis is an uncommon manifestation of human listeriosis, Nyfeldt was convinced that he had isolated the causative organism of infectious mononucleosis. Burn[9] first demonstrated that this organism could be a serious pathogen in the neonate. Since that time, the organism has been shown to produce several distinct, recognizable clinical syndromes in patients and above all has a predilection for the fetoplacental unit. The latter was brought to the fore by the work of Reiss and coworkers,[68] who described 15 cases of perinatal listeriosis. Their presentation of the clinical manifestations and diagnostic advice are erudite and have not really been improved on since 1951. They called the condition *granulomatosis infantiseptica* because of the presence of generalized tiny granulomata in many organs, including the placenta. The basic lesions are pinhead whitish areas that on histologic study reveal well-circumscribed nodules in an otherwise normal parenchyma or diffuse foci of necrosis with infiltration by mononuclear cells and nuclear debris. These studies were conducted in Halle in a bombed-out hospital in a ruined city, with only one power point of any use in the laboratory. It is a great credit to them that the disease was recognized as a separate entity and the descriptive term *granulomatosis infantiseptica* coined. The isolation in pure culture of a gram-positive bacillus from a case of granulomatosis infantiseptica by these investigators was proof of the infectious nature of the disease.

Biologic Features

Although there are eight species in the genus *Listeria,* according to McLaughlin[52] only *L. monocytogenes, L. ivanovii,* and *L. seeligeri* have been isolated from human infections. Recently Andre and Genicot,[1] however, reported the isolation of *L. welshimeri* from patients with an influenza-type illness. Rocourt and Seeliger[70] state that *L. monocytogenes* is the principal pathogen in both humans and animals, and the other species are generally considered to be nonvirulent.

Morphology

Listeria species are microaerophilic, facultatively anaerobic, nonsporulating, nonencapsulated, motile, gram-positive bacilli that are ubiquitous in nature. *Listeria monocytogenes* is a flagellated, opportunistic, intracellular pathogen, and from that point of view it resembles brucellae, salmonellae, and mycobacteria. It is a short, non-acid-fast rod measuring 0.5 to 2.0 μm in length and grows readily on media containing serum or blood. This microorganism grows within a temperature range of 4 to 45°C with optimal growth at 35 to 37°C. It may grow as either smooth or rough colonies on sheep-blood agar; the smooth variety seems to be the more pathogenic. Young cultures consist of small, translucent gray colonies surrounded by a narrow band of beta-hemolysis. These cultures contain predominantly coccoid organisms; whereas young cultures are gram positive, after a few days the bacteria tend to become gram variable. Colonies of *Listeria* can be readily disregarded in the laboratory as they can be mistaken for diphtheroids and regarded as contaminants, unless the microbiology personnel are alert to the possible presence of this organism. It can be readily differentiated from corynebacteria by its characteristic tumbling motility at 25°C but not at 37°C. In Gram stains of young cultures where coccoid forms are commonly seen, *Listeria* may be confused with streptococci. *Listeria* organisms are catalase and bile-esculin positive, and these features can be of assistance in identification of the organism (Table 16-1). This microorganism closely resembles *Erysipelothrix,* which is a slender rod. *Listeria* can be differentiated from it by the presence of its flagella, tumbling motility, and catalase production. Bottone and Sierra[5] consider that the colony morphologic size can aid in differentiating *Listeria* as the colonies are larger and more opaque.

Cultural Characteristics

When *L. monocytogenes* is cultured on clear tryptose-agar, the colonies have a characteristic blue-green appearance in oblique light. The majority of clinical specimens allow for easy isolation of the organism by the utilization of routine culture media. Doyle and Schoeni[15] reported that *L. monocytogenes* can be difficult

Table 16-1 Characteristics of *Listeria Monocytogenes*

Gram-positive bacillus
Length 0.8 to 2.5 μm
Microaerophilic
Asporogenous
Growth at 4°C
Tumbling motility at 22°C
Small, round colonies
Beta-hemolysis—positive
Catalase production—positive
Salicin fermentation—positive
Trehalose fermentation—positive
Bile-esculin hydrolysis—positive
Hippurate hydrolysis—positive
Voges-Proskauer test—positive

Data partially derived from Kontnick C, Von Graevenitz A, Piscitelli V. Differential diagnosis between *Streptococcus agalactia* and *Listeria monocytogenes*. Ann Clin Lab Sci 1977; 7:269–276.

to isolate from mixed cultures such as fecal specimens or food samples that may contain other microorganisms. In such instances the yield may be enhanced by enrichment techniques and the use of selective media. In the technique of "cold enrichment," the cultures are incubated in tryptose broth and stored at 4°C for at least 4 weeks, and subcultures are obtained at weekly intervals. If the specimen contains mixed bacterial flora, 25 units of polymyxin B sulfate may be added to the broth as a selective ingredient. *Listeria* will, as already mentioned, grow at 4°C, but growth at this temperature is slow; identifying the organism may take several weeks.

Antigenic Structure and Serotypes

On the basis of their somatic (O) and flagellar (H) antigens, the genus *Listeria* can be grouped into different serotypes. Seeliger and Jones[79] state there are 16 recognized serotypes of *Listeria monocytogenes* on the basis that there are at least 15 different somatic antigens and 5 flagellar antigens. Most of the isolates from patients with listeriosis of late have been serotype 4b. Hall and associates,[31] in discussing the marked increase in incidence in England and Wales, stated that it would appear to be more than the result of increased awareness and reporting, as it has been linked with a disproportionate increase in serotype 4b. The largest food-borne outbreak of listeriosis in North America occurred in Los Angeles County, California, and Linnan and associates[47] reported that of the *L. monocytogenes* isolates available for study 82 percent (86 of 105) were serotype 4b. This serotype is the main cause of perinatal infection. An interesting phenomenon pertaining to serologic typing is that Seeliger[78] found from large-scale studies of cultures isolated in Germany in the early 1950s that the predominant serotype was type 1. In 1958, 75 percent of 108 cultures from human infections and 58 percent of 29 cultures from animals were type 1. For some unexplained reason, this investigator discovered in the latter part of 1960 that most of the isolates were serotype 4b. Although there is no explanation for this change in pattern, it was not associated with any alteration in the severity or clinical characteristics of the disease.

Pathogenicity

This microorganism produces no exotoxin. Many potential virulence factors have been identified in the literature, but, as pointed out by Ralovich,[66] they may or may not be important to the overall pathogenicity of *L. monocytogenes*. Issekutz and associates,[37] in their discussion of the virulence factors associated with this microorganism, include the ability to survive within macrophages and the production of at least two hemolysins. On blood agar, beta-hemolysis distinguishes *L. monocytogenes* from nonpathogenic species. Lamont and associates[44] reported that different strains of this microorganism show variations as regards hemolysin production. The hemolysins are alpha-listeriolysin, which is related to streptolysin O and beta-listeriolysin. Mutants of this pathogen that did not produce alpha-listeriolysin were found to be not virulent in mice. According to Gaillard and associates,[23] strains that are made listeriolysin negative by means of transposon mutagenesis are no longer virulent. Listeriolysin appears to facilitate the survival of this pathogen inside host cells rather than encourage its entry. Excessive production of listeriolysin is not associated with increased virulence. Likewise, hemolytic activity varies among strains isolated from patients with listeriosis and does not correlate with the severity of the infection. To date no direct correlation between virulence and total hemolysin production has been demonstrated. Stanley[85] reported the presence of an extractable lipid in *L. monocytogenes* that was responsible for the production of monocytosis in rabbits and rodents, but it did not act like a monocytosis-producing agent in humans. Godfrey and Wilder[26] reported the production of cytotoxic substances such as hydrogen peroxide and superoxide by *L. monocytogenes*, but again their role as virulence factors has not been demonstrated to affect the pathogenicity of the organism.

Otokunefor and Galsworthy[61] reported that a component of the cell envelope of *L. monocytogenes* produces nonspecific activation of B cells as well as immunosuppression, but there is no evidence to demonstrate that either effect is of importance in the pathogenesis of listeriosis.

The ability of the microorganism to cause keratoconjunctivitis in guinea pigs was one of the original tests for pathogenicity of *L. monocytogenes*. Anton,[2] who first described this test, also reported that instillation of the organism into the conjunctival sac of a pregnant rabbit unintentionally caused the death of the animal. The same procedure was the cause of abortion in another gravid rabbit. The author was primarily interested in the ability of the organism to produce conjunctivitis and infiltration of the cornea and conjunctiva with monocytes and paid no particular attention to the fact that such a procedure could result in abortion. However, it clearly demonstrates that a pre-existing defect in an epithelial barrier is not essential for the pathogen to become invasive.

Ecology

Listeria monocytogenes has a broad environmental niche and is known to be saprophytic on organic decaying matter. The microorganism can be isolated from a variety of sources, including dust, cultivated and uncultivated soils, mud, water, raw and treated sewage, vegetation, poor-quality silage, abattoir waste, milk of cows with or without mastitis, and numerous species of wild and domestic animals. Watkins and Sleath[87] reported that not only is *L. monocytogenes* found in considerable numbers in sewage but also it survives longer than salmonellae when sewage sludge is sprayed on agricultural land. In his review of the presence of this microorganism in food and water, Brackett[7] stated that it had been isolated from fish, crustaceans, and insects. Fenlon[21] reported the isolation of this bacterium from the intestinal tract of wild birds and stated that this was in keeping with the fact that healthy intestinal carriers have been identified among poultry, swine, and rodent populations. Kampelmacher and Van Noorle-Jansen[40] reported that up to 70 percent of the human population can carry the organism in the gut at any one time. They considered the asymptomatic fecal carriage rate would be higher in poultry and abattoir workers, as well as laboratory personnel who dealt with the organism on a regular basis.

Although reservoirs of *L. monocytogenes* have been identified in feral animal populations, no mechanism for its transfer to domestic animals and humans has been elucidated, and attempts to demonstrate carrier states in close human or animal contacts of patients afflicted by listeriosis have usually been unsuccessful. The source for sporadic human infections has in general remained unidentified and difficult to investigate because of the ubiquitous nature of the organism.

The epidemiology of listerial infections is discussed in a later section, but it is essential here to recognize that listeriosis is a worldwide problem. Furthermore, in view of social evolution and changes in dietary habits associated with increasing urbanization, it may assume a greater importance in developing countries.

Pathogenesis

Despite the ubiquitous nature of the organism, the severity of the disease in the fetus and neonate, and its recognition as an important public health problem, there are still only limited data available on the pathogenesis. Why the bacterium *L. monocytogenes* has a particular tropism for the central nervous system and the fetoplacental unit remains to be elucidated.

In many instances listeriosis appears as an opportunistic infection in individuals with impaired cell-mediated immunity. Schwartz and associates[76] reported that one-third of listerial infections are perinatal, and the remainder are in elderly or immunosuppressed patients.

Table 16-2 Clinical Conditions with an Increased Susceptibility to Listerial Infections

Gravid patients
Fetus
Cancer
Immunosuppression
Chronic renal disease
Long-term hemodialysis
Transplant recipients
Diabetes mellitus
Drug abuse
Hepatitis
Alcoholism

The individuals who are at greatest risk to listerial infections include patients who are on long-term hemodialysis as well as those on corticosteroid or immunosuppressive therapy (Table 16-2). Fauci and associates[20] reported that corticosteroids diminished the cell-mediated immune response and noted that individuals receiving such therapy had an increased susceptibility to infections caused by certain pathogens.

Listeria monocytogenes is one of the facultative intracellular pathogens that can persist in the cells of the monocyte-macrophage system. Hahn and Kaufmann[30] reported that in mice protective immunity to this pathogen relies on T lymphocytes and only a minor role is played by antibodies. The T cells attract monocytes to the site of listerial invasion and activate listeriocidal measures in the tissue macrophages and blood-derived monocytes. As a result of these processes, a granuloma is formed, and as a consequence local elimination of the pathogen occurs. Despite the ability of *L. monocytogenes* to replicate within nonactivated macrophages, experimental listeriosis is an acute infection, and when specific T cells have been generated the pathogen is rapidly eliminated. Hahn[29] demonstrated that macrophages can be eliminated in mice by treatment with a high-molecular dextran sulfate, and by this means the animals are rendered highly susceptible to listerial infections because they lack the proper effector cell in their defense. These studies reinforce the work of Mackaness,[49] who demonstrated almost 30 years ago the importance of T cell–mediated immunity to this opportunistic pathogen. Miller and Hedberg[54] found that when hydrocortisone acetate was administered to mice it enhanced their susceptibility to listerial infections and therapy demonstrated in an animal model that corticosteroids depress the levels of T cells and impair macrophage activity.

Cell-Mediated Immunity

For some time it has been conjectured that pregnancy depresses cellular immunity because of the well-recognized thymic involution that occurs during pregnancy in animals. However, there must be some modification in immune function in the gravid patient to allow for survival of the fetus. During normal pregnancy, cell-mediated immunity is significantly depressed, and as a result there is decreased resistance to infection by intracellular pathogens such as *L. monocytogenes*. The fundamental mechanisms of this immune defect have not been elucidated, although Weinberg[88] in his review considers that there is increased T-suppressor activity in pregnancy. As both humoral and cellular immune responses may be depressed by T-suppressor lymphocytes, there has been much speculation that this class of cells may play a role in the immunologic aspects of pregnancy. Regulation of maternal immune reactions by suppressor cells could in theory arise in several ways. Soluble factors of fetal origin may activate maternal suppressor cells, or soluble suppressor-cell products representing the actual suppressive signal could act on maternal cells responsible for immune responses. The placental transfer of regulatory fetal cells could also affect maternal immune responses.

Our understanding of the specificity of suppressor cells in pregnancy is limited. Although they may serve to protect the fetus from immunologic reaction against paternal antigens, their effects may extend to other reactions, such as immune responses against infectious agents. Because the pregnant host appears less well equipped to protect the fetoplacental unit in mid-pregnancy against listerial infection, an immunologic alteration must be present, but whatever its exact nature, it is a phenomenon limited to relatively few organisms. Further investigation of host defense in obstetric patients may result in better methods for the identification of defects in resistance to infectious processes and the development of measures to augment the natural defenses of the host.

Neonates infected with *L. monocytogenes* are considered to have a poor immunologic response to the pathogen, although to date the only support for such a concept is derived from murine studies. Issekutz and associates[37] noted little if any cell-mediated or persistent humoral immunity in infants 1 year after they had had listerial infections.

Virtually nothing is known apropos the infectious dose of this pathogen for humans. Likewise, there are no reliable quantitative data pertaining to the amount of contaminated food that must be ingested for an individual to be at risk of acquiring the disease. It is conceivable that the infectious dose may be related to host susceptibility.

Listeria monocytogenes, as has been discussed, is known to invoke a predominantly cell-mediated immune response, and many of the conditions associated with increased susceptibility (see Table 16-2) are characterized by altered T-cell function. Stamm and associates[84] reported more than a hundred cases of listeriosis among renal transplant recipients; in the majority the central nervous system was involved. Hotson and Pedley[34] reported that this pathogen was the most common cause of bacterial meningitis in patients who were cardiac transplant recipients. Similar findings were reported by Louria and associates[48] in patients with hematologic malignant disease.

What is surprising is that this pathogen is not commonly encountered in patients with the acquired immunodeficiency syndrome (AIDS). Such patients should be highly susceptible to listerial infections. Mascola and associates[51] in their review stated that AIDS patients have defective cellular-mediated immunity and many similarities to patients with malignant disease; they would have expected to see cases of listeriosis more frequently, but they considered listerial infections may be substantially underreported. They also suggested that avoidance of certain foods, prior antimicrobial therapy, and decreased exposure to this pathogen could account for the infrequent occurrence of listeriosis in AIDS patients. Kales and Holzman[38] agree that *L. monocytogenes* is an unusual opportunistic pathogen in AIDS patients, but they have noted an increase in the number of infections caused by this pathogen in such patients. They consider that AIDS patients possess some resistance to infection. All their patients responded to therapy, and no relapses were observed. Although the mechanism of their resistance to infection is unknown, these investigators considered that T cell–independent factors may be involved. To date, no such factors have been defined. Much remains to be elucidated pertaining to the pathogenesis of listerial infections, especially why the pathogen has a particular tropism for the central nervous system.

Epidemiology

The precise nature of the epidemiology of listerial infections has not been elucidated. Although it has been speculated that animals and birds comprise a major reservoir for the organism, it is difficult to decipher the sporadic nature of the disease. Person-to-person transmission has rarely been documented, and isolated cases are the rule. Domestic animals have been considered prime sources for human infections because they are encountered in rural environments. In reporting isolation of the organism from healthy chickens, Schwartz[77] suggested that poultry could be an important reservoir in respect to human infections. Surprisingly, no widespread studies were conducted in the poultry industry during the subsequent 15 years, especially as the vast majority of listerial infections in the United States occurred in urban residents.

In addition to animal sources, the role of vegetation as a reservoir for human infection is well documented (Fig. 16-2). More than 30 years ago Gray[27] reported that sheep and cattle could acquire listerial infection by the ingestion of contaminated silage. However, only during the past decade has the epidemiologic linkage between vegetation, animals, and human infection been investigated.

Sources of Infection

Food-borne Listeriosis

Schlech[74] speculated that gastrointestinal exposure or colonization is the prime source of infection in susceptible individuals. In their review of recent data pertaining to human listeriosis, the World Health Organization Working Group[89] considered that food-borne infection is predominantly transmitted by monozootic means. Furthermore, although soil may be the source, transmission to humans is primarily from the environment via animals and food surfaces. This microorganism must be consid-

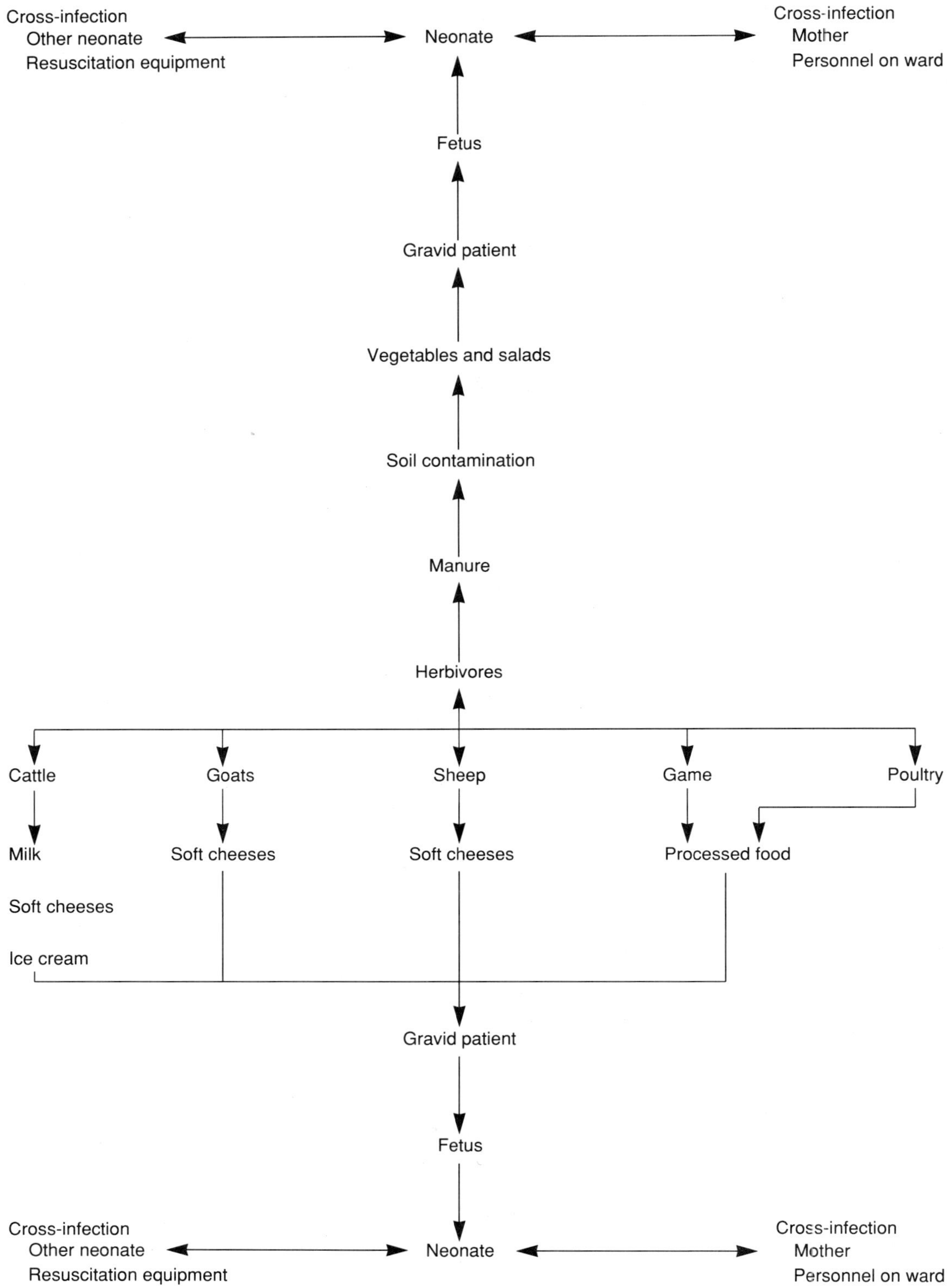

Figure 16-2 Vehicles of spread of listerial infections to gravid patient and neonate.

ered an environmental bacterium whose primary method of transmission to humans is by foods that have during processing and production been contaminated.

An implication from major outbreaks reported in the literature is that if listeriosis is caused by food-borne transmission in epidemics it may even result to a major degree from the same route in sporadic cases. Such a supposition is in accord with anecdotal case reports associating listeriosis with the isolation of the identical phage type of the organism from an ingested food.

Schlech and associates[75] reported an outbreak of listeriosis in the maritime provinces of Canada. The investigations conclusively documented for the first time food-borne transmission of the pathogen. The study comprised 34 cases of perinatal infection and 7 nongravid adults who developed listeriosis. The case fatality rate in infants born alive was 27 percent, and there were 19 intrauterine deaths. None of the seven nongravid patients had any evidence of immunosuppression, yet two of the patients died. The outbreak did not become apparent until the infection rate affected 1.3 percent of the obstetric patients in the regional hospital. When the laboratory data were reviewed for the previous year, it became evident that a small cluster of cases had been missed from the epidemiologic aspect of listerial infections. A case-control study of the reported outbreak implicated a locally produced coleslaw as the probable vehicle of transmission of the pathogen. The strain of *L. monocytogenes* responsible for the epidemic was subsequently isolated from an unopened package of this vegetable product. The cabbage in it was supplied by a local farmer who had fertilized his cabbage fields with raw sheep manure from a flock that had had ovine listeriosis the previous year.

Dairy Products

Fleming and associates[22] furnished the first solid evidence that dairy products could transmit the pathogen and be responsible for outbreaks of human infection. Their study comprised 42 immunosuppressed adults, of whom approximately one-third developed listerial meningitis and seven perinatal infections. The case fatality rate for all patients afflicted by the pathogen was 29 percent. The epidemiologic studies indicated that pasteurized milk was probably the vehicle of transmission of the infection. Although no isolates of the organism were recorded from the milk cultures, it was known that bovine listeriosis had been present in the herd that supplied the dairy. The excretion of the pathogen in cow's milk is well known, and animals with listerial mastitis may yield normal-appearing milk that contains large numbers of bacteria in the monocytes present.

Pasteurization of Milk

Improperly performed pasteurization of milk and contamination after the process are the most likely explanations for the presence of pathogens in pasteurized milk. Some of the bacteria in the milk supplied by cows with bovine mastitis may survive pasteurization and replicate at refrigerator temperatures. Even when pasteurized milk is shown to be contaminated by bacteria, it may be difficult to determine the mode and source of such contamination. Doyle and associates[14] consider this pathogen to be more resistant to pasteurization processes when it is inside a bovine phagocyte than when it is freely suspended in milk. High-temperature, short-time (HTST) pasteurization, a temperature of 71.7°C for 15 seconds or 62.5°C for 30 minutes may allow *L. monocytogenes* to survive and replicate. The World Health Organization Working Group[89] concluded from the information at its disposal that "pasteurization is a safe process which reduces the number of *Listeria monocytogenes* occurring in raw milk to levels that do not pose an appreciable risk to human health." Such a statement only gives cause for concern to gravid patients as the organism has a predilection for the fetoplacental unit.

Role of Antacids

The epidemiologic connection between the animal reservoir and the transmission of the pathogen to humans has not been settled. This fact is aptly demonstrated by the studies of Ho and associates,[33] who described an outbreak of *L. monocytogenes* serotype 4b infections in Boston area hospitals in which several foods were directly implicated as vehicles of transmission. They noted during their analysis of the patient histories that many of the individuals had been treated with cimetidine or antacids. These investigators considered that such medications could increase the risk of listerial infections because the pathogen may not be destroyed in the stomach when the gastric pH is at a higher level than normal. The report states that the majority of the afflicted had gastrointestinal symptoms before and subsequent to the onset of their febrile illness. The symptoms noted by the patients included nausea, vomiting, abdominal pain, and diarrhea. These observations were accompanied in several of the patients with the presence of numerous fecal leukocytes and monocytes. The authors pointed out that ulceration of the intestine has been documented in neonates as well as in sheep and rabbits with listeriosis.

The role of gastric defenses against infection or colonization is unclear. A proportion of the cases of listeriosis are found among previously healthy individuals where there is no discernible predisposing cause. The role of intercurrent infection in altering a carrier state to a clinically infectious illness by reduction in resistance requires further investigation. The same applies to any differences in dietary factors. By such investigations it should be feasible to assess different exposures in various risk groups.

Virtually nothing is known about the infectious dose of *L. monocytogenes* for humans. Likewise, there is no reliable quantitative information on the amount of contaminated food that must be ingested to risk acquiring the disease. It is conceivable that the infectious dose may be related to host susceptibility. A further possible factor that requires investigation is the food substrate.

As regards surveillance, at present the major indications for defining an outbreak are an increase in the number of cases over that expected and the isolation of a common strain from the majority of such cases. Detection of the former demands a sensitive and reliable system for monitoring infections that are due to *L. monocytogenes*. Such a system requires the availability of laboratory facilities for phage typing, isoenzyme typing, or subtyping by gene restriction techniques. To accomplish such surveillance studies, a network of reference laboratories at both national and international levels is essential.

Soft Cheeses

Linnan and associates[47] reported an outbreak of listeriosis in southern California in which 93 gravid women or their progeny were afflicted, together with 49 nongravid patients. This outbreak was associated with the consumption of Mexican-style cheeses. The evaluation of this outbreak implied that cheese contamination was frequently the result of the utilization of raw milk in its production. Raw milk is an inherently dangerous product and as such should never be added to the pasteurized product. Ho and associates[33] also implicated cheese in addition to raw vegetables as conveyors of the outbreak of listeriosis they studied. Of all foods, cheeses have been found to be frequently contaminated, especially those with white mold. Such cheeses have a higher pH than the majority of cheeses in the later ripening stages, and consequently they appear to be more liable to contamination by this bacterium. Surveys have indicated that up to 10 percent of such cheeses may be contaminated by *L. monocytogenes*. Pini and Gilbert[63] examined 222 samples of British and imported soft cheeses and found that 10 percent of the cheeses contained *L. monocytogenes* in numbers ranging from less than 10^2 to 10^5 colony-forming units per gram. These investigators considered such levels unacceptable, and it is obvious, as is discussed later, that gravid patients should not include soft cheeses in their diet. The risk of contamination of other dairy products depends on many factors. Acidified dairy products, for example, cottage cheese, are free of this pathogen. Postprocess contamination of ice cream has been reported, but the quantitative data are very limited. Azadian and associates[3] have reported a case of listerial meningitis associated with the ingestion of cheese made from goat's milk.

Meat and Meat Products

Besides dairy products, up to 30 percent of raw, ready-to-eat meat products have been reported to contain this pathogen. This is not surprising, considering the fecal carriage rate of *L. monocytogenes* by many animals and birds and the potential for contamination in abattoirs. The organism has been isolated from beef, pork, lamb, and ground meat as well as poultry. Depending on the method of sampling, from 15 to 80 percent of retail poultry has been reported to be contaminated with this pathogen. Pini and Gilbert[63] reported that of 100 composite samples of raw chicken 60 were found to contain *L. monocytogenes* and 28 percent contained other *Listeria* species. These investigators recorded increases in the number of organisms in refrigerated retail poultry during storage, as freezing apparently has no detrimental effect on this pathogen. *Listeria monocytogenes* can survive and replicate at the temperatures used in domestic and commercial refrigerators, which has naturally been a matter of concern in supermarkets where refrigerated food might be a source of infection. Sizmur and Walker[82] isolated this organism from prepacked salads and drew attention to the fact that the trend toward food products with a longer shelf life could enable this organism to attain high levels in certain foods. Such potential problems should be addressed now by the food and catering industries as well as their regulatory bodies and not postponed until the incidence of listerial infections increases in an exponential manner.

Seafood

There is some evidence that cooked fish and other seafoods may be contaminated with this pathogen. During an epidemic of perinatal listeriosis in Auckland, New Zealand, no cause for the outbreak was discovered, although Lennon and associates[46] in their report considered that shellfish as well as raw fish may have been involved.

From the studies cited, there is obvious support for the concept that *L. monocytogenes* is an enteric pathogen that is transmitted by contaminated food. Ho and associates[33] consider that in many respects listerial infections have a resemblance to salmonella enteritis. The latter disease has a propensity to afflict the very young, the old, and the debilitated, and the causative organism, *Salmonella enteritidis,* is widely distributed in domestic animals as well as being food borne.

Gastrointestinal Carriage

What has to be determined in respect to *L. monocytogenes* is why transient gastrointestinal carriage for the organism is common and invasive infection rare. Several studies have documented the isolation of pathogenic strains of *L. monocytogenes* from the gastrointestinal tract of asymptomatic individuals, including subjects who are at high risk, such as gravid patients and those who have had renal transplantation. Lamont and Postlethwaite[43] consider from the results of their studies that pregnancy does not affect the fecal carriage rate of *L. monocytogenes* and closely related species. Six of 110 pregnant and nonpregnant patients in their study were fecal carriers of *Listeria* spp. Only one gravid and two nongravid patients had *L. monocytogenes* in their fecal samples. These investigators in addition obtained pharyngeal and cervicovaginal cultures from their patients, and in no instance did they isolate the pathogen. They concluded that the increased susceptibility of pregnant women to infection is probably not due to a higher carriage rate of the organism.

Lennon and associates[46] surveyed 750 consecutive asymptomatic gravid patients for rectal and vaginal carriage of *L. monocytogenes*. Only one of the patients had a positive isolate from a vaginal culture. Positive rectal swabs were found in 25 (3.3 percent) of the patients. All isolates were serotype 1b. Infants delivered to the 25 patients with positive rectal swabs appeared to be unaffected by listerial infection. Furthermore, the patients were not treated because they were asymptomatic. Cord blood cultures were negative in all 11 of the 11 cases tested, and rectal cultures were negative in 14 of 14 tested. What is worthy of note is that 24 of the patients with positive rectal cultures were found among 300 prenatal patients attending a clinic serving the southern part of the city of Auckland. Consequently, the incidence of positive rectal cultures was 8 percent in that particular clinic.

Bojsen-Møller[4] reported that the organism can be isolated from the feces of at least 1 percent of adults in Denmark at any time but considered that the duration of carriage was short, lasting only for a matter of days. This communication demonstrated that healthy individuals who dwell in the same household as patients with listeriosis had a rectal carriage rate of 26 percent. This was a much higher carriage rate than the 4.8 percent recorded for the other groups, including individuals who worked in abattoirs.

Fecal carriage rates of 25 percent have been observed in poultry workers. Kampelmacher and Van Noorle-Jansen[39] reported a carriage rate of 77 percent in laboratory personnel involved in the isolation and culture of this organism. These investigators state that such studies support the concept that many individuals may be exposed to this pathogen but remain free of symptoms and disease. Kampelmacher and associates[39] in a later report demonstrated rectal carriage rates of up to 30 percent in gravid patients who had had serial fecal cultures during their pregnancy. They found that contact with domestic or farm animals did not result in carriage rates that differed significantly from gravid women who had had no contact with animals and lived in urban areas.

Outbreaks of Food-Borne Infection

A review of the literature over the past decade indicates that it is likely that most people are colonized by and excrete this pathogen for short periods of time following ingestion of contaminated food. Person-to-person transmission has rarely been documented. Sporadic cases rather than epidemics are the rule. It is the well-documented reports of outbreaks of food-borne listeriosis that have had extensive media coverage and as a result have caused concern to both the food industry and the lay public. At the same time such measures have banished the inertia on the part of public health and governmental authorities.

The extent to which listerial infections are sporadic or part of source outbreaks and how they are associated with food remain to be determined. This lack of information makes it mandatory for regulatory bodies to label those foods that require no further processing prior to consumption and state that they are free of pathogens that could have a detrimental effect on a pregnancy. Withdrawal of contaminated foods would have marked economic implications. Such a measure could result in the food industry financing studies that would clarify the extent of food-borne infections such as those due to *L. monocytogenes*, *S. enteritidis*, and *Campylobacter*.

Salmonella enteritidis

In the decade from 1976 to 1986, infections due to *S. enteritidis* showed a sixfold increase in the United States, and the report of St. Louis and associates[72] indicated that this *Salmonella* serotype is associated with the ingestion of food containing eggs. Telzak and associates[86] investigated the largest nosocomial outbreak of *S. enteritidis* to have occurred in the United States. In one hospital 404 of the 965 patients (42 percent) were afflicted by the infection, and 9 patients succumbed. These investigators by means of epidemiologic studies found that raw eggs used in low-sodium tuna-macaroni salad were responsible for the outbreak. Such a conclusion was derived from the fact that raw eggs in the hospital at the time of the outbreak when cultured in pooled batches were positive for the organism. In addition, 555 hens' ovaries from the farms that supplied the eggs on culture were found to be positive in 383 (69 percent) instances for the pathogen. All isolates were phage type B, and all except one of the clinical isolates had an identical pattern of antibiotic susceptibility. As a result of the epidemiologic data, the New York State Department of Health recommended that all the health care facilities under its jurisdiction eliminate raw or undercooked eggs from the diets of elderly or immunocompromised patients. It also placed an embargo on eggs from the farms and distribution centers implicated in the outbreak until extensive bacteriologic studies had been concluded.

Campylobacter

Members of the genus *Campylobacter* have attained prominence in recent years because they are the most common cause of bacterial enteritis. Microbiologists are also more aware of this genus of gram-negative, microaerophilic, curved, motile rods because it requires selective media and incubation at 40 to 42°C for optimal growth. Campylobacteriosis usually manifests a bacteremic phase, and although it is transient in the gravid patient it can cause infection of the fetoplacental unit. In a review of campylobacteriosis in pregnancy Simor and associates[81] furnished summaries of 20 cases of intrauterine fetal infection. Eleven of the cases ended in second-trimester abortion or stillbirth, and the placentas demonstrated evidence of inflammation, infarction, and necrosis. The obstetrician should be alert to the fact that members of the genus *Campylobacter* not only have a predilection to invade the placental and fetal structures of ungulates but also probably cause similar problems in human pregnancies. Campylobacteriosis infections are food borne; like listeriosis and *Salmonella* infections, chickens may be important vectors.

Sporadic Listeriosis

Pini and Gilbert[63] reported that *L. monocytogenes* contaminated about 60 percent of fresh and frozen chickens in the United Kingdom. Kerr and associates[41] stated that this organism is present in small numbers in commercially available cooked chicken products that are ready for ingestion. In a population-based case-control study of risk factors for sporadic listeriosis, Schwartz and associates[76] emphasized the importance of certain foods. It was estimated that uncooked hot dogs and undercooked chicken contributed to only 20 percent of the total risk of listerial infection, but 80 percent of the risk of sporadic infection remains to be elucidated. The study must be repeated, but it does indicate that uncooked hot dogs and undercooked chicken should be included on the list of food commodities associated with listeriosis.

I can only endorse a 1989 editorial that included the following statement:

> What is very clear is that as produced, processed and finally cross-contaminated in chicken packing plants, very nearly all chicken carcasses are contaminated with listeria, as well as with *Campylobacter jejuni* and Salmonellae. In the past two or three years infections due to these microbes have increased almost exponentially: they are all sporadic in distribution, and all three organisms are frequently introduced into the environment of the domestic kitchen via chicken meat. . . . There is always complacency in the livestock industry when infective agents do not cause significant economic losses in flocks or herds: listeria, salmonellae, campylobacters all fail to do this. Surely it is time to think of the effect on human beings.[18]

At the same time the food industry has to modify its

Table 16-3 Spectrum of Listerial Infection

Patients	Illnesses
Pregnant women	Influenza-type syndrome Infrequently meningitis
Fetuses	Granulomatosis infantiseptica Nonimmune hydrops fetalis
Neonates	Early onset—septicemia Late onset—meningitis
Adults	Bacteremia Meningitis Nonmeningitic parenchymal cerebritis Endocarditis Pneumonia Acute respiratory distress syndrome Cholecystitis Hepatitis Liver abscess Peritonitis Septic arthritis Osteomyelitis Conjunctivitis Endopthalmitis

attitude toward potential pathogens. For example, other factors that enable *L. monocytogenes* to survive in food must be addressed:

1. It is resistant to alkaline conditions.
2. It has the ability to replicate under microaerophilic and anaerobic conditions.
3. It can grow in certain foods in which the salt concentration may be as high as 10 percent.
4. The concentrations of sodium nitrite that are allowed for food preservatives fail to inhibit replication of the organism.

All too obviously, much remains to be elucidated as regards the epidemiologic aspects of listeriosis as it is an evolving public health problem. The role of autoinfection, direct acquisition of the organism from the environment, and the role of various foods as a vehicle of infection require further study. A concerted effort on the part of the microbiologist, clinician, and epidemiologist is essential. The obstetrician must also become involved as the initial subjects to be afflicted are all too often the gravid patient and her intrauterine fetus.

Clinical Manifestations

There is conflicting and inconclusive evidence of the vagaries of the infection expressed in different risk groups. Usually clinical expression does not appear to differ in sporadic cases from that in outbreak situations, which supports the concept that many sporadic cases are the consequence of food-borne transmission.

Only a few individuals actually acquire listeriosis, and in healthy subjects the infection is apparently contained by activated macrophages. However, occasionally a clinical illness develops. The range of listerial infectious illnesses extends from asymptomatic to life-threatening entities, such as septicemia and meningitis (Table 16-3). In a review of the cases of listeriosis reported in the English literature in the decade 1968 to 1978, Nieman and Lorber[58] noted that the most common presentations in adults were central nervous system infections, bacteremia, and endocarditis. Less common manifestations are hepatitis, arthritis, local abscess formation, osteomyelitis, conjunctivitis, oculoglandular disease, and endophthalmitis, the majority of which involve elderly patients or individuals who are immunosuppressed.

Gravid Patients

Pregnant women with listeriosis present with a mild illness that resembles influenza. The clinical findings in most cases are nonspecific, and as a result maternal listeriosis cannot be readily distinguished from other entities that complicate pregnancy, such as pyelitis and influenza. Many gravid women with listerial infection are not seriously ill, and in retrospect a large proportion of them cannot remember any symptoms suggestive of an infection. There appears to be an increased susceptibility to listeriosis in the second half of pregnancy. Listerial infections are encountered in the first trimester; although they are reported to have an adverse effect on the gestation, Cruickshank and Warenski[12] recorded such a case with a normal neonatal outcome. Their patient at the thirteenth week of gestation had a febrile illness with signs and symptoms of chorioamnionitis. Blood culture was positive for *L. monocytogenes,* and the patient was treated with intravenous ampicillin and gentamicin and subsequently with trimethoprim-sulfamethoxazole (TMP-SMX). Fifteen days after commencement of therapy, an amniocentesis was performed, and the fluid obtained was sterile on culture. Despite uterine tenderness for several weeks, the gestation continued to term, and the patient was delivered of a healthy, culture-negative infant.

The pregnant patient may present in the second trimester with an acute febrile illness associated with chills, malaise, pharyngitis, conjunctivitis, myalgia, and back or flank pain. Diarrhea or other gastrointestinal symptoms are far less commonly noted in gravid patients with listerial infections. When the patient is first seen, the illness is frequently diagnosed as pyelonephritis, as the kidneys may be involved in the listeric process. In about 40 percent of cases, there is no marked febrile episode, whereas in many a swinging fever is observed. Bacteremia caused by *L. monocytogenes* does not produce any clinical features that distinguish it from other causes of bacteremia. It should always be considered as a cause of pyrexia in gravid patients. The organism when it is the cause of bacteremia can be isolated by the utilization of standard blood culture media. Blood cultures of a patient with an influenza-type illness and fever during pregnancy are important because it is during the bacteremic phase of the illness that the fetoplacental unit is infected. Infection of the intrauterine conceptus can, depending on the duration of the pregnancy, terminate in abortion, stillbirth, or preterm delivery. Relier[69] has emphasized that untreated maternal listeriosis invariably results in a poor prognosis for the fetus.

It is easy to see why a clinical picture compatible with an influenza type of illness could be ignored by the patient and her physician, especially as the symptoms disappear in many instances with or without therapy. The disease is usually self-limited in the mother, for many such individuals have conceived at some future date and had uneventful pregnancies and healthy infants.

Some gravid patients who have listerial infections have headaches, photophobia, and some difficulty with neck movements but no other visual disturbances. Although listerial meningitis should be considered in the differential diagnosis, this form of listeriosis, as pointed out by Boucher and Yonekura,[6] is rarely observed in the gravid patient.

Host Susceptibility

Some pregnant women are at greater risk to develop listerial infections, more specifically individuals who are being treated with immunosuppressive drugs. Fan and associates[19] reported a case of maternal death due to *L. monocytogenes* septicemia in a woman on immunosuppressive therapy for lupus nephritis. They also recorded a pregnant woman with AIDS who developed listerial septicemia. From these cases they emphasized that *L. monocytogenes* may be an important, unrecognized pathogen in pregnant women with impaired immunity. Dick and associates[13] reported the case of a patient who had a renal transplant from her brother and during the twentieth week of pregnancy developed a 3-day illness characterized by headache, listlessness, and fever. The headache was of subacute onset and the fever reached 38.5°C. The illness was not associated with upper respiratory, gastrointestinal, or urinary tract symptoms. The symptoms abated, although she felt listless for the subsequent 2 weeks. At the twenty-fourth week of gestation she was admitted to the hospital on account of fever, severe bifrontal headache, neck stiffness, photophobia, a mucopurulent vaginal discharge, and a swinging temperature up to 39.8°C. Fundoscopic examination revealed no abnormality. There were no signs of meningism. No abdominal tenderness was elicited, and the uterine fundus was equivalent in height to a gestation of 24 weeks' duration. Fetal movements had ceased 24 hours prior to admission, and no fetal heart sounds were audible. Culture of the cerebrospinal fluid was sterile. *Listeria monocytogenes* was isolated from the blood but not from cervicovaginal cultures. Ampicillin therapy was prescribed. Uterine contractions commenced, and a macerated fetus was in due course delivered. The swinging fever settled after the delivery. The placenta on histologic examination revealed marked inflammatory changes affecting the chorion and villi. Microabscesses were noted among the villi. Similar abscesses were also observed in the fetal lungs and liver. The distribution of the abscesses was in accord with hematogenous origin of the infection.

This case agrees with the opinion of Relier[69] that listeriosis in gravid patients is associated with two or more febrile episodes. The first is the primary, and all too frequently it is recognized only in retrospect. There is no doubt that the gravid patient who is on immunosuppressive therapy has a more fulminant infection. Likewise, the greater the febrile response during the bacteremic phase, the worse the prognosis for the intrauterine patient.

Rudolph and associates[71] reported that spontaneous abortion is more common in transplant recipients than in the normal female population. O'Donnell and associates[60] found that the abortion rate in renal transplant recipients is related to the degree of immunosuppression. The higher dosage of immunosuppressive agents prescribed may be associated with an abortion rate in excess of 20 percent.

The high rate of spontaneous abortion in such patients may be related to an increased incidence of listerial infection, although no mention was made of any febrile illnesses in the report of O'Donnell and coworkers.[60] The products of conception from spontaneous abortions in women who are transplant recipients or on immunosuppressive therapy should have cultures to provide a clearer definition of the incidence of listeriosis in such cases.

Recurrent Abortion

Listeria monocytogenes has been implicated as a cause of recurrent abortion. Rappaport and associates[67] reported a series of patients with repeated abortions or stillbirths in whom they were able to obtain repeated positive cultures of the organism from the cervix. They treated these individuals with penicillin and a sulfonamide and discovered that the cervical cultures were again positive from 1 to 6 weeks after the therapy had been completed. They concluded that such patients should be kept on prophylactic sulfonamide therapy. In the few patients so treated, they claimed a reduction in pregnancy wastage from what they considered to be chronic genital listeriosis. These results and their claim that such infections may be sexually transmitted have never been substantiated.

Route of Infection

Halliday and Hirata[32] suggested an ascending infection as the means by which intrauterine involvement occurs, as they assumed listerial infections could be caused by sexual contact or fecal-vaginal contamination. An argument against these routes of infection is the fact that most cases of perinatal listeriosis have intact membranes until shortly before delivery. Fecal-vaginal contamination also seems unlikely, as Kampelmacher and Van Noorle-Jansen[40] found that none of the mothers or neonates demonstrated any evidence of infection, despite the fact that 44 percent of the 137 prenatal patients had positive fecal cultures for *L. monocytogenes*. Further support for such a concept is the finding of Lennon and coworkers[46] that vaginal carriage of *L. monocytogenes* was found in only 1 of 750 consecutive asymptomatic gravid patients during the time of an epidemic of perinatal listeriosis. Driscoll and associates[16] in their placental studies found an inflammatory reaction in all layers of the placenta. They observed diffuse deciduitis with microabscesses where there was focal destruction of placental barriers and entrapment of chorionic villi, and they concluded that this was the site where pathogens could enter the fetus. Yamazaki and coworkers[90] in their studies of the placental pathology found evidence of chorioamnionitis, umbilical vasculitis, and funisitis but failed to demonstrate any organisms in the placenta. They agree that villositis lesions imply transplacental infection but then state that chorioamnionitis may represent an ascending infection from the lower genital tract. The finding of purulent chorioamnionitis in their study provides evidence, in their opinion, that congenital listeriosis may be acquired as the result of an ascending infection. The debate as to the mode of transmission to the intrauterine patient has not been resolved, but most authors consider that the majority of fetal infections are transplacental.

Fetal Cardiotocography

The maternal infection is self-limiting and readily responds to antibiotic therapy if the physician is aware of the significance of the febrile episode associated with an influenza-like syndrome. If the infection passes unrecognized, soon after the febrile episode there is a reduction in fetal movements, followed by premature delivery or intrauterine demise of the fetus during the subsequent 7 to 10 days. It is of interest that on occasion before the onset of fever fetal tachycardia is discernible by means of cardiotocography. On several occasions I have obtained a record of the baseline fetal heart rate in patients with an influenza-like syndrome in the second half of pregnancy; when the heart rate is between 170 and 180 beats per minute, a diagnosis of listeriosis must be considered.[10]

The following case is illustrative. A 24-year-old patient in the thirty-fourth week of her first pregnancy noted lethargy, myalgia, conjunctivitis, and decreased fetal movements during the previous 24 hours. She was afebrile and normotensive. On physical examination the height of the uterine fundus was compatible with the duration of the gestation. No uterine tenderness was elicited, but contractions of moderate intensity were noted. The cervix was partially effaced and 4 cm dilated, and the fetal membranes were intact. Ultrasonography showed a normal fetus with growth parameters compatible with a gestation of 34 weeks. Tocolysis was commenced by the use of an intravenous infusion of ritodrine, but even at a dose of 300 μg per minute the labor was not arrested. An amniocentesis was performed, and the amniotic fluid obtained was murky and discolored. A Gram's stain of the fluid revealed the presence of gram-positive coccobacilli. A diagnosis of listeriosis was formulated, and the patient was given intravenous ampicillin and gentamicin. Tocolysis was discontinued. The fetal tachycardia persisted at 170 beats per minute, but no decelerations were observed. After 6 hours of antibiotic therapy, amniotomy was performed; the amniotic fluid had a grumous appearance and was greenish brown. The patient was delivered of a male infant weighing 2,275 g. Cultures from the placenta, fetal membranes, and amniotic fluid yielded colonies of *L. monocytogenes*. The pediatrician treated the infant with ampicillin and tobramycin after aspirating the upper respiratory tract. Cultures of the tracheal aspirate were negative. At no time was the maternal temperature above 38°C, and her postpartum course was uneventful.

This résumé has been presented to demonstrate that an influenza type of illness in the third trimester, in the absence of fever, can be associated with fetal tachycardia and premature labor. It is well established that baseline fetal tachycardia in excess of 160 beats per minute is associated with maternal fever or chorioamnionitis. In addition to the baseline tachycardia, when chorioamnionitis is present there may be loss of variability. There was no evidence of loss of variability in this case. Failure of tocolysis has often been noted in patients who go into preterm labor on account of listeriosis.

Amniocentesis

Transabdominal amniocentesis in the second half of pregnancy should be considered in patients with fever or premature labor where the differential diagnosis includes chorioamnionitis. As pointed out by Petrilli and associates,[62] such a diagnostic approach is particularly helpful to patients in whom amniorrhexis has not occurred as it provides reliable intrauterine material for Gram's stain and culture. In Gram-stained smears of the amniotic fluid sediment, *L. monocytogenes* may be intracellular or extracellular, and at times it occurs in pairs simulating pneumococci. In the Gram-stained slide, effete organisms may demonstrate gram variability and be confused with *Haemophilus* species. Likewise, in Gram-stained slides that are overly decolorized, *L. monocytogenes* may appear as gram-negative organisms and also be confused with *Haemophilus* species. Despite the occasional gram variability due to effete organisms or faulty technique, the Gram's stain of an amniotic fluid sediment can help to establish the diagnosis and allow for institution of definitive therapy. If the time interval between initiation of intravenous antibiotic therapy and delivery of the infant exceeds 6 hours, the neonatal prognosis is markedly improved. Hume[36] described a patient who at 19 weeks of gestation developed an acute febrile illness; he obtained three successive positive blood cultures of *L. monocytogenes*. The patient was treated with ampicillin, proceeded to term, and was delivered of a healthy male infant. The hospital course of both mother and infant were uneventful. Zervoudakis and Cederquist[91] presented a patient at 20 weeks with an influenza-like syndrome, and a diagnosis of listeriosis was confirmed by the isolation of the pathogen from three separate blood cultures. Treatment with penicillin for 9 days allowed the pregnancy to continue to the thirty-ninth week, when the patient was delivered of a healthy infant. These investigators performed an amniocentesis during week 37 of the pregnancy, and cultures of the amniotic fluid were negative. They consider that most cases of congenital listeriosis are secondary to low-grade maternal septicemia with involvement of the placenta and subsequent extension to the fetus. They note that fetal death often occurs in utero, and of the infants born alive many succumb shortly after birth. In their report they emphasize the importance of the early diagnosis of maternal listeriosis in reducing fetal morbidity and mortality rates. They reported that maternal antibiotic therapy results in the survival of 71 percent of infants born to such patients, compared with a 29 percent survival rate when the mother is not treated.

In the absence of vigorous maternal antibiotic therapy, intrauterine fetal demise or premature labor and delivery of an infant with congenital listeriosis are the probable sequelae of a nonspecific influenza type of illness.

Table 16-4 Distinctive Features of the Two Types of Neonatal Listeriosis

Early Onset	Late Onset
Mother may have a history of febrile illness	No obstetric complications
Meconium-stained amniotic fluid	Term labor
Premature labor	Normal birth weight
Low birth weight	Illness usually 5th to 14th day of life
Primarily septicemia	After birth
Neonatal apnea or respiratory distress	Poor feeding
Hepatosplenomegaly	Irritability
Rash	Tense anterior fontanelle
Positive blood culture	Meningitis or meningoencephalitis
	Infection from environment or cross-infection
	Blood culture often negative

Intrauterine Fetal Infection

Intrauterine fetal infection is primarily a septicemia, as evidenced by hepatosplenomegaly and a widespread macular-papular skin eruption of a red or violaceous hue, together in some instances with petechiae, which may involve mainly the trunk and lower extremities. The first description of the pathologic changes in perinatal listerial infection stressed the occurrence of multiple granulomatous lesions, and as a result the disease was referred to as *granulomatosis infantiseptica*. Most fatal cases have evidence of systemic infection, but not all have visceral lesions. In some instances the latter, when present, are not widely disseminated, and microscopic studies reveal abscesses rather than granulomas. The lesions are found predominantly in the liver, spleen, and adrenals. The last site is in accord with the septicemic nature of the intrauterine disease.

If the listeriosis infection does not result in intrauterine fetal death, premature delivery of an infant with congenital listeriosis ensues. The neonatologist must be alerted for any case in which meconium or brown-discolored amniotic fluid is noted at the time of amniorrhexis when gestation is of 34 weeks or less. Meconium passage is infrequently observed in the absence of a breech presentation in premature labors. Buchdahl and associates[8] state that it has been reported to be a sign of listerial infection. They consider that a high index of suspicion is necessary for the early detection and prompt treatment of this life-threatening perinatal infection. The presence of small gram-positive coccobacilli in meconium is excellent evidence of congenital listeriosis.

Placenta

In all cases where perinatal listeriosis is considered in the differential diagnosis, the placenta and membranes should be cultured for the pathogen as well as submitted for histologic studies. Placental studies reveal that normal as well as abnormal macroscopic features may be present. Small lesions are not always discovered, as in most institutions the routine processing of the well-fixed placenta involves cutting serial blocks of about 1 cm in width. Microscopic examination, however, may confirm the diagnosis. McLaughlin and coworkers[53] have identified *L. monocytogenes* in placental tissue samples by the utilization of monoclonal antibodies. This technique confirms the diagnosis when histologic studies demonstrate lesions that are suggestive of listeriosis. No study of the placenta is complete unless a search has been made for evidence of funisitis, umbilical vasculitis, and amnionitis in these cases

Neonatal Infection

If listeric infection of the neonate is a consequence of fetal infection, this congenital infection is referred to as *early-onset* disease, as occurs in group B streptococcal infection. In fact, neonatal listerial infection simulates group B streptococcal infection in many ways, including "late onset" disease (Table 16-4). Neonatal listeriosis is clinically indistinguishable from any other severe infection. The difference in the early- and late-onset forms of neonatal listeriosis are shown in Table 16-4.

Early Onset

The early-onset or "septicemic" form is associated with prematurity and increased neonatal mortality. The most frequent initial clinical sign in such infants is respiratory distress. This manifestation of listeriosis may go undetected if adequate cultures are not obtained. In such infants at the time of birth, cultures should be obtained from the external auditory canal and throat. Apnea, cyanosis, hypothermia, and bradycardia are often noted. Other clinical features that may be present include hepatosplenomegaly, conjunctivitis, cutaneous lesions, and a petechial rash. If the etiology of the infection is not rapidly established, a bad prognosis is to be expected. In addition to early, intensive antibiotic therapy, aggressive ventilatory and pharmacologic support is essential for survival of the neonate.

Late Onset

The late-onset form of neonatal listeriosis has a lower mortality rate than the early-onset form of the disease. There is no history of obstetric complications, and the infant is of normal birth weight. This latter form of the disease appears after the fifth day of life, and the prominent feature is meningitis. It is ushered in by fever, poor feeding, irritability, and a tense anterior fontanelle. The clinical course is often fulminant, and the suppurative meningitis may result in hydrocephalus. This form of the disease cannot be distinguished clinically from any other bacterial meningitis. *Listeria monocytogenes* can readily be isolated from the cerebrospinal fluid but blood, nasopharyngeal, and external auditory canal cultures are usually negative. This form of neonatal listeriosis may in many instances be a nosocomial infection and appear in clusters in some hospitals. Larsson and colleagues[45] reported that the use of the same rectal thermometer in a nursery without disinfecting between cases was responsible for neonatal late-onset disease in two of their patients. Nelson and associates[57] reported the nosocomial transmission of the pathogen in the delivery room from a neonate born with early-onset disease to a second neonate, which resulted in late-onset infection in the form of meningitis. They considered that the spread of the infection was due to the utilization of the same resuscitation equipment for the two infants. They underscored the fact that all equipment used for the resuscitation of neonates, such as emergency resuscitation bags and laryngoscopes, must be thoroughly disinfected. The author has recommended to regional hospital centers that equipment used for the neonate in the delivery room should be disposable. Simmons and colleagues[80] have also reported cases where cross-infection occurred in an obstetric operating theater. Such reports support the concept that late-onset infection may be due in some instances to nosocomial transmission. It has been suggested that in some cases colonization of the neonate occurs at birth, although the onset of the disease is delayed until the second or third week of life.

Diagnosis of the affected neonate is the province of the pediatrician. Neonatal listeriosis is a significant cause of morbidity and mortality and in this regard is outranked only by group B streptococcal and coliform infections. Greater attention to this aspect of the infection is covered in Chapter 27 that addresses infections in the neonate.

Treatment

Moellering and associates[55] stated almost 20 years ago that "there is no consensus among various authors as to which antibiotic regimen is most effective." This statement remains true today. In their study they demonstrated that when therapeutic concentrations are attained, penicillin and ampicillin exert only a bacteriostatic rather than a bactericidal action on *L. monocytogenes,* although both agents have been successfully employed in the treatment of listeriosis. These investigators recommended combination therapy in the form of penicillin or ampicillin with an aminoglycoside such as gentamicin. The rationale for the use of combination therapy was based on occasional reports of therapeutic failures with penicillin and ampicillin.

The primary function of the clinical microbiology laboratory is to identify clinically significant microorganisms from body fluids and tissues and determine their susceptibility to antimicrobial agents. The clinician generally believes that the antibiotic susceptibility of a pathogen bears some semblance to the organism's response to the drug in a clinical situation. This fact is well illustrated by *L. monocytogenes,* which is tolerant to the action of ampicillin; consequently the sensitivity of the isolate must be ascertained, as occasionally resistant strains may be encountered. Bactericidal activity of the agent is achieved only at a high concentration in spite of a low minimum inhibitory concentration, and frequently the antibiotic is in vivo only bacteriostatic. The discrepancy between in vitro activity and therapeutic efficacy is due to the fact that *L. monocytogenes* is a facultative intracellular parasite, and in the phagolysosome of macrophages it is barely accessible to antibiotics.

Cephalosporins should never be considered as first-choice drugs as the organism is frequently resistant to this group of agents. The therapeutic efficacy of acylureido-penicillins and piperacillin has as yet not been delineated. Erythromycin and chloramphenicol have been used in the treatment of listeriosis, but they are bacteriostatic rather than bactericidal agents, which could be a marked drawback in treating severe infections. Rifampin is an agent to which the organism has shown no resistance, and this compound is also intracellularly active; however, there is minimal information pertaining to its use in the treatment of listeriosis. The quinolones, based on their intracellular effectivity and pharmacokinetic properties, would appear to be efficacious for the treatment of listeria infections, but to date no available clinical data address this issue.

Trimethoprim-sulfamethoxazole (TMP-SMZ) is a safe, effective antimicrobial combination that has been shown to be highly active and bactericidal in vitro against *L. monocytogenes*. Scheer and Hirschman[73] reported that TMP-SMZ was efficacious in the treatment of both bacteremia and meningitis caused by this pathogen. Spitzer and associates[83] reported that this antimicrobial combination proved highly efficacious in the treatment of a patient with bacteremia caused by *L. monocytogenes* who was allergic to penicillin. Although TMP-SMZ has not been extensively used in the treatment of listeriosis, it should be considered suitable for patients who have a penicillin allergy.

Despite the ever-increasing number of new antibiotics available, the therapy of listeriosis remains ampicillin alone or combined with gentamicin or tobramycin. Marget and Seeliger, in their discussion of the therapy of listeriosis, state:

> The most widely used and clinically used and certainly the most effective therapy up to now, ampicillin, often merely attains bacteriostatic concentrations *in vivo;* furthermore, it is neither intracellularly effective nor synergistic in combination with the frequently used aminoglycosides.[50]

The optimal therapeutic regimen for listeriosis has not

been found, and consequently prevention of listeriosis in the gravid patient and the intrauterine patient must be a major goal in reproductive medicine.

Prevention

Although the source of most listeria infections is unknown, the evidence of food-borne transmission in humans is now quite convincing. Food-borne transmission can be responsible for epidemics, clusters, and sporadic cases.

It is important to keep the problem of listeriosis in perspective when talking to patients by pointing out that the incidence of perinatal listeriosis is low and that only a few gravid patients actually acquire listeriosis. The latter fact is of no consolation to patients who go on to have a handicapped or stillborn child.

During their initial prenatal visit pregnant women should be advised to avoid eating soft, ripened cheeses and to wash thoroughly salads, fruits, and vegetables. Furthermore, retail cook-chill meals and ready-to-eat poultry should not be eaten cold. If they are including such foods in their diet, they should ingest them only if they are heated to above 75°C. They should be informed that cooked foods should be stored in the refrigerator in a separate compartment from cheeses and raw foods. It should be emphasized that such foods should be kept for as short a time as possible, and the expiration date on the labels observed. Similarly, when utilizing a microwave oven, the patients may pay due heed to the manufacturers' instructions to ensure an even temperature in the food. Likewise, leftover reheated food should be discarded. It is important that the patient is aware of these facts, although the extent to which cases of listeriosis are sporadic or part of source outbreaks and how often they are associated with food remain to be determined.

Because of the lack of information on the rate of contamination of foods and on the risk of invasive disease among susceptible gravid patients exposed to the organism, it is difficult to recommend avoidance of a series of foods. However, the gravid patient should be told of the ability of the pathogen to replicate in refrigerated foods and possibly even in some heat-treated products.

If obstetricians were to consider the possibility of an infection due to *L. monocytogenes* in all gravid patients with a fever or an influenza-like syndrome and include it as a possible diagnosis in preterm labor, the perinatal prognosis would be greatly improved.

As pointed out earlier in this chapter, listeriosis is an emerging public health problem, and a concerted diagnostic and research effort by clinicians, microbiologists, and epidemiologists is essential. Progress in this area must not be by accident but by necessity.

In conclusion, I add the title of an article I wrote more than a decade ago: "Listeriosis: not rare, but rarely diagnosed."[10]

References

1. Andre P, Genicot A. First isolation of *Listeria Welshimiri* from human beings. Zentralbl Bakteriol Mikrobiol Hyg A 1987; 263:605–606.
2. Anton W. Kritsch—Experimenteller beitrag zur Biologie des Bakterium Monocytogenes. Zentralbl Bacteriol Mikrobiol Hyg A 1934; 131:89–103.
3. Azadian BS, Finnerty GT, Pearson AD. Cheese-borne listeria meningitis in immunocompetent patient. Lancet 1989; 1:322–323.
4. Bojsen-Møller J. Human listeriosis. Diagnostic, epidemiological and clinical studies. Acta Pathol Microbiol Immunol Scand 1972; 229:1–157.
5. Bottone EJ, Sierra MF. *Listeria monocytogenes:* another look at the "Cinderella among pathogenic bacteria." Mt Sinai J Med 1977; 44:42–59.
6. Boucher M, Yonekura ML. *Listeria* meningitis during pregnancy. Am J Perinatol 1984; 1:312–318.
7. Brackett RE. Presence and persistence of *Listeria monocytogenes* in food and water. Food Technology 1988; 42:162–164.
8. Buchdahl R, Hird M, Gamsu H, et al. Listeriosis revisited: the role of the obstetrician. Br J Obstet Gynaecol 1990; 97:186–189.
9. Burn CG. Clinical and pathological features of an infection caused by a new pathogen of the genus *Listerella*. Am J Pathol 1936; 12:341–348.
10. Charles D. Listeriosis: not rare but rarely diagnosed. Contemporary Ob/Gyn 1980; 15:111–115.
11. Cotoni L. A propos des bacteries denommes *Listerella* rappel d'une observation ancienne de meningite chez l'homme. Annals de Microbilogie Paris 1942; 68:92–95.
12. Cruickshank DP, Warenski T. First trimester maternal *Listeria monocytogenes* sepsis and chorioamnionitis with normal neonatal outcome. Obstet Gynecol 1989; 73:469–471.
13. Dick JP, Palframann A, Hamilton DV. Listeriosis and recurrent abortion in a renal transplant recipient. J Infect 1988; 16:273–277.
14. Doyle MP, Glass KA, Beery JT, et al. Survival of *Listeria monocytogenes* in milk during high-temperature short-time pasteurization. Appl Environ Microbiol 1987; 53:1433–1438.
15. Doyle MP, Schoeni JL. Selective-enrichment procedure for isolation of *Listeria monocytogenes* from fecal and biological specimens. Appl Environ Microbiol 1986; 51:1127–1129.
16. Driscoll SG, Gorbach A, Feldman D. Congenital listeriosis: diagnosis from placental studies. Obstet Gynecol 1962; 20:216–223.
17. Dumont J, Cotoni L. Bacille semblance à celui du rouget de porc recontré dans le LCR d'un meningitique. Annals de L'Institute Pasteur 1921; 35:625–627.
18. Editorial: Listeriosis. Lancet 1989; 1:83–84.
19. Fan YD, Pastorek JG, Janney FA, Saunders CV. Listeriosis as an obstetric complication in an immuno-compromised patient. South Med J 1989; 82:1044–1045.
20. Fauci AS, Dale AC, Balow JE. Glucocorticosteroid therapy: mechanisms of action and clinical considerations. Ann Intern Med 1976; 84:304–315.
21. Fenlon DR. Wild birds and silage as reservoirs for *Listeria* sp in the agricultural environment. J Appl Bacteriol 1985; 59:537–543.

22. Fleming DW, Cochi SL, MacDonald KL, et al. Pasteurized milk as a vehicle of infection in an outbreak of listeriosis. N Engl J Med 1985; 312:404–407.
23. Gaillard JL, Berche P, Sansonetti P. Transposon mutagenesis as a tool to study the role of hemolysin in the virulence of *Listeria monocytogenes*. Infect Immun 1986; 52:50–55.
24. Gilbert RJ, Miller KL, Roberts D. *Listeria monocytogenes* and chilled foods. Lancet 1989; 1:383–384.
25. Gill DA. Circling disease: a meningoencephalitis of sheep in New Zealand. Notes on a new species of pathogenic organism. Veterinary Journal 1933; 89:258–270.
26. Godfrey RW, Wilder MS. Generation of oxygen species and virulence of *Listeria monocytogenes*. Infect Immun 1985; 47:837–839.
27. Gray ML. A possible link in the relation between silage feeding and listeriosis. J Am Vet Med Assoc 1960; 136:205–208.
28. Gray ML, Killinger AH. *Listeria monocytogenes* and listeric infections. Bacteriologie Review 1966; 30:309–382.
29. Hahn H. Effects of dextran sulfate 500 on cell-mediated resistance to infection with *Listeria monocytogenes* in mice. Infect Immun 1974; 10:1105–1109.
30. Hahn H, Kaufmann SHE. Role of cell-mediated immunity in bacterial infections. Rev Infect Dis 1981; 3:1221–1250.
31. Hall SM, Crofts N, Gilbert RJ, et al. Epidemiology of listeriosis, England and Wales. Lancet 1988; 2:502–503.
32. Halliday HL, Hirata T. Perinatal listeriosis: a review of twelve patients. Am J Obstet Gynecol 1979; 133:405–410.
33. Ho JL, Shands KN, Friedland G, et al. An outbreak of type 4b *Listeria monocytogenes* infection involving patients from eight Boston hospitals. Arch Intern Med 1986; 146:520–524.
34. Hotson JR, Pedley TA. The neurological complications of cardiac transplantation. Brain 1976; 99:673–694.
35. Hulphers G. Lefvernekos hos kanin orsakad af en ej forut beskrifven bakterie. Svensk Vetinar Tidskrift 1911; 2:265–273.
36. Hume OS. Maternal *Listeria monocytogenes* septicemia with sparing of the fetus. Obstet Gynecol 1976; 48:33S–34.
37. Issekutz TB, Evans J, Bortolussi R. The immune response of human neonates to *Listeria monocytogenes* infection. Clin Invest Med 1984; 7:281–286.
38. Kales CP, Holzman RS. Listeriosis in patients with HIV infection: clinical manifestations and response to therapy. J Acquir Immune Defic Syndr 1990; 3:139–143.
39. Kampelmacher EH, Huysinga WT, Van Noorle-Jansen LM. The presence of *Listeria monocytogenes* in feces of pregnant women and neonates. Zentralbl Bakteriol Mikrobial Hyg A 1972; 222:258–262.
40. Kampelmacher EH, Van Noorle-Jansen LM. Further studies on the isolation of *Listeria monocytogenes* in clinical healthy individuals. Zentralbl Bakteriol Mikrobiol Hyg A 1972; 221:70–77.
41. Kerr K, Dealler SF, Lacey RW. Listeria in cook-chill food. Lancet 1988; 2:37–38.
42. Kontnick C, Von Graevenitz A, Piscitelli V. Differential diagnosis between *Streptococcus agalactia* and *Listeria monocytogenes*. Ann Clin Lab Sci 1977; 7:269–276.
43. Lamont RJ, Postlethwaite R. Carriage of *Listeria monocytogenes* and related species in pregnant and non-pregnant women in Aberdeen, Scotland. J Infect 1986; 13:187–193.
44. Lamont RJ, Postlethwaite R, MacGowan AP. *Listeria monocytogenes* and its role in human infection. J Infect 1988; 17:7–28.
45. Larsson A, Cederberg A, Ivarsson S, et al. *Listeria monocytogenes* causing hospital-acquired enterocolitis and meningitis in newborn infants. Br Med J 1978; 2:473–474.
46. Lennon D, Lewis B, Mantell C, et al. Epidemic perinatal listeriosis. Pediatr Infect Dis J 1984; 3:30–34.
47. Linnan MJ, Mascola L, Lou XD, et al. Epidemic listeriosis associated with Mexican-style cheese. N Engl J Med 1988; 319:823–828.
48. Louria DB, Hensle T, Armstrong D, et al. Listeriosis complicating malignant disease: a new association. Ann Intern Med 1967; 67:260–281.
49. Mackaness GB. Cellular resistance to infection. J Exp Med 1962; 116:381–406.
50. Marget W, Seeliger HPR. *Listeria monocytogenes* infections: therapeutic possibilities and problems. Infection 1988; 16(suppl 2):S175–177.
51. Mascola L, Lieb L, Chiu J, et al. Listeriosis: an uncommon opportunistic infection in patients with acquired immunodeficiency syndrome. Am J Med 1988; 84:162–164.
52. McLaughlin J. *Listeria monocytogenes:* recent advances in the taxonomy and epidemiology of listeriosis in humans. J Appl Bacteriol 1987; 63: 1–11.
53. McLaughlin J, Black A, Green HT. Monoclonal antibodies show *Listeria monocytogenes* in necropsy tissue samples. J Clin Path 1988; 41:983–988.
54. Miller JK, Hedberg M. Effects of cortisone on susceptibility of mice to *Listeria monocytogenes*. Am J Clin Pathol 1965; 43:248–250.
55. Moellering RC, Medoff G, Leech I, et al. Antibiotic synergism against *Listeria monocytogenes*. Antimicrob Agents Chemother 1972; 1:30–34.
56. Murray EGD, Webb RA, Swann MBR. A disease of rabbits characterized by a large mononuclear leucocytosis caused by a hitherto undescribed bacillus. *Bacterium monocytogenes* (n sp). J Path Bacteriol 1926; 29:409–439.
57. Nelson KE, Warren D, Tomasi AM, et al. Transmission of neonatal listeriosis in a delivery room. Am J Dis Child 1985; 139:903–905.
58. Nieman RE, Lorber B. Listeriosis in adults: a changing pattern. Report of eight cases and review of the literature 1968–1978. Rev Infect Dis 1980; 2:207–227.
59. Nyfeldt A. Étiologie de la mononucléose infectieuse. C R Soc Biol (Paris) 1929; 101:590–592.

60. O'Donnell D, Sevitz H, Seggie JL, et al. Pregnancy after renal transplantation. Aust N Z J Med 1985; 15:320–325.
61. Otokunefor TV, Galsworthy SB. Immunosuppression, nonspecific B-cell activation, and mitogenic activity associated with a high molecular weight component for *Listeria monocytogenes*. Can J Microbiol 1982; 28:1373–1381.
62. Petrilli ES, D'Alaing G, Ledger WJ. *Listeria monocytogenes* chorioamnionitis: diagnosis by transabdominal amniocentesis. Obstet Gynecol 1980; 55:5S–8.
63. Pini PN, Gilbert RJ. The occurrence in the UK of *Listeria* species in raw chicken and soft food. Int J Food Microbiol 1988; 6:317–326.
64. Pirie JHH. A new disease of veld rodents. "Tiger River disease." Publication of the South African Institute for Medical Research 1937; 3:163–186.
65. Pirie JHH. Listeria: change of a name for a genus of bacteria. Nature 1940; 145:264–266.
66. Ralovich B. Listeriosis research, present situation and perspective. Budapest: Akadémiai Kiado, 1984:30–55.
67. Rappaport F, Rabinowitz M, Taoff R, Krochnik N. Genital listeriosis as a cause of repeated abortion. Lancet 1960; 1:1273–1275.
68. Reiss HJ, Potel J, Krebs A. Granulomatosis infantiseptica (eine all gemeininfektion bei neugebornen und sauglin-gen mit miliaren granulomen). Ztchr Inn Med 1951; 6:451–455.
69. Relier JP. Listeriosis. J Antimicrob Chemother 1979; 5:51–57.
70. Rocourt J, Seeliger HPR. Distribution des especes du genre *Listeria*. Zentralbl Bakteriol Mikrobiol Hyg A 1985; 259:317–330.
71. Rudolph JE, Schwizer RT, Bartus S. Pregnancy in renal transplant patients. Transplantation 1979; 21:26–29.
72. St Louis ME, Morse DI, Potter ME. The emergence of grade "A" eggs as a major source of *Salmonella enteritidis* infections: new implications for the control of salmonellosis. JAMA 1988; 259:2103–2107.
73. Scheer MS, Hirschman SZ. Oral and ambulatory therapy of *Listeria* bacteremia and meningitis with trimethoprim-sulfamethoxazole. Mt Sinai J Med 1982; 49:411–414.
74. Schlech WF. New perspectives on the gastrointestinal mode of transmission in invasive *Listeria monocytogenes* infection. Clin Invest Med 1984; 7:321–324.
75. Schlech WF, Lavigne PM, Bortolussi RA, et al. Epidemic listeriosis: evidence for transmission by food. N Engl J Med 1983; 308:203–206.
76. Schwartz B, Ciesielski CA, Broome CV, et al. Association of sporadic listeriosis with consumption of uncooked hot dogs and undercooked chicken. Lancet 1988; 2:779–782.
77. Schwartz J. Attempted isolations of *Listeria monocytogenes* from diagnostic accessions. Am J Vet Res 1969; 30:483–484.
78. Seeliger HPR. Die Ätiologische diagnose des Listeriose. Zentr Bakteriol Parasitenk Abt 1 Orig 1962; 187:267–277.
79. Seeliger HPR, Jones D. Listeria. In: Sneath PHA, Mair NS, Sharpe ME, eds. Bergley's manual of systematic bacteriology. Baltimore: Williams & Wilkins, 1986:1235–1245.
80. Simmons MD, Cockroft PM, Okubadejo OA. Neonatal listeriosis due to cross-infection in an obstetric theatre. J Infect 1986; 13:235–239.
81. Simor AE, Karmali MA, Jadavji T, Roscoe M. Abortion and perinatal sepsis associated with *Campylobacter* infection. Rev Infect Dis 1986; 8:397–402.
82. Sizmur KT, Walker CV. Listeria in prepacked salads. Lancet 1988; 1:1167.
83. Spitzer PG, Hammer SM, Karchmer AW. Treatment of *Listeria monocytogenes* infection with trimethoprim-sulfamethoxazole case report and review of the literature. Rev Infect Dis 1986; 8:427–430.
84. Stamm A, Dismukes WE, Simmons BP, et al. Listeriosis in renal transplant recipients: report of an outbreak and review of 102 cases. Rev Infect Dis 1982; 4:665–674.
85. Stanley NF. Studies on *Listeria monocytogenes:* 1. isolation of a monocytosis-producing agent-MPA. Australian Journal of Experimental Biology and Medical Science 1949; 27:123–131.
86. Telzak EE, Budnick LD, Greenberg MSWG, et al. A nosocomial outbreak of *Salmonella enteritidis* infection due to consumption of raw eggs. N Engl J Med 1990; 323:394–397.
87. Watkins J, Sleath KP. Isolation and enumeration of *Listeria monocytogenes* from sewage. Sewage sludge and river water. J Appl Bacteriol 1981; 50:1–9.
88. Weinberg ED. Pregnancy-associated depression of cell-mediated immunity. Rev Infect Dis 1984; 6:814–821.
89. World Health Organization Working Group: Foodborne listeriosis. Bull World Health Organ 1988; 66:421–428.
90. Yamazaki K, Price JT, Altshuler G. A placental view of the diagnosis and pathogenesis of congenital listeriosis. Am J Obstet Gynecol 1977; 129:703–705.
91. Zervoudakis IA, Cederquist LL. Effect of *Listeria monocytogenes* septicemia during pregnancy on the offspring. Am J Obstet Gynecol 1977; 129:465–467.

CHAPTER 17

Group B Streptococcal Disease

Lawrence C. Madoff, M.D.
Dennis L. Kasper, M.D.

In the 1930s Rebecca Lancefield developed techniques to distinguish among beta-hemolytic streptococci[67] and was first able to isolate what she termed group B streptococci from vaginal cultures of postpartum women.[68] Group B *Streptococcus* (GBS) or *Streptococcus agalactiae* was first recognized to cause human disease (it had earlier been known as an agent of bovine mastitis) by Fry in 1938,[48] who reported three fatal cases of puerperal sepsis. For reasons that remain obscure, GBS infection began to emerge in the 1960s as a recognized cause of neonatal and maternal infection. The 1970s saw a marked increase in the incidence of GBS infection in neonates so that in many geographic areas it surpassed *Escherichia coli* as the most frequent cause of bacteremia and meningitis in neonates.[47,111] This increase did not occur as a shift in the type of infection but in the setting of an overall increase in the incidence of neonatal sepsis.[47] Although progress has been made in recognizing and treating GBS infection, the mortality and serious morbidity that accompany it remain unacceptably high. Recent efforts have been directed toward understanding the pathophysiology of GBS infection and preventing infection through immunologic interventions.

Microbiology

Group B streptococci form small 3- to 4-mm gray colonies, and the vast majority of isolates from humans create a zone of clear or beta-hemolysis when grown on blood agar. Group B streptococci are commonly identified by the elaboration of CAMP factor, which creates a zone of enhanced hemolysis when group B streptococci are grown adjacent to *Staphylococcus aureus* on blood agar.[30] GBS are also identified by their hydrolysis of hippurate broth, their failure to hydrolyze bile-esculin agar, and by their antibiotic sensitivity pattern: the vast majority are resistant to trimethoprim-sulfamethoxazole and bacitracin. Many strains produce a characteristic red-orange pigment under conditions of anaerobic growth. Definitive identification of GBS is based on its phenotype and depends on serologic testing with hyperimmune antiserum to the group-specific polysaccharide antigen; however, Facklam and associates have suggested that adequate presumptive identification of a hemolytic streptococcus as group B can be made on the basis of CAMP factor, bacitracin sensitivity, and lack of bile-esculin hydrolysis.[40] In addition, commercial test kits for identification of streptococci make use of a variety of biochemical tests and appear to classify most isolates adequately.

Lancefield was able to classify the beta-hemolytic streptococci using antiserum specific to the group carbohydrates. Using innovative techniques that are now classic, she raised antisera in rabbits to acid-extracted carbohydrates produced by the streptococci.[67] She recognized that these organisms produce both a C substance, now known as the group antigen shared by all members of the species, as well as an S substance or type-specific polysaccharide. The type-specific polysaccharides, in addition to serving as identifying features of GBS, are now recognized as capsules that are important virulence determinants for the organism and are localized to the surface of the bacteria (Fig. 17-1). Six type-specific polysaccharides (Ia, Ib, II, III, IV, and V) are now identified for GBS, and several others have been presumptively identified. Current serotype classification also depends on the presence or absence of C protein seroreactivity. This group of proteins may be present in strains of any capsular polysaccharide type, and their presence is noted by the appendage of *c* to the serotype designation (for example, II/c).[55] Many GBS are lysogenic, and a phage-typing system has been developed that can assist in the tracking of otherwise identical strains for epidemiologic evaluation.[104,105]

A

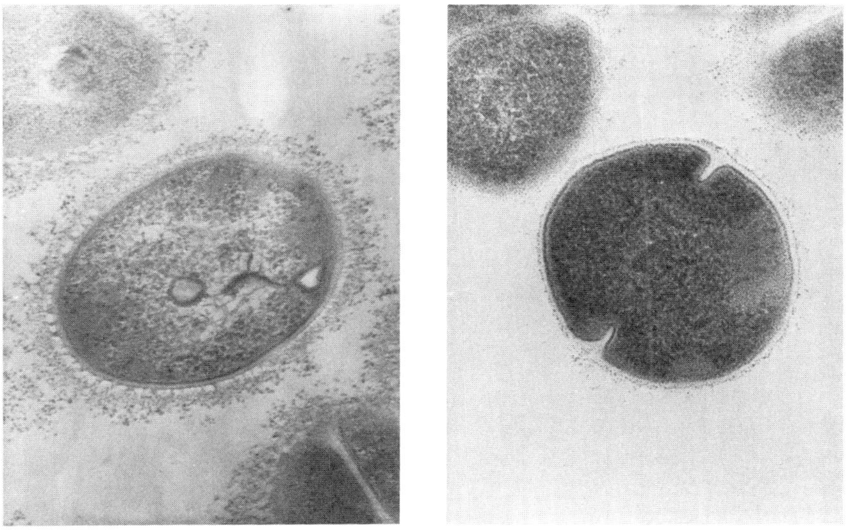

B

Figure 17-1 Transmission electron micrographs (×90,000) showing group B streptococcal surface structures.[62] **A,** Capsular polysaccharide. GBS were incubated in the presence of rabbit antiserum to the type III capsular polysaccharide. **B,** C proteins. GBS were incubated in the presence of C protein specific rabbit antiserum. Both are labeled with ferritin-conjugated antirabbit antibodies.

Antigenic Structures and Virulence Determinants

The major antigenic determinants of GBS have been the subject of extensive investigation, and some are now well characterized as virulence factors. The capsular polysaccharide is the best understood of the antigenic determinants. The structures of six of these type-specific capsular polysaccharides of GBS have now been determined.[34,56,57,113,116] Each polysaccharide, a complex structure composed of glucose, galactose, N-acetyl glucosamine, and sialic acid (N-acetyl neuraminic acid), is several hundred thousand Daltons in size and is a polymer of a repeating subunit (Fig. 17-2); each subunit contains a terminal sialic acid residue. Earlier work that depended on harsh extraction techniques altered the chemical structure of the polysaccharides. For example, the original antigen preparations used to classify the streptococci were prepared using hot extraction in 0.1 M HCl, which yielded smaller polysaccharides of approximately 10,000 MW and lacking the terminal sialic acid residues now recognized in each of the native polysaccharides. The antigenic characteristics of the native type III capsular polysaccharide have been shown to depend, in part, on the length of the polysaccharide chain through what has been described as a "conformational epitope";[114] shorter polysaccharides, although containing complete antibody binding sites, bind to antibody with lower affinity than the intact native polysaccharide, indicating that antigenicity is partially determined by the number of repeating subunits.

The structure of the group B polysaccharide has recently been determined. It has a unique, highly branched structure composed of four distinct oligosaccharides linked by phosphodiester bonds (Fig. 17-3).[79,80] Lancefield showed that antibody to the group polysaccharide, in contrast to the type-specific capsular polysaccharide, failed to protect against GBS infection in animal models.[69] Furthermore, naturally occurring human antibody to the group B antigen has been found not to corrrelate with resistance to infection.[1] Recently, however, a human monoclonal IgM antibody that reacts with the group B polysaccharide has been found to protect against infection by several GBS strains of differing capsular type in an animal model.[91]

The C protein complex of GBS represents another important antigen—and potential virulence factor—of the organism. The C proteins of GBS were originally recognized as protease-sensitive antigenic determinants that cross-reacted between Ib and "Ic" serotypes of GBS and were thus called *Ibc proteins*.[119] It is now known that this protein complex is distinct from the capsular polysaccharide and may be expressed along with any capsular type[59] (the "Ic" serotype is actually Ia capsule type with C proteins or serotype "Ia/c"). One or more of the determinants is present in approximately 60 to 80 percent of clinical isolates.[31,59] Lancefield and coworkers recognized that antibodies to the C proteins were protective against infection in a mouse virulence model.[70] Early work showed two distinct C protein antigens in the prototype Ia/c strain of GBS: one of these was resistant to trypsin (now called *alpha*).[119] The other, now called *beta*, was susceptible to degradation by trypsin. Recent work has begun to characterize these two antigens more fully. It is now recognized, for example, that they can be expressed independently on different strains.[59] The alpha-C protein antigen is protective and appears to be a polymorphic protein with a regularly varying molecular weight that appears as a "ladder" on Western blot.[75] It also appears to be phenotypically distinct in different strains of GBS, varying both in quantity and in the molecular weight of the largest component pro-

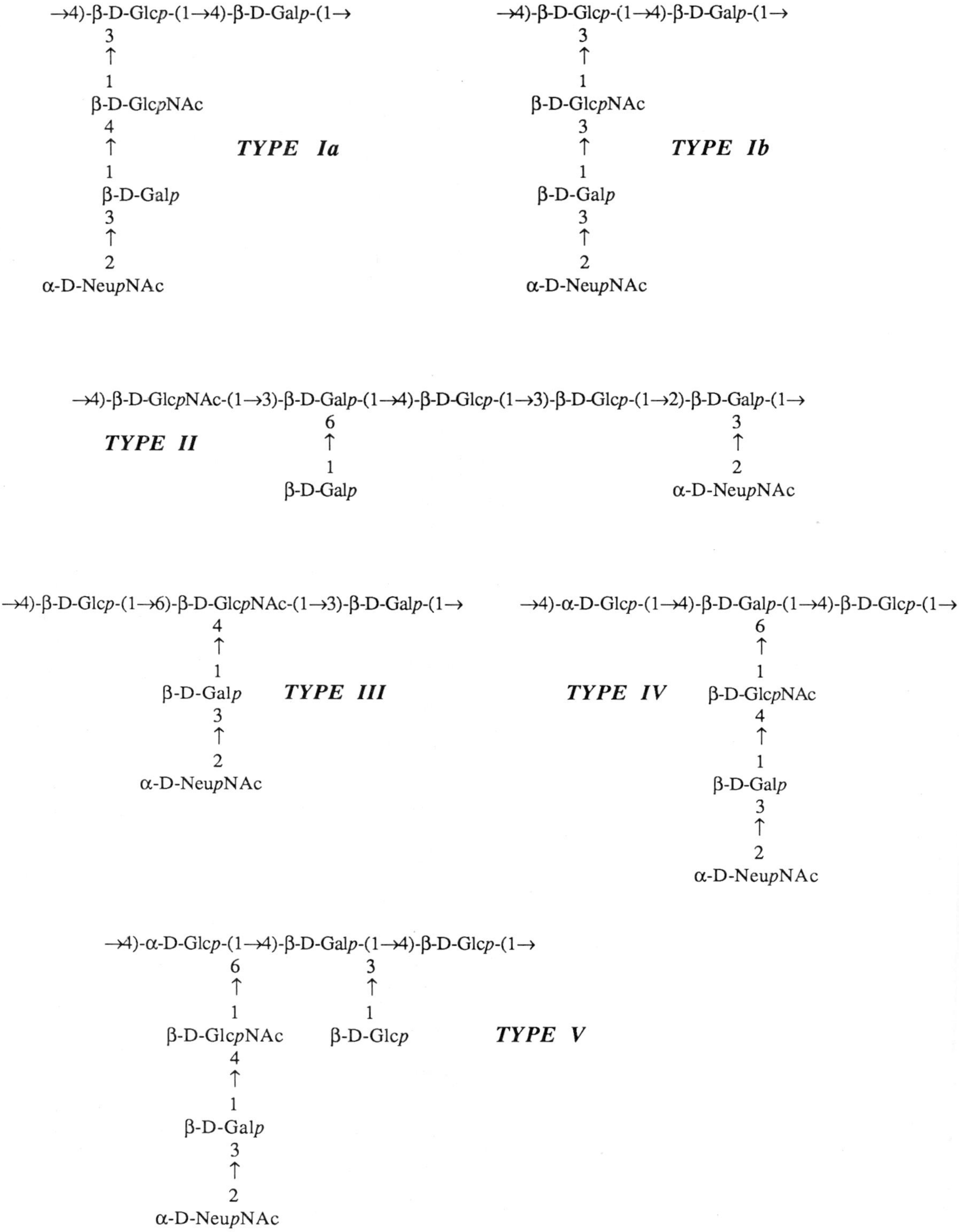

Figure 17-2 Repeating unit structure of group B streptococcal capsular polysaccharides type Ia,[56] type Ib,[56] type II,[57] type III,[116] type IV,[34] and type V.[113] (From Wessels MR, DiFabio JL, Benedi V-J, et al. 1991.[113])

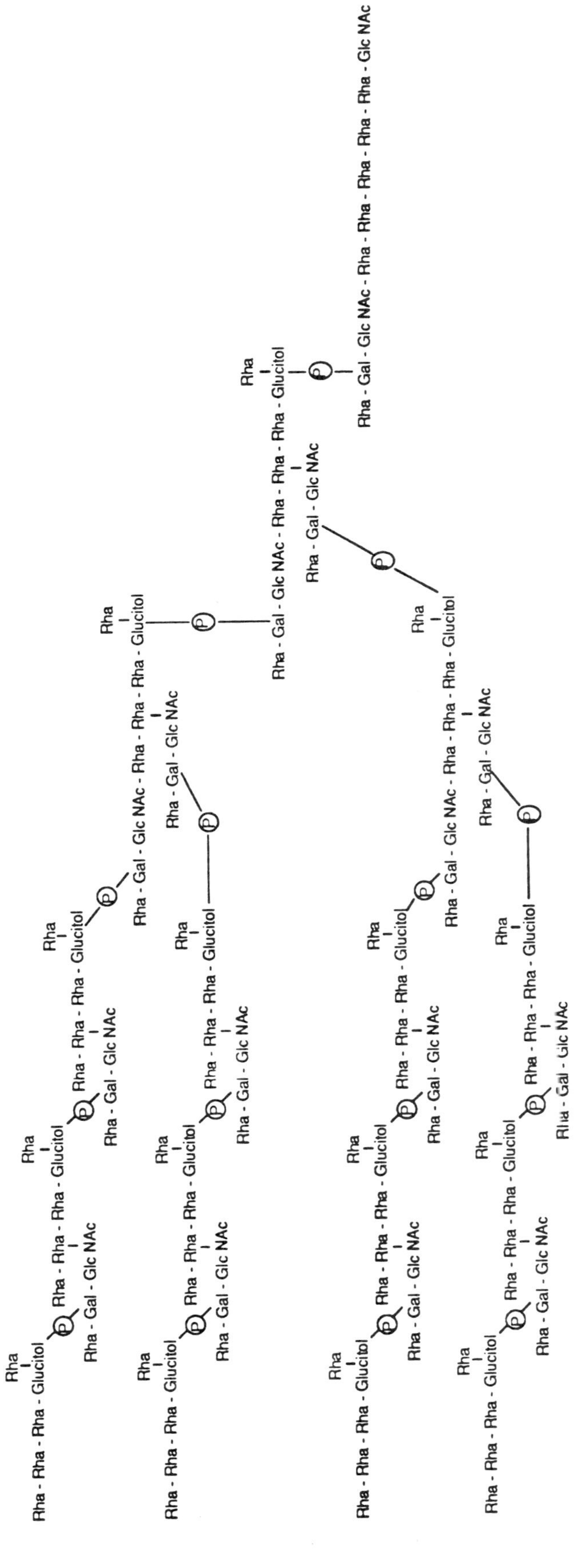

Figure 17-3 Proposed structure of the group polysaccharide of group B *Streptococcus*.[79]

tein.[74] No biologic function has yet been ascribed to this protein, but it may enhance the evasion of complement-mediated opsonization in the absence of specific antibody.

The beta-C protein appears as a single protein of molecular mass of 130 kD when extracted with detergent.[74,94] This protein has been shown to bind specifically to the Fc region of human IgA, suggesting a possible virulence property. Smaller subunits of the beta-C protein have been reported to be secreted into broth by the organism.[22]

Both alpha- and beta-C protein genes have been cloned,[32,78] and their products, expressed in *E. coli*, are able to elicit protective antibody in an animal model. The sequence of the beta-C protein gene has been determined and shows a hydrophobic membrane anchor region and a C-terminal, proline-rich cell wall spanning region characteristic of surface proteins of gram-positive cocci.[58]

The number of C proteins, their structure, virulence properties, and regulation remain incompletely known. Recently, two additional C protein antigens, gamma and delta, have been proposed on the basis of immunochemical evidence.[23] The gamma antigen appears to be present only in some isolates that express the alpha C protein. The delta antigen appears to be common in serotype III isolates, in contradistinction to the other C proteins, which are rarely present in type III strains.[31] It is not known at present whether these epitopes are protective, and their structures remain undefined.

R proteins[28] and X proteins,[44] also present in group A streptococci, are found in some GBS isolates, usually type III strains. Although these appear to be surface-localized determinants,[110] their role in pathogenesis, if any, is not known.

Secreted Products

The CAMP factor, an acronym for the authors Christie, Atkins, and Munch-Petersen who first described it in 1944,[30] is a polypeptide of 25 kD[60] that causes an enhanced zone of beta-hemolysis when GBS are cocultured with *S. aureus* on blood agar. The gene encoding this protein has been cloned and expressed in *E. coli*.[98] Although it is immunogenic, no role in virulence or immunity has been determined for this protein.

GBS also elaborate pigment, hippuricase, nucleases, and lipoteichoic acid into the extracellular milieu.[43] These secreted products of GBS have been studied in L-forms, or cell wall–defective variants.[46] The group B streptococcal hemolysin has characteristics similar to streptolysin S of group A streptococci and appears to be cell bound.[76] Although hemolysins have been shown to be major virulence factors in other organisms, nonhemolytic isogenic transposon mutants of group B streptococci were not less virulent than parent strains in an animal model.[112] Soluble, secreted forms of both the type-specific capsular polysaccharide[25] and the beta-C protein[22] have been described. Neuraminidases (enzymes that cleave sialic acid from polysaccharides) have been studied in some detail in GBS. Neuraminidase production is generally higher in type III strains than in other serotypes and appears to correlate with the virulence of the organism.[24,120] Whether this relationship is causal or based on some other association has not been determined.

Clinical Syndromes

Asymptomatic Carriage in Adults

Group B streptococci are now well established as a part of the vaginal microflora in many adult women. Because maternal colonization is an important risk factor for neonatal exposure and therefore neonatal invasive disease, the rate of asymptomatic carriage is important for determining this risk. The rate of colonization has been extensively studied and appears to be highly dependent on culture technique.[120] One of the major factors in determining the colonization prevalence is the number of cultures obtained from each patient. Serial cultures increase the yield of positive cultures.[8] The culture conditions appear to affect the rate of positivity as well, with higher rates being obtained with selective broth inoculation than with agar plates. The site of culture also influences the yield, with higher rates of vaginal colonization detected when multiple sites are cultured.

The prevalence of colonization with GBS appears to increase after beginning sexual intercourse.[8] It does not appear to be a sexually transmitted agent in the traditional sense but may, instead, be transferred from the colorectal to the vaginal flora by vaginal penetration. Other risk factors for colonization include being in the first half of the menstrual cycle, using an intrauterine device, and being younger than 20 years of age. Ethnicity has been reported to affect carriage rates. One recent, large, multicenter survey of pregnant women found the highest rates in Hispanics from New York City (predominantly Caribbean), followed by blacks, whites, and other (predominantly Mexican) Hispanics, with an overall prevalence of 18.6 percent.[92] Factors found not to be associated with GBS colonization include number of sexual partners, use of oral contraceptive agents, acute infection with *Neisseria gonorrhoeae,* and presence of gynecologic symptoms such as vaginal discharge.

Concurrent colonization with *Candida* species but not with *Chlamydia trachomatis, Ureaplasma urealyticum, Trichomonas vaginalis,* or *Mycoplasma hominis* appears to increase the rate of colonization in pregnant women.[92] Baker and Edwards have extensively reviewed these data and state that in order to best predict the risk of exposure of the neonate both vaginal and anorectal cultures should be obtained on more than one occasion during pregnancy.[7] The reported rates of colonization of the genital or the lower GI tract have ranged nearly 10-fold, from less than 5 percent to greater than 40 percent among pregnant women in different studies.[92] Along with the technical differences, these rates also probably reflect true differences in the rate of colonization among different demographic groups in different geographic locations and different time periods.

Transmission to Neonates

Transmission to the neonate has been well documented to occur during passage through the birth canal

Table 17-1 Distinguishing Features of Early- and Late-Onset GBS Disease

	Early	Late
Age at onset (mean)	0-5 days (20 hours)	5 days-3 months (24 days)
Risk factors	Prematurity Prolonged rupture of membranes Maternal fever/chorioamnionitis Low birth weight Multiple gestation	
Major clinical features	Sepsis Pneumonia Meningitis	Sepsis Meningitis Septic arthritis Osteomyelitis
Major serotypes causing disease	Ia, Ib, II, III	III
Mortality	13-55%	5-23%

or prior to birth by infection ascending from the vagina. Thus infection of the neonate depends on the presence and the quantity of GBS present in the mother at the time of birth. Infection may also occur in utero by ascending through the cervix through either ruptured or compromised membranes. The apparent rate of transmission is highly variable among studies ranging from 29 to 72 percent[5,85,120] but averaging approximately 60 percent. These differences may reflect several factors: technical differences in the methods of culturing specimens from both mother and neonate, including the site, timing, and culture method; differences in the inoculum; and differences in the actual birth. The rate of transmission, for invasive infection[16] as well as asymptomatic colonization,[85] appears to depend, in part, on the quantity of bacteria present in the maternal genital tract at the time of birth, with a higher inoculum leading to a higher rate of transmission. Cultures of specimens from the oropharynx, skin, urine, rectum, and external auditory canal have all been used in an attempt to determine colonization rates of newborns. The presence of GBS at multiple sites increases the risk for invasive infection in the neonate.[35,85]

Neonatal Disease

Two distinct syndromes of neonatal disease, early onset and late onset, were described in the early 1970s as group B streptococcal sepsis began to emerge as an important clinical entity.[6] They differ in presentation, prevalence of serotypes, risk factors for acquisition, mortality, and probably pathogenesis (Table 17-1). Early-onset disease occurs within 5 days of birth, and most disease occurs in the first day. Late-onset disease generally occurs between 6 days and 3 months of age.[2] As shown in Figure 17-4, early-onset disease is more common, and the vast majority of cases occur on the first day of life. Early-onset disease tends to occur in premature and low-birth-weight babies (although most cases still occur in term infants) and those born of pregnancies complicated by premature rupture of membranes, prolonged labor, or maternal chorioamnionitis.[2,6] In contrast, late-onset disease occurs more often in the products of uncomplicated pregnancies. The serotype distribution of GBS strains causing early-onset disease reflects the serotype distribution of colonizing strains (approximately one-third type Ia and Ib, one-third type II, and one-third type III strains, most are C protein positive), whereas late-onset disease is far more frequently caused by type III strains.[2,6] Early-onset disease is characterized clinically by a predominance of pneumonitis and septicemia, whereas late-onset disease is frequently associated with meningitis.

Early-Onset Infection

The reported attack rates for early-onset group B streptococcal infection (defined as invasive group B streptococcal disease within 5 days of birth) vary from 0.7 to 3.7 per 1,000 live births, with the lower attack rates in the more recent reports.[85,107] The mean age at onset for early-onset disease is 20 hours; in utero infection through grossly or microscopically compromised membranes probably accounts for the fact that half of early-onset infection is clinically apparent at the time of birth.[16] Bacteremia is the most frequent manifestation, either without localized infection (approximately one-third of cases) or with pneumonia or meningitis. The signs of early-onset group B streptococcal infection are not specific for this entity and include fever, lethargy, jaundice, respiratory distress, and hypotension.[2,6] Infants with meningitis may not initially be distinguishable from those with other foci of infection. Seizures develop in up to 50 percent of infants with meningitis, but lumbar puncture is indicated in all infants with suspected infection with GBS regardless of the specific clinical findings.

Pulmonary involvement occurs in approximately 40 percent of neonates with early-onset presentation, and almost all of them have signs of acute respiratory disease within hours of birth (including labored or grunting respirations, apnea, or tachypnea). Chest x-ray may show discrete infiltrates suggesting bacterial pneumonia but may be indistinguishable from hyaline membrane disease.[63] Less common clinical manifestations of GBS

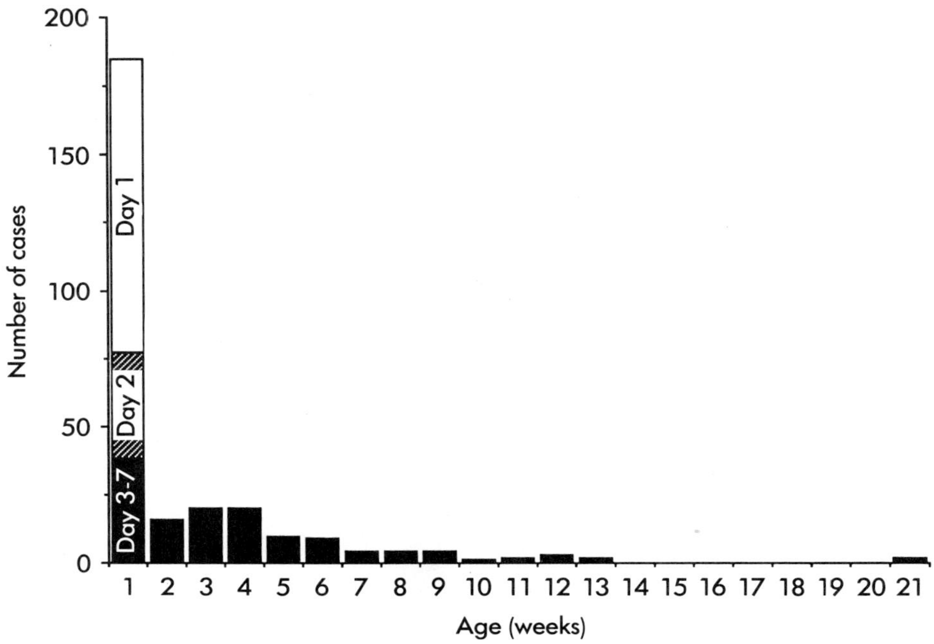

Figure 17-4 Age at onset of neonatal group B streptococcal sepsis in 286 cases between 1962 and 1976.[2] (Adapted, with permission, from Anthony BF, Okada DM. The emergence of group B streptococci in infections of the newborn infant. Annu Rev Med 1977; 28:355–69. © 1977 by Annual Reviews Inc.)

early-onset infection include arthritis, endocarditis, peritonitis, cellulitis, and conjunctivitis.[54] The mortality for early-onset infection is higher than that for late-onset disease and was initially reported to be as high as 55 percent.[2] This rate appears to have declined with improved recognition and early presumptive treatment of the disease, and more recent rates have ranged from 13 to 37 percent.[35] Low birth weight appears to have a major impact on mortality; one report showed an overall mortality of 61 percent but only 14 percent for infants of more than 1,500 g.[90]

Late-Onset Infection

Late-onset group B streptococcal infection is generally defined as invasive disease occurring after day 6 of life.[2,6] Almost all cases occur within the first 3 months of life, but occasional cases may occur after 3 months (Fig. 17-4). The attack rates for late-onset disease have been less extensively studied than those for early-onset disease but usually have been found to range from 0.9 to 1.9 per 1,000 live births, a slightly lower rate than for early-onset disease.[35] Late-onset disease is distinguished from early-onset disease by the extremely high proportion of meningitis associated with bacteremia (more than 85 percent of cases) and the overwhelming preponderance of serotype III strains of GBS (more than 90 percent). Other features that distinguish late-onset infection are the generally unremarkable obstetric history, absence of maternal complications, and the fact that disease usually occurs in term infants.

Infants with late-onset sepsis, meningitis, or both typically present with nonspecific symptoms and signs: fever, lethargy, and poor feeding. Presentation may also be fulminant, with overwhelming sepsis and meningitis characterized by obtundation, hypotension, and seizures. Because infants may progress rapidly from a relatively benign and nonspecific picture to fulminant disease, all infants in this age group with fever (temperature of 38° C or higher) require aggressive workup and immediate presumptive therapy with antibiotics. The workup should include blood culture and lumbar puncture; in fulminant disease, a Gram's stain of CSF may reveal gram-positive cocci. Bacteremia without any apparent source of infection may also occur in late-onset disease, as can osteomyelitis and septic arthritis. Less frequent manifestations of late-onset infection include peritonitis,[26] endocarditis,[14] and urinary tract infection.[103]

The prognosis for late-onset infection is somewhat better than for early-onset infection and may be improving. Although initial mortality rates were reported as high as 23 percent,[2] a more recent report indicated a mortality rate of only 5 percent,[35] possibly a reflection of greater awareness of the syndrome and appropriate early presumptive treatment. Because of the high incidence of meningitis in late-onset group B streptococcal disease, permanent neurologic sequelae occur in many of the survivors. Among all patients with group B streptococcal meningitis (both early- and late-onset disease), as many as half have neurologic complications that include deafness, blindness, mental retardation, and more subtle cognitive deficits.[27,39] Several prognostic features that portend an unfavorable outcome are the presence of hypotension, coma, or persistent seizures. Laboratory findings associated with death or permanent neurologic sequelae include leukopenia, a CSF leukocyte count in excess of 1,000 per cubic millimeter, or CSF protein of greater than 300 mg per dl.

Group B streptococcal osteomyelitis and septic arthritis are less serious forms of late-onset infection that do not carry the dismal prognosis of GBS meningitis.[36] These forms of disease are frequently unaccompanied by fever or indications of systemic involvement. Signs of painful joint mobility may be the only indication of the presence of disease. The outcome of patients with these types of infection appears to be favorable; permanent dysfunction of the affected limb is unusual.

Maternal Infection

The first cases of group B streptococcal infection in humans were reported in postpartum women,[48] and group B streptococcal infection continues to be an important source of morbidity and occasional mortality in this group. As with neonatal infection, the incidence of group B streptococcal maternal infection has risen dramatically since the early 1970s. Reports of blood culture isolates among women on obstetric services from the 1970s show that between 11 and 21 percent of positive isolates were group B streptococci.[3,71] The most common clinical syndrome is endometritis characterized by fever and uterine tenderness, with positive blood cultures occurring in approximately one-third of cases.[41] Endometritis in which GBS plays a role has been found to complicate deliveries at a rate of 1.3 per 1,000 deliveries (strikingly similar to the rate of early-onset neonatal infection). GBS is estimated to be responsible for one-fifth of postpartum endometritis, approximately 45,000 cases per year in the United States.[4] There is a marked association with cesarean section; 94 percent of cases in one series occurred following this procedure.[84] Most obstetric cases of GBS infection respond rapidly to antimicrobial therapy; however, there are reports of maternal mortality as a consequence of GBS endometritis and complicating conditions such as necrotizing fasciitis.[106] Urinary tract infection with GBS may complicate pregnancy, most commonly as asymptomatic bacteriuria but also accompanied by dysuria or occasionally pyelonephritis.[84] The role of urinary tract infection in more serious maternal and neonatal infection remains undefined.

Other Infections in Adults

In one report from 1988, GBS bacteremia in a general hospital population occurred more frequently in adults than in infants,[82] at a rate of over 0.1 per 1,000 hospital admissions. Adults with group B streptococcal sepsis that is not related to obstetric complications are generally elderly or in some way immunocompromised and therefore at risk for this infection. Reported underlying conditions include diabetes mellitus, malignancy, hepatic insufficiency, corticosteroid use, and HIV infection.[82,88] Some cases occur in apparently normal adults. A mortality rate as high as 40 percent has been reported in adults with nonobstetric group B streptococcal bacteremia. Endocarditis has been a well-documented complication of maternal infection, particularly in the preantibiotic era, when it occurred most frequently as an acute endocarditis. More recently GBS endocarditis has become a disease of more elderly patients with underlying valvular heart disease and without sex predilection. It remains a disease with a high mortality rate and frequently complicated by large vegetations and embolization.[49,72] Other nonobstetric infections in adults include pneumonia, which occurs primarily in bedridden, elderly patients;[109] skin and soft tissue infections (cellulitis, cutaneous abscesses, secondary infection of decubitus ulcers); osteomyelitis; septic arthritis; and meningitis. Unlike meningitis in the neonate, adult GBS meningitis is usually not caused by serotype III strains but has a more even distribution among serotypes, with type II strains the most frequently reported isolates.[118] Most adults have underlying conditions, and there is a high rate of mortality and serious morbidity, although the majority of adults survive with antibiotic therapy.[15]

Diagnosis

The diagnosis of colonization or asymptomatic infection (which are synonymous terms) has been discussed previously. It is apparent that reliable antepartum diagnosis of GBS colonization in pregnant women depends on obtaining more than one culture, preferably from different sites and at different times during gestation. Intrapartum detection of colonization, which might allow the selective prophylaxis or presumptive treatment of high-risk infants, has been attempted. Results of these attempts have thus far been less than ideal. Gram's stain of vaginal and cervical swabs in high-risk women have yielded sensitivity of greater than 90 percent but with low specificity (approximately two-thirds) when compared to routine culture techniques.[42,52] Yet another study of Gram's stain detection failed to confirm this high detection rate and reported only 38 percent sensitivity.[96] Rapid latex agglutination and immunofluorescence techniques using vaginal samples have been reported as nonculture methods for rapidly obtaining colonization information. When used directly on vaginal material, these methods appear to have a low sensitivity (33 to 58 percent). These results can be enhanced by preincubation of the sample in selective media to approximately 90 percent sensitivity.[95,102] However, this methodology introduces a delay of 8 to 18 hours in the time required to obtain a result. Another recent report underscores the critical importance of these diagnostic tests. Towers and associates[108] evaluated 131 high-risk patients with rapid ELISA and Gram's stain. These methods had a reported sensitivity of 60 and 45 percent, respectively, when compared to culture, and the sensitivity increased with increasing colony counts. However, two cases of fatal early-onset GBS sepsis occurred in the infants of patients with low colony counts and negative ELISAs.

The definitive diagnosis of invasive disease depends upon the isolation of group B streptococci from a normally sterile body fluid or focal collection. Because of the need to begin empiric therapy before culture results are available, several rapid indirect methods of diagnosing infection have been developed. These methods, which take advantage of the presence of the group B polysaccharide in body fluids (blood, urine, and CSF) that can be detected with use of hyperimmune antiserum, include countercurrent immunoelectrophoresis, latex particle agglutination, staphylococcal co-agglutination, and ELISA, all of which can give results in minutes to hours. Recently, two commercially available systems for

Table 17-2 Antimicrobial Therapy

Condition	Agent(s)	Dose (IV)	Usual Duration
Asymptomatic infection	Treatment not indicated		
Neonatal sepsis	Ampicillin plus gentamicin followed by penicillin G	200 mg/kg/day 2.5 mg/kg q8-12 h 200,000 u/kg/day	Until culture diagnosis 10 Days
Neonatal meningitis	Ampicillin plus gentamicin followed by penicillin G	200-400 mg/kg/day 2.5 mg/kg q8-12 h 200,000-500,000 u/kg/day	Until CSF sterile 14 Days
Neonatal osteomyelitis	Penicillin G	200,000 u/kg/day	4 Weeks
Adult bacteremia/endometritis	Penicillin G*	12 million u/day	10 Days
Adult endocarditis	Penicillin G*	20 million u/day	4 Weeks

*Vancomycin or a first-generation cephalosporin may be used as alternatives for the adult.

latex particle agglutination have become available. Both of these, Wellcogen (Burroughs-Wellcome) and Directigen (Becton-Dickinson), have levels of sensitivity greater than 90 percent, which is comparable to research laboratory techniques when specimens from two sites (urine plus blood or CSF) are measured.[11,93]

Therapy

Group B streptococci have remained universally susceptible to penicillin G, which remains the drug of choice for invasive disease. Because the etiologic agent of neonatal sepsis is rarely known with certainty at the time therapy is initiated, intravenous therapy with a combination of either penicillin G or ampicillin and gentamicin is normally begun when serious infection is suspected in order to treat other potential etiologic agents of neonatal sepsis, mainly enteric gram-negative rods and *Listeria monocytogenes*. GBS is susceptible to penicillin at slightly higher concentrations than group A steptococci; minimal inhibitory concentrations (MICs) are typically in the 0.1 μg per milliliter range but can be as high as 0.4 μg per milliliter. The combination of penicillin or ampicillin and gentamicin provides in vitro synergy against GBS; the minimal bactericidal concentration (MBC) is lower for each agent when the combination is used.[33] Although the clinical significance of this phenomenon has not been established, in theory it may be important when a high inoculum is present or when drug levels may be suboptimal, such as in the CSF. In general, combination therapy is continued until a definitive diagnosis of GBS is made by culture. If therapy appears successful (clearance of CSF, clinical response), the aminoglycoside can be stopped and penicillin continued alone. In instances where positive cultures persist, the combination antimicrobial therapy is continued on theoretical grounds. Tolerance, defined as a higher-than-expected difference between the MBC and MIC, has been described in occasional strains; however, the clinical significance of this characteristic is unknown. Duration of therapy is 10 to 14 days for sepsis or meningitis. Longer durations of therapy, generally 2 to 4 weeks, are used for osteomyelitis and septic arthritis, and 4 weeks for endocarditis.

Several other agents have in vitro activity against group B streptococci, but evidence of their clinical efficacy is limited. Among these, ceftriaxone, cefotaxime,[53] and imipenem[64] achieve significant levels in CSF and might be expected to be clinically useful. However, given the long and successful clinical experience with penicillin G and ampicillin in treating group B streptococcal disease and the scant experience with other agents, alternative therapy should be considered much less desirable. Supportive therapy in a neonatal intensive care unit should be provided for any infant with GBS sepsis, pneumonia, or meningitis. Recommendations for antimicrobial therapy are summarized in Table 17-2.

Pathogenesis

An understanding of the pathogenesis of group B streptococcal infection is beginning to emerge, but many questions remain unanswered. Clearly, invasive neonatal disease depends on exposure to the organism in the vaginal flora and the size of the inoculum. Horizontal transmission of group B streptococcal infection does occur, and nursery outbreaks are occasionally reported. Because only a very small percentage of colonized infants go on to develop invasive disease, there must be other host or bacterial factors that allow for the development of clinically significant disease.

Lancefield and coworkers recognized that type-specific antiserum to the capsular polysaccharide conferred protection against invasive infection with GBS in an animal model,[70] whereas antiserum to the group B polysaccharide did not provide protection. Baker and Kasper demonstrated that the absence of antibody to the polysaccharide capsule correlates with invasive disease in human neonates.[9] Furthermore, type-specific IgG appears to transfer from mother to neonate at levels expected to confer protection. Other experimental evidence for the importance of the capsule in virulence include the findings, both in an animal model[65] and in an in vitro opsonophagocytic assay (MR Wessels, unpublished data), that increased virulence correlates with increased quantitative expression of type III capsule and that capsule-deficient or desialglated isogenic transposon mutants of type III GBS have decreased virulence in model systems.[117] Capsular polysaccharide appears to prevent the effective opsonization of bacteria by preventing the deposition of complement components on the bacterial surface.[37,38] It has been suggested that the terminal sialic acid may be important to virulence because of the resemblance of sialglated polysaccharides to those present in host glycoproteins, thus evoking tolerance to the bacteria.[61] Other bacteria with sialglated polysaccharide capsules such as *E. coli* K1 and *Neisseria meningitidis* types B and C are important causes of disease in humans and are notable causative agents of meningitis.

The C proteins of GBS have also been proposed to play a role in virulence. Payne and colleagues demonstrated that type II strains that express both alpha- and beta-C protein antigens are more resistant to opsonophagocytosis than C protein–negative strains.[86,87] We have found that GBS isolates that express alpha-C protein are more resistant to opsonophagocytic killing than alpha-negative isolates in the absence of specific antibody.[74] The beta-C protein has been shown to bind to human IgA, a fact suggesting a role in colonization of mucosal surfaces or evasion of host immunity.[94]

In contrast to many gram-negative organisms, virulent isolates of GBS are not killed in the presence of serum without polymorphonuclear leukocytes. Thus effective clearance of GBS appears to depend on the presence of type-specific antibody, functioning polymorphonuclear leukocytes, and an intact complement system.[13,99] Any or all of these immune mechanisms may be immature or inadequate in neonates.

Prevention of Disease

The mortality and serious morbidity accompanying neonatal group B streptococcal infection remain unacceptably high, despite improved recognition and therapy. Prevention of group B streptococcal infection is therefore an important goal of current research and practice. Because the risk and mortality of neonatal group B streptococcal infection increase with prematurity, low birth weight, and premature rupture of membranes, high-quality prenatal and obstetric care should decrease the risk of group B streptococcal disease as well as other morbidity. Elimination of asymptomatic carriage of GBS has never been demonstrated efficacious. Efforts at prevention of neonatal group B streptococcal sepsis have therefore been directed at preventing the acquisition of serious infection by the neonate. Two major approaches, chemoprophylaxis and immunoprophylaxis, have been suggested, each with theoretical advantages and limitations.

Chemoprophylaxis

The use of antimicrobial agents to prevent symptomatic infection has been useful in a number of areas, most notably, perhaps, in the prevention of postsurgical bacterial infection. Several strategies have been suggested for antibiotic prophylaxis of invasive group B streptococcal neonatal disease, the first being the elimination or interruption of carriage of GBS by mothers during late pregnancy, which would eliminate exposure of the newborn. Trials of oral penicillin or ampicillin therapy for 2 weeks failed both to eradicate group B streptococcal carriage in 20 to 30 percent of pregnant women[50,51] and to interrupt vertical transmission. Treatment of sexual partners with oral penicillin, in an attempt to prevent exogenous reinfection, did not greatly improve this result. Another small trial that used parenteral penicillin in asymptomatic carriers and their partners had slightly better results, with only 2 of 18 women remaining culture positive.[73] In addition to the poor response rate, another pitfall of this approach is the inability to detect colonization accurately without multiple cultures obtained throughout pregnancy, as discussed previously.

A second strategy has been the prophylactic administration of antimicrobials shortly after birth to neonates at risk for invasive group B streptococcal infection. In a large, randomized trial conducted in the late 1970s and involving more than 16,000 subjects, infants received a single dose of intramuscular penicillin G within 1 hour of birth.[100,101] The reduction in group B streptococcal sepsis relative to a control group (which received topical ocular tetracycline) was greater than 50 percent. However, an unexplained increase in infections caused by penicillin-resistant organisms, mainly gram-negative rods, was noted, and increased mortality in this group more than offset the reduced mortality from group B streptococcal infection. There is also the theoretical concern that because many early-onset group B streptococcal infections begin in utero they might be obscured rather than adequately treated by single-dose antibiotic therapy. Pyati and associates showed that penicillin prophylaxis in infants weighing less than 2 kg failed to lower the incidence or reduce the mortality of GBS early-onset infection.[89]

The most promising chemoprophylactic approach to date is the intrapartum administration of antibiotics to the mother. This approach was first investigated in 1977 by Yow and colleagues,[121] who showed that a single dose of ampicillin administered to pregnant women at the onset of labor effectively blocked the vertical transmission of GBS as assessed by colonization of the newborns. Similar findings were obtained when attempts to eradicate carriage of GBS used antibiotics that were continued until term, effectively maintaining intrapartum levels of antibiotics.[77] Since that time Boyer and others[16-21] have continued to refine this approach to interruption of the vertical transmission of GBS. In the most important and best-conducted study of chemoprophylaxis thus far,[20] colonization of women was detected by culture of vaginal swabs obtained at a single time point during pregnancy; selected women at high risk for delivery of infants with early-onset infection (using such factors as premature labor, prolonged rupture of membranes, or intrapartum fever) were then randomized to treatment with ampicillin versus no treatment. Treatment consisted of a single dose of ampicillin to the mother intrapartum, followed by four additional doses at 12-hour intervals to their babies. Colonization occurred in only 8 of 85 (9 percent) of the infants of treated mothers versus 40 of 79 (51 percent) of those who were untreated. Sepsis was entirely prevented in the neonates of treated women, whereas in the untreated group 5 (6 percent) developed sepsis. There was also a beneficial effect on the rate of postpartum endometritis.

One limitation of this approach is the difficulty in ascertaining the at-risk population: the inadequacy of both one-time culture and rapid diagnostic techniques to detect colonization have been discussed previously. In addition, fully 70 percent of early-onset group B streptococcal infection occurs in term infants, many of whom have no other identifiable risk factors[4] and thus would not receive chemoprophylaxis. Furthermore, a large number of mothers and infants would be exposed to parenteral antibiotics with the attendant risks of allergic reaction, pseudomembranous colitis, and colonization with resistant organisms. Finally, no chemotherapeutic approach currently under consideration is likely to affect the occurrence of late-onset disease.

Immunoprophylaxis

Antibody to the type-specific capsular polysaccharide effectively prevents infection with group B streptococci. This fundamental concept of pathogenesis is the basis of preventing disease through immunologic means. If sufficient levels of protective, type-specific antibody to group B streptococci could be provided to the neonate, group B streptococcal disease would be prevented. Because early-onset B streptococcal disease often begins in utero, this antibody would ideally be provided transplacentally from the mother. Unfortunately, most women of childbearing age do not have endogenous levels of type-specific antibodies to GBS. Efforts in this area have been directed toward inducing such antibodies via immunization with the capsular polysaccharide.

Thus far, the capsular polysaccharide of serotype III has been most extensively evaluated for use as a vaccine. This polysaccharide has been isolated, purified, and characterized as a vaccine in human volunteers. A single subcutaneous dose of 50 μg of capsular polysaccharide has been shown to elicit protective levels of immunity in 60 percent of recipients.[10] To demonstrate that pregnant women would respond similarly, Baker and Kasper showed that the type III polysaccharide was able to elicit protective antibody levels in 63 percent of pregnant women, including 57 percent of those with previously low levels of antibody. They also demonstrated that most of the antibody was IgG and that 80 percent of the infants born to vaccine responders had protective levels of antibody (at least 2 μg per milliliter) at 1 month of age.[10] Because the most important target population for a vaccine is those women who are colonized with GBS but have low levels of type-specific antibody, it has been argued that perhaps this group has a selective inability to respond to immunization.[29] This concern has been addressed by the same investigators[12] who studied immunization in women who had had infants with invasive group B streptococcal infection. They showed that the response to vaccination with type III capsular polysaccharide was similar for these women and a control group of nonimmune women (57.1 and 54.5 percent, respectively).

Since the purified capsular polysaccharides have failed to elicit protective levels of antibody in a substantial minority of recipients, the use of protein-polysaccharide conjugate vaccines has been proposed.[12] These vaccines have the theoretical advantage of eliciting T-cell help in antibody production and thus of improving immunogenicity; conjugate vaccines have been used successfully to improve the efficacy of vaccines for *Haemophilus influenzae* type b in young children. Recently, vaccines composed of purified capsular polysaccharide of type III GBS covalently coupled to tetanus toxoid have been synthesized, tested in animals, and shown to elicit protective antibody in a T cell–dependent manner.[66,115] Similar vaccines composed of oligosaccharides of the type III capsule attached to tetanus toxoid have also been developed and shown to be immunogenic in animals.[83] Although type III GBS is responsible for somewhat more than half of group B streptococcal disease in neonates, a successful vaccination strategy will need to encompass the remaining significant serotypes. Purified capsular polysaccharides to type Ia and II GBS have been tested in human volunteers with response rates of 40 and 88 percent, respectively.[10] Conjugate vaccines employing these polysaccharides are currently under development. An interesting alternative strategy involves the use of a vaccine composed of the type III capsular polysaccharide coupled to a C protein. Such a vaccine, using a single hybrid molecule, could elicit antibody protective against more than 90 percent of clinical GBS isolates. The C protein would serve the dual purposes of acting as a carrier for the polysaccharide in augmenting the immune response and of eliciting protective antibodies to the strains that are not type III, most of which express C proteins. Theoretical disadvantages of active immunization include the failure to protect very premature infants (born prior to transplacental passage of antibody) and the difficulties of fully reaching and immunizing the population at risk, particularly in disadvantaged groups. Nonetheless, this strategy appears the most desirable and will require large-scale clinical trials to document its safety and efficacy.

Whereas active immunization carries the advantage of long-term immunity, passive immunization has also been studied as a strategy for the prevention of GBS infection. This approach would allow the administration of protective antibody to patients not previously immunized or to infants born prior to transplacental antibody acquisition. Type-specific antibody, either monoclonal or from pooled immune serum, could be administered to mothers and/or neonates at risk for GBS infection. Although the use of pooled human intravenous immune globulin (IVIG), and a human monoclonal antibody against GBS have each been shown to prevent GBS infection in neonatal rats,[45,91,97] their efficacy in humans has not been documented.

It is likely that no single type of intervention will eliminate group B streptococcal disease of the newborn. Ultimately, reduction in the mortality and morbidity due to this pathogen will depend on multiple approaches: improved prenatal and obstetric care, better recognition of the population at risk for GBS infection, and a combination of chemotherapeutic and immunologic modalities for the prevention and treatment of invasive group B streptococcal disease.

References

1. Anthony BF, Concepcion NF, Concepcion KF. Human antibody to the group-specific polysac-

charide of group B Streptococcus. J Infect Dis 1985; 151:221–226.
2. Anthony BF, Okada DM. The emergence of group B streptococci in infections of the newborn infant. Annu Rev Med 1977; 28:355–369.
3. Baker CJ. Group B streptococcal infections. Adv Intern Med 1980; 25:475–501.
4. Baker CJ. Group B streptococcal infection in newborns: prevention at last? N Engl J Med 1986; 314:1702–1704.
5. Baker CJ, Barrett FF. Transmission of group B streptococci among parturient women and their neonates. J Pediatr 1973; 83:919–925.
6. Baker CJ, Barrett FF, Gordon RC, Yow MD. Suppurative meningitis due to streptococci of Lancefield group B: a study of 33 infants. J Pediatr 1973; 82:724–729.
7. Baker CJ, Edwards MS. Group B streptococcal infections. In: Remington JS, Klein JO, eds. Infectious diseases of the fetus and newborn. Ed 3. Philadelphia: WB Saunders, 1990:742–811.
8. Baker CJ, Goroff DK, Alpert S, et al. Vaginal colonization with group B streptococcus: a study in college women. J Infect Dis 1977; 135:392–397.
9. Baker CJ, Kasper DL. Correlation of maternal antibody deficiency with susceptibility to neonatal group B streptococcal infection. N Engl J Med 1976; 294:753–756.
10. Baker CJ, Kasper DL. Group B streptococcal vaccines. Rev Infect Dis 1985; 7:458–467.
11. Baker CJ, Rench MA. Commercial latex agglutination for detection of group B streptococcal antigen in body fluids. J Pediatr 1983; 102:393–395.
12. Baker CJ, Rench MA, Kasper DL. Response to type III polysaccharide in women whose infants have had invasive group B streptococcal infection. N Engl J Med 1990; 322:1857–1860.
13. Baltimore RS, Kasper DL, Baker CJ, Goroff DK. Antigenic specificity of opsonophagocytic antibodies in rabbit anti-sera to group B streptococci. J Immunol 1977; 118:673–678.
14. Barton CW, Crowley DC, Uzark K, Dick M. A neonatal survivor of group B beta-hemolytic streptococci endocarditis. Am J Perinatol 1984; 1:214–215.
15. Bayer AS, Chow AW, Anthony BF, Guze LB. Serious infections in adults due to group B streptococci. Clinical and serotypic characterization. Am J Med 1976; 61:498–503.
16. Boyer KM, Gadzala CA, Burd LI, et al. Selective intrapartum chemoprophylaxis of neonatal group B streptococcal early-onset disease. I. Epidemiologic rationale. J Infect Dis 1983; 148:795–801.
17. Boyer KM, Gadzala CA, Kelly PD, Gotoff SP. Selective intrapartum chemoprophylaxis of neonatal group B streptococcal early-onset disease. III. Interruption of mother-to-infant transmission. J Infect Dis 1983; 148:810–816.
18. Boyer KM, Gadzala CA, Kelly PD, et al. Selective intrapartum chemoprophylaxis of neonatal group B streptococcal early-onset disease. II. Predictive value of prenatal cultures. J Infect Dis 1983; 148:802–809.
19. Boyer KM, Gotoff SP. Strategies for chemoprophylaxis of GBS early-onset infections. Antibiot Chemother 1985; 35:267–280.
20. Boyer KM, Gotoff SP. Prevention of early-onset neonatal group B streptococcal disease with selective intrapartum chemoprophylaxis. N Engl J Med 1986; 314:1665–1669.
21. Boyer KM, Gotoff SP. Antimicrobial prophylaxis of neonatal group B streptococcal sepsis. Clin Perinatol 1988; 15:831–850.
22. Brady LJ, Boyle MD. Identification of non-immunoglobulin A-Fc-binding forms and low-molecular-weight secreted forms of the group B streptococcal beta antigen. Infect Immun 1989; 57:1573–1581.
23. Brady LJ, Daphtary UD, Ayoub EM, Boyle MD. Two novel antigens associated with group B streptococci identified by a rapid two-stage radioimmunoassay. J Infect Dis 1988; 158:965–972.
24. Brown JG, Straus DC. Characterization of neuraminidases produced by various serotypes of group B streptococci. Infect Immun 1987; 55:1–6.
25. Carey RB, Eisenstein TK, Shockman GD, et al. Soluble group- and type-specific antigens from type III group B *Streptococcus*. Infect Immun 1980; 28:195–203.
26. Chadwick EG, Shulman ST, Yogev R. Peritonitis as a late manifestation of Group B streptococcal disease in newborns. Pediatr Infect Dis 1983; 2:142–143.
27. Chin KC, Fitzhardinge PM. Sequelae of early-onset group B hemolytic streptococcal neonatal meningitis. J Pediatr 1985; 106:819–822.
28. Christensen KK, Christensen P. The R-proteins. Antibiot Chemother 1985; 35:114–118.
29. Christensen KK, Christensen P, Lindberg A, Linden V. Mothers of infants with neonatal group B streptococcal septicemia are poor responders to bacterial carbohydrate antigens. Int Arch Allergy Appl Immunol 1982; 67:7–12.
30. Christie R, Atkins NE, Munch-Peterson E. A note on a lytic phenomenon shown by group B streptococci. Australian Journal of Experimental Biology and Medical Science 1944; 22:197–200.
31. Chun CS, Brady LJ, Boyle MD, et al. Group B streptococcal C protein–associated antigens: association with neonatal sepsis. J Infect Dis 1991; 163:786–791.
32. Cleat PH, Timmis KN. Cloning and expression in *Escherichia coli* of the Ibc protein genes of group B streptococci: binding of human immunoglobin A to the beta antigen. Infect Immun 1987; 55:1151–1155.
33. Cooper MD, Keeney RE, Lyons SF, Cheatle EL. Synergistic effects of ampicillin-aminoglycoside combinations on group B steptococci. Antimicrob Agents Chemother 1979; 15:484–486.
34. Di Fabio JL, Michon F, Brisson J-R, et al. Structure of the capsular polysaccharide antigen of type IV group B *Streptococcus*. Canadian Journal of Chemistry 1989; 67:877–882.
35. Dillon HJ, Khare S, Gray BM. Group B strepto-

coccal carriage and disease: a 6-year prospective study. J Pediatr 1987; 110:31–36.
36. Edwards MS, Baker CJ, Wagner ML, et al. An etiologic shift in infantile osteomyelitis: the emergence of the group B streptococcus. J Pediatr 1978; 93:578–583.
37. Edwards MS, Kasper DL, Jennings HJ, et al. Capsular sialic acid prevents activation of the alternative complement pathway by type III, group B streptococci. J Immunol 1982; 128:1278–1283.
38. Edwards MS, Nicholson-Weller A, Baker CJ, Kasper DL. The role of specific antibody in alternative complement pathway-mediated opsonophagocytosis of type III, group B *Streptococcus*. J Exp Med 1980; 151:1275–1287.
39. Edwards MS, Rench MA, Haffar AA, et al. Long-term sequelae of group B streptococcal meningitis in infants. J Pediatr 1985; 106:717–722.
40. Facklam RR, Padula JF, Wortham EC, et al. Presumptive identification of group A, B, and D streptococci on agar plate media. J Clin Microbiol 1979; 9:665–672.
41. Faro S. Group B beta-hemolytic streptococci and puerperal infections. Am J Obstet Gynecol 1981; 139:686–689.
42. Feld SM, Harrigan JT. Vaginal gram stain as an immediate detector of group B streptococci in selected obstetric patients. Am J Obstet Gynecol 1987; 156:446–448.
43. Ferrieri P. GBS enzymes, hemolysin, toxins and other products. Antibiot Chemother 1985; 35:57–70.
44. Ferrieri P. Surface-localized protein antigens of group B streptococci. Rev Infect Dis 1988; S363–366.
45. Fischer GW, Hunter KW, Wilson SR. Modified human immune serum globulin for intravenous administration: in vitro opsonic activity and in vivo protection against group B streptococcal disease in suckling rats. Acta Paediatr Scand 1982; 71:639–644.
46. Flores AE, Ferrieri P. Biochemical markers of the penicillin-induced L phase of a group B, type III *Streptococcus* sp. J Clin Microbiol 1983; 18:961–967.
47. Freedman RM, Ingram DL, Gross I, et al. A Half century of neonatal sepsis at Yale: 1928 to 1978. Am J Dis Child 1981; 135:140–144.
48. Fry RM. Fatal infections by haemolytic streptococcus group B. Lancet 1938; 1:199–201.
49. Gallagher PG, Watanakunakorn C. Group B streptococcal bacteremia in a community teaching hospital. Am J Med 1985; 78:795–800.
50. Gardner SE, Yow MD, Leeds LJ, et al. Failure of penicillin to eradicate group B streptococcal colonization in the pregnant woman. A couple study. Am J Obstet Gynecol 1979; 135:1062–1065.
51. Hall RT, Barnes W, Krishnan L, et al. Antibiotic treatment of parturient women colonized with group B streptococci. Am J Obstet Gynecol 1976; 124:630–634.
52. Holls WM, Thomas J, Troyer V. Cervical Gram stain for rapid detection of colonization with beta-streptococcus. Obstet Gynecol 1987; 354–357.
53. Hoogkamp KJ. Activity of cefotaxime and ceftriaxone alone and in combination with penicillin, ampicillin and piperacillin against neonatal meningitis pathogens. J Antimicrob Chemother 1985; 16:327–334.
54. Howard JB, McCracken GJ. The spectrum of group B streptococcal infections in infancy. Am J Dis Child 1974; 128:815–818.
55. Jelinkova J, Motlova J. The nomenclature of GBS. Antibiot Chemother 1985; 35:49–52.
56. Jennings HJ, Katzenellenbogen E, Lugowski C, Kasper DL. Structure of the native polysaccharide antigens of type Ia and type Ib group B Streptococcus. Biochemistry 1983; 22:1258–1263.
57. Jennings HJ, Rosell KG, Katzenellenbogen E, Kasper DL. Structural determination of the capsular polysaccharide antigen of type II group B Streptococcus. J Biol Chem 1983; 258:1793–1798.
58. Jerlstrom PG, Chhatwal GS, Timmis KN. The IgA binding beta antigen of the c protein complex of group B streptococci: sequence determination of its gene and detection of two binding regions. Mol Microbiol 1991; 5:843–849.
59. Johnson DR, Ferrieri P. Group B streptococcal Ibc protein antigen: distribution of two determinants in wild-type strains of common serotypes. J Clin Microbiol 1984; 19:506–510.
60. Jurgens D, Shalaby FY, Fehrenbach FJ. Purification and characterization of CAMP-factor from *Streptococcus agalactiae* by hydrophobic interaction chromatography and chromatofocusing. J Chromatogr 1985; 348:363–370.
61. Kasper DL. Bacterial capsule: old dogmas and new tricks. J Infect Dis 1986; 153:407–415.
62. Kasper DL, Baker CJ. Electron microscopic definition of surface antigens of group B *Streptococcus*. J Infect Dis 1979; 139:147–151.
63. Katzenstein A, Davis C, Braude A. Pulmonary changes in neonatal sepsis due to group B beta-hemolytic streptococcus: relation to hyaline membrane disease. J Infect Dis 1976; 133:430–435.
64. Kim KS. Efficacy of imipenem in experimental group B streptococcal bacteremia and meningitis. Chemotherapy 1985; 31:304–309.
65. Klegerman ME, Boyer KM, Papierniak CK, et al. Type-specific capsular antigen is associated with virulence in late-onset group B streptococcal type III disease. Infect Immun 1984; 44:124–129.
66. Lagergard T, Shiloach J, Robbins JB, Schneerson R. Synthesis and immunological properties of conjugates composed of group B streptococcus type III capsular polysaccharide covalently bound to tetanus toxoid. Infect Immun 1990; 58:687–694.
67. Lancefield RC. A serological differentiation of human and other groups of hemolytic streptococci. J Exp Med 1933; 57:571–595.
68. Lancefield RC. The serological differentiation of

pathogenic and nonpathogenic strains of hemolytic streptococci from parturient women. J Exp Med 1935; 61:335–349.
69. Lancefield RC. Antigens of group B streptococci relation to mouse-protective antibodies and immunity. In: Robbins JB, et al, eds. New approaches for inducing natural immunity to pyogenic organisms. Bethesda, Md: National Institutes of Health, 1975:145–151.
70. Lancefield RC, McCarty M, Everly WN. Multiple mouse-protective antibodies directed against group B streptococci. Special reference to antibodies effective against protein antigens. J Exp Med 1975; 142:165–179.
71. Ledger WJ. Bacterial infections complicating pregnancy. Clin Obstet Gynecol 1978; 21:455–475.
72. Lerner PI, Gopalakrishna KV, Wolinsky K, et al. Group B streptococcus *(S. agalactiae)* bacteremia in adults: analysis of 32 cases and review of the literature. Medicine (Baltimore) 1977; 56:457–473.
73. Lewin EB, Amstey MS. Natural history of group B streptococcus colonization and its therapy during pregnancy. Am J Obstet Gynecol 1981; 139:512–515.
74. Madoff LC, Hori S, Michel JL, et al. Phenotypic diversity in the alpha C protein of group B streptococcus. Infect Immun 1991; 59:2638–2644.
75. Madoff LC, Michel JL, Kasper DL. A monoclonal antibody identifies a protective C-protein alpha-antigen epitope in group B streptococci. Infect Immun 1991; 59:204–210.
76. Marchlewicz BA, Duncan JL. Properties of a hemolysin produced by group B streptococci. Infect Immun 1980; 30:805–813.
77. Merenstein GB, Todd WA, Brown G, et al. Group B beta-hemolytic streptococcus: randomized controlled treatment study at term. Obstet Gynecol 1980; 55:315–318.
78. Michel JL, Madoff LC, Kling DE, et al. Cloned alpha and beta C-protein antigens of group B streptococci elicit protective immunity. Infect Immun 1991; 59:2023–2028.
79. Michon F, Brisson JR, Dell A. Multiantennary group-specific polysaccharide of group B *Streptococcus*. Biochemistry 1988; 27:5341–5351.
80. Michon F, Katzenellenbogen E, Kasper DL, Jennings HJ. Structure of the complex group-specific polysaccharide of group B *Streptococcus*. Biochemistry 1987; 26:476–486.
81. Milligan TW, Baker CJ, Straus DC, Mattingly SJ. Association of elevated levels of extracellular neuraminidase with clinical isolates of type III group B streptococci. Infect Immun 1978; 21:738–746.
82. Opal SM, Cross A, Palmer M, Almazan R. Group B streptococcal sepsis in adults and infants. Contrasts and comparisons. Arch Intern Med 1988; 148:641–645.
83. Paoletti LC, Kasper DL, Michon F, et al. An oligosaccharide-tetanus toxoid conjugate vaccine against type III group B *Streptococcus*. J Biol Chem 1990; 265:18278–18283.
84. Pass MA, Gray BM, Dillon HJ. Puerperal and perinatal infections with group B streptococci. Am J Obstet Gynecol 1982; 143:147–152.
85. Pass MA, Gray BM, Khare S, Dillon HJ. Prospective studies of group B streptococcal infections in infants. J Pediatr 1979; 95:437–438.
86. Payne NR, Ferrieri P. The relation of the Ibc protein antigen to the opsonization differences between strains of type II group B streptococci. J Infect Dis 1985; 151:672–681.
87. Payne NR, Kim YK, Ferrieri P. Effect of differences in antibody and complement requirements on phagocytic uptake and intracellular killing of "c" protein-positive and -negative strains of type II group B streptococci. Infect Immun 1987; 55:1243–1251.
88. Polsky B, Gold JWM, Whimbey E. Bacterial pneumonia in patients with the acquired immunodeficiency syndrome. Ann Intern Med 1986; 104:38–41.
89. Pyati SP, Pildes RS, Jacobs NM, et al. Penicillin in infants weighing two kilograms or less with early-onset group B streptococcal disease. N Engl J Med 1983; 308:1383–1389.
90. Pyati SP, Pildes RS, Ramamurthy RS, Jacobs N. Decreasing mortality in neonates with early-onset group B streptococcal infection: reality or artifact. J Pediatr 1981; 98:625–627.
91. Raff HV, Siscoe PJ, Wolff EA, et al. Human monoclonal antibodies to group B streptococcus. Reactivity and in vivo protection against multiple serotypes. J Exp Med 1988; 168:905–917.
92. Regan JA, Klebanoff MA, Nugent RP. The epidemiology of group B streptococcal colonization in pregnancy: vaginal infections and prematurity study group. Obstet Gynecol 1991; 77:604–610.
93. Rench MA, Metzger TG, Baker CJ. Detection of group B streptococcal antigen in body fluids by a latex-coupled monoclonal antibody assay. J Clin Microbiol 1984; 20:852–854.
94. Russell-Jones GJ, Gotschlich EC, Blake MS. A surface receptor specific for human IgA on group B streptococci possessing the Ibc protein antigen. J Exp Med 1984; 160:1467–1475.
95. Ryan ME, Barrett FF. Rapid detection of group B streptococcal colonization by a direct immunofluorescent antibody technique. J Pediatr 1982; 101:993–995.
96. Sandy EA, Blumenfeld ML, Iams JD. Gram stain in the rapid determination of maternal colonization with group B beta-streptococcus. Obstet Gynecol 1988; 71:796–798.
97. Santos JI, Shigeoka AO, Rote NS, Hill HR. Protective efficacy of a modified immune serum globulin in experimental group B streptococcal infection. J Pediatr 1981; 99:873–879.
98. Schneewind O, Friedrich K, Lutticken R. Cloning and expression of the CAMP factor of group B streptococci in *Escherichia coli*. Infect Immun 1988; 56:2174–2179.
99. Shigeoka AO, Hall RT, Hemming VG, et al. Role of antibody and complement in opsonization of group B streptococci. Infect Immun 1978; 21:34–40.
100. Siegel JD, McCracken GJ, Threlkeld N, et al. Single-dose penicillin prophylaxis against neona-

tal group B streptococcal infections. A controlled trial in 18,738 newborn infants. N Engl J Med 1980; 303:769–775.
101. Siegel JD, McCracken GJ, Threlkeld N, et al. Single-dose penicillin prophylaxis of neonatal group-B-streptococcal disease. Lancet 1982; 1:1426–1430.
102. Stiller RJ, Blair E, Clark P, Tinghitella T. Rapid detection of vaginal colonization with group B streptococci by means of latex agglutination. Am J Obstet Gynecol 1989; 160:566–568.
103. St Laurent Gagnon T, Weber ML. Urinary tract streptococcus group B infection in a 6-week-old infant. JAMA 1978; 240:1269.
104. Stringer J. The development of a phage-typing system for group-B streptococci. J Med Microbiol 1980; 13:133–143.
105. Stringer J, Maxted WR. Phage typing of group B streptococci (letter). Lancet 1979; 1:328.
106. Sutton GP, Smirz LR, Clark DH, Bennett JE. Group B streptococcal necrotizing fasciitis arising from an episiotomy. Obstet Gynecol 1985; 66:733–736.
107. Teres FO, Matorras R, Perea AG, et al. Prevention of neonatal group B streptococcal sepsis. Pediatr Infect Dis J 1987; 6:874.
108. Towers CV, Garite TJ, Friedman WW, et al. Comparison of a rapid enzyme-linked immunosorbent assay test and the Gram stain for detection of group B streptococcus in high-risk antepartum patients. Am J Obstet Gynecol 1990; 163:965–967.
109. Verghese A, Berk SL, Boelen LJ, Smith JK. Group B streptococcal pneumonia in the elderly. Arch Intern Med 1982; 142:1642–1645.
110. Wagner M, Wagner B, Kubin VR. Immunoelectron microscopic study of the location of group-specific and type-specific polysaccharide antigens on isolated walls of group B streptococci. J Gen Microbiol 1980; 369–376.
111. Walsh JA, Hutchins S. Group B streptococcal disease: its importance in the developing world and prospect for prevention with vaccines. Pediatr Infect Dis J 1989; 8:271–277.
112. Weiser JN, Rubens CE. Transposon mutagenesis of group B streptococcus beta-hemolysin biosynthesis. Infect Immun 1987; 55:2314–2316.
113. Wessels MR, DiFabio JL, Benedi V-J, et al. Structural determination and immonochemical characterization of the type V group B *Streptococcus* capsular polysaccharide. J Biol Chem 1991; 266:6714–6719.
114. Wessels MR, Kasper DL. Molecular size affects antigenicity of type III, group B *Streptococcus* capsular polysaccharide. Trans Assoc Am Physicians 1985; 98:384–391.
115. Wessels MR, Paoletti LC, Kasper DL, et al. Immunogenicity in animals of a polysaccharide-protein conjugate vaccine against type III group B *Streptococcus*. J Clin Invest 1990; 86:1428–1433.
116. Wessels MR, Pozsgay V, Kasper DL, Jennings HJ. Structure and immunochemistry of an oligosaccharide repeating unit of the capsular polysaccharide of type III group B *Streptococcus*. A revised structure for the type III group B streptococcal polysaccharide antigen. J Biol Chem 1987; 262:8262–8267.
117. Wessels MR, Rubens CE, Benedi VJ, Kasper DL. Definition of a bacterial virulence factor: sialylation of the group B streptococcal capsule. Proc Natl Acad Sci U S A 1989; 86:8983–8987.
118. Wilkinson HW. Group B streptococcal infection in humans. Annu Rev Microbiol 1978; 32:41–57.
119. Wilkinson HW, Eagon RG. Type-specific antigens of group B streptococcus. Infect Immun 1971; 4:596–604.
120. Yow MD, Leeds LJ, Thompson PK, et al. The natural history of group B streptococcal colonization in the pregnant woman and her offspring. I. Colonization studies. Am J Obstet Gynecol 1980; 137:34–38.
121. Yow MD, Mason EO, Leeds LJ, et al. Ampicillin prevents intrapartum transmission of group B streptococcus. JAMA 1979; 241:1245–1247.

CHAPTER 18

Urinary Tract Infections

Susan M. Cox, M.D.
F. Gary Cunningham, M.D.

Urinary tract infections, including asymptomatic bacteriuria, cystitis, and acute pyelonephritis, are the most common bacterial infections that complicate pregnancy. Their significance has become apparent over the last 30 years; realization of their impact followed the original work of Edward Kass, who in 1960[35] reported that 40 percent of pregnant women with untreated asymptomatic bacteriuria developed pyelonephritis. This observation led to studies that demonstrated that eradication of bacteriuria decreased this complication significantly and represents one of the more important contributions to preventive medicine. Kass[36] also reported that the incidence of low-birth-weight infants was increased in women with bacteriuria and that eradication of silent infection reduced the frequency of this complication. The latter finding has been the subject of considerable debate,[69] as have the associations of bacteriuria with anemia and pregnancy-induced hypertension.

The purpose of this chapter, which is dedicated to the late Dr. Kass, is to review current concepts, clinical presentation, diagnosis, evaluation, and treatment of urinary infections during pregnancy.

Epidemiology

Incidence

Urinary tract infections are more common in women than in men, and approximately 15 percent of women experience at least one infection during their lifetime.[37,52] In females, bacteriuria acquisition begins early in life, and 5 percent of high school girls[40] and 8 percent of nulliparous married women[56] have bacteriuria. The increased incidence in women is largely explained by the anatomic differences between the sexes.

Etiology

The female urethra is approximately 3 to 4 cm in length, with its external opening in close proximity to the vaginal canal, which in turn borders the anus and rectum. The vagina is normally colonized with organisms from the lower gastrointestinal tract, and the distal urethra frequently is colonized with these potential uropathogens.[6,7,23,29] Enterobacteriaceae, especially *Escherichia coli, Klebsiella,* and *Enterobacter* account for 85 to 90 percent of urinary infections during pregnancy. Most recurrent infections in young women are caused by *E. coli,* and Fowler and Stamey[18] have shown that these women are likely to have introital colonization with bacteria capable of adherence. Other organisms, including *Citrobacter, Proteus,* and *Pseudomonas* spp., are uncommon urinary tract pathogens during pregnancy.

Associations

A number of factors during pregnancy are associated with the development of symptomatic urinary infection. Paramount among these is asymptomatic, or covert, bacteriuria, which is identified in 2 to 10 percent of pregnant women.[64] Whalley reported that when bacteriuria is identified during pregnancy, it is almost invariably present at the first prenatal visit, and fewer than 1 percent of women with sterile screening cultures acquire bacteriuria during pregnancy. About two-thirds of cases of acute pyelonephritis during pregnancy are in women with preexisting bacteriuria, whereas the other third are in women who did not have bacteriuria when tested earlier during pregnancy.[20] Although the pathogenesis of asymptomatic bacteriuria is probably the same in pregnant and nonpregnant women, the former are much more likely to develop symptomatic infection. The pathogenesis of acute cystitis is not clear, although it is presumed that these infections are related in part to ascending bacterial contamination. Factors associated with acute pyelonephritis during pregnancy include physiologic urinary tract obstruction, which leads to stasis. Hydroureter and hydronephrosis are thought to be caused principally by mechanical compression from the enlarging uterus, but smooth-muscle relaxation induced by progesterone may also play a role. Although their significance is not known for certain, pregnancy-induced glucosuria and aminoaciduria provide an excellent milieu for bacterial proliferation.

Another important component in the pathogenesis of symptomatic infection is that of bacterial virulence. Indeed, "virulence factors" may explain why some women with covert infections develop symptomatic infections and others do not. The capacity of some pathogens to adhere to uroepithelium is considered an important factor related to bacterial virulence. Bacterial adherence is mediated by adhesins located on the cell surface. Different strains of uropathogenic *E. coli* express combinations of surface adhesins known as *pili* or *fimbriae*.[60] These adhesins reversibly bind to oligosaccharide receptors on the surface of different cell types, including erythrocytes and uroepithelial cells. Most *E. coli* express so-called type I pili, which bind to the mannose-containing mucin of uroepithelial cells.[16,49] However, such binding results in poor attachment, and these bacteria are effectively washed out of the urinary tract along with mucin. It is thus not surprising that these type I pili are not strongly associated as a virulence factor for symptomatic infections.

More recently, other adhesins called *P-fimbriae* were described. They specifically bind to the disaccharide galactose-alpha-(1-4)-galactose-beta component of globoseries glycolipids.[31,42] These glycolipids serve as receptors on the uroepithelial cell surface, and they are virulence markers for urinary infections.[14,17,32,44,45,59,62] Whereas P-fimbriae are expressed on only 10 to 20 percent of *E. coli* strains isolated from women with cystitis or asymptomatic bacteriuria,[32,63] nearly 90 percent of strains that cause acute nonobstructive pyelonephritis express P-fimbriae.[14,17,32,44,45] The exact role that bacterial adherence has in the pathogenesis of urinary infections during pregnancy is unclear at this time; however, Stenquist and colleagues[59] report a preponderance of P-fimbriated *E. coli* in pregnant women with acute pyelonephritis compared with *E. coli* isolated from women with asymptomatic bacteriuria.

Asymptomatic Bacteriuria

Definition

Asymptomatic bacteriuria is defined by persistent, actively multiplying bacteria within the urinary tract in the absence of specific symptoms. Because pregnancy does not predispose bacteriuria acquisition, its prevalence essentially is the same in both pregnant and nonpregnant women. The incidence of bacteriuria during pregnancy approximates 5 to 6 percent but may be as high as 10 percent in high-risk populations.[64] Prevalence generally is dependent on socioeconomic status, and the incidence is higher in indigent than in other women.[62] Neither race nor ethnic background had been linked to bacteriuria,[62,64] and most studies have not demonstrated significant differences in bacteriuria incidence between black and white women when socioeconomic status was controlled. Other conditions unequivocally associated with an increased frequency of covert bacteriuria, in both pregnant and nonpregnant women, include diabetes and sickle-cell trait.[64] The association of age and parity with pregnancy bacteriuria is unclear.

Clinical Significance

Asymptomatic bacteriuria in nonpregnant women carries minimal health risks, and thus it is neither necessary nor cost-effective to perform routine screening. To the contrary, during pregnancy covert bacteriuria clearly represents a significant health risk, and most recommend that screening be performed. As discussed, although pregnancy per se does not predispose to bacteriuria acquisition, it does predispose to acute pyelonephritis if bacteriuria exists. It has been well established that about a third of pregnant women with untreated covert infection develop acute pyelonephritis.[64] Fortunately, bacteriuria eradication during pregnancy reduces the incidence of pyelonephritis to 3 to 4 percent.[64]

Other than acute symptomatic infection, adverse effects that have been attributed to bacteriuria in pregnancy are controversial. Some of these complications include anemia, pregnancy-induced hypertension, preterm labor, and low-birth-weight infants.[36] In a prospective study, Gilstrap and coworkers[22] compared these outcomes in bacteriuric women with those of nonbacteriuric controls to determine whether covert infection was associated with adverse sequelae. Although, as shown in Table 18-1, they documented no increased incidence of adverse sequelae, salutary effects of bacteriuria treatment could not be quantified. Certainly, significant controversy continues to surround the association between bacteriuria and preterm birth.

Diagnosis

Because by definition these women have no symptoms, asymptomatic bacteriuria is identified by demonstrating significant bacteriuria. Kass[33] developed the

Table 18-1 Adverse Pregnancy Outcomes

Pregnancy Complication	Bacteriuria RENAL (%) (N = 114)	Bacteriuria BLADDER (%) (N = 134)	No Infection (%) (N = 248)
Hematocrit less than 30	2.6	3.7	2.1
Hypertension	12	15	14
Low-birth-weight infants	10	13	13
Fetal growth retardation	8	8	8
Preterm delivery	4	8	5

From Gilstrap et al. 1986.[21]

Table 18-2 Antimicrobial Agents Commonly Used to Treat Asymptomatic Bacteriuria During Pregnancy

Sulfonamides	500 mg four times daily
Nitrofurantoin	50-100 mg four times daily
Cephalosporins	250 mg four times daily
Ampicillin	250 mg four times daily
Nitrofurantoin	100 mg daily at bedtime

most commonly accepted definition of significant bacteriuria as the presence of at least 100,000 colonies of a single uropathogen per milliliter of urine. The most frequently used collection method is the midstream clean-catch technique. The accuracy of a single culture obtained via this technique is about 80 percent, compared with 96 percent when urine is obtained by catheterization.[34-36] Unless obtained by catheterization, counts of less than 100,000 organisms per milliliter or specimens that contain more than one organism are generally thought to represent contamination. Recently, however, Stamm and colleagues[58] reported that lower colony counts also may represent active infection, and this has been our experience.

Urinary screening should be performed at the initial prenatal visit. Because only about 1 percent of women acquire bacteriuria during pregnancy, repeat cultures later are unnecessary.

Treatment

Numerous antimicrobial agents have been proven safe and effective to treat asymptomatic pregnancy bacteriuria. Most of these regimens utilize Food and Drug Administration (FDA) category B drugs as those shown in Table 18-2. Although no one regimen is necessarily best for all patients, a simple regimen with which we have considerable experience is nitrofurantoin 100 mg given orally once a day at bedtime for 10 days. It has been shown as effective as ampicillin, sulfamethoxazole, or cephalexin given four times daily for 21 days. Various single-dose regimens have also been investigated during pregnancy, and success rates ranged from 50 to 88 percent.[3,28,30,46] Although such cure rates are helpful for poorly compliant women, a more efficacious regimen is preferred.

For women with recurrent or persistent infections following therapy, continuous bacterial suppression with an antimicrobial for the remainder of pregnancy should be considered. A useful regimen for this is nitrofurantoin, 100 mg given at bedtime.

Follow-up

Regardless of the antimicrobial agent selected or the duration of therapy—unless continuous—approximately one-third of bacteriuric women experience either persistent or recurrent infection during pregnancy. Thus, after initial treatment, it is important to perform follow-up urine cultures. For those women with persistent or recurrent episodes of bacteriuria, suppressive therapy can be given as outlined previously.

Cystitis

Despite the numerous studies concerning asymptomatic bacteriuria and acute pyelonephritis during pregnancy, there is a paucity of information that addresses acute cystitis and pregnancy. During a 6-year period, Harris and Gilstrap[27] reported 126 cases of cystitis out of 9,734 deliveries for an incidence of 1.3 percent. Others have reported cystitis in as few as 0.3 percent of pregnant women.[59] Importantly, two-thirds of women with acute cystitis initially had sterile urine cultures,[27] and therefore cystitis frequently appears to arise de novo in most pregnant women.

Clinical Significance

Although there is no evidence that acute cystitis is associated with an increased risk of acute pyelonephritis, because nearly 40 percent of women with acute pyelonephritis have accompanying cystitis symptoms, we as-

Table 18-3 Common Symptoms in Pregnant Women with Acute Cystitis

Dysuria—most reliable
Urgency
Frequency
Suprapubic discomfort

sume that they are related. Other adverse pregnancy effects such as hypertension, anemia, or preterm labor have not been causally related.

Although one might expect that risk and complications of acute cystitis, including pyelonephritis, would be similar for bacteriuria during pregnancy, this may not be the case. During a surveillance program to eradicate bacteriuria in pregnancy, Harris and Gilstrap[27] found a marked reduction in the incidence of pyelonephritis, but none was noted with cystitis. They also localized the site of bacteriuria with antibody-coated bacteria and found that bacteria recovered from women with acute cystitis were localized to the bladder in 95 percent of cases. They concluded that cystitis in pregnant women was a different entity from either asymptomatic bacteriuria or pyelonephritis.

Diagnosis

Women with acute cystitis during pregnancy have the same signs and symptoms as nonpregnant patients (Table 18-3). Unfortunately, urinary frequency, urgency, and suprapubic discomfort are common in pregnant women without infection. The diagnosis of cystitis during pregnancy is based on either significant dysuria or gross hematuria, along with a positive urine culture and no systemic symptoms. Signs of upper urinary tract involvement, such as costovertebral angle pain and tenderness, are invariably absent. Fever or other systemic signs signal renal involvement.

Urinalysis usually shows microscopic pyuria and bacteriuria. However, the diagnostic gold standard is a positive urine culture because 10 to 15 percent of pregnant women without infection may manifest pyuria. *Escherichia coli* is the most common uropathogen isolated from these women. Other pathogens include *Proteus mirabilis, Klebsiella pneumoniae,* and occasionally *Streptococcus agalactiae*.[47,68]

Treatment and Follow-up

Pregnant women with acute cystitis can be treated with oral antimicrobials as outpatients and have an excellent response to any of the several regimens described for treatment of bacteriuria in Table 18-2. The length of therapy is generally 5 to 7 days; however, a shorter course of therapy is reasonable. A number of investigators recommend single-dose antimicrobials for acute cystitis during pregnancy. Amoxicillin, 3 g orally with 1 g of probenecid, or trimethoprim (480 mg) and sulfamethoxazole (2.4 g) orally have reported cure rates of nearly 90 percent. Although these regimens are cost-effective and safe, we are reluctant to recommend single-dose therapy for pregnant women at present because if these regimens fail the woman may develop pyelonephritis. The patient may actually have early pyelonephritis at the time of initial therapy. Thus we recommend that pregnant women with acute cystitis be treated for at least 3 days.

Harris and Gilstrap[27] reported that 18 percent of women with acute cystitis subsequently had recurrently positive urine cultures during pregnancy. Because the majority of these women were asymptomatic, follow-up cultures are recommended.

Acute Pyelonephritis

Antepartum pyelonephritis is identified in 1 to 2 percent of all pregnancies and is the most common serious medical complication of pregnancy.[20] In the United States in 1985, more than 85,000 pregnant women were hospitalized for this complication. The population incidence varies and depends on the prevalence of asymptomatic bacteriuria and on whether treatment is given. In untreated populations, two-thirds of cases arise from women with preexisting bacteriuria while one-third are in women who do not have bacteriuria early in pregnancy. The reported incidence of pyelonephritis has decreased subsequently over the last 20 years largely because of the widespread acceptance of screening for bacteriuria. At Wilford Hall USAF Hospital, Harris[25] reported a decrease from 4 percent to 0.8 percent during a 20-year period. He attributed this decline to the identification and eradication of bacteriuria as well as to frequent culture follow-up. At Parkland Hospital, 80 percent of women attend antenatal clinics, and bacteriologic screening of the urine is routine. For nearly 30 years, 8 percent of these women have had asymptomatic bacteriuria, and for at least 20 years, treatment has been initiated promptly. Prior to the introduction of screening, nearly 3 percent of pregnancies at our hospital were complicated by pyelonephritis; however, universal screening and treatment for bacteriuria has reduced this incidence to about 1 percent.

Associations

Pregnancy significantly increases the risk of developing acute pyelonephritis. As discussed, the principal reason for this predisposition is obstructive uropathy with resultant urine stasis. Late in pregnancy there is a pressure gradient of approximately 15 ml of water between the lower and upper ureter.[21] Although antepartum pyelonephritis is associated with several predisposing factors previously reviewed, preexisting asymptomatic bacteriuria is a prime concern.

Clinical Findings

The majority of cases of acute pyelonephritis occur during the second and third trimesters.[11,20] In a review of 656 obstetric patients with pyelonephritis from our hospital, Gilstrap and colleagues[20] reported that 73 percent were identified antepartum, 19 percent postpartum, and 8 percent intrapartum. Of the 482 antepartum cases, 9 percent were identified during the first trimester, and the remainder were evenly divided between the second and third trimesters. The higher incidence of pyelonephritis later in pregnancy is related to increasing urinary obstruction as pregnancy progresses.

Signs and symptoms of pyelonephritis are shown in Table 18-4. They include fever, chills, nausea and vomiting, and costovertebral angle tenderness. Nearly 40 percent of women also complain of lower urinary tract symptoms such as urgency, frequency, and dysuria. Fever may be quite high, reaching 40°C in many women, and is generally spiking in nature. In the 656 women from Parkland Hospital,[20] 85 percent had a temperature of at least 38°C (100.4°F) and 12 percent had temperatures higher than 40°C (104°F). Moreover, 54 percent had right-sided costovertebral tenderness, 27 percent had bilateral tenderness, and 16 percent had left-sided tenderness.

Diagnosis

Acute pyelonephritis is diagnosed primarily by systemic signs and symptoms, along with a positive urine culture that invariably yields more than 100,000 colonies per milliliter of a single organism (Table 18-5). Blood cultures are positive in approximately 15 percent of cases. Cultures may be negative because urinary tract infections tend to recur and woman may take leftover medications when they feel an infection may be beginning. Even a single oral dose of an antibiotic may render the urine culture negative.

Treatment

General guidelines for the management of pregnant women with pyelonephritis are summarized in Table 18-6. These women should be hospitalized for close observation. They frequently have severe nausea, vomiting, and anorexia combined with fever that leads to significant dehydration. Careful monitoring is necessary to detect life-threatening complications, and close observation with frequent assessment of vital signs is central to the care of these women.

Initial treatment is directed toward restoration of the contracted blood volume. Administration of intravenous crystalloids, either physiologic saline or lactated Ringer's solution, along with antimicrobial agents is essential. Initially, fluids are given rapidly in order to establish a urinary output of at least 30 to 50 ml per hour. Laboratory assessment should include a complete blood cell count, serum electrolytes, and creatinine, as well as urine and blood cultures. Additional laboratory work usually is unnecessary at this time unless the diagnosis is uncertain or the woman develops a complication.

The choice of antimicrobial agent is empiric; however, in women who have had a previous urinary tract infection or asymptomatic bacteriuria during pregnancy, prior in vitro sensitivities may be used to select therapy. At our hospital for the last 20 years, ampicillin was used successfully for treatment of uncomplicated pyelonephritis. However, during the past decade many uropathogens that cause community-acquired pyelonephritis have been found resistant to ampicillin by in vitro sensitivities. Additionally, Duff[15] reported therapeutic failures thought to be due to resistant organisms in 27 percent of 131 women treated with ampicillin alone.

Concerns for the increasing ampicillin resistance of bacteria that cause these infections have prompted many investigators to add an aminoglycoside for treatment of those women. This procedure is worrisome because 20 percent have transient renal dysfunction resulting from the infection itself. Additionally, in pregnant women without renal dysfunction, therapeutic aminoglycoside levels are not easily obtained with standard formulas. Finally, synergistic nephrotoxicity from endotoxin and aminoglycoside is of particular concern with such therapy. We perform serial monitoring of serum creatinine, but some investigators recommend measurement of peak and trough aminoglycoside concentrations.[15] For cost-effectiveness, simplicity, and for reasons outlined previously, therapy with a single agent that is deemed to be safe during pregnancy is preferable. The extended-

Table 18-4 Clinical Presentation of Pregnant Women with Acute Pyelonephritis

Fever
Chills
Nausea and vomiting
Lower urinary tract symptoms
Costovertebral angle tenderness

Table 18-5 Bacteria Most Commonly Isolated from Pregnant Women with Pyelonephritis

E. coli	77%
Klebsiella-Enterobacter	15%
Proteus spp.	4%
Other genera	4%

Adapted from Cox SM and Cunningham FG. 1988.[8]

Table 18-6 Guidelines for the Management of Pregnant Women with Acute Pyelonephritis

Hospitalization
Intravenous fluid hydration
Intravenous antimicrobials
Frequent monitoring of urine output and vital signs
Urine and blood cultures
Complete blood count and serum creatinine

spectrum penicillins are ideally suited for these ill women. The ureidopenicillins, mezlocillin and piperacillin, are broad-spectrum, semisynthetic, penicillinase-resistant penicillins that are classified as FDA category B and are thus relatively safe for use during pregnancy. We recently treated more than 190 women with these penicillins, and the cure rate exceeded 95 percent.[7] Moreover, we identified no adverse maternal or fetal outcomes attributable to these drugs. In only a small percentage of these patients was the addition of an aminoglycoside considered necessary. Guidelines for adding aminoglycoside to primary therapy include a follow-up positive urine culture 24 hours after initiation of antibiotics, poor clinical response after 72 hours of therapy, evidence of continuing sepsis, previous screening cultures showing resistance to penicillin or cephalosporins, and recurrent disease.

Recurrent Pyelonephritis

Recurrent pyelonephritis is common during the same pregnancy. Gilstrap and coworkers[20] reported it to be 23 percent, half occurring antepartum and the remainder postpartum. In their earlier report, Harris and Gilstrap[26] reported a recurrence rate of about 20 percent. In general, the same organisms that caused the initial episode of pyelonephritis caused the subsequent infection. As indicated, it is often helpful to review the culture and sensitivity report from the initial infection. Harris and Gilstrap[26] found that when women with acute pyelonephritis were treated with suppressive antimicrobial therapy for the remainder of the pregnancy, the recurrence rate was only 2.7 percent, compared to 60 percent in nonsuppressed patients. Although Cunningham and associates[11] reported an incidence of 10 percent for recurrent pyelonephritis, they found that 30 percent of their patients had a subsequent positive urine culture.

These data indicate that the pregnant woman who is not given antimicrobial suppression is at substantial risk for recurrent infection, either asymptomatic bacteriuria or acute pyelonephritis. Monitoring of urine cultures is therefore recommended for those women not maintained on suppressive therapy. An effective, relatively inexpensive suppression regimen utilized at Parkland Memorial Hospital is nitrofurantoin, 50 to 100 mg once daily at bedtime. Protracted suppressive therapy with other antibiotics, such as ampicillin or cephalosporins, generally is not recommended because these agents may induce increased resistance.

Response to Treatment

With appropriate intravenous hydration and antimicrobial treatment, pregnant women with pyelonephritis usually show rapid clinical improvement. Cunningham and colleagues[11] have shown that 85 percent of women with pyelonephritis who were given ampicillin, cephalothin, or chloramphenicol were afebrile after 48 hours. From our recent experiences at Parkland Hospital,[8] of 190 women given either piperacillin or mezlocillin, almost 80 percent were clinically well after 48 hours, and only 4 percent required parenteral therapy for longer than 96 hours. Failure to improve within the first 2 to 3 days suggests a complication that is frequently associated with underlying obstruction, such as urolithiasis or an anatomic anomaly.

Evaluation of Nonresponders

In the absence of a prompt clinical response, women with pyelonephritis should be evaluated for urinary tract obstruction. In many cases, it is caused by renal calculi, but some women have serious sequelae without any evidence for obstruction.[51] If obstruction is identified, passage of a double-J ureteral stent usually relieves it;[38,50] if the stent fails, surgical removal of the stones usually is followed by rapid resolution of infection.

For the woman who remains substantively febrile after 72 hours of appropriate therapy, a plain abdominal radiograph is indicated because nearly 90 percent of renal stones are radiopaque. Possible benefits far outweigh any minimal fetal risk from radiation exposure. If negative, then intravenous pyelography, modified by the number of radiographs taken after contrast injection, usually provides adequate imaging of the collecting system so that stones or structural anomalies can be detected. Occasionally a second or even a third x-ray examination may be indicated. In some women, there is nonvisualization of the collecting tract with intravenous pyelography, and further workup is necessary. Retrograde pyelography may disclose an end-stage obstructed kidney with pyonephrosis as a cause of continuing sepsis. In these cases, calculi frequently coexist, and removal of the infected kidney may be lifesaving.

Some physicians prefer renal sonography to detect underlying lesions.[5] Pyelocaliceal dilatation, urinary calculi, and possibly an intrarenal or perinephric abscess may be visualized. In our experience, sonar has not always been successful in localizing these lesions, and a negative examination is not reason to cease the workup of a woman with continuing urosepsis.

Although the procedure is promising, we have had little experience with computed tomography images taken at the kidney level. Its use is encouraged if a perinephric abscess is suspected. Finally, magnetic resonance imaging techniques can be used to characterize these lesions. It is probably safe, but not widely available.

Complications of Pyelonephritis

Acute pyelonephritis during pregnancy can be devastating, both for the mother and her fetus. Approximately 25 percent of women with severe infection demonstrate clinical evidence of multiple organ system derangement.[21] These complications are more common in women who appear clinically ill or "toxic" and are apparently mediated by bacterial endotoxin or lipopolysaccharide (LPS).

Septicemic Shock

Although up to 15 percent of women with severe antepartum pyelonephritis have bacteremia, fortunately, septic shock is rare. Hypotension and diminished per-

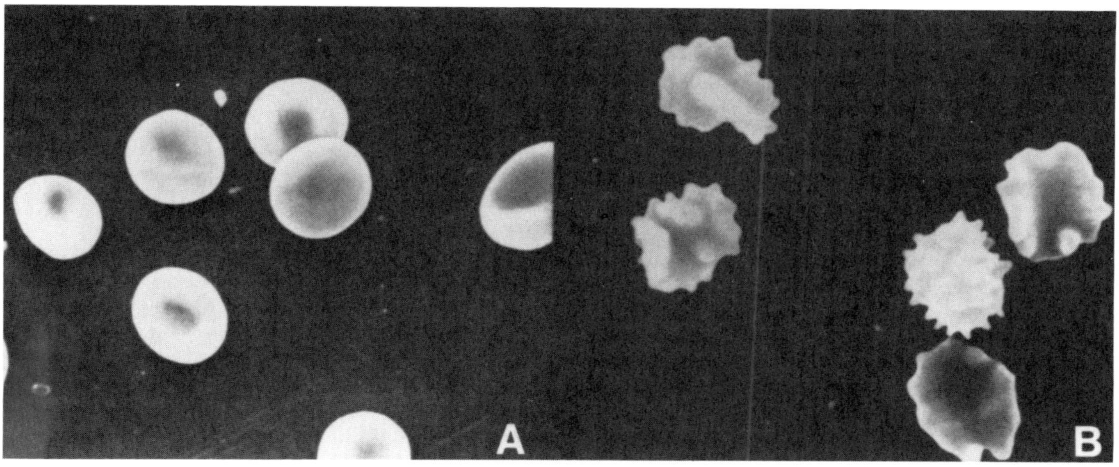

Figure 18-1 A, Scanning electron microscopy of peripheral blood taken from a woman at the time of admission for acute antepartum pyelonephritis. Normal discocytes shown constituted 97 percent of the erythrocytes. **B,** Peripheral blood from the same woman 24 hours later and showing echinocytes that constituted 7 percent of erythrocytes (schistocytes were noted in 6 percent).

fusion as a consequence of endotoxemia must be differentiated from hypotension caused by dehydration from nausea, vomiting, and fever. Even though many of these women have other evidence of endotoxemia, only a few have continuing evidence of hypotension after fluid resuscitation. In women who are severely ill with septicemia, capillary endothelial damage and severely diminished systemic vascular resistance with low cardiac output are the full-blown clinical manifestations. Generally cardiac output is restored with aggressive intravenous fluid resuscitation, and vasopressor drugs are rarely required.

Renal Dysfunction

In a prospective study of 220 women with antepartum pyelonephritis, 25 percent had seriously diminished glomerular filtration rates defined by a creatinine clearance of less than 80 ml per minute.[65] Pragmatically, renal dysfunction is identified when the serum creatinine concentration exceeds 1 mg per deciliter after hydration.[8] Renal dysfunction usually is transient and returns to normal within several days. It is thought that these pathologic changes are mediated by LPS, which is known to be nephrotoxic. Management includes observation with continued intravenous fluids and antimicrobials and with serial monitoring of serum creatinine levels. Attention should be given to selection of antimicrobials that have no nephrotoxicity or to appropriate reduction in the dosage of those that do.

Hematologic Changes

Although hematologic aberrations with acute pyelonephritis have been reported, they are seldom of clinical importance. Although there is abundant evidence that endotoxemia causes hemolysis that may result in moderate to severe anemia, erythrocyte transfusions are seldom indicated. Cox and Cunningham[8] reported that 25 percent of pregnant women with pyelonephritis had anemia as defined by a hematocrit less than 30 percent. Further studies have shown that anemia is accompanied by alterations in erythrocyte morphology, and the subsequent echinocytosis (Fig. 18-1) is also thought to be caused by LPS.[9]

Overt severe thrombocytopenia is an uncommon manifestation in these women; when it does occur, however, it is an ominous finding.[24] Rarely, endotoxin may activate the coagulation cascade to produce clinically apparent disseminated intravascular coagulation. Women in whom this develops are usually seriously ill, and treatment for consumptive coagulopathy is directed toward eliminating the focus of infection.

Pulmonary Injury

Perhaps 2 percent of women with severe pyelonephritis develop some manifestation of respiratory insufficiency.[10] Endotoxin alters the permeability of the alveolar-capillary membrane, with subsequent development of pulmonary edema.[1,5] Pulmonary injury is clinically similar to other variants of adult respiratory distress syndrome (Fig. 18-2). Fortunately, in most women with antepartum pyelonephritis, clinical aberrations are transient and respond to increased oxygen delivered by face mask. Occasionally, however, tracheal intubation with mechanical ventilation and positive end-expiratory pressure is required. Thus, in addition to close monitoring of blood pressure, pulse, and urinary output, attention must be given to the respiratory rate and development of dyspnea. Tachypnea should be promptly investigated by chest radiograph and arterial blood gas analysis. Prompt recognition and appropriate respiratory therapy ought to prevent the severe hypoxemia that may cause fetal death or preterm labor.

Pulmonary injury, like other endotoxin-mediated complications, frequently coexists with evidence of other

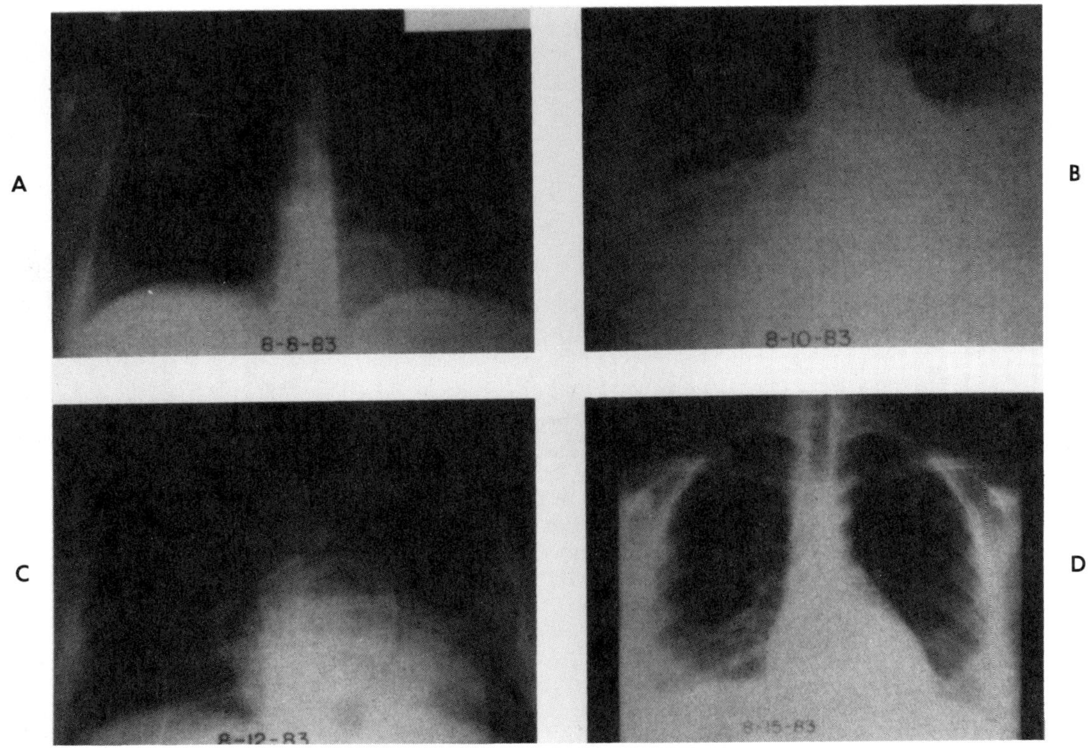

Figure 18-2 **A,** An 18-year-old multipara at 20 weeks' gestation had a normal radiograph at admission on September 8, 1983. **B,** Respiratory distress 20 hours later was accompanied by a left-sided pulmonary infiltrate, which progressed to bilateral infiltrates on September 10, despite normal cardiovascular function. **C** and **D,** The infiltrates improved, and she had a normal x-ray film by September 12. (From Cunningham FG, Lucas MJ, Hankins GDV. 1987.[10])

organ injury. For example, it is not unusual for a woman with evidence of pulmonary capillary injury to have associated hematologic aberrations, renal dysfunction, or other abnormalities. Moreover, these symptoms are more likely in women with proven bacteremia and those with infections caused by *K. pneumoniae*.

Hypothalamic Instability

Pregnant women with acute pyelonephritis frequently show wide ranges of daily temperature. Fever as high as 104°F may be followed by periods of hypothermia. This aberration is mediated by endotoxin effects. The LPS of bacterial endotoxin is a potent exogenous pyrogen,[4,54] and very small quantities are capable of producing a febrile response.[48,67] The resulting increase in body temperature results from an alteration in the set point of the thermoregulatory center in the hypothalamus.[12] This effect of bacterial endotoxin on the hypothalamic thermoregulatory center is complex and appears to be mediated via both a direct exogenous pyrogenic action and an indirect mechanism that involves endotoxin-stimulated host cell release of various endogenous pyrogens, such as interleukin-1, tumor necrosis factor, interleukin-6, and interferon.[2,12,13,55]

Adverse Effects During Pregnancy

Several investigators have reported an association of symptomatic urinary tract infection with pregnancy-induced hypertension. This finding is controversial. Although Sever and colleagues[53] affirmed it, Gilstrap and coworkers[22] reported that the incidence of hypertension was actually higher in control women than in those who suffered pyelonephritis during the pregnancy studied. Acute pyelonephritis has been reported to be associated with an increased incidence in low-birth-weight infants and preterm delivery that are probably due to an increased incidence of preterm labor caused by pyelonephritis. In a large study from Parkland Hospital,[22] 15 percent of infants born to mothers who had antepartum pyelonephritis weighed less than 2,500 g; however, their mean birth weight was not significantly different from that of infants born to uninfected women.

Long-Term Prognosis

Women who have acute pyelonephritis or frequent urinary tract infections during pregnancy may have a urinary tract abnormality. Indeed, as many as 37 percent of these women when nonpregnant have either recurrent infection or radiographic urinary anomalies.[43,64] In an 8- to 13-year follow-up of 208 women with acute pyelonephritis,[20] 41 percent were treated for one or more episodes of symptomatic urinary tract infections when not pregnant, and 38 percent of those with subsequent pregnancies had another infection during pregnancy. Fortunately, despite risks for frequent recurrences and the presence of urinary tract abnormalities, it is uncommon for these women to develop end-stage renal insufficiency.[19]

References

1. Asbaugh DG, Bilelow DB, Petty LY, et al. Acute respiratory distress in adults. Lancet 1967; 2:319–323.
2. Atkins E. Pathogenesis of fever. Physiol Rev 1960; 40:580–646.
3. Bailey RR. Single-dose antibacterial treatment for bacteriuria in pregnancy. Drugs 1984; 27:183–186.
4. Bennett IL Jr, Cluff LE. Bacterial pyrogens. Pharmacol Rev 1957; 9:427–475.
5. Benson M, LiPuma JP, Resnick MI. The role of imaging studies in urinary tract infection. Urol Clin North Am 1986; 13:605–612.
6. Cox CE. The urethra and its relationship to urinary tract infection: the flora of the normal female urethra. South Med J 1966; 59:621–626.
7. Cox CE, Lacy SS, Hinman F Jr. The urethra and its relationship to urinary tract infections. II. The urethral flora of the female with recurrent urinary infection. J Urol 1968; 99:632–638.
8. Cox SM, Cunningham FG. Ureidopenicillin therapy for acute antepartum pyelonephritis. Curr Ther Res 1988; 44:1029–1034.
9. Cox SM, Shelburne P, Mason R, et al. Mechanisms of hemolysis and anemia associated with acute antepartum pyelonephritis. Am J Obstet Gynecol 1991; 164:587–590.
10. Cunningham FG, Lucas MJ, Hankins GDV. Pulmonary injury complicating antepartum pyelonephritis. Am J Obstet Gynecol 1987; 156:797–807.
11. Cunningham FG, Morris GB, Mickal A. Acute pyelonephritis of pregnancy: a clinical review. Obstet Gynecol 1973; 41:112–117.
12. Dinarello CA, Cannon JG, Wolff SM. New concepts on the pathogenesis of fever. Rev Infect Dis 1988; 10:168–189.
13. Dinarello CA, Wolff SM. Pathogenesis of fever. In: Mandell AL, Douglasss Jr RG, Bennett JE, eds. Principles and practice of infectious diseases. Ed 3. New York: Churchill Livingston, 1990:462–467.
14. Dowling K, Roberts JA, Kaack MB. P-fimbriated *Escherichi coli* urinary tract infection: a clinical correlation. South Med J 1987; 80:1533–1536.
15. Duff P. Pyelonephritis in pregnancy. Clin Obstet Gynecol 1984; 27:17–31.
16. Duguid JP, Gilles RR. Fimbriae and adhesive properties in dystentery bacilli. J Pathol Bacteriol 1957; 74:397–411.
17. Elo J, Tallgren LG, Väisänen V, et al. Association of P and other fimbriae with clinical pyelonephritis in children. Scand J Urol Nephrol 1985; 19:281–284.
18. Fowler JE, Stamey TA. Studies of introital colonization of women with recurrent infections. VII. The role of bacterial adherence. J Urol 1977; 117:472–473
19. Freedman LR. Chronic pyelonephritis at autopsy. Ann Intern Med 1967; 66:697–710.
20. Gilstrap LC, Cunningham FG, Whalley PJ. Acute pyelonephritis in pregnancy: an anterospective study. Obstet Gynecol 1981; 57:409–413.
21. Gilstrap LC, Hankins GDV, Snyder RR, Greenberg RT. Acute pyelonephritis in pregnancy. Compr Ther 1986; 12:38–42.
22. Gilstrap LC, Leveno KJ, Cunningham FG, et al. Renal infection and pregnancy outcome. Am J Obstet Gynecol 1981; 141:709–716.
23. Guze LB, Beeson PB. Observations on the reliability and safety of bladder catheterization for bacteriologic study of the urine. N Engl J Med 1956; 255:474–475.
24. Hankins GDV, Whalley PJ. Acute urinary tract infection in pregnancy. Clin Obstet Gynecol 1985; 28:266–278.
25. Harris RE. The significance of eradication of bacteriuria during pregnancy. Obstet Gynecol 1979; 53:71–73.
26. Harris RE, Gilstrap LG. Prevention of recurrent pyelonephritis during pregnancy. Obstet Gynecol 1974; 44:637–641.
27. Harris RE, Gilstrap LC. Cystitis during pregnancy: a distinct clinical entity. Obstet Gynecol 1981; 57:578–580.
28. Harris RE, Gilstrap LC, Pretty A. Single-dose antimicrobial therapy for asymptomatic bacteriuria during pregnancy. Obstet Gynecol 1982; 59:546–549.
29. Helmholz HF. Determination of the bacterial content of the urethra: a new method, with results of a study of 32 men. J Urol 1950; 64:158–166.
30. Jakobi P, Neiger R, Merzbach D, Paldi E. Single-dose antimicrobial therapy in the treatment of asymptomatic bacteriuria in pregnancy. Am J Obstet Gynecol 1987; 156:1148–1152.
31. Källenius G, Möllby R, Svensson B, et al. The P^k antigen as receptor for the haemagglutinin of pyelonephritic *Escherichia coli*. FEMS Microbiol Lett 1980; 7:297–302.
32. Källenius G, Svenson SB, Hultberg H, et al. Occurrence of P-fimbriated *Escherichia coli* in urinary tract infections. Lancet 1981; 2:1369–1372.
33. Kass EH. Asymptomatic infections of the urinary tract. Trans Assoc Am Physicians 1956; 69:56–60.
34. Kass EH. Bacteriuria and the diagnosis of infections of the urinary tract. AMA Arch Intern Med 1957; 100:709–714.
35. Kass EH. Bacteriuria and pyelonephritis of pregnancy. AMA Arch Intern Med 1960; 105:194–198.
36. Kass EH. Pyelonephritis and bacteriuria: a major problem in preventive medicine. Ann Intern Med 1962; 56:46–53.
37. Kass EH. Savage W, Santamarina BAG. The significance of bacteriuria in preventive medicine. In: Kass EH, ed. Progress in pyelonephritis. Philadelphia: FA Davis, 1965:3–10.

38. Krieger JN. Complications and treatment of urinary tract infections in pregnancy. Urol Clin North Am 1986; 13:685–693.
39. Kunin CM. Initial significance of bacteriuria visualized in the unstrained urinary sediment. N Engl J Med 1961; 265:589–590.
40. Kunin CM. Urinary tract infections in children. Hosp Pract 1976; 11:91–98.
41. Latham RH, Running K, Stamm WE. Urinary tract infections in young adult women caused by *Staphylococcus saprophyticus*. 1983; JAMA 250:3063–3066.
42. Leffler H, Svanborg-Edén C. Chemical identification of a glycosphingolipid receptor for *Escherichia coli* attaching to human urinary tract epithelial cells and agglutinating human erythrocytes. FEMS Microbiol Lett 1980; 8:127–134.
43. Leigh DA, Gruneberg RN, Brumfitt W. Long-term follow-up of bacteriuria of pregnancy. Lancet 1968; 1:603–605.
44. Lidfelt KJ, Bollgren I, Källenius G, Svenson SB. P-fimbriated *Escherichia coli* in children with acute cystitis. Acta Paediatr Scand 1987; 76:775–780.
45. Lomberg H, Hanson LA, Jacobsson B, et al. Correlation of P blood group, vesicoureteral reflux and bacterial attachment in patients with recurrent pyelonephritis. N Engl J Med 1983; 308:1189–1192.
46. McFadyen IR, Campbell-Brown M, Stephenson M, Seal DV. Single dose treatment of bacteriuria in pregnancy. Eur Urol 1987; 13:22–25.
47. Mead PJ, Harris RE. The incidence of group B beta hemolytic streptococcus in antepartum urinary tract infections. Obstet Gynecol 1978; 51:412–414.
48. Miche HR, Manogue KR, Spriggs DR, et al. Detection of circulating tumor necrosis factor after endotoxin administration. N Engl J Med 1988; 318:1481–1486.
49. Ofek I, Mirelman D, Sharon N. Adherence of *Escherichia coli* to human mucosal cells mediated by mannose receptors. Nature 1977; 265:623–625.
50. Rinaldo JE, Rogers RM. Adult respiratory distress syndrome: changing concepts of lung injury and repair. N Engl J Med 1982; 306:900–909.
51. Rodriguez PN, Klein AS. Management of urolithiasis during pregnancy. Surg Gynecol Obstet 1988; 166:103–109.
52. Schaeffer AJ. Recurrent urinary tract infections in women: pathogenesis and management. Postgrad Med 1987; 81:51–58.
53. Sever JL, Ellenberg JH, Edmonds D. Urinary tract infections during pregnancy: maternal and pediatric findings. In: Cass EH and Brumfield W, eds. Infections of the upper tract. Chicago: University of Chicago Press, 1975:19–21.
54. Siebert FB. Fever producing substances found in some distilled water. Am J Physiol 1923; 67:90–104.
55. Skarnes RC, Brown SK, Hull SS, McCraken JA. Role of prostaglandin E in the triphasic fever response to endotoxin. J Exp Med 1981; 154:1212–1224.
56. Sleigh JD, Robertson JG, Isdale MH. Asymptomatic bacteriuria in pregnancy. J Obstet Gynaecol Br Commonw 1964; 71:74–81.
57. Stamey TA, Sexton CC. The role of vaginal colonization with enterobacteriaceae in recurrent urinary infections. 1975; J Urol 113:214–217.
58. Stamm WE, Counts CW, Running K, et al. Diagnosis of coliform infection in acutely dysuria women. N Engl J Med 1982; 307:463–468.
59. Stenquist K, Sanberg G, Lidin-Janson F, et al. Virulence factors of *Escherichia coli* in urinary isolates from pregnant women. J Infect Dis 1987; 156:870–877.
60. Svanborg-Edén C. Bacterial adherence in urinary tract infections caused by *Escherichia coli*. Scand J Urol Nephrol 1986; 20:81–88.
61. Svanborg-Edén C, Hagberg L, Leffler H, Lomberg H. Recent progress in the understanding of the role of bacterial adhesion in the pathogenesis of urinary tract infection. Infection 1982; 10:327–332.
62. Turck M, Goff BS, Petersdorf RG. Bacteriuria in pregnancy: relation to socioeconomic factors. N Engl J Med 1962; 266:857–860.
63. Väisänen V, Tallgren LG, Makela PH, et al. Mannose-resistant haemagglutination and P antigen recognition are characteristic of *Escherichia coli* causing primary pyelonephritis. Lancet 1981; 2:1366–1369.
64. Whalley P. Bacteriuria of pregnancy. Am J Obstet Gynecol 1967; 97:723–738.
65. Whalley PJ, Cunningham FG, Martin FG. Transient renal dysfunction associated with acute pyelonephritis of pregnancy. Obstet Gynecol 1974; 46:174–177.
66. Whalley PJ, Martin RG, Pritchard JA. Sickle cell trait and urinary tract infection during pregnancy. JAMA 1964; 189:903–906.
67. Wolff SM. Biological effects of bacterial endotoxins in man. J Infect Dis 1973; 128:S5259–5264.
68. Wood EG, Dillon HC. A prospective study of group B streptococcal bacteriuria in pregnancy. Am J Obstet Gynecol 1981; 140:515–520.
69. Zinner SH, Kass EH. Long-term (10 to 14 years) follow-up of bacteriuria of pregnancy. N Engl J Med 1971; 285:820–824.

CHAPTER 19

Clinical Intra-Amniotic Infection

Ronald S. Gibbs, M.D.

Intra-amniotic infection is a clinically detectable infection arising in the uterus and its contents during pregnancy. Various investigators have used alternative terms including *clinical chorioamnionitis, amnionitis, amnionic fluid infection,* and *intrapartum infection* to refer to this same condition.

Intra-amniotic infection is to be distinguished from histologic chorioamnionitis, defined histopathologically by polymorphonuclear infiltrates in the placenta and its membranes. Histologic chorioamnionitis occurs far more frequently than does clinically evident intra-amniotic infection.[7] At term, histologic chorioamnionitis occurs in approximately 20 percent of pregnancies but is infrequently associated with clinically evident intra-amniotic infection. Prior to term, histologic chorioamnionitis occurs much more frequently, recently being reported as high as 60 percent in pregnancies with birth weights between 1,000 and 1,500 g.[25]

Definition

Usually the diagnosis of intra-amniotic infection is made clinically upon the findings of fever, often with membrane rupture, maternal tachycardia, fetal tachycardia, uterine tenderness, foul odor to the amniotic fluid, and maternal leukocytosis.[11,13] Few patients show all of these signs and symptoms.

Incidence

In the past, retrospective studies reported the incidence of this condition at approximately 1 to 2 percent.[11,28] However, two recent prospective studies have reported incidences of 4.2 and 10.5 percent.[32,39] The incidence may have truly increased due to increased use of invasive techniques during labor, or the former rates may have underestimated the occurrence of the disease.

Pathways for Infection

Most commonly, intra-amniotic infection results from an ascending process, such as after prolonged rupture of the membranes or prolonged labor.

An infrequent route for intra-amniotic infection is hematogenous. *Listeria monocytogenes* has been the most reported cause of blood-borne intra-amniotic infection, and other reported cases have been due to Group A streptococci and *Campylobacter spp.*[20,30]

A third pathway for the development of intra-amniotic infection is introduction of bacteria during an invasive procedure. The risk of acute intra-amniotic infection is approximately 1 in 1,000 after diagnostic amniocentesis; after intrauterine transfusions, the risk may be as high as 5 percent.[5,33] Intraamniotic infection may also be a complication of cervical cerclage. Although the risk after placement of a cervical cerclage is usually 1 to 2 percent,[1] the risk of intrauterine infection may be as high as 25 percent with advanced cervical dilation and membrane prolapse.[6]

Risk Factors for Infection

Two recent large studies of risk factors for intra-amniotic infection have appeared.[32,39] Based upon their logistic regression analysis, these studies identified features of complicated labors as independent risk factors. These features are low parity, multiple vaginal examinations, and increasing duration of membrane rupture, of labor, and of internal fetal monitoring.

Amniotic Fluid Inhibitors

Several investigators have reported amniotic fluid antibacterial factors. One group reported a low-molecular-weight peptide with a zinc cofactor that inhibited bacterial growth.[35] Subsequently, Blanco and coworkers reported that amniotic fluid from patients with intra-amniotic infection (IAI) was significantly less likely to inhibit the growth of *E. coli* and of group B streptococci,[2,3] but we were unable to isolate a specific amniotic fluid bacterial inhibitor once we corrected for the effects of pH and osmolality.[36] At present, it is unclear whether there are specific bacterial inhibitors in amniotic fluid and whether they are clinically relevant.

Microbiology

Similar to several other obstetric infections, IAI is most often a polymicrobial infection. In a case-control study, 70 percent of the patients with intra-amniotic infection had more than 10^2 colony-forming units per milliliter of virulent organisms compared with only 8 percent of control patients ($p < 0.001$).[11] *Mycoplasma hominis* is also more comon in the fluid of patients with intra-amniotic infection than in controls (35 versus 8 percent; $p < 0.001$).[4]

The most common organisms in patients with intra-amniotic infection are anaerobes, mycoplasmas, *Gardnerella vaginalis,* group B streptococci, and aerobic gram-negative rods (Table 19-1).[40]

Table 19-1 Common Organisms in Intra-Amniotic Infection

In Amniotic Fluid	In Maternal/Neonatal Blood
Ureaplasma urealyticum	Group B streptococci
Mycoplasma hominis	*E. Coli*
Gardnerella vaginalis	
Bacteroides bivivus	
Group B streptococci	
Anaerobic streptococci	
E. coli	
Other aerobic gram-negative rods	

Bacterial vaginosis has been associated with IAI. First, in cases of IAI, *G. vaginalis, M. hominis,* and anaerobes appeared to be associated with each other in the amniotic fluid.[37] When one of these organisms was present in the amniotic fluid, it was significantly more likely that another member would be present. Second, in a set of very-high-risk patients for IAI, Silver and associates reported a significant association between bacterial vaginosis and IAI.[37] Third, patients with bacterial vaginosis are more likely to have anaerobes and *G. vaginalis* in the amniotic fluid.[37]

Compared with pregnancies yielding normal-birth-weight infants, those resulting in low-birth-weight infants (heavier than 2,500 g) were more likely to have anaerobes in the amniotic fluid.[40] *Bacteroides bivivus* was more common in the amniotic fluid from infected low-birth-weight pregnancies (45.9 versus 27.9 percent; $p = 0.035$), as were *Fusobacterium spp.* (21.6 versus 3.8 percent; $p < 0.001$). We found no differences in the isolation rates of Group B streptococci, *E. coli* or other aerobic organisms, *M. hominis,* or *Ureaplasma urealyticum.* Thus it is possible that subclinical anaerobic infection may cause preterm labor or preterm premature rupture of the membranes and consequently is more likely to be isolated in low-birth-weight pregnancies complicated by clinically evident intra-amniotic infection.

Because multiple organisms are often isolated in the amniotic fluid in cases of intra-amniotic infection, we have performed serologic studies to help determine which ones may be pathogenic. We presumed that pathogenic organisms would elicit a specific maternal antibody response. Patients with intra-amniotic infection and with *M. hominis* in the amniotic fluid have a significantly greater antibody response than do appropriate controls.[12] Similar significant antibody changes have been observed with *B. bivivus.*[15] By contrast, no significant antibody changes were identified for either *G. vaginalis* or *Chlamydia trachomatis.*[16,17]

Whereas Group B streptococci, *E. coli,* or both are present in only 20 percent of cases of intra-amniotic infection, they account for fully 67 percent of perinatal bacteremia.[37,40] When group B streptococci and *E. coli* are isolated in the amniotic fluid from cases of intra-amniotic infection, maternal or neonatal bacteremia with the corresponding organism occurs in 25 and 33 percent of cases, respectively. Among 408 cases of intra-amniotic infection, there were 28 cases of maternal bacteremia (group B streptococci, 11; *E. coli,* 7; *Staphylococcus aureus,* 2; *L. monocytogenes,* 2; *Bacteroides spp.*, 2; and one each enterococci, *Streptococcus viridans, S. pneumoniae,* and *Pseudomonas aeruginosa).* Blood stream isolates from newborns in these cases were as follows: group B streptococci, 4; *E. coli,* 5; *S. aureus,* 2; other streptococci, 3; enterococci, 2; *Enterobacter sp.*, 1, *Haemophilus influenzae,* 1; *H. parainfluenzae,* 1; and microaerophilic streptococci, 1. Anaerobes were unlikely to cause bacteremia as there were no cases of anaerobic neonatal sepsis documented and only 1 percent of cases of maternal anaerobic sepsis. Current techniques may be able to detect anaerobic bacteremia, especially with small inoculum size. Alternatively, anaerobes may be active locally and not markedly invasive organisms.

Clinical and Laboratory Diagnosis

The diagnosis of intra-amniotic infection is suggested by fever, maternal tachycardia, fetal tachycardia, uterine tenderness, and foul odor to the amniotic fluid, often, but by no means always, with prolonged membrane rupture. Because it is unusual for patients to have all of these findings, laboratory findings may assist in confirming the diagnosis. Of these laboratory measures, maternal peripheral blood leukocyte count is the most readily available. Several investigators over the past decade have evaluated other diagnostic techniques, including amniotic fluid Gram's stain, gas liquid chromatography, amniotic fluid leukocyte esterase, and amniotic fluid glucose.

In a case-control study, Gibbs and colleagues reported leukocytosis (greater than 15,000) in 63 percent of cases with intra-amniotic infection and in 21 percent of matched controls.[11] Hoskins and coworkers found leukocytosis (greater than 12,000 per cubic millimeter) to be a test with 67 percent sensitivity, 86 percent specificity, 82 percent positive predictive value, and 72 percent negative predictive value.[26]

Gram's stain and culture of amniotic fluid are of value in confirming the diagnosis of chorioamnionitis in symptomatic patients, when amniotic fluid is obtained through the intrauterine pressure catheter.[11] In a case-control study, organisms were observed in 67 percent (35 of 52) cases of IAI versus only 12 percent (6 of 52) of controls ($p < 0.001$), and 81 percent of IAI cases had detectable leukocytes on direct smear compared with only 29 percent of control cases ($p < 0.001$).

A simple chemical test for the presence of one of the leukocyte esterase enzymes has been developed. The esterase activity can be measured in the absence of intact cells and is not affected by changes in the pH, protein concentration, or bacterial content of the fluid specimen. Hoskins and coworkers evaluated the leukocyte esterase reagent strip in amniotic fluid from 21 patients with suspected chorioamnionitis and 21 controls.[26] The leukocyte esterase test showed excellent sensitivity (91 percent), specificity (95 percent), and positive and negative predictive values (95 and 91 percent, respectively).

Gravett and colleagues first described use of gas-liquid chromatography (GLC) for the diagnosis of chorioamnionitis.[19] Gas-liquid chromatography was used to identify abnormal organic acids (that is, acids other than actate) in the amniotic fluid specimens. Abnormal organic acids were found in only 1 of 22 control specimens compared with 15 of 16 samples from infected patients ($p < 0.0005$). These abnormal acids (such as acetate, propionate, and butyrate) were believed to be products of bacterial metabolism. Despite the impressive results achieved by the Gravett group, GLC analysis is not a test that can be readily used in practice for diagnosis of intra-amniotic infection.

Low amniotic fluid glucose (less than approximately 10 to 14 mg/ml) has been evaluated as a rapid predictor of IAI, but results are too preliminary to be applied to practice.

Outcome

Complications of IAI are summarized in Table 19-2. Older retrospective studies demonstrated that intra-amniotic infection was accompanied by a two- to three-fold increase in cesarean section rate. Also, with a relatively short time from diagnosis of intra-amniotic infection to delivery, no "critical interval" (after which maternal-neonatal complications might increase) was noted. Although perinatal mortality has increased in cases of intra-amniotic infection, nearly all of the excess perinatal mortality was directly due to prematurity, and little attributable to infection per se.[13,23,28,29]

Table 19-2 Complications of Intra-Amniotic Infection

Bacteremia in mother or neonate in 10 percent
Protraction of labor, decreased response to oxytocin
Increased cesarean section rate
Increased perinatal death, respiratory distress syndrome, and total infections in low-birth-weight infants

Effect on Labor

Controlled investigations have found that intra-amniotic infection in low-birth-weight pregnancies is significantly more likely to result in poor outcome than noninfected pregnancies at the same gestational age. Garite and colleagues compared pregnancies with and without amnionitis at 28 to 34 weeks' gestation.[10] Those with amnionitis ($n = 47$) had significantly more perinatal deaths, respiratory distress syndrome (RDS), and total infections than those without amnionitis ($n = 204$). In another case-control study (with more than 70 percent of the cases with low-birth-weight infants), Ferguson and coworkers reported no statistically significant differences in outcome in the chorioamnionitis cases that were accompanied by a higher perinatal mortality rate (20 percent versus 11 percent), higher sepsis rate (6 percent versus 2 percent), and higher asphyxia rate (27 percent versus 16 percent).[9] With all of these adverse effects being higher in chorioamnionitis group, it is possible that there may be a substantial error in this study in not detecting true adverse effects. In a larger study of similar design, Morales reported significant increases in the group with chorioamnionitis ($n = 92$) in mortality, RDS, intraventricular hemorrhage, and clinically diagnosed sepsis compared with controls of similar gestational age ($n = 606$).[31] We have compared outcome characteristics in cases of intra-amniotic infection leading to low-birth-weight versus normal-birth-weight infants.[40] In the low-birth-weight group, there was more frequent maternal bacteremia (13.5 percent versus 4.9 percent, $p = 0.06$), more frequent early neonatal bacteremia (16.2 percent versus 4.1 percent, $p = 0.005$), and more frequent neonatal death from sepsis (10.8 percent versus none, $p < 0.001$). These studies collectively demonstrate beyond doubt the adverse effect of intra-amniotic infection in low-birth-weight pregnancies.

Recent studies have addressed the effect of intra-amniotic infection on labor. Duff and colleagues reported that women with clinically evident intra-amniotic infection were most often primigravidas and that approximately 80 percent had been receiving oxytocin at the time of diagnosis of intra-amniotic infection.[8] Asymptomatic patients who had positive amniotic fluid cultures (considered to be subclinical intra-amniotic infection) required a higher dose of oxytocin to achieve adequate uterine activity.[38] Then, even with adequate uterine activity, these patients showed slow dilation that could not be explained by excessive fetal size, abnormal pelvis, anesthetics, or other drugs. The authors speculated that infection per se may adversely affect cervical collagen tissue.

Treatment

With the exception of a few highly unusual instances,[34] delivery is essential to cure of the mother and fetus. Until recently, there has been debate as to when the antibiotics should be administered. Many had supported intrapartum treatment in order to begin treatment promptly and to protect the mother from complications such as septicemia and shock, whereas others deferred treatment until after delivery so that "more thorough cultures of the neonate" were obtained. No optimal antibiotic regimen has been established for intra-amniotic infection, but studies to date have employed a penicillin, usually ampicillin, and usually in combination with an aminoglycoside. Because of the high failure rate of the ampicillin-aminoglycoside combination in patients with chorioamnionitis *and* with cesarean delivery, we have also advocated the empiric addition of clindamycin after cord clamping.[14] Studies are currently underway to evaluate other regimens. In view of the organisms causing intra-amniotic infection, it is likely that many of the newer penicillins, cephalosporins, or combinations of penicillin plus beta-lactamase inhibitor may be equally effective. These alternative regimens may offer pharmacokinetic advantages over gentamicin and may obviate the need to add clindamycin in patients having cesarean delivery in the presence of intra-amniotic infection.

Three recent studies have concluded that intrapartum treatment of intra-amniotic infection leads to a lower rate of neonatal sepsis than immediate postpartum treatment. In 1987 we reported a nonrandomized allocation as to timing of treatment (intrapartum versus immediate postpartum).[41] All mothers received penicillin G (5 million units intravenously every 6 hours) plus gentamicin (1.5 mg per kilogram every 8 hours). Neonates had blood cultures and chest x-rays performed and were treated with ampicillin plus gentamicin for 72 hours. When neonatal sepsis or pneumonia occurred, antibiotics were continued for 10 days. Eighty percent of mothers were treated intrapartum, with postpartum treatment being used mainly in patients who were likely to deliver within an estimated 2 hours afer the diagnosis of intra-amniotic infection. Maternal outcome was not different between the two groups, but more importantly neonatal sepsis (0.3 percent versus 20 percent, $p = 0.001$) and neonatal death from sepsis (0.9 percent versus 4.3 percent, $p = 0.07$) were both decreased in the group receiving intrapartum treatment.

In another retrospective study, bacteremia occurred in 1.5 percent of intrapartum versus 5.7 percent of no intrapartum treatment groups with gestational ages at least 35 weeks ($p = 0.06$).[18] The authors concluded that these observations were consistent with the concept that intrapartum treatment would decrease neonatal bacteremia.

In 1988, we published a randomized trial of intrapartum versus immediate postpartum treatment in women with intra-amniotic infection.[14] By randomization, all mothers received ampicillin (2 g intravenously every 6 hours) plus gentamicin (1.5 mg per kilogram every 8 hours). When cesarean delivery was performed, clindamycin was added postpartum. After delivery, neonates had blood cultures and a chest x-ray performed. Neonatal treatment consisted of ampicillin (75 mg per kilogram intravenously every 12 hours) plus gentamicin (2.5 mg per kilogram every 12 hours), begun within 2 hours of birth. Antibiotics were continued for at least 72 hours in all cases and for 10 days when sepsis or pneumonia was diagnosed.

In well-matched groups maternal outcome measures (maximum postpartum temperature, hospital stay postpartum, and number of febrile days) were all significantly improved in mothers with intrapartum treatment ($p = 0.05$). More importantly, early neonatal sepsis was reduced to 0 in the intrapartum treatment group from 21 percent of the postpartum treatment group ($p = 0.03$). If we consider sepsis or pneumonia, then these complications occurred in none of the intrapartum treatment group versus 32 percent of the postpartum treatment group ($p = 0.003$). The decrease in neonatal infections was accompanied by a hospital stay that was 2 days shorter (3.8 ± 1.1 versus 5.7 ± 3.0, $p = 0.02$).

On the basis of these three studies, we may conclude that intrapartum treatment begins to treat the fetus in utero, and it clearly outweighs any theoretical disadvantage such as interference with neonatal cultures.

In the presence of intra-amniotic infection, cesarean delivery should be reserved for cases with standard obstetric indications for abdominal delivery. The cesarean section rate is increased, however, to approximately 35 to 40 percent because of an increased likelihood of dystocia and fetal distress. When abdominal delivery is necessary, a transperitoneal (low transverse cervical) approach is nearly always used, and the results are excellent. Cesarean hysterectomy should be used when there are additional indications for hysterectomy, such as refractory uterine atony.[24] Extraperitoneal cesarean section, although championed by some, has little advantage.[21,27,43] (See Table 19-3 for a summary of the treatment of IAI.)

Long-Term Outcome

Two recent studies have reported the influence of clinical chorioamnionitis on the long-term prognosis of the infants. In 1985 Hardt and colleagues reported that low-birth-weight infants born from pregnancies complicated by chorioamnionitis had lower mental development index scores than did control infants.[22] Morales and colleagues reported scores for preterm infants born from pregnancies complicated by chorioamnionitis and from controls.[31] The mental development and physical development scores did not show significant differences, but cases of chorioamnionitis were matched with controls on the basis of severity of RDS and intraventricular hemorrhage. Because both of these complications were significantly increased in cases of chorioamnionitis, it appears to us to be inappropriate to match on the basis of these complications. Thus, although clinical chorioamnionitis per se may not adversely affect mental and physical development, it may indirectly lead to lower

Table 19-3 Summary of Treatment of Intra-Amniotic Infection

1. Obtain amniotic fluid culture (or cervical, if former not available) and blood cultures.
2. Begin intrapartum treatment with ampicillin plus gentamicin. Alternative single-drug therapies have not been evaluated formally but may be equally effective if broad-spectrum agents are used.
3. Monitor mother and fetus closely.
4. Anticipate vaginal delivery in most cases, but the cesarean section rate is increased (to approximately 40 percent).
5. Reserve cesarean delivery for standard obstetric indications such as dystocia or fetal distress.
6. When abdominal delivery is indicated, a low transverse cervical procedure (transperitoneal) is nearly always used. Cesarean hysterectomy is necessary only for additional indications such as hemorrhage. Extraperitoneal cesarean section appears to offer no advantage. After cesarean delivery, add antibiotic coverage for anaerobes with clindamycin.

development scores by increasing other serious complications.

References

1. Aarnoudse JG, Huisjes HJ. Complications of cerclage. Acta Obstet Gynecol Scand 1979; 58:255–257.
2. Blanco JD, Gibbs RS, Krebs LF. Inhibition of group B streptococci by amniotic fluid from patients with intraamniotic infection and from control subjects. Am J Obstet Gynecol 1983; 147:247–250.
3. Blanco JD, Gibbs RS, Krebs LF, Castaneda YS. The association between the absence of amniotic fluid bacterial inhibitory activity and intra-amniotic infection. Am J Obstet Gynecol 1982; 143:749–756.
4. Blanco JD, Gibbs RS, Malherbe H, et al. A controlled study of genital mycoplasmas in amniotic fluid from patients with intraamniotic infection. J Infect Dis 1983; 147:650–653.
5. Burnett RG, Anderson WR. The hazards of amniocentesis. Journal Iowa Medical Society 1968; 58:130–137.
6. Charles D, Edwards WR. Infectious complications of cervical cerclage. Am J Obstet Gynecol 1981; 141:1065–1070.
7. Driscoll SG. The placenta and membranes. In Charles D, Finland M, eds. Obstetric and perinatal infections. Philadelphia: Lea & Febiger, 1973:532.
8. Duff F, Sanders R, Gibbs RS. The course of labor in term patients with chorioamnionitis. Am J Obstet Gynecol 1983; 147:391–395.
9. Ferguson MG, Rhodes PG, Morrison JC, et al. Clinical amniotic fluid infection and its effect on the neonate. Am J Obstet Gynecol 1985; 151:1058–1061.
10. Garite TJ, Freeman RK. Chorioamnionitis in the preterm gestation. Obstet Gynecol 1982; 59:539–545.
11. Gibbs RS, Blanco JD, St. Clair PJ, Castaneda YS. Quantitative bacteriology of amniotic fluid from patients with clinical intraamniotic infection at term. J Infect Dis 1982; 145:1–8.
12. Gibbs RS, Cassell GH, Davis JK, et al. Further studies on genital mycoplasmas in intra-amniotic infection: blood cultures and serologic response. Am J Obstet Gynecol 1986; 154:717–726.
13. Gibbs RS, Castillo MS, Rodgers PJ. Management of acute chorioamnionitis. Am J Obstet Gynecol 1980; 136:709–715.
14. Gibbs RS, Dinsmoor MJ, Newton ER, Ramamurthy RS. A randomized trial of intrapartum versus immediate postpartum treatment of women with intra-amniotic infection. Obstet Gynecol 1988; 72:823–828.
15. Gibbs RS, Forman J, St Clair PJ, Baseman J. Detection of serum antibody response to *Bacteroides bivivus* by enzyme-linked immunosorbent assay in women with intra-amniotic infection. Obstet Gynecol 1987; 69:208–213.
16. Gibbs RS, Schachter J. Chlamydial serology in patients with intra-amniotic infection and controls. Sex Transm Dis 1987; 14:213–215.
17. Gibbs RS, Weiner MH, Walmer K, St Clair PJ: Microbiologic and serologic studies of *Gardnerella vaginalis* in intra-amniotic infection. Obstet Gynecol 1987; 70:187–190.
18. Gilstrap LC, Leveno KJ, Cox SM, et al. Intrapartum treatment of acute chorioamnionitis: impact on neonatal sepsis. Am J Obstet Gynecol 1988; 159:579–583
19. Gravett MG, Eschenbach DA, Speigel-Brown CA, Holmes KK. Rapid diagnosis of amniotic fluid infection by gas-liquid chromatography. N Engl J Med 1982; 306:725–728.
20. Halliday HL, Hirata T. Perinatal listeriosis: a review of twelve patients. Am J Obstet Gynecol 1979; 133:405–410.
21. Hanson H. Revival of the extraperitoneal cesarean section. Am J Obstet Gynecol 1978; 130:102–103.
22. Hardt NS, Kostenbauder M, Ogburn M, et al. Influence of chorioamnionitis on long-term prognosis in low birth weight infants. Obstet Gynecol 1985; 65:5–10.
23. Hauth JC, Gilstrap LC, Hankins GDV, et al. Term maternal and neonatal complications of acute chorioamnionitis. Obstet Gynecol 1985; 66:59–62.
24. Hayashi RH, Castillo MS, Noah ML. Management of severe postpartum hemorrhage with a prostaglandin F_2 analogue. Obstet Gynecol 1984;

63:806–808.
25. Hillier SL, Martius J, Krohn M, et al. A case-control study of chorioamnionic infection and histologic chorioamnionitis in prematurity. N Engl J Med 1988; 319:972–978.
26. Hoskins IA, Johnson TRB, Winkel CA. Leukocyte esterase activity in human amniotic fluid for the rapid detection of chorioamnionitis. Am J Obstet Gynecol 1987; 157:730–732.
27. Imig JR, Perkins RP. Extraperitoneal cesarean section: a new need for old skills. A preliminary report. Am J Obstet Gynecol 1976; 125:51–54.
28. Koh KS, Chan FH, Monfared AH, et al. The changing perinatal and maternal outcome in chorioamnionitis. Obstet Gynecol 1979; 53:730–734.
29. Looff JD, Hager WD. Management of chorioamnionitis. Surg Gynecol Obstet 1984; 158:161–166.
30. Monif GRG. Antenatal group A streptococcal infection. Am J Obstet Gynecol 1975; 123:213–214.
31. Morales WJ. The effect of chorioamnionitis on the developmental outcome of preterm infants at one year. Obstet Gynecol 1987; 70:183–186.
32. Newton ER, Prihoda TJ, Gibbs RS. Logistic regression analysis of risk factors for intraamniotic infection. Obstet Gynecol 1989; 73:571–575
33. Queenan JT. Modern management of the Rh problem. Ed 2. Hagerstown, Md: Harper & Row, 1977:180.
34. Romero R, Scioscia AL, Edberg SC, Hobbeno JC: Use of parenteral antibiotic therapy to eradicate bacterial colonization of amniotic fluid after rupture of membranes. Obstet Gynecol 1986; 67:155–175.
35. Schlievert P, Johnson W, Galask RP. Isolation of a low molecular weight antibacterial system from human amniotic fluid. Infect Immun 1976; 14:1156–1166.
36. Silver HM, Siler-Khodr T, Prihoda TJ, Gibbs RS. The effects of pH and osmolality on bacterial growth in amniotic fluid. Am J Perinatol (in press).
37. Silver HM, Sperling RS, St Clair PJ, Gibbs RS. Evidence relating bacterial vaginosis to intraamniotic infection. Am J Obstet Gynecol 1989; 161:808–812.
38. Silver RK, Gibbs RS, Castillo M. Effect of amniotic fluid bacteria on the course of labor in nulliparous women at term. Obstet Gynecol 1986; 68:587–592.
39. Soper DE, Mayhall CG, Dalton HP. Risk factors for intraamniotic infection: a prospective epidemiologic study. Am J Obstet Gynecol 1989; 161:562–568.
40. Sperling RS, Newton E, Gibbs RS. Intra-amniotic infection in low-birth-weight infants. J Infect Dis 1988; 157:113–117.
41. Sperling RS, Ramamurthy RS, Gibbs RS. A comparison of intrapartum versus immediate postpartum treatment of intra-amniotic infection. Obstet Gynecol 1987; 70:861–865.
42. Word BM, Klein JO. Therapy of bacterial sepsis and meningitis in infants and children: 1989 poll of directors of programs in pediatric infectious diseases. Pediatr Infect Dis J 1989; 8:635–637.
43. Yonekura ML, Wallace R, Eglinton G. Amnionitis—optimal operative management: extraperitoneal cesarean section vs low cervical transperitoneal cesarean section. Paper presented at the third annual meeting of the Society of Perinatal Obstetricians, San Antonio, January 1983, Abstract 24A.

CHAPTER 20

Gonorrhea

David Charles, M.D.

Gonorrhea is an infectious disease that is almost always transmitted by sexual exposure. It is an entity that seems to have existed in Europe from classical times. The satyric poets give hints about the existence of conditions that might be interpreted as gonorrhea, but they are so vague that no definite conclusion can be drawn about the existence of the disease. This is more remarkable, owing to the sexual mores of both the Greeks and Romans, as one would have expected that this disease would have figured in their fast life-style. However, it was Galen, one of the many Greek-trained doctors in Rome in the second century, who used the term *gonorrhea* to describe the urethral discharge associated with this disease in the male. Another migrant Greek physician to Rome was Soranus of Ephesus. He is the most renowned obstetrician of antiquity, and he may well have been conversant with gonococcal infections in that he recommended bathing the eyes of the neonate, in all probability to prevent ophthalmia neonatorum. Neither Galen nor Soranus furnished an unmistakable description of gonorrhea. In fact, no such description was available until the twelfth century, when the surgical writers differentiated "chaude pisse" from the general term *gonorrhea,* which included any form of urethral discharge. Chaude pisse ("the burning") was a well-recognized entity from that time on.

At the end of the fifteenth century, there was a great epidemic of the disease called *syphilis,* and until the latter part of the nineteenth century confusion reigned because gonorrhea and syphilis were viewed as one and the same disease. Paracelsus, the Swiss physician, thought gonorrhea was the initial symptom of syphilis. Ambroïse Paré, who is often referred to as "the father of surgery," also believed syphilis and gonorrhea were one disease, and because of his great reputation his error halted advances that could have led to the establishment of gonorrhea and syphilis as separate diseases. In fact, confusion reigned until the nineteenth century, when Philip Ricord[40] in Paris finally proved by innumerable inoculation experiments that they were separate diseases.

It was not until the science of bacteriology took charge that it was possible to state definitely that gonorrhea, syphilis, and chancroid were separate diseases caused by three different organisms. Albert Neisser[30] described the causative organism of gonorrhea in 1879, and subsequently the pathogen was named *Neisseria gonorrhoeae* (Fig. 20-1). In fact, a genus of aerobic gram-negative diplococci that includes the important pathogens of gonorrhea and meningococcal meningitis was given the name *Neisseria.* The name of Albert Neisser is associated in the mind of the clinician with the term *Neisserian infection,* which is the eponymic euphemism for gonococcal infection. Five years after Neisser's description of the gonococcus, Hans Gram described his method of staining bacteria and identified the gonococcus tinctorially, and this method is still used today for the presumptive diagnosis of gonorrhea.

Epidemiology

Gonorrhea is encountered in all parts of the world. In the United States estimates place the incidence of this infection as approximately 2 million cases a year. This infection confers no immunity to subsequent gonococcal

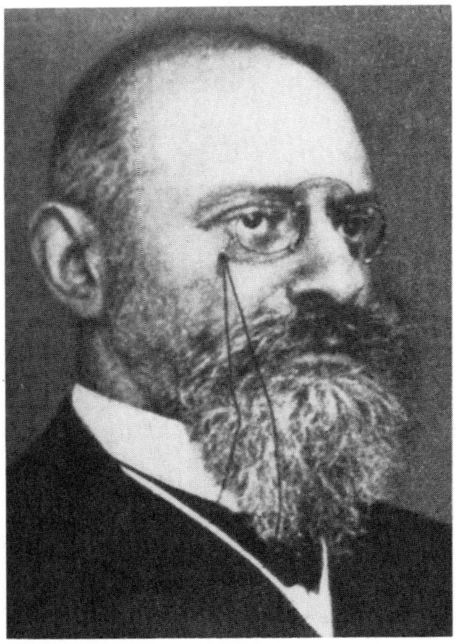

Figure 20-1 Albert Ludwig Siegmund Neisser: 1855–1916.

disease. From the early 1960s through the early 1970s, the annual incidence of gonorrhea increased because of the liberalization of sexual practices; as pointed out by Cates and Rauh,[4] this was also the time when sexual maturation of the children born after the Second World War occurred.

As gonorrhea was recognized as an increasing public health problem, a control program was instituted to curtail continued escalation in the incidence of this disease. Public education, clinical screening, and contact tracing were introduced, and these measures did have a beneficial effect and, no doubt, played an important role in the reduction of the incidence between 1975 and 1985. Despite these efforts, the incidence of gonorrhea increased in 1985 for the first time in almost a decade. At the same time, there was a marked increase in both the number and variety of antibiotic-resistant strains of the pathogen. The resurgence of gonorrhea in many areas of the world is in marked contrast to the story of many other communicable diseases.

Incidence

Adler[1] found that in England and Wales between 1966 and 1977 the rate of gonorrhea in women rose by 130 percent and the number of cases of acute salpingitis increased by 50 percent during the same period of time.

In the mid-1970s the reported number of cases of gonorrhea in the United States was 1 million. One must remember that reported cases account for only about 50 percent of actual cases, but the reported incidence of this disease is important, as it allows one to monitor trends over a period of years. During the decade 1975 to 1984 the incidence of gonorrhea reported by the Centers for Disease Control[5] declined from about 1 million cases per year to 878,000. This decline produced a corresponding reduction in the morbidity rates from 468 to 375 per 100,000 total population. During this period of time there was little change in the rates of gonorrhea among teenage females.

Environmental Factors

In the past gonorrhea has been viewed as a disease that increased at times of social distress and was considered to be related to poverty. There was no social distress when there was a reversal of the trend in 1985. In fact, that year was a time of relative peace and growing economic prosperity. What it implies is that the morbidity rate due to gonorrhea is a by-product of how a society is structured and functions. Premarital sexual activity for the female as well as the male is now widely regarded in Western societies as a norm. The trend in sexual freedom has been augmented by the innovations embodied in modern contraceptive regimens. By removing the fear of pregnancy, woman's equality in sex is assured, and consequently many women can find no reason why they should curtail their sexual activity. The forces of restraint imposed by marriage, family, customs, and neighbors have been rejected because the secular reasons for constraints, such as fear of pregnancy and the problems of illegitimacy, have been greatly diminished by currently available contraceptive regimens. In excess of 80 percent of cases occur in the age group 15 to 30 years. Of all the at-risk groups, the most blatant attitudinal and behavioral changes have occurred among women in the 15- to 20-year age group. What is of some importance is that gonorrhea in women is frequently asymptomatic. Nielson and coworkers[31] found the asymptomatic period of gonorrhea in women to be twice that in men and can vary from 4 to 180 days.

Transmission of Infection

Gonorrhea is almost always sexually contracted, except for conjunctivitis in the neonate and infrequent cases of gonococcal vulvovaginitis in preadolescent girls. One must also mention gonococcal pharyngitis, especially as oral sex appears to have become increasingly popular among homosexuals and heterosexuals in Western industrialized societies. Positive pharyngeal cultures are noted most often in homosexual males and then in heterosexual women. It is now well recognized, as pointed out by Weisner,[49] that pharyngeal gonococcal infections are no longer medical curiosities.

By contrast, transmissions of the gonococcal infection via toilet seats, towels, bed linen, mattresses, chairs, bathing beaches, or drinking glasses are face-saving myths or figments of the imagination. It would be as factual as a person stating:

It is no good standing on the seat
As pox in this city jumps six feet.

It seems clear that infectivity rates are currently influenced by partner change rates, percentage of partners infected, the duration of the asymptomatic state of the contact, and the precautions taken. The behavioral aspects of gonorrhea in an inner city sexually transmitted disease clinic are highlighted in the report of Upchurch and associates,[47] who found that more than a third of the individuals continued to engage in sexual activity after onset of symptoms or knowledge of sexually transmitted disease exposure. The reported prevalence of cervical gonorrhea among gravid patients varies from study to study and, according to Edwards and associates,[15] ranges from 1.0 to 7.5 percent. Of 1.7 million prenatal cultures for gonorrhea carried out in the United States in 1979, about 3 percent were positive. Many pregnant patients in industrialized countries have a history of gonorrhea, which, even after therapy, frequently recurs. Gonorrhea in gravid patients can be considered in most instances as reinfections and, as pointed out by MacDonald and associates,[26] the prevalence among gravid women has not been found to be any higher than among women who are not pregnant. To date there are no reliable data pertaining to the frequency of symptomatic versus asymptomatic infection in women. It is probable that asymptomatic infection may result in infection of the infant during parturition. Rothenberg[41] estimated that approximately one-third of neonates born to infected mothers will acquire gonococcal infection during descent through the birth canal. Consequently it is essential that all gravid patients be screened by history, physical examination, and appropriate cultures for *N. gonorrhoeae*.

Microbiology

Neisseria gonorrhoeae is an aerobic, nonmotile, gram-negative, bean-shaped coccus that is generally arranged in pairs and consequently is referred to as a diplococcus. It is also known as an intracellular diplococcus, as in smears containing pus the pathogen is seen ingested by polymorphonuclear leukocytes.

Humans are the definitive hosts for this pathogen. The organism is sensitive to desiccation and survives in a moist environment. Consequently, the gonococcus shows a distinct predilection for columnar and transitional epithelium. The stratified epithelia of the vulva and vagina are resistant to invasion by this pathogen.

Cultural Requirements

It has fastidious growth and survival requirements. The organism grows best in a medium that is mildly alkaline with a pH of 7.2 to 7.6 and is destroyed on exposure to acid media. Maximal growth occurs at 36 to 37° C in a moist environment containing 5 to 10 percent carbon dioxide. It will not readily grow on culture media if there are many competing organisms. The organism is most readily identified when grown on an enriched culture medium (Table 20-1). The first such medium was described by McLeod and associates[28] and was a form of chocolate agar that contained heated blood. This medium absorbs inhibitors to the growth of the diplococcus. Thayer and Martin[45] introduced a selective agar medium that contains vancomycin, colistin, and nystatin to suppress the growth of other bacteria as well as fungi. The gonococci on such media appear as smooth, round, translucent gray colonies of approximately 2 mm in diameter. Such media have in the past two decades revolutionized the isolation of the diplococcus not only from endocervical cultures but also from such highly contaminated sites as the pharynx and rectum.

Table 20-1 Microbiologic Features of *Neisseria Gonorrhoeae*

Aerobic, nonmotile gram-negative
Bean-shaped, generally in pairs
Humans are the definitive hosts
Predilection for columnar or pseudostratified epithelium
Energy requirements
Glucose
Pyruvate
Lactate
Growth requirements
pH 7.2 to 7.5
Temperature 36-37°C
Moist environment
Avoid desiccation
Atmosphere containing 5-10 percent CO_2
Enriched culture medium
Bacterial colonies
Smooth and round
Gray and translucent
Diameter about 0.5 to 2 mm
Colonies enlarge with age
Specific reactions
Oxide positive
Ferments glucose with production of acid
Does not ferment fructose or mannose

Biochemical Reaction

Colonies that are suspected to be *N. gonorrhoeae* can be identified by Gram's stain, oxidase reaction, and pattern of carbohydrate metabolism. The enzyme cytochrome is a feature of many bacteria, and it assists in the oxidation of reduced cytochrome by molecular oxygen. To detect if oxidase is present, a few drops of a 0.5 percent solution of the chemical tetramethyl paraphenylene diamine hydrochloride are added to the culture plate. If the bacterial colonies are oxidase positive, they have a purple appearance. The oxidase test is nonspecific, yet with the colonial appearance and Gram's stain it narrows the field to the genus *Neisseria*. The carbohydrate pattern can be determined by the ability of the organism to produce acid from sugars. The gonococcus is only capable of producing acid from glucose. It should be noted that occasionally distinctive colonies of the organism that are gram negative and oxidase positive may fail to ferment glucose or other sugars such as sucrose and maltose.

Colony Morphology and Serotypes

Kellogg and coworkers[25] demonstrated that the virulence of the diplococcus was associated with specific colony types and identified four morphologically distinct types of the pathogen. Colony types 1 and 2 were present on initial isolation from infected patients, whereas types 3 and 4 emerged on nonselective subculture media in the laboratory. Only types 1 and 2 were capable of causing infection in volunteers. The virulent strains belonging to colony types 1 and 2 were shown by Jephcott and coworkers[23] as well as Swanson and associates[43] to possess pili, which are protein projections of the outer membrane and allow for attachment of the pathogen to epithelial cells. Colony types 3 and 4 organisms, which are avirulent, lack pili. It is also recognized that antibodies directed against the pili inhibit cellular attachment and as a result enhance phagocytosis by the polymorphonuclear leukocytes. Johnston and coworkers[24] demonstrated that the outer membrane of the gonococcus contains several proteins—referred to as proteins 1, 11, and 111—which have antigenic specificity. These investigators detected 16 different serotypes of the gonococcus by utilizing antibodies directed against the outer membrane proteins. Serotyping of the gonococcus has been useful in epidemiologic studies. Hook and Holmes[21] consider that protein 1 is involved in the early stages of a gonococcal infection and that proteins 11 and 111 mediate attachment of the organism as well as susceptibility to the bactericidal activity of human serum.

Gonococcal Antibodies

Numerous bacteria generate proteases and nucleases, presumably to provide nutrients. It is of interest how the gonococcus, which normally resides on mucous membranes, elaborates IgA1-specific protease, which may be important in allowing the pathogen to colonize where it would otherwise be bound by secretory IgA. It must be borne in mind that local antibodies are not the result of extravasation of serum antibodies but a local response at the area of stimulation. *Neisseria gonorrhoeae* colonizes and infects mucosal surfaces and is adept at surviving in the genitourinary tract. Gonococcal infection results in the production of gonococcal antibodies, which are predominantly IgG and IgA in the serum and mucosal secretions. Gonococcal antibody is opsonic and is known to block adherence to epithelial cells, activate the classic complement pathway, and form immune complexes. The role of the gonococcal antibody in modifying the course of the infection remains to be delineated.

Despite antibody production in the genital tract, other factors must play a role in gonococcal infections. It is recognized that *N. gonorrhoeae* may cause repeated infections despite circulating humoral immunity, cell-mediated immunity, and local antibody. Additional studies are required on the host-parasite interactions of the genital tract epithelia so as to comprehend adequately this infection.

Clinical Manifestations

The majority of gonococcal infections affect predominantly the genital tract, the urethra in the male, and the endocervix in the female. Such infections may remain localized to the primary site, and in women this means that about 75 percent of those with gonococcal cervicitis may be asymptomatic. Consequently, in the female it is difficult if not well-nigh impossible to ascertain when the infection occurred. The incubation period in both males and females is between 2 and 5 days.

About 50 percent of women become infected with the diplococcus after a single exposure but, as pointed out by Platt and associates,[35] infection is far more prevalent after multiple exposures. Although it has long been recognized that women may be asymptomatic carriers of the diplococcus, physicians fail to recognize that men also can be healthy carriers. Consequently, it is not surprising that gonorrhea has been referred to as the uncontrolled and uncontrollable disease.

Sites of Infection

Although the cervix is usually the primary site of gonococcal infection in women, the urethra, Skene's glands, and Bartholin's gland can also be involved. The symptoms that evolve are referable to the affected structure. A few women have dysuria associated with frequency of micturition and state that they frequently notice such symptoms after coitus or that such symptoms come and go without adequate explanation. In fact women with gonococcal cervicitis may complain of only a vaginal discharge, and all too frequently because of a concomitant vaginal trichomoniasis a diagnosis of gonococcal endocervicitis is not considered.

Rectal infection occurs in at least one-third of female patients with gonococcal cervicitis. This is usually the result of direct spread from the leukorrhea associated with the endocervicitis or of genitorectal exposure. Such an infection may be asymptomatic or present as mild pruritus ani. In some instances rectal infections present with pain and bleeding, and proctoscopic examination reveals the presence of inflammation and mucopus.

Oral sex appears to be increasingly popular in Western societies, and consequently there has been a great deal of attention directed to pharyngeal gonorrhea. Wallin and Siegel[48] consider that pharyngeal infection is more prevalent in gravid women. Corman and associates[9] obtained pharyngeal cultures from 723 gravid women and had positive cultures in 12 (1.7 percent) Such pharyngeal infections are generally asymptomatic.

Clinically gonorrhea in women is usually asymptomatic, and symptoms noted initially (Table 20-2) tend to be of short duration. A latent phase supervenes, and an asymptomatic carrier state may persist for months or even years. Such patients are liable, if not treated, to contaminate their infants during parturition. Edwards and associates[15] have emphasized the lack of symptoms and recurrent positive cultures among gravid patients with gonococcal infections. They reported that the prevalence of gonorrhea among gravid women in studies has varied from 1 to 7.5 percent.

Disseminated Gonococcal Infection

Gonococcal septicemia has been variously described as disseminated gonococcal infection, metastatic gonorrhea, and gonococcemia. This entity is most commonly associated with occult genital infections in women, and the clinical manifestations include fever, arthritis, cutaneous lesions, and endocarditis (Table 20-3). Although distinct bacteremic and arthritic phases

Table 20-2 Symptoms of Uncomplicated Gonococcal Infections in Gravid Women

Endocervical infections
- Majority are asymptomatic
- Mucopurulent discharge
- Urinary tract symptoms (dysuria, urgency, frequency)

Rectal infections
- Majority are asymptomatic
- Mild pruritus ani
- Anal discharge
- Anorectal pain
- May coexist with perianal warts

Pharyngeal infections
- Majority are asymptomatic
- Sore throat
- Acute tonsillitis

1. Whatever the symptoms, they are short-lived.
2. The existence of gonococcal infection is derived from the laboratory rather than the symptomatology.
3. Asymptomatic gonococcal infections are found in the majority and form an important segment of the lottery of sexually transmitted diseases.

have been described, they often overlap. Infected gravid patients have, according to Holmes and associates,[20] an increased risk of disseminated infections, especially in the second and third trimesters.

Gonococcal Arthritis

Acute migratory polyarthritis similar to that found with rheumatic fever and involving the large joints during the second or third trimester of pregnancy should alert the physician to the possibility of a gonococcal infection. Gonococcal arthritis involves the knee joint four times as often as the shoulder; depending on the severity of the joint infection, erosion of the cartilage and atrophy of the adjacent bony structure may occur. If untreated, osseous adhesions and crippling ankylosis ensue. Gonococcal arthritis of the monoarticular or polyarticular type may be encountered in untreated patients. Such joint involvement may be accompanied by tenosynovitis, particularly at the wrist or dorsum of the hands. Gonococcal infection is currently the principal cause of pyogenic arthritis in women during reproductive life.

Brown[3] reported 11 women with gonococcal arthritis during pregnancy and underscored the necessity of early diagnosis and treatment. He stated that joint aspirates yielded positive cultures in only 25 percent of the patients. Why gonococci should be difficult or impossible to isolate in 75 percent of affected joints is unclear.

Chapman and Fernandez-Rocha[7] reported that over a 10-year period 32 gravid patients were admitted to their hospital with gonococcal arthritis. They consider that although arthritis develops in only 1 percent of patients with gonococcal infection the gravid patient is at particular risk. In a review of hospital records for a 5-year period they found no pregnant women with nongonococcal arthritis. They noted that gonococcal arthritis was predominantly associated with the third trimester of pregnancy.

Table 20-3 Clinical Manifestations of Gonococcemia (Disseminated Gonococcal Infection)

- Most common in late second or third trimester
- Frequently no symptoms of genital or pharyngeal infection
- Fever 38-39°C
- Chills

Joint involvement
- Migratory polyarthralgia
  - Knees
  - Ankles
  - Wrists
  - Metacarpophalangeal
- Polyarthritis
- Tenosynovitis
- Synovial effusions

Cutaneous lesions
- Predominently on volar aspects
  - Hands
  - Wrists
  - Arms
  - Ankles
  - Feet
- Maculopapular
  ↓
- Pustules
  ↓
- Necrotic center
  ↓
- Fade and leave no scar

Acute endocarditis

Myocarditis

Meningitis

Mehta and Wright[29] describe a patient who during the first trimester of pregnancy presented with pain in the right groin together with limitation of movement of the right hip. Radiologic examination of the joint demonstrated some soft-tissue swelling, loss of cartilage space, and generalized demineralization of the femur and acetabulum. Joint exploration revealed the joint capsule to be thickened and edematous and containing a semipurulent exudate. Lytic lesions of the femoral head and synovial membrane were biopsied; both specimens and the aspirated fluid yielded *N. gonorrhoeae,* as did a vaginal culture. The patient received intravenous penicillin in a daily dosage of 8 million units for 6 days, followed by ampicillin 500 mg by mouth every 6 hours for 2 weeks. She had a normal obstetric course and was delivered of a healthy infant at term. Two years after the gonococcal arthritis, she developed early degenerative osteoarthritic changes in the right hip. This report illustrates that gonococcal arthritis may be encountered in the first trimester of pregnancy.

Cutaneous Lesions

The skin lesions associated with gonococcemia originate as erythematous macules of a violaceous hue on the distal extremities. They are often noted on the volar aspects of the arms, wrists, hands, ankles, and feet. The lesions are 1 to 5 mm in diameter and progress from the macular stage to vesicles and pustules with necrotic centers. The central core may have a hemorrhagic base and be associated with petechiae. Cultures from the skin lesions are frequently negative, and it is essential to obtain cultures from the endocervix, rectum, and oropharynx. The last site must never be forgotton when gonococcemia is considered, as in about 20 percent of such cases the oropharynx is the only site from which the diplococcus is recovered.

Effects of Gonorrhea on Pregnancy Outcome

The effects of gonococcal infection on early pregnancy have not been well studied. Postabortal gonococcal salpingitis has been recognized with increased frequency following pregnancy termination. Some women seeking a pregnancy termination have life-styles that place them in a high-risk category, and physicians should never procure an abortion before excluding or treating a gonococcal infection.

An ascending infection from gonococcal endocervicitis resulting in endomyometritis, salpingitis, or septic abortion can occur in the first trimester of pregnancy. This is in accord with the fact that it is not until about the twelfth week of gestation that the decidua parietalis and decidua capsularis fuse to obliterate the endometrial cavity and impede the spread of the organism from the lower genital tract. The vagaries of gonococcal infections associated with pregnancy are highlighted by the report of Genadry and associates,[18] who described a case of acute purulent salpingitis that presented with acute abdominal pain in a patient with a gestation of 14 weeks' duration. Laparotomy revealed that both fallopian tubes were hyperemic, with a purulent exudate issuing forth from the fimbriated ends. Gram's stain of the purulent material revealed the presence of gram-negative intracellular diplococci, and culture subsequently confirmed the diagnosis of acute gonococcal salpingitis. The patient received intensive antibiotic therapy for 5 days, had an uneventful postoperative course, and went on to deliver at term a healthy male infant. Blanchard and associates[2] cite evidence that gonococcal pelvic inflammatory disease may be more common than is generally supposed, and they suggest that pathogenetic mechanisms other than ascending infection from the lower genital tract probably exist.

Gonococcal infections in the second and third trimesters of pregnancy can result in serious sequelae. Edwards and associates[15] summarized the evidence for adverse perinatal complications, including chorioamnionitis, premature rupture of the membranes, preterm labor and delivery, and intrauterine growth retardation. Such complications were noted to be markedly increased in women who had positive gonococcal cultures at the time of parturition. Handsfield and associates[19] from a retrospective study concluded that maternal diplococcal infection in late pregnancy is associated with perinatal infection of the fetus as well as maternal peripartum pyrexia and puerperal sepsis (Table 20-4).

Table 20-4 Potential Pregnancy Hazards as a Result of Gonorrhea

In first trimester
Endomyometritis
Salpingitis
Abortion
Later in pregnancy
Chorioamnionitis
Premature rupture of fetal membranes
Preterm labor
Postpartum
Puerperal sepsis
Neonate
Eye infections
Oropharyngeal infections
Gonococcemia—septic arthritis

Unless gonorrhea is specifically sought at the initial prenatal visit and in the latter weeks of pregnancy, perinatal gonococcal infections will continue to plague the practice of obstetrics. Although most neonatal gonococcal infections occur during parturition, contamination of the fetus may occur in utero following amniorrhexis. Thompson and associates[46] documented gonococcal ophthalmia neonatorum in infants delivered by cesarean section after the fetal membranes had ruptured. Oppenheimer and Winn[32] reported the presence of gonococcal infection in the deep tissue of a stillborn infant. Thadepalli and associates[44] recorded a case of gonococcal amnionitis that was followed by neonatal sepsis subsequent to intrapartum fetal heart rate monitoring. Scalp abscesses have been reported more frequently since the advent of widespread use of fetal scalp electrodes. Plavidal and Werch[36] recorded a fetal scalp abscess due to the gonococcus subsequent to the application of a scalp electrode for fetal heart monitoring. The mother was known to have had a positive cervical culture in early pregnancy but had failed to report for treatment. This case supports the concept that the maternal lower genital tract is the major source of organisms that can be inoculated into the fetal scalp at the time an electrode is applied for monitoring the fetal heart.

In developing nations gonococcal infections appear to be responsible for a substantial proportion of premature births in obstetric units. Elliott and associates[16] in a study from Nairobi found that premature rupture of the fetal membranes and gonococcal infection were independently associated with preterm labor and delivery. They stated that if these associations are causal they accounted for up to 51 percent of the prematurity they observed in their study population. The pathogenesis of gonococcal-associated prematurity remains to be delineated, but Elliott and associates[16] estimate that control of maternal gonococcal infection in Kenya may reduce the prematurity rate by about one-seventh.

Gonococcal ophthalmia neonatorum still accounts for about 50 percent of the cases of neonatal conjunctivitis in the developing world. Even in the industrial nations of the world, it still remains the most common manifestation of gonococcal infection in the neonate. It is an acute purulent conjunctivitis that appears predominantly

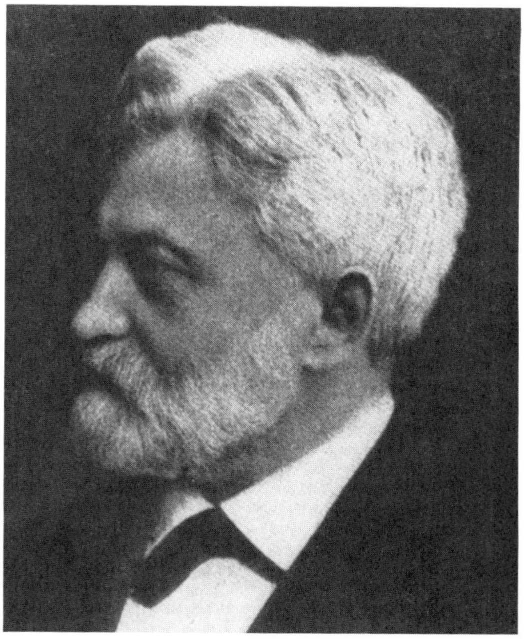

Figure 20-2 Karl Siegmund Franz Credé: 1819–1892.

during the first week of life; as pointed out by Dillon,[12] there is a marked risk of serious ophthalmic sequelae because of corneal injury, and if therapy is delayed anterior synechiae and panophthalmitis may occur. Podgore and Holmes,[37] however, reported gonococcal ophthalmia neonatorum without any signs of inflammation. Gonococcal ophthalmia must be ruled out in every case of conjunctivitis in a neonate. Similarly, because of the continued high annual incidence of gonorrhea in the United States and the evolution of resistant organisms, there is no room for complacency about this disease, which is still the most serious cause of conjunctivitis in the newborn.

The name of Credé is associated eponymically with the prophylaxis of gonococcal ophthalmia neonatorum, which was one of the most important advances in obstetric practice in the nineteenth century (Fig. 20-2). Credé[10] in 1881 reported that instillation of a few drops of a weak solution of silver nitrate (1:50) into each eye immediately after birth prevented gonococcal ophthalmia. Silver nitrate is still effective, and a 1 percent aqueous solution is one of the regimens recommended by Centers for Disease Control.[6] The other regimen that is recommended is a single application of erythromycin 0.5 percent ophthalmic ointment. One of these agents should be instilled into the eyes of neonates as soon as possible following delivery and at the latest within an hour of birth. The recommendation that single-use tubes or ampules be used in preference to multiple-use tubes is sound advice and should be heeded.

Any form of ophthalmia neonatorum that persists for 2 to 3 days or one that appears more severe than the usual chemical conjunctivitis that is common after silver nitrate instillation should be investigated. Although the presence of gram-negative diplococci on a Gram's stain furnishes a presumptive diagnosis, one should be aware, as reported by Denison and associates,[11] that *N. gonorrhoeae* can be confused with morphologically similar *Neisseria* species that are not pathogenic.

Diagnosis

All gravid patients should be cultured at their initial visit for evidence of gonococcal cervicitis, a measure that is imperative in view of the high incidence of asymptomatic infection. Routine screening must include endocervical cultures on selective media, which should be immediately dispatched to the laboratory. In obtaining material for culture, no vaginal lubricant should be used because lubricants may have bactericidal properties that can inhibit the growth of the diplococcus. Furthermore, specimens for culture should be collected on synthetic fiber swabs, which are free of such inhibitors as the unsaturated fatty acids found in cotton swabs. After the removal of the cervical mucus plug, the swab is inserted into the endocervical canal and rotated for about 10 seconds to allow absorption of endocervical secretions. The specimen so obtained should be inoculated in Transgrow bottles that contain Thayer-Martin medium with a carbon dioxide–enriched atmosphere and then sent to the laboratory as expeditiously as possible. A cultural diagnosis of *N. gonorrhoeae* is established by the presence of gram-negative diplococci that are oxidase positive and ferment glucose.

A microscopic study of a Gram's stain of material from the endocervix could be of assistance in attaining a presumptive diagnosis because cultural identification of the pathogen requires about 48 hours. One must remember, however, that other gram-negative cocci such as *Acinetobacteria,* which are morphologically indistinguishable from *N. gonorrhoeae,* may be present in endocervical and vaginal preparations. The absence of gram-negative diplococci in such preparations does not rule out gonococcal infection. It is imperative that all cases of gonorrhea be confirmed by culture, both to obtain a definitive diagnosis and to facilitate antimicrobial susceptibility testing.

Rectal Cultures

It has become common practice to obtain rectal cultures from women as gonococcal proctitis is sufficiently common in women to warrant such procedures. To obtain suitable cultures the swab should be inserted about 1 inch into the anal canal to reach the crypts where the infection is usually located. The omission of rectal cultures results in an incidence of missed diagnoses of almost 5 percent. An anoscope is neither necessary nor desirable, but if the swab is contaminated by feces it should be discarded and a further specimen obtained. One should bear in mind that a single set of negative cultures does not exclude the diagnosis of gonorrhea.

Follow-Up Cultures

Gravid patients who have had therapy for gonococcal infections should have repeat cultures in the third trimester. Sexual partners of such women should be treated.

If the sexual partners of the woman remain untreated, she should have repeated cultures at monthly intervals for the remainder of the pregnancy.

Treatment

Paradoxically for many years it was easier to treat gonorrhea in the gravid patient than to diagnose the gonococcal infection. The standard treatment of uncomplicated gonorrhea was for many years the intramuscular administration of 4.8 million units of aqueous procaine penicillin G in two separate sites, along with the oral administration of 1 g of probenecid. The latter agent was incorporated in the therapeutic regimen in order to reduce rapid tubular elimination of the antibiotic.

Antibiotic Resistance

Over the last two decades there has been a noticeable decrease in the susceptibility of the gonococcus to penicillin. Gonococcal resistance to antimicrobial agents has been evolving since the availability of sulfonamides in the 1930s and penicillin in the 1940s. Reyn[38] in 1963 reported that more than 50 percent of the strains of *N. gonorrhoeae* then isolated were less sensitive to penicillin than those isolated 20 years earlier. This investigator documented steady increases in chromosomal penicillin resistance accompanied by the requisite increasing doses of penicillin to treat infections. Chromosomally mediated resistance is not limited to penicillin but, as pointed out by Rice and associates,[39] is a more general phenomenon that includes tetracycline and cefoxitin. Easmon[13] has suggested that the underlying mechanism for chromosomally mediated resistance may involve changes in one or more of the penicillin-binding proteins. Gonococcal resistance to spectinomycin and to other aminoglycosides is also chromosomally mediated, but is expressed phenotypically at the level of the ribosome. Hook and Holmes[21] consider that alterations occur in the 30s ribosomal subunit. The first therapeutic failures due to a chromosomally mediated penicillin-resistant strain of the gonococcus in the United States occurred in North Carolina in 1983. Faruki and associates[17] stated that the isolates were unusually resistant to penicillin, and 15 of their 16 patients who were treated with 4.8 million units of procaine penicillin plus 1 g of probenecid failed to respond to therapy. They emphasized that chromosomally mediated resistant *N. gonorrhoeae* could become a major problem if surveillance and control measures were not utilized.

In 1976 high levels of penicillin resistance in gonococci due to plasmid-related production of the enzyme beta-lactamase was described by Phillips[34] as well as by Percival and associates.[33] This aspect of antibiotic resistance overshadowed problems encountered with chromosomal resistance. Since 1980 penicillinase-producing strains of *N. gonorrhoeae* (PPNG) have increased in a dramatic manner in the United Kingdom because of indigenous spread. McCutchan and colleagues[27] suggested that in areas with a prevalence of such strains in excess of 5 percent, spectinomycin or a cephalosporin should be adopted as first-line therapy. Jaffe and associates[22] at the same time reported that the incidence of PPNG strains had increased in the United States and indicated that in some areas there were endemic foci. Easmon and associates[14] stated that widespread use of cephalosporins for gonococcal infections would increase the rate of nonenzyme resistance in gonococci. Between 1981 and 1984 they isolated 40 strains of the diplococcus that were highly resistant to spectinomycin, and only some of the strains produced penicillinase. They report they have not encountered such resistant strains since 1984. Recently chromosomally resistant strains of *N. gonorrhoeae* were prevalent in their institution, and many of them had reduced sensitivity to cefuroxime, cefotaxime, and ceftriaxone. These observations were derived from a populace in which cephalosporins were rarely prescribed. These investigators have been able to transform gonococci resistant to penicillin, cefuroxime, and cefotaxime into diplococci sensitive to these antibiotics by DNA from donor chromosomally resistant strains of *N. gonorrhoeae*. They were also able to demonstrate a close relationship between the transfer of penicillin and cephalosporin resistance.

The continued ability of gonococci to evade antibiotic therapy is a matter of concern. The increasing levels of chromosomal resistance and a possible link between resistance to penicillin and the other beta-lactam agents necessitate regular reviews and reassessment of the treatment of gonococcal infections. Schwarcz and associates,[42] in reporting the Gonococcal Isolate Surveillance Project, support such a concept. They demonstrated that there is a wide distribution of antimicrobial-resistant *N. gonorrhoeae* in the United States. These data resulted in the national treatment policy revisions by the Centers for Disease Control.[6] Consequently penicillin, ampicillin, and amoxicillin are no longer recommended for the treatment of gonococcal infections. The treatment of gonococcal infections in both gravid patients and infants currently utilizes ceftriaxone (Table 20-5). Concomitant therapy with erythromycin is recommended for gravid patients who require treatment for gonorrhea because of the likelihood of co-infection with *Chlamydia trachomatis*. More important, no single-dose regimen currently recommended for gonorrhea is reliably effective against *C. trachomatis*. Christmas and associates,[8] in their study pertaining to concomitant infection in pregnancy with *C. trachomatis* and the gonococcus, found that erythromycin 500 mg four times a day provided a high cure rate of chlamydial cervicitis. Doxycycline and the quinolines, because of potential adverse effects on the fetus, should not be prescribed in pregnancy.

Hypersensitivity to Penicillin

Gravid patients with gonococcal infections who are allergic to beta-lactam antibiotics should be treated with spectinomycin.

Disseminated Gonococcal Infection

Patients with suspected disseminated infections should be admitted to hospital so as to rule out serious complications such as endocarditis and meningitis and to permit assessment of the therapeutic response. The majority of patients demonstrate a marked improvement

Table 20-5 Treatment of Gonorrhea in Pregnancy

Infection	Recommended Therapy	Alternative Therapy
Uncomplicated endocervical, rectal, or pharyngeal infections	One intramuscular injection of ceftriaxone 250 mg, followed by a 7-day course of erythromycin base 500 mg four times a day for possible coexisting *C. trachomatis* infection	Patients allergic to beta-lactams should receive one injection of spectinomycin 2 g followed by erythromycin
Gonococcemia	Ceftriaxone 1 g by intramuscular or intravenous injection every 24 hours or ceftizoxime 1 g by intravenous injection every 8 hours or cefotaxime 1 g by intravenous injection every 8 hours for 7 days	Patients allergic to beta-lactams should receive spectinomycin 2 g every 12 hours for 7 days

From Centers for Disease Control, 1989.[6]

within 48 hours of the institution of appropriate antibiotic therapy. In fact, failure to improve in a couple of days may force the clinician to reconsider the diagnosis. In the management of such patients, repeated cardiac evaluation is essential, as gonococcal endocarditis occurs in about 1 to 2 percent of patients with gonococcemia. The diagnosis must be given due consideration if the patient exhibits a new heart murmur.

Ophthalmia Neonatorum

Treatment of gonococcal ophthalmia neonatorum with topical antimicrobial agents is inadequate therapy. Ceftriaxone in a single dose of 25 mg per kilogram of body weight has been shown to be highly efficacious. The use of highly protein-bound ceftriaxone should, however, be avoided in icteric infants. Coexisting neonatal conjunctivitis due to *C. trachomatis* must always be entertained if there is no amelioration of the infant's clinical status.

Summary

The gonococcus remains an important pathogen in perinatal medicine. The vagaries of the clinical presentation and diagnostic difficulties in gravid patients are matters of concern, and the therapy requires constant review.

There has been a great deal of interest in the pathogenesis and immunology of gonococcal infections during the past decade. Research endeavors have been directed at the production of an effective vaccine. The diplococcus continues to evolve and adapt itself to evade the host's immune system. A vaccine will be a necessity in the future if the diplococcus continues to develop plasmid or chromosomally mediated antimicrobial resistance. The increasing number and proportion of resistant strains have produced clinical and public health as well as fiscal dilemmas. There is no doubt that this pathogen will acquire resistance to an ever-increasing number of antibiotics. The success witnessed with penicillin therapy in the past may well prove impossible to duplicate with other therapeutic agents in the future. Such salutary opinions only stress the potential problems that may arise i empiric therapy is prescribed for gonococcal disease Clinicians must be aware of local resistance patterns an heed data derived from surveillance projects.

The solution to the gonococcal revival requires increased cooperation by all the specialties involved wit sexually transmitted diseases.

References

1. Adler MW. Trends for gonorrhea and pelvic inflammatory disease in England and Wales and for gonorrhea in a defined population. Am J Obstet Gynecol 1980; 138:901–904.
2. Blanchard AC, Pastorek JG, Weeks T. Pelvic inflammatory disease during pregnancy. South Med J 1987; 80:1363–1365.
3. Brown D. Gonococcal arthritis in pregnancy. South Med J 1973; 66:693–695.
4. Cates W, Rauh JL. Adolescents and sexually transmitted diseases: an expanding problem. J Adolesc Health Care 1985; 6:257–261.
5. Centers for Disease Control: Sexually transmitted disease statistics, 1984. Washington: US Department of Health and Human Services, Public Health Service, 1985.
6. Centers for Disease Control: Sexually transmitted diseases treatment guidelines. MMWR 1989; 38:S1–43.
7. Chapman DR, Fernandez-Rocha L. Gonococcal arthritis in pregnancy: ten year review. South Med J 1975; 63:1333–1336.
8. Christmas JT, Wendel GD, Bawdon RE, et al. Concomitant infection with *Neisseria gonorroeae* and *Chlamydia trachomatis* in pregnancy. Obstet Gynecol 1989; 74:295–298.
9. Corman LC, Levison ME, Knight R, et al. The high frequency of pharyngeal gonococcal infections in a prenatal clinic population. JAMA 1975; 230:568–570.

10. Credé CSF. Die Verkutüng der Augenentzündung der Neugeborenen. Arch F Gynäk 1881; 17:50–53.
11. Denison MR, Perlman S, Andersen RD. Misidentification of *Neisseria* species in a neonate with conjunctivitis. Pediatrics 1989; 81:877–878.
12. Dillon HC Jr. Prevention of gonococcal ophthalmia neonatorum. N Engl J Med 1986; 315:1414–1415.
13. Easmon CSF. Gonococcal resistance to antibiotics. J Antimicrob Chemother 1985; 16:409–417.
14. Easmon CSF, Ison CA, Woodford N. Spectinomycin and resistant *Neisseria gonorrhoeae*. N Engl J Med 1988; 318:325–326.
15. Edwards LE, Barrada MI, Hamann AA. Gonorrhea in pregnancy. Am J Obstet Gynecol 1978; 132:637–641.
16. Elliott B, Brunham RC, Laga M, et al. Maternal gonococcal infection as a preventable risk factor for low birthweight. J Infect Dis 1990; 161:531–536.
17. Faruki H, Kohmescher RN, McKinney D, Sparling FP. A community based outbreak of infection with penicillin resistant *Neisseria gonorrhoeae* not producing penicillinase (chromosomally mediated resistance). N Engl J Med 1985; 313:607–611.
18. Genadry RE, Thompson BH, Niebyl JR. Gonococcal salpingitis in pregnancy. Am J Obstet Gynecol 1976; 126:512–513.
19. Handsfield HH, Hodson WA, Holmes KK. Neonatal gonococcal infection: I. Orogastric contamination with *Neisseria gonorrhoeae*. JAMA 1973; 225:697–701.
20. Holmes KK, Counts LW, Beatty HN. Disseminated gonococcal infection. Ann Intern Med 1971; 74:979–993.
21. Hook EW, Holmes KK. Gonococcal infections. Ann Intern Med 1985; 102:229–233.
22. Jaffe HW, Biddle JW, Johnson SR, Weisner PJ. Infections due to penicillinase-producing *Neisseria gonorrhoeae* in the United States, 1976-1980. J Infect Dis 1981; 144:191–197.
23. Jephcott AE, Reyn A, Birch-Andersen A. *Neisseria gonorrhoeae* 111 demonstration of assumed appendages to cells from different colony types. Acta Path et Microbiol Scand 1971; 79B:437–439.
24. Johnston KH, Holmes KK, Gotschlich EC. The serological classification of *Neisseria gonorrhoeae* 1: isolation of the outer membrane complex responsible for serotype specificity. Journal of Experimental Medicine 1976; 143:741–745.
25. Kellogg DS, Peacock WL, Deacon WE, et al. *Neisseria gonorrhoeae* 1: virulence genetically linked to clonal variation. J Bacteriol 1963; 85:1274–1279.
26. MacDonald P, Alexander R, Catz C, Edelman R. Summary of a workshop on maternal genitourinary infections and the outcome of pregnancy. J Infect Dis 1983; 147:596–605.
27. McCutchan JA, Adler MW, Berrie JRH. Penicillinase-producing *Neisseria gonorrhoeae* in Great Britain 1977-1981: alarming increase in incidence and recent development of endemic transmission. Br Med J 1982; 285:337–340.
28. McLeod JW, Coates JC, Happold FC, et al. Cultivation of gonococcus as method in diagnosis of gonorrhea with special reference to oxidase reaction and to value of air re-enforcement and its carbon dioxide content. J Path Bacteriol 1934; 39:221–231.
29. Mehta A, Wright TA. Gonococcal arthritis in pregnancy. Can Med Assoc J 1977; 117:1190–1191.
30. Neisser A. Ueber eine der Gonorrhoe eigentümliche Micrococcus-form. Centralbl f d Med Wissensch 1879; 17:497–500.
31. Nielson R, Sondergaard J, Ullman S. Asymptomatic male and female gonorrhea. Acta Derm Venereol (Stockh) 1975; 53:499–501.
32. Oppenheimer EH, Winn KJ. Fetal gonorrhea with deep tissue infection *in utero*. Pediatrics 1982; 69:74–76.
33. Percival A, Corkhill JE, Ayra OP, et al. Penicillinase-producing gonococci in Liverpool. Lancet 1976; 2:657–658.
34. Phillips I. β-Lactamase producing penicillin-resistant gonococci. Lancet 1976; 2:656–657.
35. Platt R, Rice PA, McCormack WM. Risk of acquiring gonorrhea and prevalence of abnormal adnexal findings among women recently exposed to gonorrhea. JAMA 1983; 250:3205–3207.
36. Plavidal FJ, Werch A. Gonococcal fetal scalp abscess: a case report. Am J Obstet Gynecol 1977; 127:437–438.
37. Podgore JK, Holmes KK. Ocular gonococcal infection with minimal or no inflammatory response. JAMA 1981; 246:242–243.
38. Reyn A. Current problems in the diagnosis and therapy of gonorrhoea from a laboratory point of view. Acta Dermatol Venereol (Scand) 1963; 43:380–393.
39. Rice RJ, Biddle JW, Jean Louis YA, et al. Chromosomally mediated resistance in *Neisseria gonorrhoeae* in the United States: results of surveillance and reporting 1983-84. J Infect Dis 1986; 153:340–345.
40. Ricord PH. A practical treatise on venereal disease. Ed 2. Doane AS, trans. New York: JS Redfield Clinton Hall, 1844.
41. Rothenberg R. Ophthalmia neonatorum due to *Neisseria gonorrhoeae:* prevention and treatment. Sex Transm Dis 1979; 6:S187–191.
42. Schwarcz SK, Zenilman JM, Schnell D, et al. National surveillance of antimicrobial resistance in *Neisseria gonorrhoeae*. JAMA 1990; 264:1413–1417.
43. Swanson J, Kraus SJ, Gotschlich EC. Studies of gonococcal infection 1: pili and zones of adhesions: their relation to gonococcal growth patterns. J Exp Med 1971; 134:886–906.
44. Thadepalli H, Rambhatla K, Maidman JE. Gonococcal sepsis secondary to fetal monitoring. Am J Obstet Gynecol 1976; 126:510–512.
45. Thayer JD, Martin JE. Improved medium selective for cultivation of *Neisseria gonorrhoeae*. Public Health Rep 1966; 81:559–562.
46. Thompson TR, Swanson RE, Weisner J. Gonococcal ophthalmia neonatorum relationship of time

of infection to relevant control measures. JAMA 1974; 228:186–188.
47. Upchurch DM, Brady WE, Reichart CA, Hook EW. Behavioral contributions to acquisition of gonorrhea in patients attending inner city sexually transmitted disease clinic. J Infect Dis 1990; 161:938–941.
48. Wallin J, Siegel M. Pharyngeal *Neisseria gonorrhoeae:* colonizer or pathogen? Br Med J 1979; 1:1462–1463.
49. Weisner PJ. Gonococcal pharyngeal infection. Clin Obstet Gynecol 1975; 18:121–129.

CHAPTER 21

Syphilis

David Charles, M.D.

Osler had a profound influence on the teaching and practice of medicine on both sides of the Atlantic. He was, above all, an astute clinician who referred to syphilis as the "great imitator" because of the numerous guises with which it was attired. On account of the vagaries of the infection, he stated that the individual who "knows syphilis knows medicine." In previous years it was true to say that there was hardly any medical specialty on which syphilis did not impinge. The incursions of this disease bore a semblance to Quixote charging at windmills.

Today, however, many physicians in practice have never encountered a case of syphilis and its ramifications. The infection can affect and infect all age groups, but the most disconcerting manifestations of this affliction are those resulting from intrauterine involvement of the conceptus. Although the threat of syphilis and the attendant problem of congenital syphilis declined for several years because of the control of the disease by public health measures, the extensive use of serologic testing, and the fact that the pathogen remained susceptible to penicillin, the disease still wends its way through society. There is no evidence that it will soon be banished from clinical practice. In fact, after a marked decline in the early 1970s there has been a noteworthy resurgence in the number of infants affected by congenital syphilis in the past decade. Physicians must recognize that syphilis hovers in the wings of their practice on a global scale; although it has been down, it has never been out.

Historical Introduction

Syphilis came upon the scene at a critical time in the history of Western Europe. Medieval society was in decadence. Feudal kings—the Tudors in England, the Valois in France, the Hapsburgs in Spain and Germany—were engaged in chronic, bloody, and dynastic struggles that drained their lands of treasure and exhausted their peoples. To the evils of the old dying order were added new evils stemming from the age of exploration and the appearance, among merchants and townsmen, of the profit motive as the mainspring of life and conduct. The sudden appearance and rapid dissemination of syphilis in France and Italy at this time in history came as a surprise as well as a difficult problem for Renaissance medicine. Whether this disease had existed in Europe before this time or was the gift of the crew who sailed with Columbus from the New World is still a matter of debate. Some consider it to be of long standing in Europe, but unrecognized or cloaked and included under the general term *leprosy,* which is known to have sheltered many conditions. There has always been a penchant to consider it as a new disease introduced from the New World by the sailors who returned with Columbus from his second voyage of discovery. The evidence is partly negative, when evaluated in a chronologic manner, and partly positive.

Ancient Times

The negative evidence is that there is no indication whatsoever that syphilis was prevalent in ancient times in either Europe or Africa. Many cemeteries have been examined by the Survey Department of the Egyptian Government, the burials in them ranging over a period of 5,000 years, but in no instance have the bones revealed unmistakable evidence of syphilis. Egyptian antiquities have long been a source to which inquirers have appealed for links with the pathology of the past because of the evidence that mummification affords.

A careful reading of the satyric and comic poets, as well as the classical medical writers, fails to trace any mention of those disfiguring effects of syphilis that would certainly have been commented upon by the Greeks and Romans had they existed. In like manner, no medical writer before 1493 alludes to any disease resembling syphilis. The history of syphilis is unique in that its occurrence is recorded in the medical literature not in a stepwise manner but with dramatic aplomb.

Middle Ages

Columbus left Seville to make his second voyage to the New World on August 2, 1493. He landed on the island of Hispaniola and arrived in Palos in Andalusia on his return journey after first paying a visit to Lisbon. One of the ships under his command was driven north and entered the French port of Bayonne. It is now well documented that various crew members disseminated the infection in Paris, Rome, and Naples. In fact, war provided the means for the international spread of syphilis when Charles VIII of France dispatched an army of mercenaries that included men who had sailed with Columbus to attack Naples. An initial victory was turned into defeat, and the French army, rendered impotent by a raging epidemic, retreated ignominiously and was disbanded. The mercenaries, after returning from Italy, moved around Europe, and as a result many more people became infected. This infectious entity was not long in obtaining a name; in France it was referred to as the *Neapolitan disease,* and in Italy and the Holy Roman Empire as *il morbo Gallico,* the French disease. It was known at a later date as the *great pox.*

Historians agree that an epidemic raged in Europe from the final quinquennium of the fifteenth century to the midsixteenth century, resulting in thousands of deaths. There was no effective therapy; only prayer was available. Fear of the disease led to the enlistment of one of the Church's 14 emergency-duty saints. As a result Saint Denis became the patron saint of syphilitics. A short prayer of intercession to Saint Denis can still be seen in the Bavarian State Library in Munich. In each lower corner a pockmarked penitent is depicted with head upturned in supplication.

Fracastoro of Verona, who was a poet, geologist, humanist, and physician, in 1530 wrote a poem "Syphilis sive Morbus Gallicus" ("Syphilis or the French Disease"). In ancient mythology Syphilius was a shepherd who decided to worship the king and not the gods, and as a result Apollo infected the air with noxious vapors. From the latter Syphilius contracted a disease associated with a marked ulcerous skin eruption. The poem presents the various symptoms and signs of the disease as well as its treatment by the use of mercury or guaiac, a "holy wood" used by the American Indians. From the eponymous hero of the poem came the word that now has a definite scientific meaning.

Bard of Avon

Whether Shakespeare was, in fact, acquainted with the medical literature of his time is a question that will probably never be answered, but there is no doubt whatsoever that he was conversant with the current medical opinions of his day. The Bard of Avon never used the word *syphilis,* although his references to sexually transmitted diseases appeared about 90 years after the publication of Fracastoro's poem. As pointed out by Kail,[37] he referred to "the malady of France" in at least seven of his plays, and his observations on this disease were not only accurate but in many instances far ahead of his time. No more vivid clinical picture of the late stages of syphilis has ever been written than when Timon advises the two courtesans on how to take their revenge on men:

Consumptions sow
In hollow bones of man; strike their sharp shins,
And mar men's spurring. Crack the lawyer's
voice,
That he may never more false title plead,
Nor sound his quillets shrilly. Hoar the flamen,
That scolds against the quality of flesh
And not believes himself. Down with the nose,
Down with it flat, take the bridge quite away
Of him that, his particular to foresee,
Smells from the general weal. Make curl'd-pate
ruffians bald,
And let the unscarr'd braggarts of the war
Derive some pain from you. Plague all,
That your activity may defeat and quell
The source of all erection. There's more gold.
Do you damn others, and let this damn you,
And ditches grave you all!

Timon of Athens 4.3

The classification of sexually transmitted diseases was in hopeless disarray during the eighteenth century, and they were thought to be due to a single poisonous agent modified by the constitution of the patient. John Hunter was determined to clarify the matter and ascertain whether the agent that caused gonorrhea was identical with that producing syphilis. He inoculated himself in

May of 1767 with material obtained from a patient suffering from gonorrhea. The patient, as is now well known, also had syphilis, and Hunter contracted the disease. This not only wrecked his own life but also delayed progress because he maintained that both gonorrhea and syphilis were caused by the same agent. His experiment led to the initial lesion of syphilis being called the *Hunterian sore* but it also prevented for many years the attainment of factual information pertaining to the disease and its therapy.

Modern Times

It was not, however, until the early years of the twentieth century that the causative organism was identified. In 1905, Fritz Schaudinn,[51] who was a protozoologist, pointed out to Paul Ehrlich Hoffman in the Berlin Health Institute the presence of a minute spirillum in the exudation of a lesion from a patient who was undergoing treatment for the disease. The name *Treponema pallidum* was assigned to the organism, and it was found to accord with Koch's postulates. Its life history was studied at the Pasteur Institute in Paris, and it was soon recognized as the pathogen responsible for syphilis in man, apes, and rabbits.

In 1906, the complement fixation test was reported by Wassermann, Neisser, and Bruck.[54] One year later Michaelis[43] described a flocculation test that eventually replaced the Wassermann test to a large extent because of its simplicity, speed, and low cost. The methodology was now available to confirm by laboratory tests the clinical diagnosis of syphilis. More important, however, the blood tests made it feasible to detect hitherto unsuspected cases in the latent or asymptomatic stages of the disease in the absence of lesions and prior to progression to the late symptomatic stages.

The discovery of the pathogen led Paul Ehrlich in his laboratory in Frankfurt to do a series of experiments to discover some substance that would be poisonous to the spirochete without being deleterious to its host. In 1910 he introduced the organic arsenical Salvarsan, the first drug with any pretension to specificity in the treatment of syphilis. Ehrlich and Hata[20] published their results with this compound, and although somewhat primitive by present-day standards it was efficacious for the treatment of syphilis. This was the era of therapeutic discoveries and the dawn of antimicrobial therapy. In 1928, Fleming isolated penicillin, but it was not until 1940 that Florey and his associates demonstrated the antimicrobial activity of this compound in man. In 1943 Mahoney and associates[40] demonstrated the effectiveness of penicillin in the treatment of syphilis.

Epidemiology

Although the incidence of infectious syphilis decreased with the introduction of antibiotics, it is a long way from being eradicated and remains a disease with a worldwide distribution. The classic Hunterian chancre is seen today just as it was in early times. Likewise, the early lesions of secondary syphilis still appear in most patients as they did in former years. As a general rule diseases do not change; when they do, they alter primarily as a result of environmental factors, new knowledge, and therapeutic advances. Syphilis appears to have changed from the original virulent form to a less fulminant and predictable infection.

During the past few decades there has been a change in the clinical presentation of the disease because of an increased number of patients with extragenital chancres. Changes in sexual mores may be responsible, but with such changes the physician encounters more subtle manifestations of the great imitator. Indiscriminate use of antimicrobial agents may account for some of the atypical features of the disease. It is also possible that corticosteroids and other immunosuppressive agents may alter the course of this infection. In the past syphilis has been portrayed as occurring in stages: primary, secondary, or tertiary. Some of the clinical manifestations are so different that they were once considered to be unrelated clinical entities. Syphilis may be one of the best-known sexually transmitted diseases, but much remains to be learned about the manifestations of this infection.

Incidence

There is no room for complacency, as the Centers for Disease Control[10] reported that in the United States in 1985 the rates of primary and secondary syphilis began to increase, following a 5-year period of steady reduction in the incidence of this infection. In 1987 the Centers for Disease Control[12] reported that the incidence was 14.6 cases per 100,000 population, the highest rate since 1950. An increase in primary and secondary syphilis was followed shortly thereafter by an increase in the morbidity and mortality associated with congenital syphilis. Confirmation of this fact was included in the report by the Centers for Disease Control,[12] which revealed that in the second half of 1987 the rate of congenital syphilis in the United States had increased by 21 percent to 10.5 cases per 100,000 live births. Two-thirds of these cases occurred in the states of California, Florida, and New York. In a further report the Centers for Disease Control[14] revealed that in the State of New York the incidence of congenital syphilis rose to 357 cases in 1988, which represented more than half of the reported cases in the United States. In view of these figures, New York introduced a program to screen all neonates for congenital syphilis.

These increases in adult and congenital syphilis took place despite concurrent changes in the epidemiology of the disease that would have led one to believe that there should have been a decrease in the rates of infection. Syphilis was disproportionately more common among homosexual and heterosexual males in the 1970s but in the quinquennium 1977 to 1982 the incidence in this segment of the population decreased on account of the marked reduction in unsafe sexual practices among homosexual males. Consequently, as the incidence of the disease increased, it reverted to being predominantly a heterosexual disease. In 1988 the rates increased dramatically in females and heterosexual males. What is of interest is that the rates for early syphilis have increased in the United States when the rates for the other reportable sexually transmitted disease, gonorrhea, have declined. The reason for this aberration is unknown.

The increased incidence of this disease is most

Table 21-1 Measures That Can Significantly Reduce or Eradicate Congenital Syphilis

Prevention of the spread of syphilis in the heterosexual community through rapid and thorough epidemiologic investigations
The education of females at risk to infection about the need to seek early and continuous prenatal care
Encourage medical care providers to perform routine serologic tests on patients in the third as well as the first trimester

marked in women regardless of ethnic background. Although these changes in incidence are noted in black and heterosexual women living in urban areas, there has also been an alteration in the male to female ratios of the disease to just below 2:1.

Drug Abuse

In some areas the increased incidence of syphilis has been linked to individuals who use illegal drugs. This is a specific segment of society in which disease intervention is difficult, but such individuals are not the only ones who have had an impact on the increase of syphilis in the population. Crack cocaine use along with the intense dependence it fosters forces many users to trade sex for drugs. Such females are a reservoir for syphilis and AIDS to both their clients and families. Adams and associates[1] in a report for the National Institute for Drug Abuse have estimated that 3 million individuals in the United States in 1986 regularly used cocaine. Minkoff and associates[44] reported that among a group of inner city parturient women detection of cocaine derivatives in urine samples was significantly associated with syphilis and HIV infections. They intimated that cocaine use may increase the need to consider more aggressive surveillance from the point of view of perinatal medicine because such gravid patients fail to utilize the benefits offered by prenatal care services.

Congenital Syphilis

Experience reveals that even in the absence of drug abuse women who deliver infants with congenital disease have failed to avail themselves of prenatal services. In some areas the urban clinics are understaffed, and the resources prevent the delivery of adequate prenatal care. It is unlikely that the rate of congenital syphilis will decrease until the incidence of the disease is reduced in women during reproductive life. Epidemiologists are of the opinion that there are at least three unreported cases for every one detected. The Centers for Disease Control[11] in their guidelines for the prevention and control of congenital syphilis indicate that the majority of family planning clinics as well as prenatal services require serologic tests for syphilis. In addition to New York the states of Texas and Florida demand cord blood serology studies for syphilis in view of the demographics of the disease. Queries about the true incidence of congenital syphilis have been moot because of false-positive diagnoses in noninfected seropositive neonates who had passive transfer of maternal antibody and similarly false-negative serology in the infants of mothers. The latter demonstrated no antibody titer when initially screened, but later in the pregnancy had undergone seroconversion. Congenital syphilis can be eliminated or greatly reduced by the adoption of simple measures as listed in Table 21-1. In high-risk groups serologic testing should be instituted in each trimester of pregnancy.

Prenatal Screening

In the United Kingdom congenital syphilis is currently no longer a major public health problem. The low incidence is to a large extent due to the universal policy of screening gravid patients and the prompt treatment of early acquired syphilis. Bowell and associates[7] in a retrospective survey found that 62 of 76,519 pregnancies were noted to have positive serology. Their study revealed that positive sera were present in 1 in 1,234 gestations. These investigators reported that prenatal screening identified 13 patients with previously unrecorded acquired syphilis, and 11 of the women subsequently received antibiotic therapy in the course of their pregnancy. In the 62 pregnancies associated with positive serology, there were six fetal losses, but in no instance was there any evidence of congenital syphilis, and none of the liveborn infants had any stigmata of congenital syphilis. These investigators state that despite the current low incidence of syphilis in the United Kingdom it is imperative that prenatal serologic screening of all patients continue and that by such means it is possible to institute adequate therapy early in a gestation. Williams[58] indicated that despite the low incidence of syphilis in the United Kingdom standard screening for the disease in the first trimester of pregnancy is cost-effective, even when the medicolegal aspects and the strong possibility of recrudescence in the absence of continued vigilance are taken into account. Clay[16] states that apart from the notable exception of male homosexuals and bisexuals there is no evidence of behavioral changes among sexually active individuals since the appearance of human immunodeficiency virus (HIV). She notes that reported cases of most sexually transmitted diseases in heterosexuals continue to increase, especially in young people. This investigator reaffirms that failures in first-trimester screening are important and arise because of late booking, failure of treatment, reinfection, omission of testing or treatment, laboratory error, or failure to retest individuals at high risk in the third trimester. Optimal therapeutic regimens for eradicating treponemes in late pregnancy have not been determined even for penicillin, and failure with alternative agents such as erythromycin is well documented. Repeat serologic testing will not identify all infected patients, as some remain free of antibodies against the organism even at the time of parturition. Clay[16] considers that prenatal screening for syphilis is essential and wisely answers the critics—who consider it not cost-effective and of questionable benefit because of the low incidence of syphilis in the United Kingdom—by her concluding sentence: "Perhaps if we learnt to take pride in an achievement that has been

Table 21-2 Factors That Prevent Eradication of Congenital Syphilis

Socioeconomic deprivation	
	Late attendance at clinic
	Drug abuse of all kinds
	Delays in communication
Lack of resources	
	Lack of trained personnel
	Overcrowded clinics
	Delays from screening to follow-up
	Delays in treatment
	Failure to repeat serology in late pregnancy in high-risk groups
	Failure to treat sexual partners
	Failure to recognize infections acquired late in pregnancy*

*Repeat testing should be carried out but will not identify all infected subjects, as some will have developed antibodies against *Treponema pallidum*

laboriously and quietly attained we would recover the enthusiasm necessary for continued commitment to screening for syphilis."

In contradistinction to the low incidence of congenital syphilis in the United Kingdom, Ricci and associates[49] reported that the overall rate for congenital syphilis in a tertiary care center in Florida was 18.4 cases per 10,000 live births and that 67 percent of the mothers of these infants lacked prenatal care. These investigators emphasize that the prevention of congenital syphilis necessitates demographic studies of the populace involved. In their study, in addition to the involved population being predominantly black Americans, it was noted that the majority of the mothers of infants afflicted with congenital syphilis had been substance abusers. The report reveals that there was a highly significant association of crack cocaine use by the mothers of infants with congenital syphilis compared with the matched control group in the study. The investigators consider that the disease in the infants can be prevented if measures are adopted to address the demographic factors exhibited by the population studied. Stringent prenatal care and frequent serologic studies will not attain their aim of preventing congenital syphilis because cocaine is the most addictive drug known, and intensive psychosocial support and screening for recidivism are essential. The problem is that traditional criteria of risk for the disease may not accurately account for a particular outbreak, or if they do they may encompass only a minority core group.

Tropical Africa

In tropical countries venereal syphilis continues to be a serious health hazard. The prevalence rate among gravid patients may be of the order of 10 to 20 percent. De Muylder and colleagues[18] found active syphilis in almost 10 percent of a group of randomly selected gravid patients in a provincial hospital in Zimbabwe. They stated that their incidence was similar to that found in other studies from southern Africa. This report indicates that this disease plays a major role in the high perinatal mortality in these countries. Hira and associates[32] reported that in selected urban, semiurban, and rural areas of Zambia 12.8 percent of the pregnant women were seropositive, and about one-sixth of these infections are acquired during the pregnancy. Consequently there is a high incidence of congenital syphilis as well as abortions and stillbirths attributed to this infection. These investigators agree that adverse pregnancy outcomes due to syphilis are preventable through routine serologic screening and treatment during pregnancy. Although 90 percent of pregnant patients attend prenatal services in Zambia and serologic screening is mandatory, there are several reasons why the system breaks down, as shown in Table 21-2. It is thus obvious that in communities or countries with a high incidence of syphilis that stricter control of sexually transmitted diseases is essential. Furthermore, maternal and child health programs should pool their resources in an endeavor to see that the disease is controlled, which is the first step toward its eradication.

Microbiology

The causative agent of syphilis is a spirochete that is a member of the genus *Treponema*. Spirochetes are flexible, helical bacteria that are grouped together because of common structural features and a unique type of motility. All are slow growing, which may be a factor that plays a role in assessing the duration of therapy.

Members of the genus *Treponema* are the cause of four diseases, only one of which, namely, syphilis, is sexually transmitted. The other three diseases—pinta, yaws, and endemic syphilis—are referred to as the nonvenereal treponematoses. None of the pathogenic treponemes is morphologically distinguishable, and none has been satisfactorily propagated on artificial media.

The treponeme responsible for syphilis is called *T. pallidum,* so named because of its pale white appearance when seen by dark-ground microscopy. In its appearance and movement it is regular, sylphlike, and graceful. The organism has a spiral shape and tapered ends. It measures 7 to 14 μm in length and 0.25 μm in width. The spirals are evenly spaced about 1 μm apart. The average length of the spirochete is about the same as the diameter of a red blood cell.

The basic structure of the *Treponema* is a prokaryotic cellular mass surrounded by trilaminar membranous structures. The unique spiral structure of the pathogen is maintained by six fibrils, which overlap near the middle of the cell. They lie between the central protoplasmic core, which contains cytoplasm, ribosomes, and mesosomes and is bounded by a cell wall and outer envelope. The cell wall contains muramic acid and N-acetyl glucosamine, in a similar way to other bacteria, and thereby rendering it sensitive to certain antibiotics such as penicillin.

This organism is a natural pathogen only for humans, but unlike many organisms that afflict humankind *T. pallidum* cannot be satisfactorily cultured in vitro. Fieldsteel and colleagues[22] demonstrated that limited replication does occur in cell cultures, but successful subculturing has not been reported. The life of the organism is tenuously poised, because outside the human host it is very susceptible to drying, to sunlight and heat above body temperature, and to mild antiseptics. The organism is very susceptible to cold and dies when chilled to refrigerator temperatures. The latter is of practical impor-

Table 21-3 Characteristic Movements of *Treponema Pallidum* Observed on Dark-Field Microscopy

Rotates rapidly on its long axis like a corkscrew
Opening and closing of coils in a springlike manner with alternating flexion about its midpoint
Has a slight backward and forward motion—true motion or progression
Does not exhibit unidirectional motility, as frequently seen in saprophitic treponemes

tance in relation to blood transfusion, as no viable *T. pallidum* have ever been recovered from blood stored at refrigeration temperatures for 48 hours. It replicates every 30 to 36 hours, which accounts for its comparatively prolonged incubation period of between 10 and 90 days with an average of approximately 30 days. *Treponema pallidum* is not anaerobic as was once considered, and it does appear to thrive in vitro in atmospheres that contain 5 percent oxygen. Moisture is essential for its survival, so that it flourishes in the mouth and anogenital region.

This pathogen is believed to enter the body through minute abrasions in the skin or mucosal surface. Older views that the corkscrewlike configuration of the spirochete enabled it to penetrate unbroken epithelium are not currently accepted, although specific proof as to its mode of entry is unavailable. Once it has invaded, local replication ensues, which can result in an obliterative endarteritis and ulceration of the skin or mucous membrane. *Treponema pallidum* can be isolated from such lesions and propagated by the intratesticular injection of rabbits that are free from rabbit syphilis caused by *T. cuniculi*. The latter is not a human pathogen but closely resembles *T. pallidum* on dark-field microscopy. The rabbits should be housed at 16 to 20°C because the infection is aborted at higher temperatures. The testicular fluid is subsequently examined by dark-field microscopy for the presence of spirochetes.

The *T. pallidum* can be identified in a dark-field preparation not only by its size and spiral shape but also by its characteristic motility (Table 21-3).

Pathophysiology

The numerous unusual features of treponemal infections furnish a never-ending challenge to clinicians as well as microbiologists and immunologists. Syphilis has long been known to be one of the most complex infectious diseases, and much remains to be determined about its protean manifestations.

The pathogenesis involves acute and chronic manifestations, as well as the capacity for long-term acute latent infections. From the point of view of the parasite, syphilis represents an ideal host-parasite relationship. The pathogen can cause both acute infectious lesions, which are important in the dissemination of the disease in the host, as well as its transmission via sexual contact in the early stages of the infection. The pathogen can in

Table 21-4 Classifications of Syphilis

A.	Primary	Earliest clinical lesion
	Secondary	Disseminated infection Mucocutaneous lesions Lymphadenopathy Constitutional symptoms
	Tertiary	Gummatous, osseous Cardiovascular Neural
	Congenital	Early—before 2 years —after 2 years
B.	Early	Includes incubating and infection of less than 1 year and thereby disseminated disease
	Late	All infections of more than 1 year
	Congenital	Neonate Postneonate

the absence of treatment persist in the host for many years despite demonstrable resistance to infection. The longer syphilis remains untreated in a woman before she conceives, the more likely it is that when she becomes pregnant the pathogen will be held in check, and consequently her fetus will be less liable to intrauterine demise or born with congenital luetic infection.

Classification

It was standard practice until recently to describe syphilis as occurring in stages: primary, secondary, and tertiary. This classification, despite its clinical utility, could give a false impression that the primary stage is merely the localized chancre; the secondary stage involves the cutaneous tissues and dissemination of the organism through the body, resulting in systemic symptoms and signs; and the tertiary stage is involvement of the central nervous system, cardiovascular system, and deep organs. The last stage is the one that exhibits cutaneous lesions such as the gumma, which can ulcerate and masquerade as some other clinical entity. The gumma is a granulomatous lesion consisting of a necrotic center and small-vessel obliterative endarteritis. The late stages of syphilis are not seen in gravid patients. A classification that is important from the point of view of therapy as well as the epidemiology of the disease merely divides the infection into early, which is the infectious phase of the disease, and late (Table 21-4). It is immaterial which classification one adopts as long as one realizes that *T. pallidum* is disseminated by the bloodstream and lymphatics throughout the body within minutes of infection. The number of infecting treponemes probably also affects the incubation period.

Host Response

During the early phases of the disease, antibody and cellular responses develop in the host. In the natural

Sexual contact with individual with infectious syphilis
↓
Incubating syphilis ← Only 30–50 percent develop disease even if no therapy
↓
Clinical lesion—chancre
Overlap ↓
Disseminated syphilis
↓
Recurrent exacerbations in 25 percent
↓
Latency
↓
20–30 percent
↓
Late (tertiary) syphilis

Figure 21-1 Algorithm showing the natural course of syphilis.

course of the disease (Fig. 21-1), treponemes are not consistently eliminated, and the disease progresses to a later phase. Baseman and Hayes[4] demonstrated that there is a humoral response to a variety of treponemal proteins during infectious syphilis, yet in many instances the disease continues to progress. It is apparent from their studies that cell-mediated immunity is altered during early infection and thereby provides a mechanism by which virulent organisms avoid selective host defense mechanisms. Several antibodies against treponemal antigens have been identified, but the disease progresses, even with high antibody titers. In fact, the humoral response does little to curtail the disease, which is in accord with the fact that most infected patients seeking treatment have evidence of antibody production, which is measured by the majority of serologic tests for syphilis. Some antibodies persist throughout the life of the host, yet reinfection may take place. Clinical experience suggests that superimposed infection in patients with persisting or late infection is a rare event.

Syphilis does not cause generalized immunosuppression that can lead to opportunistic infections. Both clinical and experimental observations demonstrate that in untreated syphilitic patients new lesions do not develop at sites of challenge, but this state wanes with varying rapidity subsequent to therapy, depending on how early in the course of the disease treatment is instituted, as well as other unknown factors. A specific antibody directed against the treponeme can be detected by the fluorescent treponemal antibody test following absorption (FTA-ABS) or the hemagglutination test. It is not known whether these antibodies are protective. An antibody capable of immobilizing the treponeme develops after the chancre has healed but is always present when the cutaneous lesions appear. In the presence of complement in vitro, this antibody actually inactivates the pathogen, leading to the important and as-yet unanswered question of why syphilis persists and in some instances progresses in vivo despite the presence of antibody. Attempts to confer passive humoral immunity in rabbits with either whole serum or IgG from chancre-immune animals have produced surprising results, namely, that chancres develop late and have an atypical appearance. The fact that they occur despite infusion of large amounts of immune serum indicates that the classical humoral immune mechanisms are not protective. An interesting quantitative difference between passive humoral immunity and active immunity has been noted. Immune serum or IgG protects recipients against only a relatively small inoculum of the organism, whereas active chancre immunity is protective against a much larger inoculum. It is not known whether the antibodies that confer partial protection are opsonizing or treponemacidal.

The interaction between treponemes and macrophages or polymorphonuclear leukocytes needs to be clarified in light of observations that antibody prevents attachment of the organisms to cells in tissue culture. Some studies indicate that the antibody synthesis may be suppressed during syphilitic infections. Perhaps, despite the presence of several antibodies, production of the most appropriate and specific treponemacidal antibody is suppressed. In fact, the humoral response does little to control the disease process.

The primary lesion—the chancre—heals spontaneously within 4 to 6 weeks, accompanied by a local mononuclear infiltrate, lymphadenopathy, and the beginning of a systematic humoral response. The clearance of the organism from the local nidus of infection indicates that the local immune response is effective in eradicating the organism. It is therefore something of a paradox that the local reaction is followed by a rapidly disseminated infection, according to Tabor and colleagues,[53] in about 25 percent of untreated cases. The inability of the host to prevent widespread dissemination of the treponeme in these cases is apparently due to a delay in the transition from local to systemic immunity, whereas the balance may be altered in favor of systemic resistance in those individuals who do not exhibit secondary lesions.

Clinical Manifestations

Within a few hours of infection, the treponeme is disseminated by the blood stream and by the lymphatics to the regional lymph nodes long before the appearance of any lesion. The time interval from the initial inoculation to the appearance of the chancre is dependent on the size of the infecting inoculum. *Incubating syphilis* is a term often used for the interval between the time of infection and appearance of the clinical lesion. If the patient is pregnant, the fetus can become infected as a result of placental transmission of the organism.

Early Syphilis

The chancre is a painless, shallow ulcer that forms at the site of inoculation, and the lesion is accompanied by firm, nontender, nonsuppurative regional lymphadenopathy. The labia are the most common sites but the lesion may appear on the cervix or at the fourchette, urethra, or perineum. Some chancres may be inconspicuous or may, because of location, escape notice. Although most chancres appear on the vulva or cervix, they may be seen on the lips, oropharynx—specifically tongue and tonsil—breast, or anorectal area.

In all women who acquire a painless indurated ulcer of the vulva, the physician's first objective is to diagnose or exclude the chancre of early contagious syphilis. In eliciting the patient's history, the physician must take into account the realities of human sexual behavior and experimentation and consider the possibility of oral and anal ulceration due to the treponeme. An attempt to obtain a full history may bring forth evasiveness or denials, but these difficulties should not deflect the physician from essential investigations. This is important, especially in the gravid patient, as syphilis is a prenatal infection that may be transmitted to the intrauterine patient at any time in the course of the gestation and consequently may be associated with a variety of outcomes.

The chancre heals within 4 to 6 weeks even in the absence of therapy without leaving a scar. The adenopathy may take longer to resolve. The spontaneous healing of a suspect lesion may create a sense of false security, especially if some form of therapy, albeit inadequate, has been administered. In all cases adequate evaluation and follow-up studies are mandatory.

Two generalizations can be made concerning the early stages of infectious syphilis: (1) Any genital lesion should be considered to be due to *T. pallidum* until time and repeated evaluation prove otherwise. (2) If an indolent, painless lesion, irrespective of location but particularly if the erotic areas of the body are involved, fails to heal within 2 weeks, the great imitator should be suspected.

Disseminated Syphilis

After a period of 6 weeks to 6 months following the initiation of the infection, a systemic response, together with a mucocutaneous eruption and generalized lymphadenopathy, occurs. The patient complains of an influenza-like syndrome consisting of malaise, headache, sore throat, lacrimation, and generalized arthralgia. There may be a slight temperature elevation and weight loss. With these constitutional symptoms, a generalized lymphadenopathy is readily discernible. The lymph nodes are enlarged and have a hard, rubbery feel. The lymphadenopathy usually precedes the cutaneous eruption. This phase of the infection has often been termed *disseminated syphilis*, as it is the result of the dispersal of the pathogen from the chancre. In fact, in many instances the chancre may still be present when the cutaneous lesions appear. The skin lesions may mimic a variety of dermatologic conditions, but they are rarely associated with pruritus.

Cutaneous Lesions

Great diversity is a feature of the cutaneous lesions. They are usually symmetric and may be macular, papular, pustular, or papulosquamous. The lesions may involve the trunk and extremities, including the palms and soles of the feet. Palmar and plantar lesions are generally papulosquamous and never vesicular, as in congenital syphilis. In fact, vesicular or bullous cutaneous lesions are never observed in adults with syphilis. Follicular papules may be found in the scalp in association with alopecia areata. Lesions of the mucous membrane of the buccal cavity, tongue, and lips are either superficial ulcerated areas with grayish borders surrounded by a red areola or large gray plaques. They are most commonly recognized as "mucous patches" in the mouth, and their presence should alert the physician to a possible diagnosis of a luetic infection.

The papular lesions that occur in moist areas of the body are called *condylomata lata* and are essentially hypertrophic granulomatous tissue. These moist areas correspond with the flexion creases of the body. They are nontender but often coalesce when they occur at sites liable to friction, such as the perianal and axillary areas. Such lesions are often exuberant, reddish brown, flat-topped, moist, and highly infectious. Both the condylomata lata and the mucous patches in the mouth contain large numbers of the parasite, as is evident when dark-field microscopic studies are conducted. This phase of the disease may be evanescent and disappear with or without appropriate therapy. The lesions usually resolve over a period of 3 to 6 weeks, but if no treatment is prescribed about 25 percent of the patients have one or more exacerbations of the lesions in the subsequent 2 to 4 years.

Disseminated syphilis must always be considered as a systemic disease, and therefore it is not surprising that it may cause hepatitis, a nephrotic syndrome, meningitis, periostitis of the long bones, iridocyclitis, and anterior uveitis. During this phase of the disease, a host response, as elicited by tests for lymphocytic transformation evoked by treponemal antigens and serologic studies for antibodies, is always present.

Latent Syphilis

After the stage of disseminated syphilis, there is a phase with no symptoms or signs of the disease. There is only serologic evidence of the infection at this stage, and although it has been termed *latent* it should not be assumed that the disease process does not progress. It can be associated with exacerbations of spirochetemia and clinical manifestations of disseminated syphilis. As indicated in Table 21-4, early syphilis comprises all stages from the inception of the infection to the latent stage. Early syphilis is accompanied with spirochetemia. This fact is important from the point of view of the intrauterine patient because congenital syphilis results from maternal spirochetemia during pregnancy. It is uncommon for women with late syphilis to give birth to a child with congenital syphilis, and the incidence of stillbirths in such individuals is comparable to that in the general population.

Syphilis and Pregnancy

The clinical manifestations of infection due to *T. pallidum* in gravid patients are very similar to those seen in nongravid women. Pregnancy per se has little if any effect on the natural course of the disease, but early syphilis can affect pregnancy outcome.

Traditionally, syphilis was not considered a cause of abortion. Most investigators considered that the fetus was protected from transplacental infection for the first 4 to 5 months of the pregnancy by an effective barrier function of the cytotrophoblast. Harter and Benirschke,[29] however, showed that the treponeme was present in material obtained from abortions where the duration of the pregnancies was between 9 and 10 weeks.

Thus despite the fact that syphilis is primarily of concern as a cause of congenital stigmata in liveborn infants, the transmission of the spirochete to the fetus at an early age suggests that spontaneous abortion due to this pathogen is possible. No data are available to indicate the prevalence of abortion attributable to spirochetal infection, although the majority of clinicians would consider that the number is very small. The available methods of disease control applied to congenital infection are also appropriate for the prevention of abortion due to treponemal infection.

Congenital syphilis remains a significant health problem. The severity of the fetal infection tends to be related to the time of the maternal disease, as this affects the number of organisms invading the conceptus as well as the maternal immune response. If the maternal infection is acquired in the last trimester of pregnancy, the relatively high numbers of spirochetes present in the blood stream can easily traverse the placenta. At this stage relatively little treponemicidal IgG crosses the placenta, as the humoral response of the mother has only recently been initiated. Such intrauterine patients are liable to massive dissemination of the pathogen, and as a result severe early congenital syphilis ensues.

If the maternal infection occurs prior to conception or early in the gestation, the immune response exhibited by the mother is partially protective, and the majority of the spirochetes are cleared from the conceptus. Infants infected in this manner in general have a far less severe infection at birth because of the presence of maternal IgG, but they have signs of congenital syphilis. It is now recognized that surviving fetuses most liable to be seriously afflicted at birth are those infected at or after the twenty-fourth week of the pregnancy.

Pregnancy does not prevent exacerbation of the cutaneous manifestations and spirochetemia of disseminated syphilis. Under such circumstances overwhelming fetoplacental infection and intrauterine fetal death can occur. Fetal infection can result in low birth weight, premature labor, or hydrops fetalis. The physician must be alert to the fact that if the spirochetemia is not severe or happens very late in the gestation, the neonate may not have any stigmata of syphilis.

Congenital Syphilis

The resurgence of syphilis in the population of childbearing age has produced renewed interest in congenital syphilis. Clinically affected neonates demonstrate evidence of disseminated syphilis because the infection is the result of the placental transmission of the pathogen. If, as already stated, the maternal infection is acquired in the latter weeks of the pregnancy or the spirochetemia is not marked, evidence of congenital disease may not be recognized at birth and will be manifest only several weeks later. Consequently, persistent infection may be symptomatic or asymptomatic, and its expression may be present at birth or delayed for several weeks or months. Clinical manifestations appearing within the first 2 years of life are often designated as *early* congenital syphilis and those occurring after this time interval are referred to as *late* congenital syphilis, but there may be an overlap in the clinical features. Hira and associates[33] noted several significant differences in the manifestations of congenital syphilis in neonates and infants between 4 weeks and 6 months of age. The neonates had a higher mortality and jaundice. The most common clinical observations in the neonates were hepatosplenomegaly, cutaneous lesions, anemia, and jaundice. The older infants were more often afflicted by snuffles and joint swellings with pseudoparesis (Table 21-5).

Table 21-5 Clinical and Radiologic Features of Early Congenital Syphilis

Feature	Neonate (Percent)	Older Than 28 Days (Percent)
Hepatosplenomegaly	91	88
Jaundice	49	7
Anemia	64	89
Cutaneous eruption	31	55
Snuffles	12	50
Joint swelling	3	34
Metaphyseal dystrophy	95	91
Periosteal reaction	38	79
Osteitis-type changes	30	40
Cerebrospinal fluid changes	44	38
Positive serology (FTA-ABS)	99	99

Adapted from Hira, et al, 1985.[32]

Early Congenital Syphilis

Early congenital syphilis may be clinically indistinguishable from other entities, particularly other congenital infections. The diagnosis may be difficult because the clinical presentation is highly variable. The clinical signs of early congenital syphilis are seldom seen at birth but usually manifest themselves 2 to 4 weeks after delivery. The cutaneous lesions may be maculopapular or papular, and a bullous eruption also occurs. The latter is sometimes referred to as *syphilitic pemphigus* and may be present at birth. The lesions consist of vesicular or bullous lesions on the palms and soles and occasionally on other parts of the body. It is only in early congenital syphilis that bullous vesicular eruptions are observed. Such lesions contain spirochetes, are highly contagious, and when ruptured leave a denuded area that usually undergoes crusting. Fluid from these lesions, when studied by dark-field microscopy, usually reveals the presence of spirochetes. Many such infants have rhinitis and respiratory distress during the neonatal period. Later in the first weeks of life, the mucous membranes of the nasopharynx are involved and produce the heavy infectious mucoid discharge that is usually termed *snuffles*. Periostitis and osteochondritis of the long bones resulting in the pseudoparalysis of Parrot's disease are frequently noted. Meningitis and CSF abnormalities are also frequently observed in neonatal congenital syphilis. The diagnosis of early congenital syphilis is usually not difficult when clinical lesions are apparent, but this is not always the case.

Humoral Immune Response

In the case of congenital syphilis, there is an inability to identify accurately the infected but asymptomatic infant. The problem stems from the inability to distinguish the humoral immune response of the mother, whose IgG antibodies traverse the placenta to the fetus, from the specific antibody response of the infant. The assessment of total IgM levels has been one approach as an aid to obtain a diagnosis of congenital syphilis, but elevated total fetal serum IgM levels can result from a variety of congenital entities, making the diagnosis of congenital syphilis by this nonspecific criterion equivocal.

Sanchez and associates[50] examined by Western blot analysis the fetal IgM response to antigens of *T. pallidum* in 39 pairs of maternal-infant sera and included in the study 12 mothers and infants with active syphilis. A fetal IgM response to treponemal antigens with apparent molecular masses of 72, 47, 45, 42, 13, 17, and 15 kDa (kilodaltons) was recorded in sera of infants with congenital syphilis. By means of high-performance liquid chromatography (HPLC) they fractionated the sera into IgG and IgM components and demonstrated that in every case the fetal IgM antibodies were directed specifically against a 47 kDa antigen. Their results suggest that fetal IgM reactivity with the 47-kDa antigen of *T. pallidum* can be adopted as an important marker for the diagnosis of congenital syphilis. Wicher and associates,[57] however, showed that except for minor differences *T. pallidum* infection produces very similar specific humoral responses in humans, rabbits, and guinea pigs. They found no marked differences between the three species in their response to critical pathogen epitopes. *Treponema pallidum* was found to contain few if any pathogen-specific peptides. In addition, these investigators could not identify any IgM antibodies specific for the pathogen at any stage of the disease.

Early congenital syphilis may exemplify an entity in which non-immunologic mechanisms may play a role in its pathogenesis. Delayed hepatic development and osteochondritis are not easily attributable to the immune response and are most likely the direct results of the treponemal infection. The presence of lymphocytic infiltrates in many of the tissues, together with IgM antitreponemal antibodies generated by the fetus or infant, is indicative of an active, be it ineffectual, perinatal immune response. More information pertaining to the pathogenic mechanisms involved may be generated by the animal models developed by Fitzgerald[23] and Kajdacsy-Balla and coworkers.[38]

It is difficult to describe the natural history of untreated congenital syphilis, but affected children have stigmata of early lesions as exemplified by dental problems as well as lesions that emanate from the chronic infection.

Late Congenital Syphilis

Late congenital syphilis appears in children after the second year of life and in the majority of cases is asymptomatic, but serologic studies are invariably positive. It is a multisystem disease, but it may be remarkably mild and pass unnoticed, so that it may be several years or decades before the congenital infection reveals itself.

The most common manifestations noted by Fiumara and Lessell[26] and Mascola and associates[42] include periostitis of the frontal and parietal bones, short maxilla, high arch to the palate, dental abnormalities such as "mulberry molars" that are the result of infection of the dental pulp, peg-shaped notched central incisors known as Hutchinson's teeth, and saddle nose due to destruction of the nasal septum and bone. Interstitial keratitis, eighth-nerve deafness, saber shins, and rhagades were less frequently observed. Clutton's joints were rarely noted in the late stages of congenital syphilis. Fiumara and Lessell[26] reported that eighth-nerve deafness usually occurred in the first decade of life but might not be apparent until the third or fourth decade. When present, it is always found in conjunction with other manifestations of late congenital syphilis.

The striking destructive nature of the untreated disease and its vertical transmission are embodied in the aide-mémoire, handed down from generation to generation of medical students, pertaining to the syphilitic family:

There once was a man from Torbay,
Who thought that the syph went away,
So now he has tabes,
And saber-shinned babies,
And thinks he is Queen of the May.

Laboratory Diagnosis

Visualization of the treponeme by dark-field microscopic examination is the most accurate method of substantiating a clinical diagnosis of syphilis. The test can be applied to material obtained from moist lesions or a regional lymph node. Overlaying a gently abraded lesion with a couple of drops of normal saline often provides an adequate specimen. However, the removal of any pus or scab is often necessary in order to achieve an adequate specimen. The injection of 0.5 ml of normal saline into a regional lymph node allows for an aspirate to be evaluated for the presence of the pathogen. False-positive results almost never occur if the test is conducted by personnel experienced in dark-field microscopy. The use of this diagnostic test has been limited because of the lack of dark-field microscopes as well as individuals trained in the interpretation of such preparations. Many physicians in clinical practice have never seen *T. pallidum* in a dark-field preparation. Cutaneous lesions from disseminated as well as congenital syphilis can be examined in this manner if the crust has been removed and the base of the lesion abraded. When dark-field microscopy is unavailable to the physician, direct fluorescent antibody testing can be utilized as an alternative method for detecting the spirochete. The serum from a lesion is pressed under a slide, allowed to dry, and then stained with fluorescein-labeled antibody to *T. pallidum*. In order to attain specific *T. pallidum* antibody, nonspecific antibodies are removed by absorption by nonpathogenic treponemes.

Dark-field microscopic identification of *T. pallidum* from suspected lesions is still the best and most expeditious way to diagnose infectious syphilis. It should be remembered that in approximately 25 percent of females with syphilis the lesion develops on the cervix. Symptomless female contacts of males with the infection should therefore have dark-field microscopy of material obtained from the endocervix.

A practiced eye is necessary for confident identification of *T. pallidum*. The organism has to be differentiated from the spirochetes commonly seen in inflammatory genital conditions of both sexes. These include *T. balanitides, T. gracilis, T. refringens,* and such human saprophytes as *T. macrodentium*. As saprophytic, nonpathogenic treponemes are common around the gingival margins, a dark-field evaluation of intraoral lesions may be difficult to interpret. Similarly, direct visualization of the pathogen may be impeded by any antiseptic solutions or topical ointments applied by the patient. If the examination of a lesion is found initially to be negative, dark-field microscopy should be repeated the following day. The patient, in the meantime, should be instructed not to use ointments or antibiotics and not to wash the lesions with soap or antiseptic solutions. If the dark-field examination is still negative, serologic methods of diagnosis should be utilized.

Serologic Tests

Serologic tests for syphilis are intended to enable the clinician to diagnose and treat the disease. The ideal test should be technically simple to conduct, furnish consistently reproducible results, and produce no false-positive or false-negative data. Currently there is no test that fulfills these requirements.

Nonspecific Antibody Tests

The first serologic test for the diagnosis of syphilis was devised in 1906 by Wassermann, Neisser, and Bruck.[54] This test was a complement fixation reaction in which the antigenic reagent was an aqueous extract of fetal liver obtained from a syphilitic infant. It was later shown that the reactive reagent in the liver extract was actually a component of normal tissues and not of treponemal origin. The Wassermann test nevertheless proved capable of distinguishing individuals with syphilis with a fair degree of accuracy from those who were not infected, despite its lack of immunologic specificity. The Wassermann reaction has now been replaced by another nontreponemal serologic test that was developed by the Venereal Disease Research Laboratory and is commonly known as the VDRL test. It is now one of the most commonly used screening tests for syphylitic infections. The test detects reagin, a substance considered by many to be an immunologically nonspecific gamma globulin present in small and variable amounts in human blood. Tests that are used for the detection of increased levels of reagin, even when measured amounts of cardiolipin, lecithin, and cholesterol are used as antigen, are useful only for screening purposes. Apart from technical false-positive results, biologic false-positive (BFP) results occur. Acute BFP reactions are defined as lasting no longer than 6 months and are associated with a variety of clinical entities, particularly infectious mononucleosis, hepatitis, pneumonia, malaria, and immunization, as well as many bacterial and viral infections. Chronic BFP reactions are those that persist for 6 months or longer and are encountered in patients with chronic infection or connective tissue disorders such as leprosy, sarcoidoses, systemic lupus erythematosis, rheumatoid arthritis, thyroiditis, drug addiction, and lymphoma. There is no correlation between the amount of reagin in the patient's serum and the severity of the disease. Reagin is not usually detectable by the VDRL test until about 5 to 6 weeks after the infection. Therefore, a negative test does not rule out active disease. Once stimulated, reagin levels tend to climb to a maximum titer during the phase of disseminated syphilis. A fourfold or greater increase in reagin titers when paired sera are compared is suggestive evidence of syphilis. If chancres or cutaneous lesions are present and reveal on dark-field microscopy the presence of *T. pallidum*, reagin tests offer only confirmation of the diagnosis.

The anticardiolipin antibody often referred to as the *nonspecific* antibody can be measured by the rapid plasma reagin (RPR) test, which is an abbreviated equivalent of the VDRL test. Both tests are inexpensive and sensitive. Consequently, they have been extensively used as screening procedures as well as for follow-up in immunocompetent patients to assess the response to therapy. These tests can be reported as reactive or nonreactive or as a titer that reflects the degree of current infection. The latter can be used to assess in conjunction with posttherapy titers the response to treatment.

Baseline titers are highest in disseminated syphilis. The titers as determined by RPR are usually about two dilutions higher than those noted with VDRL test, and clinicians should be aware of this fact if they attempt to correlate results from different laboratories in order to assess therapeutic results or ascertain whether reinfection has occurred in a patient.

A titer of the VDRL or RPR tests was until relatively recently utilized as a guide to therapy, and individual laboratories attempted to determine cutoff points in terms of titer to assess the need for treatment. Despite the fact that the immunologic background of these tests suggests that they are partially dependent on the presence of IgM, which is usually viewed as an indicator of disease activity, the value of this approach has limitations. As these treponemal tests produce some false-positive results, they are usually followed, if there is any doubt about the diagnosis, by more specific tests with less cross-reactivity.

Specific Treponemal Tests

The tests that measure antibody to surface antigens on *T. pallidum* are more specific and are commonly utilized to confirm infection following a positive VDRL or RPR test. The treponemal tests at present widely employed include the fluorescent antibody absorption (FTA-ABS) test, treponemal immunization (TPI) test, and the microhemagglutination assay for antibody to *T. pallidum* (MHA-TP). A modification of the FTA-ABS test, known as the FTA-ABS IgM test, has been used for the diagnosis of congenital syphilis.

The treponemal antibody tests establish a diagnosis of a spirochetal infection but do not differentiate active disease from past infection. These tests may remain positive for many years unless therapy is instituted early in the infection and therefore cannot be used to assess posttherapy progress. The VDRL test—particularly if reactive at a dilution of 16 or more and associated with a rising titer—is a better guide to the activity of the infection. The basic FTA-ABS test has a margin of error of up to 10 percent, and the source may be such factors as nonspecific group antibodies, the use of inefficient sorbent, changes of cell surface due to lyophilizing of *T. pallidum,* or the presence in the serum of antinuclear or rheumatoid factors.

The major diagnostic value of the treponemal tests is the exclusion of spirochetal infection by a negative result except at the inception of the disease. A better serologic test is a necessity because if the treponemal tests are utilized in a low-risk population the ratio of false-positive to true-positive results increases. Application of these tests to a higher-risk section of the population is associated with a decreased percentage of false-reactive results. By the use of a nontreponemal test such as the VDRL for screening purposes in low-risk populations, the small percentage of patients with a reactive serologic test can be inexpensively and accurately identified.

Baker-Zander and associates,[3] by the use of immunoblot, and Moskophidis and Müller,[46] utilizing radioimmunoprecipitation techniques, have characterized the humoral immune response to the polypeptides of *T. pallidum* during the different stages of the infection. They found serum antibodies to be present in sera from patients with different stages of the disease but absent in normal sera and sera associated with false-positive reaction in nontreponemal tests. Adequate evaluation of the serodiagnostic potential of antibody to single *T. pallidum* polypeptides has been restricted because the organism cannot be continuously grown in vitro, and as a result adequate quantities of purified antigens have been unavailable.

The solid-phase ELISA is easy to perform, relatively inexpensive, and quantitative and allows for automation. Its potential as an improved serodiagnostic test for syphilis is well recognized. The ELISA format utilizing sonicated, freshly extracted *T. pallidum* has been shown by Popsil[48] to be comparable in sensitivity and specificity to conventional tests that are available for antibodies to treponemes; antibodies to the majority of *T. pallidum* antigens appear in disseminated syphilis, whereas in the late stages of the infection antibodies to many of the polypeptides cannot be detected. The sensitivity of the recombinant antigen-based ELISA for syphilis is likely to be further improved by the inclusion of other cloned *T. pallidum* antigens that are immunogenic in all stages of the disease.

Reference laboratories make it a rule to study serum diluted and undiluted, but some nonreference laboratories conduct serologic studies on diluted samples only if on clinical evaluation the physician is suspicious of a luetic infection. In such circumstances the prozone phenomenon may conceal a positive reaction on an undiluted serum sample, as a result of antibody excess that may prevent agglutination. Berkowitz and associates[5] reported four cases of false-negative serology in gravid patients due to the prozone phenomenon. All four women were delivered of infants with congenital syphilis. One of the patients had an intrauterine fetal death at 27 weeks gestation and was delivered of a hydropic fetus. The authors recommend that, in any gravid patient with apparently negative nontreponemal tests in whom fetal compromise is suspected, the laboratory should be asked to perform prozone serum dilutions on the original serum sample.

At present the Centers for Disease Control[13] considers that all patients with syphilis be evaluated for HIV and have repeated serologic tests to determine the potential for therapeutic failure in HIV-infected patients with luetic infection.

Hass and colleagues[28] reported from their studies with male patients that treponemal tests do not reliably identify prior syphilis infection in individuals with HIV infection. This was most apparent as immune dysfunction progressed and the T4 lymphocyte count was reduced to less than 200. The loss of reactivity of the treponemal tests was related to the degree of immune dysfunction. From their studies they demonstrated that prospective studies are necessary to evaluate the sensitivity of tests for the diagnosis of syphilis in patients with HIV infection. The limitations of serologic testing for syphilis involve mainly the nontreponemal tests. False-negative results can occur with early luetic infection and in HIV-infected patients with disseminated syphilis.

Congenital Syphilis

A diagnosis of congenital syphilis should be considered in cases of stillbirth associated with placental hydrops when the maternal serology is positive. In such instances pathologic examination of the placenta, umbilical cord, and infant should be performed, as well as radiologic examination of long bones and serology. By such measures a definitive diagnosis can be attained. A positive diagnosis of congenital syphilis in such cases implies identification of the spirochete by dark-field microscopy, fluorescent antibody, or special staining techniques. Radiographic studies of the long bones can reveal osteochondritis even in severely macerated stillborn infants.

Serologic Diagnosis

The serologic diagnosis of congenital infection in the neonate can be difficult because treponemal IgG antibodies can pass from the mother across the placenta. Consequently, the demonstration of positive serology in cord serum or blood does not necessarily indicate infection, although it is likely if the titers equal or surpass those in the maternal serum. Rising titers are of greater significance. Similarly, the absence of antibodies to the treponeme at birth does not exclude syphilis because in some infected infants serologic evidence of infection may not be present for several weeks. In the case of passive transfer, nontreponemal tests usually become negative in a few weeks, but the FTA-ABS test may take several months to become negative. Maternal IgM antibodies do not cross the intact placenta, and consequently their presence in neonatal serum is convincing evidence of congenital infection and allows the distinction to be made between passive transfer of antibodies and infection. Certain antiglobulin antibodies have been found in neonatal serum, which may lead to a false-positive FTA-ABS test. Such results can be avoided by preabsorbing the sera with aggregated gamma globulin.

It was hoped that the FTA-ABS IgM test would readily detect congenital infection. This test has to be used with caution, as an infected fetus produces a good amount of IgM-anti-IgG but much less IgM antibody to *T. pallidum*. Maternal IgM in the infant's circulation following a maternal-fetal transfusion may also confuse the issue. A negative maternal test may, in early pregnancy, give a false sense that there is no risk of fetal infection. Congenial syphilis has ensued, as reported by Al-Salihi and associates,[2] after negative serologic tests early in the gestation. Dorfman and Glaser[19] reported that seven infants between 3 and 14 weeks of age were admitted to their hospital with symptomatic congenital syphilis, even though there was no suspicion at the time of delivery that either mother or neonate had luetic infection. The maternal serology was nonreactive. In four of the cases both mothers and infants had been seronegative at the time of delivery, and in these cases the mother probably acquired the infection late in the pregnancy. The authors conclude that congenital syphilis may be missed if serologic tests are not conducted on mother and infant at the time of delivery. Even when these tests are carried out, some infants will not be identified as having syphilis, probably because the infection is of recent onset and as a result there is insufficient time for an antibody response to be generated.

As previously mentioned, the difficulty in attaining a diagnosis of congenital syphilis in the neonate occurs when there are not clinical manifestations and the only finding is a reactive nontreponemal test that, compared with the maternal serology, is not significantly elevated. In this situation the neonate may be observed with monthly quantitative VDRL tests for the subsequent 8 months. Noninfected infants have a decrease in titer, which generally denotes passively transferred nontreponemal antibody, whereas a stable or rising titer is indicative of active infection. In noninfected infants, the nontreponemal test results are usually nonreactive within 3 to 4 months and only on rare occasions remain active for longer periods. A gradual fall in titer may also mean that there was an intrauterine treponemal infection but that both mother and fetus had responded to the prescribed therapy during the gestation. Again it must be emphasized, as evidenced by the report of Dormand and Glaser,[19] that a nonreactive neonatal serologic test does not exclude a diagnosis of congenital syphilis.

As pointed out in the guidelines of the Centers of Disease Control,[11] any infant delivered of a seropositive mother should be evaluated for luetic infection (Table 21–6). In addition, they recommend that such infants should have baseline CSF studies prior to therapy (Table 21–7). Amniotic fluid has not been extensively studied with respect to intrauterine spirochetal infections. Glover and associates[27] reported the presence of nonmotile treponemes in an amniotic fluid sample obtained from a patient at 30 weeks' gestation 20 hours after therapy with penicillin G benzathine. The organisms were identified by dark-field microscopy and immunofluorescent staining of the specimen. The infant was delivered 7 weeks later and exhibited no evidence of congenital syphilis. Wendel and associates[55] conducted amniocentesis on five gravid patients with untreated syphilis and intrauterine fetal death. In all instances spirochetes compatible with the motility and morphology of *T. pallidum* were observed. Autopsy studies on four of the fetuses confirmed the diagnosis of congenital syphilis, as did examination of both the fetus and placenta in the fifth case. These investigators recommend amniocentesis to improve the certainty of diagnosis of congenital syphilis, especially in cases of maternal syphilis where intrauterine demise has occurred or hydrops fetalis has been diagnosed on ultrasonography.

Table 21-6 Infants Requiring Evaluation for Congenital Syphilis

Infant of seropositive mother who
Has had no treatment
Has poor documentation of therapy
Was treated late in pregnancy
Was treated with antibiotic other than penicillin
Did not have adequate decrease in serologic titer after therapy
Had inadequate follow-up

Adapted from Centers for Disease Control, 1988.[11]

Table 21-7 Infants Who Require CSF Evaluation

Infant of seropositive mother
Clinical signs compatible with congenital syphilis
Mother had inadequate therapy
Mother treated in second half of pregnancy
Mother treated with an antibiotic other than penicillin
No assurance of maternal follow-up after therapy

Adapted from Centers for Disease Control, 1988.[11]

Treatment

The goals of therapy are (1) to halt progression of the disease in the gravid patient and (2) to terminate the potential infectivity of the patient for her fetus. Penicillin has been the antibiotic of choice for the treatment of all treponemal infections. Treponemes are very sensitive to low serum levels of penicillin, but the optimal dose is unknown. Early in vitro studies showed that 0.018 μg of penicillin per milliliter was treponemicidal, but because of the spirochetes' long generation time of about 30 hours, these levels must be sustained for 10 to 14 days. Consequently, penicillin G benzathine is a convenient and effective preparation that has been used extensively to treat treponemal infections during the past several decades. During this time *T. pallidum* has re-

Table 21-8 Treatment of Syphilis in Pregnancy

Early syphilis	Less than 1 year's duration Penicillin G benzathine 2.4 million units Intramuscular injection
Late syphilis	More than 1 year's duration Penicillin G benzathine 2.4 million units Intramuscular injection Injection weekly for 3 successive weeks

From Centers for Disease Control, 1989.[15]

Table 21-9 Adverse Penicillin Reactions

Frequent	Infrequent
Urticaria	Anaphylaxis
Pruritus	Hemolytic anemia
Erythema	Serum sickness
Maculopapular rash	Agranulocytosis
Arthralgia	Hepatitis
Asthma	Nephritis
Angioedema	Aplastic anemia

mained remarkably sensitive to penicillin with no detectable change in therapeutic efficacy.

The Centers for Disease Control[15] guidelines for the treatment of syphilis were last updated in 1989. It must be recognized that the guidelines do not guarantee a 100 percent cure rate. One must realize that their recommendations are the approach of public health authorities who desire to cure the greatest number of patients in the most efficacious manner. The treatment of this infectious disease is outlined in Table 21–8. There are some differences of opinion, however, about the optimal total dosage for disseminated syphilis. Fiumara[24] is correct in placing due emphasis on the fact that the choice of treatment is the responsibility of the physician. He recommends for early syphilis 2.4 million units of penicillin G benzathine as an intramuscular injection weekly for 2 weeks so that the patient receives a total of 4.8 million units. He reviewed the records of 138 patients who had what was termed *primary syphilis*. Using this treatment regimen, all 138 patients had rapid resolution of their lesions, and all became seronegative within 1 year. It should be noted that this investigator used both clinical and serologic cure as his criteria for therapeutic efficacy. He treated 161 patients with disseminated syphilis in an identical manner, and all were clinically cured and all attained seronegativity within 24 months.

The Centers for Disease Control[15] recommendations must be reviewed as minimum treatment standards in an effort to provide the shortest course of treatment, as many patients will not return for multiple-dose therapy.

Patients who state they have an allergy to penicillin require a careful historical review of any previous therapy where allergic manifestations were suspected.

Penicillin Allergy

Hypersensitivity reactions are the most common of the adverse reactions that are associated with penicillin therapy (Table 21–9). Serum sickness is a systemic hypersensitivity reaction characterized by fever, skin rash, and lymphadenopathy. This serum sickness type of reaction has a close resemblance to that caused by xenogeneic antisera. With penicillin therapy it usually occurs a few days after the completion of treatment; urticaria is a major feature and is indistinguishable from idiopathic urticaria.

Hemolytic anemia is occasionally encountered in patients receiving large daily intravenous dosages of penicillin. Penicillin or its metabolites bind to the surface of the red cell, creating an antigenic complex. High titers of antibody are produced, and an antigen-antibody reaction takes place on the surface of the erythrocyte, with release of chemotactic factors and activation of the complement system resulting in hemolysis. When this adverse reaction occurs, the Coombs test is positive. Recovery occurs on discontinuation of therapy.

Brown and associates[8] found that fewer than 40 percent of individuals with a history of such an allergy have a positive reaction when skin tested and fewer than 30 percent with a history of penicillin sensitivity had any reaction on subsequent therapy with the drug. This antibiotic can be administered to individuals if skin tests to major determinants are negative. If the skin tests are positive, desensitization can be carried out. The procedure should be conducted in a hospital setting because a serious IgE-mediated allergic reaction can occur. Desensitization by the protocol of Wendel and associates[56] (Table 21–10) using an oral penicillin phenoxymethyl suspension can be completed in 4 hours. In their report Wendel and associates[56] stated that after desensitization 15 women, of whom 13 were gravid and afflicted with infection by *T. pallidum*, were treated with penicillin G benzathine in a hospital setting. Two of the individuals received diphenhydramine for pruritus, but all were discharged after overnight observation. Stark and associates[52] obtained similar successes by using the same protocol. The Centers of Disease Control[15] has incorporated this protocol in its current recommended treatment guidelines. They consider that sexually transmitted disease programs should have available to them a referral center where desensitization of patients with positive skin tests can be conducted.

Alternating Antibiotics

The mainstay of therapy for syphilis in the gravid patient is penicillin. No other drug has such efficacy with so few adverse reactions. Tetracyclines produce adverse effects in both the mother and the intrauterine patient. Dose-related hepatotoxicity with fatty infiltration of the liver may occur in the mother and less frequently fatty degeneration of the renal tubular cells. Tetracyclines are readily transferred via the placenta to the fetus. In the

Table 21-10 Protocol for Penicillin Desensitization

Dose Administered Orally Every 15 Minutes	Penicillin Phenoxymethyl in Units	Cumulating Dose in Units
1	100	100
2	200	300
3	400	700
4	800	1,500
5	1,600	3,100
6	3,200	6,300
7	6,400	12,700
8	12,000	24,700
9	24,000	48,700
10	48,000	96,700
11	80,000	176,700
12	160,000	336,700
13	320,000	656,000
14	640,000	1,296,000
Observe for 30 minutes prior to penicillin therapy		

Adapted from Wendel, et al, 1985.[55]

first and second trimesters, they can cause discoloration and severe dysplasia of the teeth as well as inhibit bone growth. Congenital limb deformities and cataracts have also been noted as the result of tetracycline therapy in the first trimester. Consequently, tetracyclines should not be prescribed to gravid patients.

Erythromycin is not a reliable therapeutic agent to use in pregnancy for the treatment of treponemal infections. Philipson and associates[47] have shown that erythromycin is poorly absorbed in gravid patients, and the dosage recommended for nongravid subjects results in reduced maternal serum levels. Furthermore, there is a marked variation in maternal serum concentrations from patient to patient after oral administration of this antibiotic. Such observations would account for the cases of congenital syphilis reported by Fenton and Light[21] and Hashisaki and associates.[30] Consequently, the latest guidelines from the Centers of Disease Control[15] do not recommend erythromycin for the treatment of prenatal syphilis.

There is some evidence from reports by Hook and associates[34] that ceftriaxone is effective for the treatment of early syphilis. These investigators found that an intramuscular dose of 250 mg of ceftriaxone daily for 10 days cured 10 patients with early syphilis. They also reported a dosage of 500 mg on alternate days for five doses was successful therapy for six of their patients. Of late, several dosage regimens of ceftriaxone have been evaluated for the treatment of syphilis. To date, the optimal dose and duration of drug administration has not been established. Moorthy and associates[45] conducted a study in males with early syphilis and found that ceftriaxone in a dose of 2 g for 2 to 5 days was highly efficacious. However, in 5 patients treated with a single dose of 3 g, therapy was not successful in one of the individuals as indicated by rising VDRL titers. From such studies it does appear that multiple-dose therapy with ceftriaxone could be a satisfactory alternative to penicillin G benzathine.

Treatment Failures

Currently there is no therapeutic regimen that will prevent all cases of congenital syphilis. The report of the Centers of Disease Control[9] on congenital syphilis leaves no room for complacency as regards current therapeutic regimens.

One of the reports indicated that 70 percent of treatment failures were in patients treated with a single injection of 2.4 million units of penicillin G benzathine. The focus of attention is not the treatment of women with treponemal infection but the treatment of the intrauterine patient. The fact that the treatment of the fetus with spirochetal disease is neither from a theoretical nor a clinical standpoint completely effective needs to be stated by public health authorities and allow for other therapeutic regimens to be used. Prolonged courses of therapy, however, would lead in many cases to lack of patient compliance.

Mascola and associates[41] reported that the fetal treatment failure are usually associated with treatment in the latter weeks of pregnancy. Failure to treat established fetal spirochetal infection can result in fetal demise or preterm labor. No regimen currently used will prevent all cases of congenital syphilis, but additional therapy is required to combat severe forms of fetal infection. However, if one is treating gravid patients who are highly motivated and will comply with a longer course of treatment involving multiple injections, there will be fewer therapeutic failures.

An unsolved question as regards the treatment of syphilis is whether patients with concomitant HIV infection require more aggressive therapy than do individuals without concomitant HIV infection. On the basis of the reports of Berry and associates[6] and Johns and associates[36] of failure of recommended therapy for treponemal infection in HIV-infected patients, there appears to be a growing body of opinion that therapeutic failures are more common in these patients. Furthermore, treatment failure is often manifest as neurosyphilis. The majority of the patients with syphilis and HIV infections, however, are successfully treated for their treponemal disease with currently available therapeutic regimens. Clarification of the cause of treatment failures occurring in HIV-infected patients with disseminated syphilis may be revealed if penicillin G benzathine is administered in a dosage of 2.4 million units weekly for a total of 7.2 million units. Adequacy of therapy in such individuals cannot be assessed by reduction in the VDRL titers, as in such patients they may be decreased in the absence of therapy. All gravid patients with syphilis should routinely be evaluated for concomitant HIV infection.

Jarisch-Herxheimer Reaction

This phenomenon was first described by Jarisch[35] almost a century ago and later by Herxheimer and Krause,[31] who noted an exacerbation of the cutaneous lesions of disseminated syphilis subsequent to the commencement of treatment with mercury. It is now recognized as a systemic response that may occur within a few hours of initiation of therapy for treponemal infections. This reaction is characterized by fever, malaise, myalgia, and exacerbation of dermal lesions. It may be associated with mild hypotension and hyperventilation.

As possible mechanisms for the reaction, it has been postulated that immunologic manifestations, such as allergic reactions and immune-complex formation, that ensue from the rapid release of treponemal antigens may be responsible. Endotoxin-mediated toxicity is discounted by the fact that no detectable endotoxin has been found in purified *T. pallidum*. Young and associates[59] found no consistent correlation between the Jarisch-Herxheimer reaction and the presence of circulating immune complexes and in addition noted no evidence in the lesions of immunoglobulin or complement deposition. The strongest evidence to date of the involvement of antibodies in this entity is the ability to produce it in infected rabbits by the injection of hyperimmune serum. Further studies are required in order to elucidate the mechanism of this reaction.

Klein and associates[39] reported that 15 of 23 gravid patients treated for early syphilis experienced this phenomenon. All their patients were beyond the first trimester in their pregnancy. Evidence of the reaction began 2 to 8 hours after treatment and abated within 24 hours. The pyrexial response was most marked between 6 and 12 hours after the administration of penicillin G benzathine. Twelve of the 15 patients experienced uterine contractions and decreased fetal activity at the time of the febrile response. Transient late decelerations were observed in some of the patients who had fetal monitoring. These effects were transient, but the authors state that the patients with this reaction may go into preterm labor and that the greatest risk for this to occur is in the first 48 hours after treatment.

There is currently no way to predict which patients will undergo this reaction and consequently all patients in the second half of pregnancy who are being treated for a treponemal infection should be told to seek medical care if they note any of the manifestations of the reaction but more especially if they note a reduction in fetal activity or uterine contractions. In most instances the patient will not require admission to hospital and will only require rest and an agent such as acetaminophen as an antipyretic.

Follow-Up

Because no therapeutic regimen is known to be 100 percent effective, it is essential that those delivering prenatal care be rigorous in the follow-up of gravid patients with luetic infections. Those who have been treated require monthly serologic tests for the duration of the pregnancy. The major parameters utilized in the assessment of therapeutic response are alterations in titers determined by quantitative serologic tests such as the VDRL tests. In patients with early syphilis, titers can be expected to decline fourfold within 3 months of treatment and eightfold by 6 months. Retreatment is warranted if an adequate response is not achieved as evidenced by rising titers or failure of the nontreponemal test to decrease fourfold within 3 months. The mainstay of care for all patients who have syphilis is adequate intensive follow-up. Fiumara[25] observed that the serologic response is often delayed in patients with prior syphilitic disease who become reinfected. There is also some evidence that quantitative titers in gravid patients do not decrease as rapidly as in nongravid patients. All gravid patients who have had prior therapy for luetic infection should have serologic titers, and if elevated values are found retreatment is indicated in the form of penicillin G benzathine 2.4 million units for two doses 1 week apart.

On account of the upsurge in incidence of congenital syphilis, one must be more diligent in the application of principles that will work and not seek refuge by thinking that crack cocaine is responsible for the continued presence of congenital luetic infections in society. Cohen[17] discusses the present situation in a succinct manner. She recommends that in areas where there is a high incidence of syphilis all mothers should be screened at the time of parturition. If the maternal serology is negative, so will be that of the neonate. The reverse does not hold, and the diagnosis of congenital luetic infection may be missed if only the infant's serum is screened at the time of delivery. Treatment should be based on the maternal diagnosis and not the infant's serologic data. If the mother requires therapy, so does her progeny. If there is any dubiety as to whether the infant is infected, a conservative approach should be adopted and the infant treated. Neonates are not allergic to penicillin, and so there is no fear of anaphylaxis. No mother of a neonate should be discharged from hospital until all serologic studies have been evaluated. Positive serologic results should be communicated to the health authorities by telephone rather than by the postal service, as this allows for tracing of contacts to be initiated without delay, because as with all things procrastination is the thief of time.

Some of medicine's most notable achievements have been in the understanding of communicable diseases. Syphilis and, more significantly, congenital syphilis remain an anachronism in the scientific era of medicine. There are many reasons for this state of affairs. When disease flourishes, reserach tends to concentrate on problems of diagnosis and treatment, whereas between epidemics there is no stimulus to provide the impetus for fundamental research. Earlier beliefs that penicillin was the panacea controlling the disease have proved unjustified. The term *dying disease,* which was popular in the 1950s, is now itself dead, and syphilis, like the Phoenix, is rising again out of the ashes.

References

1. Adams EH, Gfroerer JC, Rouse BA, et al. Trends in prevalence of cocaine use. Adv Alcohol Subst Abuse 1986; 6:49–71.
2. Al-Salihi FL, Curran JP, Shteir OA. Occurrence of fetal syphilis after a nonreactive early gestational serologic test. J Pediatr 1971; 78:121–123.
3. Baker-Zander SA, Hook EW, Bonin P, et al. Antigens of *Treponema pallidum* recognized by IgG and IgM antibodies during syphilis in humans. J Infect Dis 1985; 151:264–272.
4. Baseman JB, Hayes EC. Molecular characterization of receptor binding proteins and immunogens of virulent *Treponema pallidum*. J Exp Med 1980; 151:573–576.
5. Berkowitz K, Baxi L, Fox HE. False negative screening: the prozone phenomenon, nonimmune hydrops and diagnosis of syphilis during pregnancy. Am J Obstet Gynecol 1990; 163:975–977.
6. Berry CD, Hooton TM, Collier AC, Lukehart SH. Neurological relapse after benzathine penicillin therapy for secondary syphilis in a patient with HIV infection. N Engl J Med 1987; 316:1587–1589.
7. Bowell P, Mayne K, Puckett A, et al. Serological screening for syphilis in pregnancy: results of a five year study (1983-1987) in the Oxford region. J Clin Pathol 1989; 42:1281–1284.
8. Brown BC, Price EV, Moore MB. Penicilloyl-polylysine as an intradermal test for penicillin sensitivity. JAMA 1964; 189:599–604.
9. Centers for Disease Control: Congenital syphilis—United States 1983-1985. MMWR 1986; 35:625–628.
10. Centers for Disease Control: Increases in primary and secondary syphilis: United States. MMWR 1987; 36:393–396.
11. Centers for Disease Control: Guidelines for the prevention and control of congenital syphilis. MMWR 1988; 37:S1–13.
12. Centers for Disease Control: Syphilis and congenital syphilis: United States 1985–1988. MMWR 1988; 37:486–489.
13. Centers for Disease Control: Recommendations for diagnosing and treating syphilis in HIV-infected patients. MMWR 1988; 37:601.
14. Centers for Disease Control: Congenital syphilis—New York City. MMWR 1989; 38:825–829.
15. Centers for Disease Control: 1989 Sexually transmitted diseases treatment guidelines. MMWR 1989; 38:S5-15.
16. Clay JC. Antenatal screening for syphilis. Br Med J 1989; 299:409–410.
17. Cohen DA. Congenital syphilis. N Engl J Med 1991; 324:1063–1064.
18. De Muylder X, Laga M, Tennstedt C, et al. The role of *Neisseria gonorrhoeae* and *Chlamydia trachomatis* in pelvic inflammatory disease and its sequelae in Zimbabwe. J Infect Dis 1990; 162:501–505.
19. Dorfman DH, Glaser JH. Congenital syphilis presenting in infants after the newborn period. N Engl J Med 1990; 323:1299–1302.
20. Ehrlich P, Hata S. Experimentelle chemotherapie der spirillosen (syphilis ruckfallbfieber huhnersprillose, frambosie). Berlin: J Springer, 1910.
21. Fenton LJ, Light IJ. Congenital syphilis after maternal treatment with erythromycin. Obstet Gynecol 1976; 47:492–494.
22. Fieldsteel AH, Cox DL, Moeckli RA. Cultivation of virulent *Treponema pallidum* in tissue culture. Infect Immun 1981; 32:908–915.
23. Fitzgerald T. Experimental congenital syphilis in rabbits. Can J Microbiol 1985; 31:757–762.
24. Fiumara NJ. Treatment of primary and secondary syphilis. JAMA 1980; 243:2500–2502.
25. Fiumara NJ. Reinfection primary, secondary and latent syphilis: the serologic response after treatment. Sex Transm Dis 1980; 7:111–115.
26. Fiumara NJ, Lessell S. The stigmata of latent congenital syphilis, an analysis of 100 patients. Sex Transm Dis 1983; 10:126–129.
27. Glover DD, Winter CA, Charles D, Larsen B. Diagnostic considerations in intra-amniotic syphilis. Sex Transm Dis 1985; 12:145–149.
28. Haas JS, Bolan G, Larsen SA, et al. Sensitivity of treponemal tests for detecting prior treated syphilis during human immunodeficiency virus infection. J Infect Dis 1990; 162:862–866.
29. Harter CA, Benirschke K. Fetal syphilis in the first trimester. Am J Obstet Gynecol 1976; 124:705–711.
30. Hashisaki P, Wertzberger GG, Conrad GL, Nichols CR. Erythromycin failure in the treatment of syphilis in a pregnant woman. Sex Transm Dis 1983; 10:36–38.
31. Herxheimer K, Krause D. Ueber eine bei syphilitischen vorkommende quecksilberreaktion. Dtsch Med Wochenschr 1902; 28:895–897.

32. Hira SK, Bhat GJ, Chikamata DM, et al: Syphilis intervention in pregnancy: Zambian demonstration project. Genitourin Med 1990; 66:159–164.
33. Hira SK, Bhat GJ, Patel JB, et al. Early congenital syphilis: climiceo-radiologic features in 202 patients. Sex Transm Dis 1985; 12:177–183.
34. Hook EW, Roddy RE, Handsfield HH. Ceftriaxone for incubating and early syphilis. J Infect Dis 1988; 158:881–884.
35. Jarisch A.Therapeutic veruche bei syphilis. Wien Med Wochenschr 1895; 45:721–724.
36. Johns DR, Tierney D, Felsenstein D. Alteration in the natural history of neurosyphilis by concurrent infection with human immunodeficiency virus. N Engl J Med 1987; 316:1569–1572.
37. Kail AC. The Bard and the body 3: venereal disease—the pox. Med J Aust 1983; 140:445–449.
38. Kajdacsy-Balla A, Howeedy A, Bagasra O. Syphilis in the Syrian hamster: a model of human venereal and congenital syphilis. Am J Pathol 1987; 126:599–601.
39. Klein VR, Cox SM, Mitchell MD, Wendel GD. The Jarisch-Herxheimer reaction complicating syphilotherapy in pregnancy. Obstet Gynecol 1990; 75:375–380.
40. Mahoney JF, Arnold RC, Harris A. Penicillin treatment of early syphilis: preliminary report. Vener Dis Inform 1943; 24:335.
41. Mascola L, Pelosi R, Alexander CE. Inadequate treatment of syphilis in pregnancy. Am J Obstet Gynecol 1984; 150:945–947.
42. Mascola L, Pelosi R, Blount JH, et al. Congenital syphilis revisited. Am J Dis Child 1985; 139:575–580.
43. Michaelis L. Precipitinreaktion bei syphilis. Klin Wochenschr 1907; 44:1477–1479.
44. Minkoff HL, McCalla S, Delke I, et al. The relationship of cocaine use to syphilis and human immunodeficiency virus infections among inner city parturient women. Am J Obstet Gynecol 1990; 163:521–526.
45. Moorthy TT, Lee C-T, Lin K-B, Tan T. Ceftriaxone for treatment of primary syphilis in men: a preliminary study. Sex Transm Dis 1987; 14:116–118.
46. Moskophidis M, Müller F. Molecular analyses of immunoglobulin M and G immune response to protein antigens of *Treponema pallidum* in human syphilis. Infect Immun 1984; 43:127–132.
47. Philipson A, Sabath LD, Charles D. Erythromycin and clindamycin absorption and elimination in pregnant women. Clin Pharmacol Ther 1976; 19:68–77.
48. Popsil L. A simplified ELISA method for syphilis. Dermatology 1983; 167:105–108.
49. Ricci JM, Fojaco RM, O'Sullivan MJ. Congenital syphilis: the University of Miami Jackson Memorial Medical Center experience; 1986-1988. Obstet Gynecol 1989; 74:686–693.
50. Sanchez PJ, McCracken GH Jr, Wendel GD, et al. Molecular analysis of the fetal IgM response to *Treponema pallidum* antigens: implications for improved serodiagnosis of congenital syphilis. J Infect Dis 1989; 159:508–517.
51. Schaudinn F, Hoffman PE. Ueber spirochetenbefunde im lymphdrüsensaft syphilitischer. Dtsch Med Wochenschr 1905; 31:711–714.
52. Stark BJ, Earl HS, Gross GN, et al. Acute and chronic densensitization of penicillin-allergic patients using oral penicillin. J Allergy Clin Immunol 1987; 79:523–532.
53. Tabor DR, Bagasro O, Jacobs RF. Treponemal infection specifically enhances node T-cell regulation of macrophage activity. Infect Immun 1986; 54:21–27.
54. Wassermann A, Neisser A, Bruck C. Eine serodiagnostische reaktion bei syphilis. Dtsch Med Wochenschr 1906; 32:745–751.
55. Wendel GD, Maberry MC, Christmas JT, et al. Examination of amniotic fluid in diagnosing congenital syphilis with fetal death. Obstet Gynecol 1989; 74:967–970.
56. Wendel GD, Stark BJ, Jamison RB, et al. Penicillin allergy and densensitization in serious infections during pregnancy. N Engl J Med 1985; 312:1229–1232.
57. Wicher V, Zabek J, Wicher K. Pathogen-specific humoral response in *Treponema pallidum*–infected humans, rabbits and guinea pigs. J Infect Dis 1991; 163:830–836.
58. Williams K. Screening for syphilis in pregnancy: an assessment of the costs and benefits. Community Medicine 1985; 7:37–42.
59. Young EJ, Weingarten NM, Baughn RE, Duncan WC. Studies on the pathogenesis of the Jarisch-Herxheimer reaction: development of an animal model and evidence against a role for classical endotoxin. J Infect Dis 1982; 148:606–615.

CHAPTER 22

Placenta and Membranes

Richard L. Naeye, M.D.

Many different bacteria, mycoplasmas, viruses, fungi, and parasites can infect and damage the placenta and unborn child. Those that invade the embryo frequently produce malformations and spontaneous abortions, whereas those that damage the fetus sometimes lead to stillbirth and long-term neurologic abnormalities. When the placenta is invaded, the result is often preterm birth, stillbirth, or neonatal death. Bacteria and mycoplasmas usually gain entrance to the placenta and fetus by penetrating the fetal membranes adjacent to the uterine cervix; most viruses and parasites reach the unborn infant through the placenta. Both gravida and fetus usually mount immunologic responses to the infecting agent, but in many instances the agents continue to multiply. Tissue damage from primary or recurrent infections can take many different forms including tissue necrosis, fibrosis, growth retardation, and malformations. At least one infecting agent, the rubella virus, produces growth retardation and organ malformations by elaborating products that inhibit cell multiplication.[109,126] The infecting agents that can damage the embryo, fetus, or placenta are listed in Table 22-1.

The timing of the infection has an important effect on the outcome. More details are known about the timing effects of rubella infections than about the timing effects of most other infecting agents. First-trimester maternal rubella infections almost always invade the placenta, but only about 60 percent of the associated embryos and fetuses are affected.[98] Damage to individual fetal organs depends in large part on their stage of development.[153] Eye and cardiac damage occur primarily following infections in the first 2 months of gestation, whereas hearing defects follow infections that occur throughout the first 5 months of pregnancy. The placenta is often growth retarded, but timing of this effect has not been as well documented.

The immune status of the mother is another factor in the outcome of congenital infections. With some viral agents, a primary infection results in permanent maternal immunity, so the placenta and fetus are rarely at risk if a gravida is exposed to the infecting agent a second time. Rubella is such an agent. More common are viral agents such as cytomegalovirus and herpes simplex, whose recurrences pose a risk, albeit a smaller risk to the embryo, fetus, and placenta, than did the first infection. Primary cytomegalovirus infection is passed to about 30 percent of the associated placentas and fetuses, whereas recurrent infections affect a much smaller proportion of placentas and fetuses. There are two explanations for the differences in outcome between primary and secondary infections. First, antibodies supplied by the mother during a recurrent infection often protect the placenta and fetus from becoming infected. Second, maternal viremia is usually shorter in duration with a recurrent than with a primary infection, so the placenta and embryo are less often exposed to the infectious agent during a recurrent maternal infection.

This chapter is organized by the type of infecting agent, starting with bacteria and myocoplasmas and continuing with fungi, viruses, and parasites. The space given to each type of infection and agent is usually related to its clinical importance. Thus, the most space is allotted to acute chorioamnionitis initiated by bacteria and mycoplasmas because it is the single most frequent

Table 22-1 Congenital Infections

Bacterial infections	**Viral infections**
Acute chorioamnionitis	Cytomegalovirus
Aerobic bacteria	Herpes simplex
Anaerobic bacteria	Rubella
Mycoplasmas	Varicella
Listeriosis	Smallpox, vaccinia
Syphilis	Mumps
Leprosy	Hepatitis
Lyme disease	HIV
Group B streptococcal infections	Parovirus
Fungal infections	**Parasitic infections**
Candida albicans	Malaria
Coccidiodides immitas	Toxoplasmosis
	Trypanosomes

cause of preterm birth, stillbirth, and neonatal death in most populations, and it is also responsible for more mental and motor impairments than any other type of infection.[108,112,114]

Bacterial Infections

Acute Chorioamnionitis

Acute chorioamnionitis develops when bacteria or mycoplasmas gain access to the extraplacental fetal membranes and spread into the amniotic fluid. There are several routes by which these bacteria reach the fetal membranes, but most often it is through the cervix. Usually the bacteria or mycoplasmas pass from the membranes into the amniotic fluid, overcome its antimicrobial systems, and then grow freely. Because these infections develop outside the control of health care systems and initiate labor that cannot be stopped, they pose a major unsolved public health problem. This is one of the main reasons why the frequency of preterm birth has hardly changed in many of the industrial nations in many years.[71] Acute chorioamnionitis is particularly important as a cause of poor pregnancy outcome in the poor. Gravidas living in the Third World are particularly prone to these infections, in part because the antimicrobial systems in their amniotic fluid are sometimes impaired.[5,114]

Identifying the Disorder and Its Causes

Acute chorioamnionitis manifests as an acute, sometimes diffuse inflammatory process in the extraplacental membranes, the chorionic plate of the placenta, and the umbilical cord.[112,114] There is considerable evidence that nonmicrobial substances that appear in the amniotic fluid do not cause acute chorioamnionitis. Lauweryns and associates produced all of the histologic features of acute chorioamnionitis by introducing various bacterial species into the amniotic fluid of experimental animals, but not by introducing various mixtures of meconium, gastric juice, and amniotic fluid debris into the amniotic fluid.[76] There is good evidence that viral infections do not cause acute chorioamnionitis. In a large prospective study there was no correlation between the presence of acute chorioamnionitis and increasing maternal gestational antibody titers to the 10 viruses that most often infect the placenta.[114] In recent years improved culture techniques have permitted the recovery of bacteria and mycoplasmas from up to 80 percent of placentas with acute chorioamnionitis, which is strong evidence that acute chorioamnionitis is an infectious process.[34,65] The mycoplasmas that cause the infections include *Mycoplasma hominis* and *Ureaplasma urealyticum*.[51,130] The bacteria and mycoplasmas that cause the infections are the organisms that are normally present in the vagina and cervix during pregnancy. About two-thirds of the cultures yield a single organism, nearly half of which are anaerobic bacteria. Bacteria and mycoplasmas are less often recovered from the amniotic fluid than from the fetal membranes, perhaps because the antibacterial systems in amniotic fluid are often strongly antimicrobial, particularly late in gestation.[117,138] The finding of leukoattractants in the amniotic fluid is currently the most sensitive laboratory method available for identifying the presence of acute chorioamnionitis.[124]

Several organisms that are well-known pathogens in the uterus and fallopian tubes rarely cross intact fetal membranes to cause acute chorioamnionitis. These include *Neisseria gonorrhoeae,* group B streptococci, and *Chlamydia trachomatis*.[83,152] Only one case has been reported in which the gonococcus was grown from the placenta when the fetal membranes were intact at the onset of labor.[36,152] In one study 64 percent of the newborns infected with group B streptococcus had acute chorioamnionitis, but in every case the membranes ruptured before delivery.[121] In our laboratory fetal membranes with chorioamnionitis have repeatedly been culture-negative for *C. trachomatis* when these membranes were intact at the onset of labor. The high frequencies in amniotic fluid of inhibitory activities against *C. trachomatis* may be the reason why this organism is rarely isolated from placentas and extraplacental membranes with acute chorioamnionitis when the fetal membranes were intact at the onset of labor.[165] This does not mean that it has no effect on pregnancy outcome. Some investigations have reported that premature membrane rupture and preterm delivery are more frequent when the cervix is colonized by *C. trachomatis*.[40,58,88,127,142,162] This raises the possibility that *C. trachomatis* may sometimes be a marker for factors or conditions that predispose to acute chorioamnionitis.

Bacterial vaginosis is another condition that reportedly increases the risk for developing acute chorioamnionitis and resulting preterm delivery.[58,91,150] Bacterial vaginosis is diagnosed when a Gram's stain of vaginal smears shows few lactobacilli and many *Gardnerella vaginalis* and some *Mobiluncus* species.[150] One can speculate that the presence of bacterial vaginosis is a marker for other factors that predispose to acute chorioamnionitis.

Measurements of maternal serum C-reactive protein and the products of infection in the amniotic fluid have been used to try to diagnose acute chorioamnionitis before delivery. All of these tests are expensive and time-consuming. Most lack sensitivity, and some also lack specificity.[137] This points up the need to develop an inexpensive, sensitive, selective, noninvasive test that women can use in their own homes to detect acute chorioamnionitis during its earliest stages. If such a test can be developed, it might be possible to treat acute chorioamnionitis at a very early stage and thereby prevent some preterm deliveries.

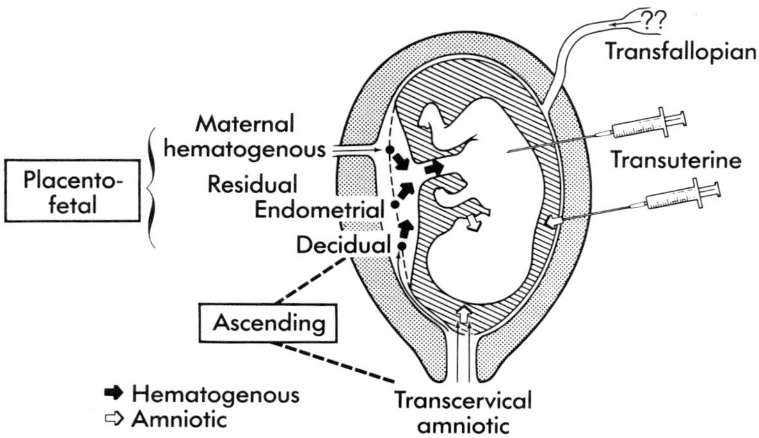

Figure 22-1 Routes of bacterial entry that produce acute chorioamnionitis. (From Blanc, 1981.[16])

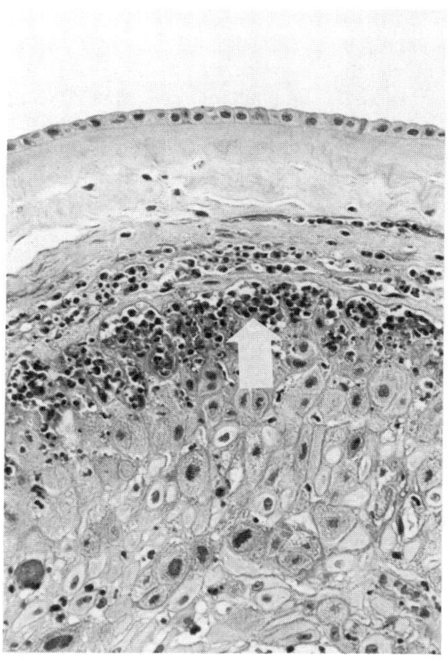

Figure 22-2 A large number of polymorphonuclear leukocytes (arrow) are infiltrating along the chorion of the extraplacental fetal membranes in a case of acute chorioamnionitis (hematoxylin and eosin; original magnification ×120).

Routes of Infection

The cervical os is the usual route through which bacteria and mycoplasmas reach the extraplacental membranes and initiate acute chorioamnionitis (Figs. 22-1 and 22-2). In rare instances diagnostic amniocentesis, fetoscopy, villous sampling, intrauterine transfusion, and a medically induced abortion introduce the bacteria or mycoplasmas into the amniotic fluid and thereby initiate acute chorioamnionitis (Fig. 22-1).[133] The infection usually starts in the membranes adjacent to the cervical os.[12,108,112-114] In vaginally delivered twins, acute chorioamnionitis usually involves the firstborn when only one member of a pair is affected, which would be expected if the infection usually originates in membranes near the cervical os because the membranes of the firstborn are adjacent to the cervical os just prior to delivery. The bacteria that follow this route must first pass through the mucous plug in the cervix, which normally resists bacterial penetration.[24]

When the organisms that cause acute chorioamnionitis have low virulence, the fetal membranes often remain intact until the start of labor. The infecting organisms spread along the surface of the chorionic cell layer in the extraplacental membranes within 12 to 24 hours after the infection has started.[108,113] Bacteria often appear to enter the amniotic fluid during this early phase of the infection. Fetal bacteremia or septicemia is a complication of bacteria in the amniotic fluid and is presumed to be the result of the fetus inhaling these bacteria.[25]

It is well documented that gravidas with asymptomic bacteriuria have an increased frequency of spontaneous preterm labors and deliveries. Treating the bacteriuria with antibiotics appears to reduce this risk.[54] Elimination of an abnormal cervicovaginal flora might be the mechanism by which the antibiotics given for bacteriuria prevent preterm births.[136] As previously noted, there is considerable evidence that an abnormal vaginal and cervical flora predisposes to acute chorioamnionitis.

Factors Predisposing to Acute Chorioamnionitis

It is not known why the frequency of acute chorioamnionitis differs so much from one population to another. Possibilities include differing levels of antimicrobial activity in the amniotic fluid, differences in the character of cervical mucous plugs, and differing bacterial floras in the cervix and vagina.[108,113,114] Normally, antimicrobial activity first appears in the amniotic fluid in the second trimester of pregnancy, progressively increases in titer to term, and is active against a wide spectrum of aerobic and anaerobic bacteria. When this antibacterial activity is absent or weak, many among the great variety of bacteria that are normally present in the vagina and cervix can grow in the amniotic fluid and lead to the development of acute chorioamnionitis. In a small study we conducted, about 5 percent of U.S. whites and blacks

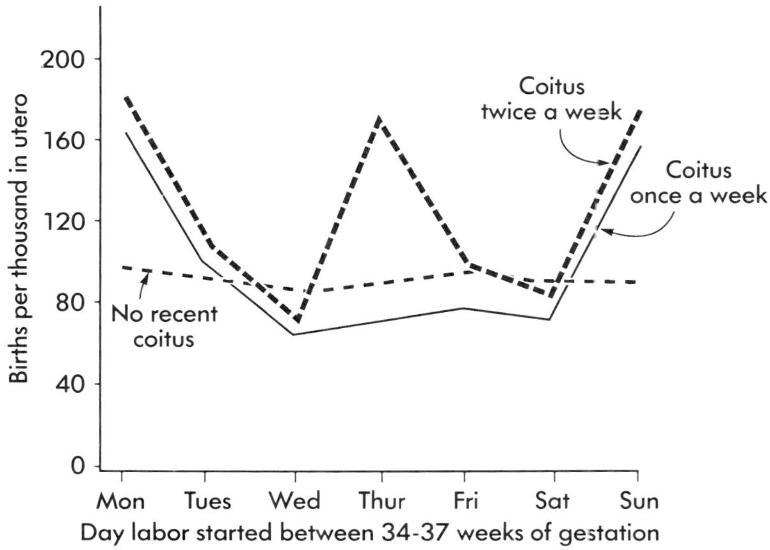

Figure 22-3 In the collaborative perinatal study (CPS) women who reported they had coitus once a week had a peak frequency of labors starting on Sunday and Monday. Women who reported coitus twice or more per week had two labor peaks, one on Sunday-Monday and the second on Thursday. Women who reported no recent coitus had no significant day-to-day fluctuations in the frequency of labor starting. (From Naeye, 1991.[108])

had abnormally low levels of antimicrobial activity in their amniotic fluid at term, whereas over 90 percent of the malnourished mothers in some Third World populations have lacked this antimicrobial activity.[5,112,114,117]

Coitus appears to have a role in the genesis of chorioamnionitis in some individuals and populations. In a large prospective study, women who discontinued coitus during pregnancy for a month or more and then resumed it before term had a high rate of preterm labors and deliveries, more than half of which were associated with acute chorioamnionitis.[108] The connection between the coitus and chorioamnionitis is a matter of speculation. Coitus could be introducing new organisms into the vagina. Another possibility is that sperm in conjunction with seminal fluid could be facilitating the passage of bacteria through the cervical mucous plug. Seminal fluid has proteolytic enzymes that faciliitiate the passage of sperm through the cervical mucous plug, but this plug normally becomes resistant to sperm penetration during pregnancy. It remains to be determined if the cervical mucus is ineffective in some gravidas in preventing sperm from reaching the fetal membranes.

In a large prospective study, women who reported they had coitus once a week during pregnancy had a peak frequency of labors starting on Sunday or Monday (Fig. 22-3). Women who reported coitus twice a week had two labor peaks, one on Sunday and Monday and the other on Thursday. Women who reported no coitus for several weeks or longer before delivery had no day-of-the-week fluctuations in the frequency with which their labors started. One explanation for the day-of-the-week fluctuations of labor onset following coitus is probably the relationship of coitus to acute chorioamnionitis. In a prospective study we found that chorioamnionitis-associated preterm labor had a time relationship to coitus. Such labors first increased in frequency about 24 hours after coitus and continued at a higher than expected frequency for nearly 2 weeks (Fig. 22-4).[113] Acute chorioamnionitis was less frequent when condoms were used than when they were not used (Fig. 22-5).

In a large prospective study the frequency of acute chorioamnionitis increased after 12 hours of membrane rupture.[11] Several other factors also predispose to the development of chorioamnionitis. Its frequency increases with the duration of labor and with the duration of internal fetal monitoring.[120] One study estimated that for each hour of increase in the duration of internal fetal monitoring or fetal membrane rupture, the probability of clinically apparent intra-amniotic infection increases 1 to 2 percent.[120]

Acute chorioamnionitis also increases in frequency with gestational age. This increase could be due to a combination of the passage of time, giving bacteria and mycoplasmas more opportunities to reach the fetal membrane, and to the effacement of the cervix in late gestation, which sometimes exposes the fetal membranes to the cervical bacterial flora. Multiparous gravidas are particularly apt to lose their cervical mucous plugs in late gestation, which exposes their fetal membranes to the cervicovaginal flora.[108,114] This is probably the reason why the frequency of late gestational chorioamnionitis increases with parity. Overdistention of the uterus, with some dilation of the cervical canal, may be the reason why acute chorioamnionitis is so much more frequent with twins after midgestation than with single fetuses.[108,114,115]

Course of Infection

Fetal neutrophils in the umbilical vessels are often attracted by chemotactic substances in the amniotic fluid to migrate out of the umbilical vessels toward the amniotic cavity (Fig. 22-6). Less often, neutrophils in the

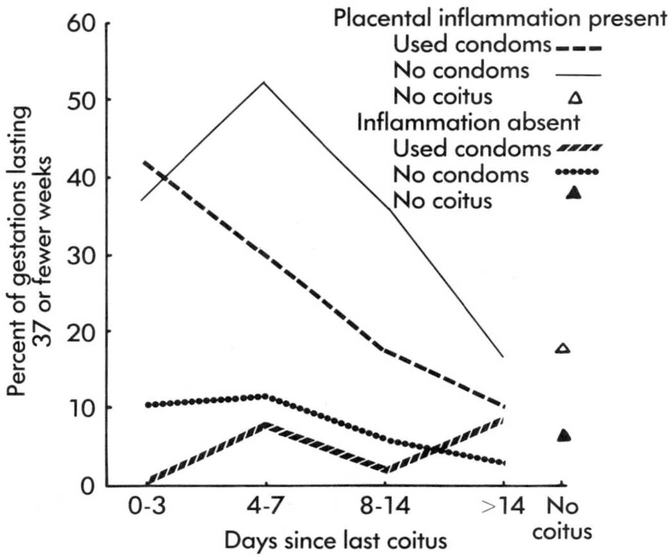

Figure 22-4 In a prospective study, preterm labor associated with acute chorioamnionitis increased in frequency 24 hours after coitus and continued at a higher than expected frequency for nearly 2 weeks. (From Naeye and Ross, 1982.[113])

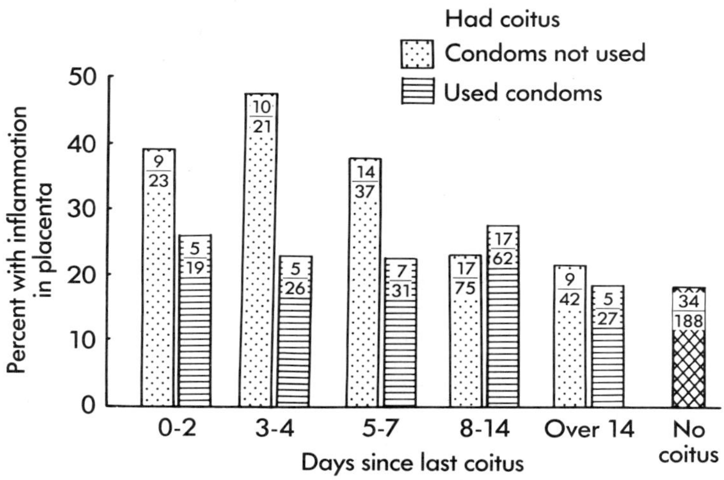

Figure 22-5 In the week following coitus, the frequency of acute chorioamnionitis in the placenta was less when condoms had been used than when they had not been used. (From Naeye and Ross, 1982.[113])

amniotic fluid migrate into the umbilical cord. These processes are termed *funisitis*. In the course of the infection, acute inflammatory cells first migrate out of the umbilical vein, and only later out of the umbilical arteries (Fig. 22-7). Even when acute chorioamnionitis is severe, some segments of the umbilical cord may be unaffected, so the absence of funisitis in several sections of an umbilical cord does not exclude the presence of acute chorioamnionitis. Neutrophils can also be absent in several sections of the extraplacental membranes when acute chorioamnionitis is present. A systematic effort should be made to look for neutrophils in the extraplacental membranes when these membranes are edematous (Fig. 22-8). The finding of just a few neutrophils in edematous membranes is a strong clue that acute chorioamnionitis will be present when the chorionic (fetal) plate of the placenta is examined. In a large prospective study, perinatal mortality was much higher in cases of acute chorioamnionitis when the extraplacental membranes were edematous than when edema was absent.[108]

The most reliable method of making the diagnosis of acute chorioamnionitis is the finding of maternal neutrophils beneath the chorionic (fetal) plate of the placenta (Figs. 22-9 and 22-10). Maternal neutrophils in the blood of the intervillous space are first attracted to attach to the chorionic plate (stage 1, Figs. 22-9 and 22-

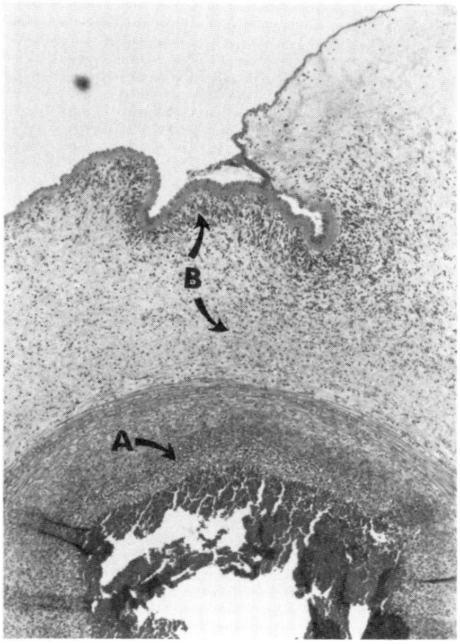

Figure 22-6 Large numbers of acute inflammatory cells are pouring out through the wall of the umbilical vein (arrow A) into Wharton's jelly (arrow B) (hematoxylin and eosin; original magnification ×60).

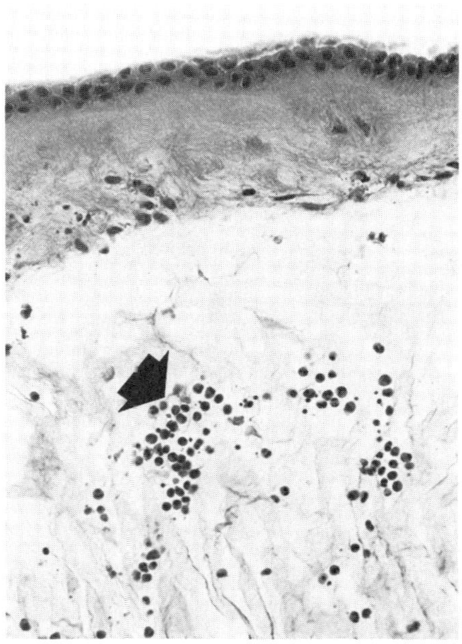

Figure 22-8 Nests of acute inflammatory cells (arrow) are present throughout edematous areas of the extraplacental fetal membranes (hematoxylin and eosin; original magnification ×120).

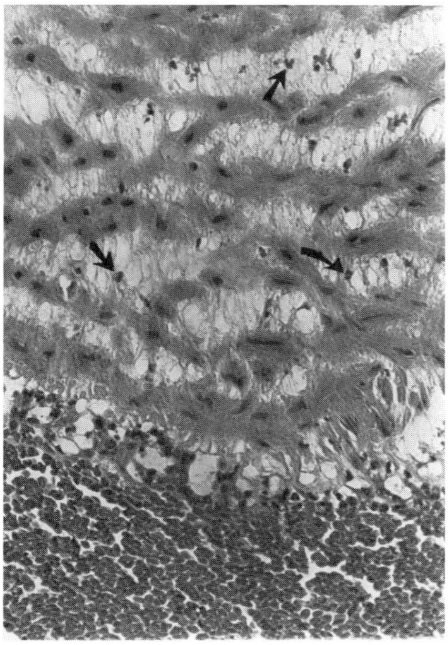

Figure 22-7 Acute inflammatory cells (arrow) are migrating from the fetal blood out into the wall of an umbilical artery (hematoxylin and eosin; original magnification ×60).

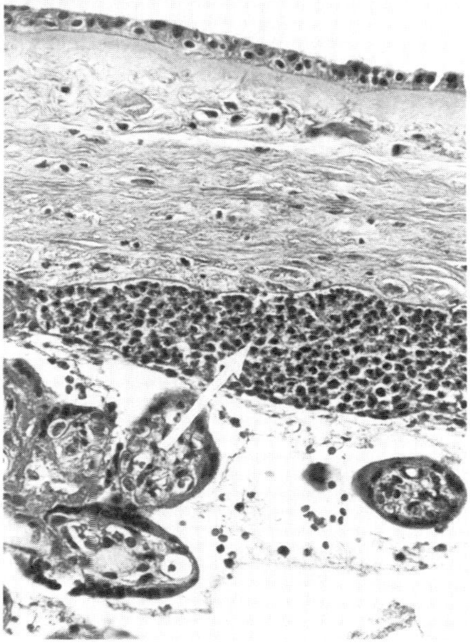

Figure 22-9 Large numbers of polymorphonuclear leukocytes (arrow) have accumulated beneath the chorionic (fetal) plate of the placenta in response to leukoattractants that have diffused through the chorionic plate from infected amniotic fluid (hematoxylin and eosin; original magnification ×120).

11).[108,112,113] Next, they migrate into the plate (stage 2). When they reach the basement membrane beneath the amnion, the process is classified as stage 3 (Figs. 22-10 and 22-11). Neutrophils do not usually pass through this basement membrane into the amniotic fluid because they do not possess a collagenase that will cleave the type V collagen that is a major constituent of this membrane.[7] When the inflammatory process is severe, it usually reaches stage 3 within 24 hours of the time of fetal membrane rupture (Fig. 22-10).[108] When the inflammation is mild, it is usually at stage 1 for the first 3 days after membrane rupture. It often reaches stage 2 by the fourth day. By the seventh day half of the mild inflammatory processes are at stage 2 and a few at stage 3.

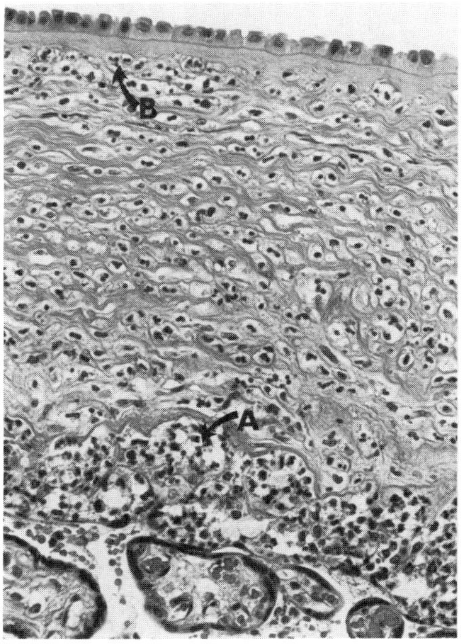

Figure 22-10 Large numbers of acute inflammatory cells have migrated from beneath the chorionic plate of the placenta (arrow A) to the basement membrane just beneath the amnion (arrow B) (hematoxylin and eosin; original magnification ×120).

In making the diagnosis of acute chorioamnionitis, the examiner should rely on the presence of acute inflammatory cells beneath a very thin area of the chorionic plate of the placenta. Thicker areas often block the passage of leukoattractants through the chorionic plate of the placenta, and hence there is no visible evidence of the infection.

Normal labor starts most frequently between midnight and morning. Cooperstock and colleagues found that this circadian peak was absent when chorioamnionitis was present, which suggests that acute chorioamnionitis initiates labor through different mechanisms from those that start normal labor.[27] Several mechanisms have been proposed to explain how acute chorioamnionitis initiates labor. Bejar and coworkers found that many of the microorganisms that cause chorioamnionitis produce phospholipase A_2. This phospholipase can cleave arachidonic acid from the fetal membranes, which could free arachidonic acid to start the prostaglandin cascade, which in turn would initiate labor.[11] Cox and associates have suggested an alternate method by which chorioamnionitis starts labor. They claim that endotoxin released by bacteria stimulates decidual cells to produce cytokines and prostaglandins.[28] Mitchell has identified increased levels of several cytokines in the amniotic fluid of women who delivered preterm with acute chorioamnionitis.[96] With any of these mechanisms the release of prostaglandin E_2 likely causes the cervix to dilate and prostaglandin F_{2a} causes the uterus to contract. Rarely if

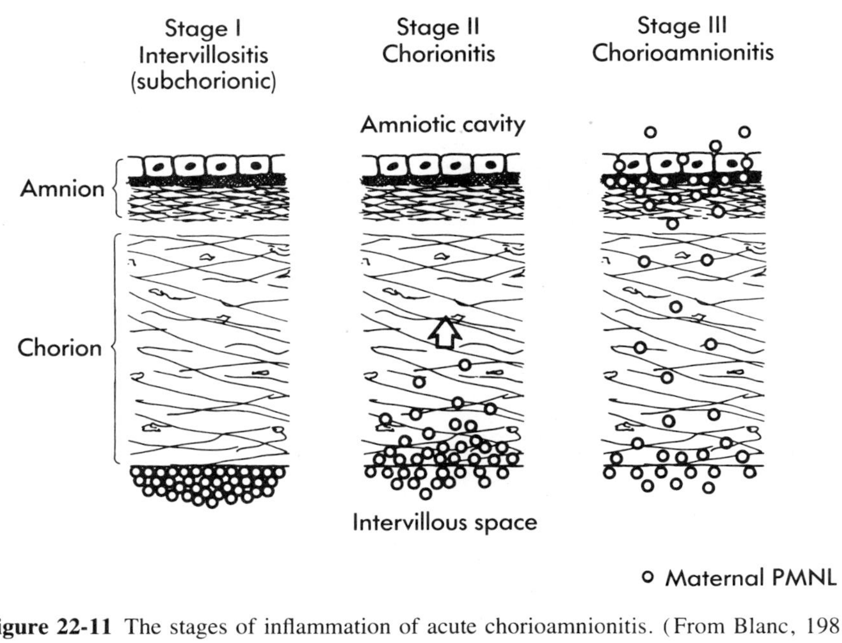

Figure 22-11 The stages of inflammation of acute chorioamnionitis. (From Blanc, 1981.[16])

ever do tocolytic agents stop the labors initiated by acute chorioamnionitis.[117]

Morbidity and Mortality

Many observers have doubted the clinical importance of acute chorioamnionitis because so many of the affected neonates appear to be healthy at birth and only about 10 percent of the gravidas have clinical evidence of infection. The most important reason for these findings is that the responsible bacteria and mycoplasmas usually have a low or limited virulence. We have recovered bacteria or mycoplasmas from nearly 80 percent of the placentas with chorioamnionitis in our medical center, and only about 10 percent are virulent strains. These virulent strains are the organisms that are usually recovered when gravidas have clinical evidence of infection.[180]

Because the clinical findings associated with acute chorioamnionitis that develops at term are so often benign, its full consequences are often not appreciated. In a large prospective study, fetal and neonatal deaths increased 2.6-fold with mild chorioamnionitis and 4.1-fold when acute chorioamnionitis was moderate or severe.[108] Most of these deaths were related to sepsis, so at no gestational period is acute chorioamnionitis completely benign.

Acute chorioamnionitis has important consequences in addition to its direct effects, namely, fetal hypoxia and preterm birth. In a large prospective study more than a third of all preterm births could be attributed to labor initiated by acute chorioamnionitis.[108,113,114] Because perinatal mortality was much higher for preterm than for full-term births, acute chorioamnionitis was the most frequent initiating cause of stillbirth and neonatal death in the study.

Immaturity is not the only reason why neonates who are born preterm as the result of acute chorioamnionitis are often ill. Often they are ill because placental edema made them hypoxic before birth (Fig. 22-12). This hypoxia presents with low 5- and 10-minute Apgar scores, the need to resuscitate vigorously at birth, the neonatal respiratory distress syndrome, and recurrent apneic episodes.[108,110,112,114] These findings correlate much more strongly with the severity and the extent of placental villous edema than with the severity and stage of the chorioamnionitis that is present.[108,110] The edema is postulated to impede the movement of oxygen and nutrients from the intervillous space into the fetal circulation by compressing capillaries and veins inside the placental villi. The severe respiratory distress experienced by many of these neonates appears due to the combined effects of lung immaturity and hypoxic damage to the lungs before birth.[108,110,114]

Funisitis often develops in the course of acute chorioamnionitis, and in a large prospective study perinatal mortality was twice as high when funisitis was present as when it was absent. In the course of funisitis, inflammatory cells invade the walls of the umbilical vein and at a later time the walls of the umbilical arteries (see Figs. 22-6 and 22-7). Stillbirth and neonatal mortality were nearly twice as high when the arteries were inflamed as when only the wall of the umbilical vein was affected.[108]

Many fetuses who are exposed to amniotic fluid bacterial infections aspirate some of the infected fluid (Fig. 22-13). Overall, only a small proportion of such infants have neonatal signs and symptoms of infection. The most frequent of these clinical findings is pneumonia. In a large prospective study this aspiration pneumonia was both less frequent and less often lethal when it arose near term than when it developed preterm, presumably because antibacterial defense mechanisms in the fetus were more mature and thus more effective at term than preterm. Neonatal pneumonia progressively increased in frequency from 14 per 1,000 in preterm neonates without chorioamnionitis to 36 per 1,000 in those with mild

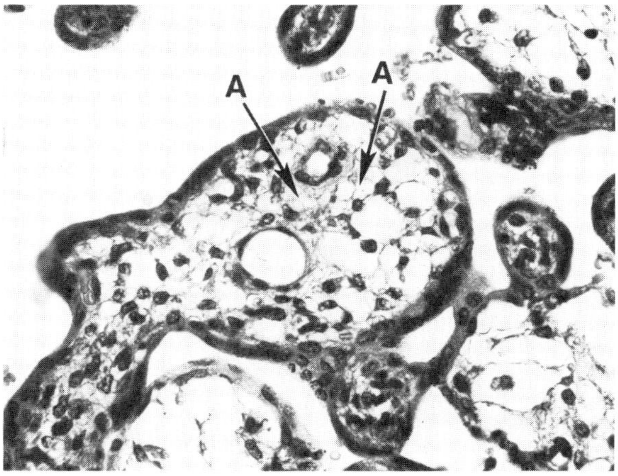

Figure 22-12 Placental villus showing large, intracellular open spaces that are occupied by edema fluid (arrows) (hematoxylin and eosin; original magnification ×600).

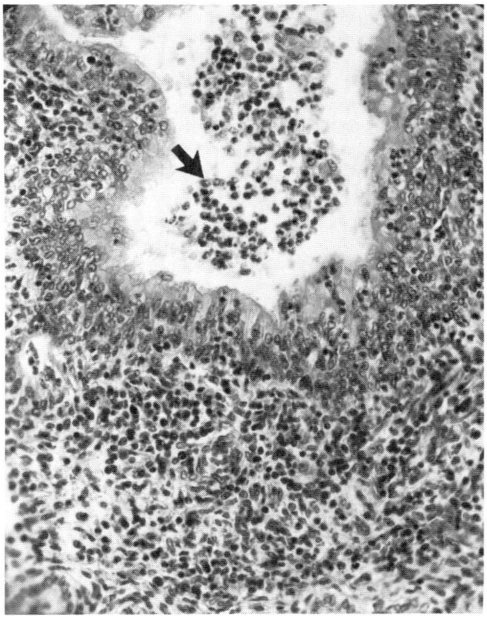

Figure 22-13 Massive aspiration of maternal polymorphs (arrow) into the lung of a premature infant during the course of acute chorioamnionitis. (hematoxylin and eosin; original magnification ×250). (From Blanc, 1981.[16])

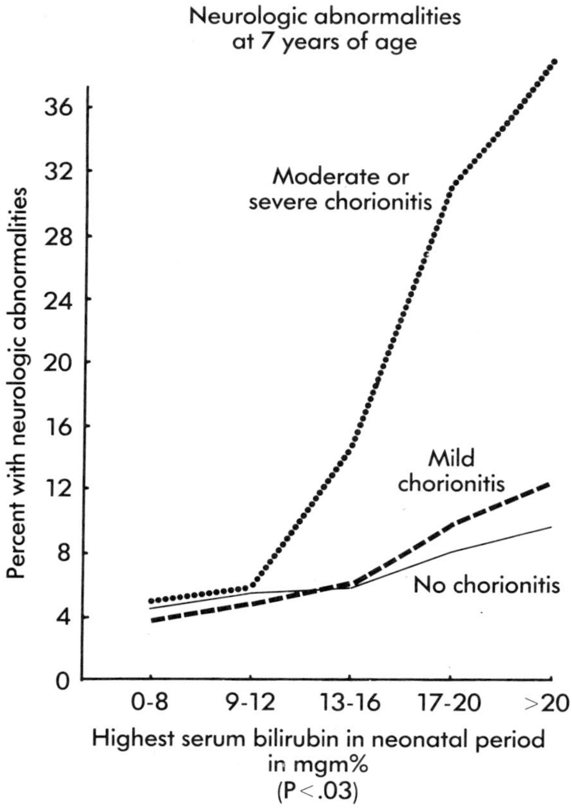

Figure 22-14 Neurologic abnormalities at 7 years of age. In a large prospective study acute chorioamnionitis was followed by long-term neurologic abnormalities at neonatal serum bilirubin levels far lower than those that usually damage neonates' brains.

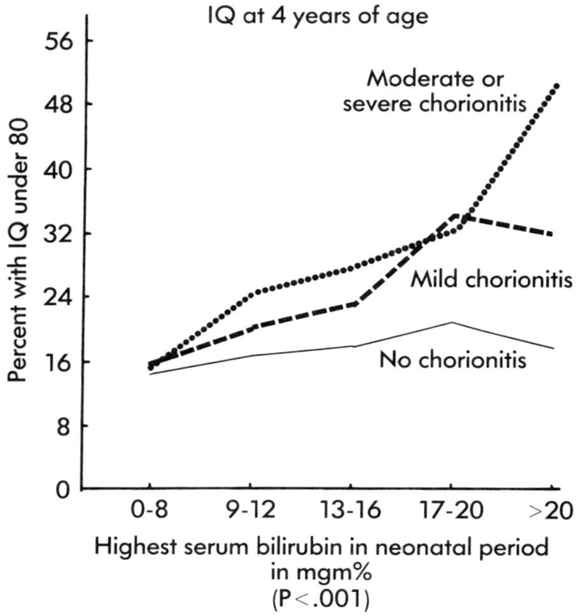

Figure 22-15 IQ at 4 years of age. Low IQ values followed the same course as neurologic abnormalities with acute chorioamnionitis and increasing serum bilirubin values in the neonate.

chorioamnionitis to 61 per 1,000 in those with severe chorioamnionitis ($p < 0.001$).[108] The comparable rates in full-term neonates were 3 per 1,000, 6 per 1,000, and 9 per 1,000 ($p < 0.02$).[108]

A small proportion of the fetuses who aspirate infected amniotic fluid develop bacteremia or septicemia. In the Collaborative Perinatal Study (CPS) the frequency of neonatal septicemia progressively increased with the severity of acute chorioamnionitis from a frequency of 3 per 1,000 in preterm children without chorioamnionitis to 9 per 1,000 in those with moderate or severe chorioamnionitis ($p < 0.001$).[108] The comparable figures in full-term children were 0.3 per 1,000 and 0.8 per 1,000 ($p < 0.001$). Septicemia was usually accompanied by pneumonia, so most of the bacteria probably entered the circulation as the result of the fetus aspirating infected amniotic fluid. A reduction in fetal breathing movements, fetal tachycardia, neonatal thrombocytopenia, and neutropenia are the most frequent manifestations of the bacteremia or septicemia.[61] Acute chorioamnionitis can also lead to fetal bradycardia or to variable and late fetal heart rate decelerations, which have often been mistakenly attributed to hypoxia.[145]

Acute chorioamnionitis is a repeating disorder in pregnancies that spontaneously end preterm. In a large prospective study its preterm appearance in one pregnancy was repeated preterm in 46 percent of the next pregnancies.[108] Neurologic abnormalities were another consequence of preterm acute chorioamnionitis in this study. Acute chorioamnionitis was followed by a 20 percent increase in the frequency of neurologic abnormalities at 7 years of age (Fig. 22-14).[108] Most of this was related to the complications of the preterm birth, the most frequent of which was diffuse placental villous edema.[110] This edema blocks gas exchange in the placenta, and the resulting fetal hypoxia damages fetal lungs and predisposes to the neonatal respiratory disease syndrome (RDS). The resulting neonatal hypoxia often impairs the autoregulation of the cerebral circulation, which sometimes leads to cerebral intraventricular hemorrhage and periventricular leukomalacia.[81] In a prospective study 16 of 17 preterm children who survived both acute chorioamnionitis and severe RDS had neurologic abnormalities at 7 years of age compared with only 34 of 668 of age-matched controls who had chorioamnionitis without neonatal respiratory distress ($p < 0.001$).[108] Other studies have produced similar results.[100] In this same prospective study, neonatal serum bilirubin levels were significantly higher at every gestational age when chorioamnionitis was present than when it was absent.[108,114] When chorioamnionitis was absent, there was no significant increase in the frequency of neurologic abnormalities and low IQ values when serum bilirubin reached levels as high as 20 mg per deciliter, whereas following chorioamnionitis neurologic abnormalities increased in frequency when peak neonatal bilirubin levels reached 12 mg per deciliter (Figs. 22-14 and 22-15).[108,114] There were further increases in the frequency of long-term neurologic abnormalities when bilirubin rose to higher levels.

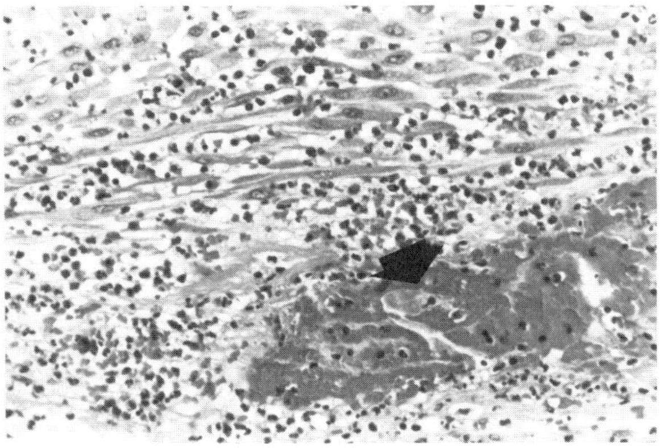

Figure 22-16 Many polymorphs have invaded the decidua basalis in a case of acute chorioamnionitis. Blood vessels have been damaged with resultant hemorrhage (arrow) and a partial placental abruption (hematoxylin and eosin; original magnification ×300).

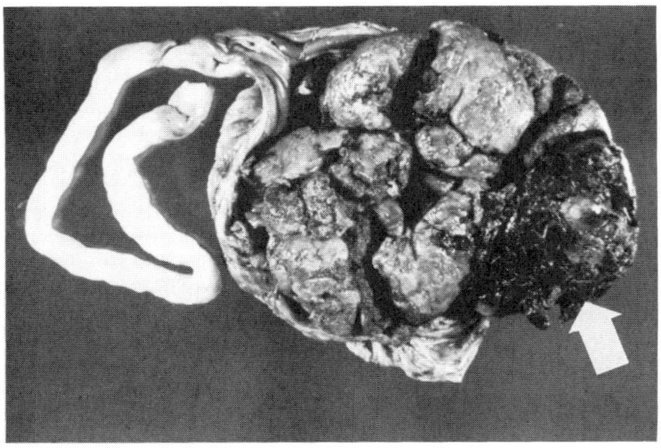

Figure 22-17 The blood clot (arrow) is the result of a chorioamnionitis associated placental abruption.

There are still other consequences of acute chorioamnionitis. The infection sometimes invades the decidua basalis, where it damages blood vessels (Fig. 22-16). Usually the blood vessels thrombose, but at times blood escapes the damaged vessels and initiates a placental abruption (Fig. 22-17).[105,108,114] A very small proportion of the neonates exposed to acute chorioamnionitis develop otitis media, meningitis, septic arthritis, or other evidence of disseminated infection. The site of bacterial entry for meningitis may often be the middle ear because middle ear infections are usually present when meningitis follows chorioamnionitis. Otitis media is often found at autopsy in the middle ears of neonates who have died after exposure to acute chorioamnionitis.

Acute chorioamnionitis reportedly has a role in the genesis of the Wilson-Mikity syndrome. In one study 30 of 35 children with the syndrome had been exposed to acute chorioamnionitis.[46] Neonatal serum IgM levels were sevenfold higher in the children who developed the Wilson-Mikity syndrome than in the children who did not develop the disorder. Emphysema is the pulmonary disorder responsible for the Wilson-Mikity syndrome, and it develops during the first weeks of life. Affected children have reportedly had large numbers of neutrophils in their amniotic fluid and significant levels of neutrophil elastase in their tracheal aspirates soon after birth.[46] The investigators in this study postulate that emphysema develops as the result of elastic tissue destruction when elastase released by inflammatory cells overwhelms the antiproteinase activity in the affected children's lungs.[46]

Acute chorioamnionitis can also affect the course of labor. Women who develop acute chorioamnionitis much more often experience slow cervical dilation and ineffective uterine contractions than uninfected gravidas.[45] These impediments are most frequent when the bacteria responsible for the chorioamnionitis have a moderate or high rather than a low level of virulence. Bacteria with low virulence have little or no effect on the rate of cervical dilation, the frequency and strength of uterine contractions, the total duration of labor, and the dose of oxytocin that is required to accelerate labor.[151] These findings are not surprising because in two of three cases of chorioamnionitis the infection extends into the myometrium, sometimes involving the entire wall of the uterus.[8]

Premature Rupture of Fetal Membranes

Premature rupture of the fetal membranes is membrane rupture before the onset of labor. In a large prospective study, chorioamnionitis was twice as frequent when fetal membranes ruptured 1 to 4 hours before the onset of labor as when the membranes ruptured just after labor began.[108,114] Thus chorioamnionitis preceded about half of the premature membrane ruptures because it usually takes more than 4 hours after membrane rupture for the microscopic findings of chorioamnionitis to appear.[108,111] In another study maternal and umbilical cord serum levels of IgM were often elevated when membranes had been ruptured for only 12 to 24 hours, an indication that infection had preceded most of these membrane ruptures because it takes more than 24 hours for IgM levels to rise after the start of infection.[67]

In our analyses of a large prospective study, acute chorioamnionitis accounted for 44 percent of the premature membrane ruptures that took place 1 to 12 hours before the onset of labor.[108] In these analyses the perinatal mortality rate was threefold higher when acute chorioamnionitis was present than when it was absent. This was true for both preterm and for full-term births.[108] When acute chorioamnionitis was taken into consideration, stillbirths and neonatal deaths were less frequent when the membranes ruptured prematurely than when labor preceded membrane rupture.[108] Premature membrane rupture was not followed by an increase in the frequency of neurologic abnormalities at 7 years of age when preterm birth and acute chorioamnionitis were taken into consideration.

What are the circumstances that permit bacteria to reach the fetal membranes and initiate acute chorioamnionitis? Normally the vaginal pH decreases during pregnancy and suppresses bacterial growth.[78] When the vaginal pH remains high, the frequency of premature membrane rupture reportedly increases several-fold, perhaps because the bacteria that initiate acute chorioamnionitis are present in larger numbers.[37] Specifically, larger number of anaerobic bacteria, mycoplasmas, *Trichomonas vaginalis,* and *C. trachomatis* are often present in the vagina when the vaginal pH is abnormally high during pregnancy.[37,63,158] Coitus can also temporarily raise vaginal pH.[43]

The bacteria and mycoplasma that initiate acute chorioamnionitis reportedly activate collagen and elastic tissue degradation by recruiting inflammatory cells that produce and stimulate the production of collagenase and elastase.[149,169,173] It is noteworthy that *Staphylococcus aureus* and *Escherichia coli* potentiate the in vitro weakening of fetal membranes, whereas group B streptococci do not.[147] This may explain why *E. coli* and *S. aureus* are common isolates from the membranes and placentas affected by acute chorioamnionitis, whereas group B streptococci rarely if ever cross intact fetal membranes and initiate acute chorioamnionitis.

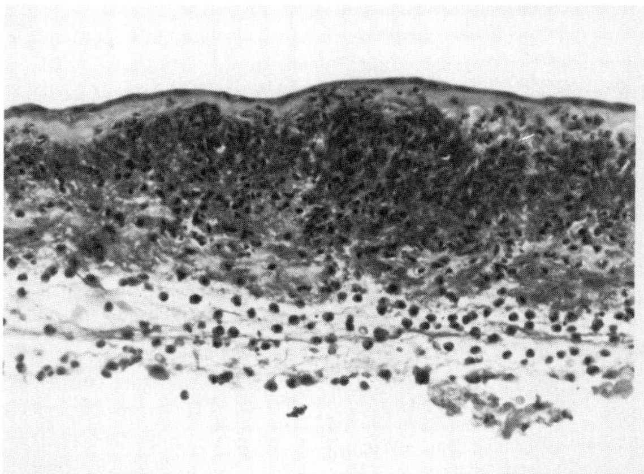

Figure 22-18 A heavy infiltrate of polymorphs is associated with necrosis immediately adjacent to the site of a spontaneous premature rupture of the fetal membranes (hematoxylin and eosin; original magnification ×300).

Acute chorioamnionitis is clearly not the only factor predisposing to premature rupture of the fetal membranes. It has been claimed that the rates of both collagen degradation and regeneration were increased in membranes that ruptured prematurely.[168]

It has been known for some years that female orgasm can induce uterine contractions, and we have postulated that fetal membranes locally weakened by infection are more likely to be ruptured by uterine contractions than are undamaged membranes (Fig. 22-18).[41,108] In a prospective study we found a strong, positive correlation between maternal orgasm and premature membrane rupture when acute chorioamnionitis was present (Fig. 22-19).[108,113] When acute chorioamnionitis was absent, orgasm was associated with a much lower frequency of premature membrane rupture.

Premature rupture of the fetal membranes before 27 weeks of gestation had a very poor prognosis in a 1984 study.[164] Only about 25 percent of the liveborns survived, and the majority of the survivors subsequently had psychomotor abnormalities.[164] Outcomes were somewhat better in a 1988 study of similar aged children.[102] In the 1988 study a third of the children survived, and only a third of these survivors had a developmental abnormality evident during the first year of life.[102] Seven of the 12 children with developmental abnormalities had cerebral palsy, and three had lesser neurologic abnormalities. Because many psychomotor impairments first appear after 1 year of age, longer-term follow-ups are needed to assess all of the impairments that follow preterm premature membrane rupture. As is the case with acute chorioamnionitis, premature membrane rupture did not increase the frequency of neurologic abnormalities at 7

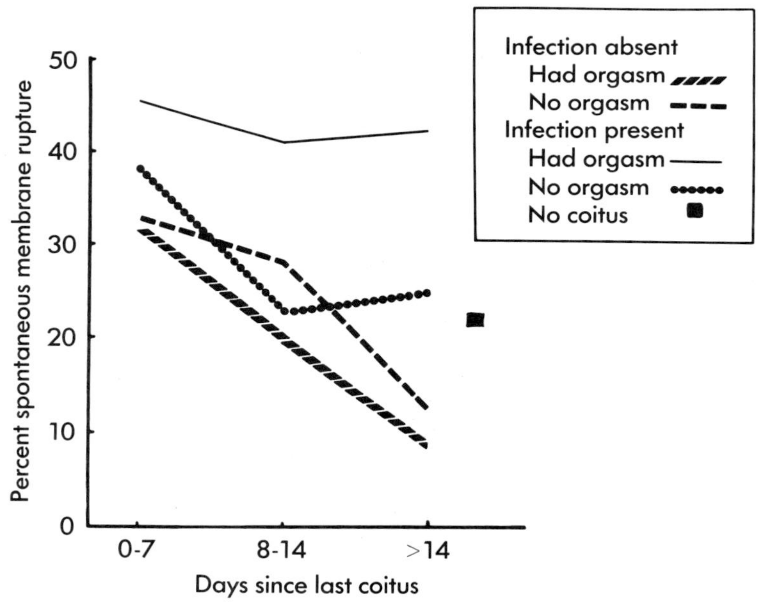

Figure 22-19 Premature rupture of the fetal membranes was most frequent in a prospective study when acute chorioamnionitis was present in conjunction with maternal coital-induced orgasm. (From Naeye and Ross, 1982.[113])

years of age when gestational age, peak neonatal serum bilirubin levels, and placental villous edema were taken into consideration.[108]

It is important to note that very few deliveries can be delayed for more than 2 to 3 weeks after the fetal membrane rupture. In one study only 7 percent of pregnancies had labor delayed beyond 48 hours following premature membrane rupture.[29] The presence of group B streptococci in the cervix at the time of rupture increases the risk of maternal endometritis and life-threatening group B streptococcal infection in the neonate.[120]

Twins and Triplets

The third most frequent cause of spontaneous preterm delivery is multiple fetuses.[108] The assumption is often made that such deliveries are the result of overdistention of the uterus by the multiple fetuses or by the hydramnios that is more frequent with multiple than with single fetuses. There are additional explanations for the high rate of preterm births with multiple fetuses. We have found that acute chorioamnionitis is present in about two-thirds of the placentas of twins who deliver spontaneously before 30 weeks of gestation. From that point in gestation until term, more than two-thirds of twin placentas either have acute chorioamnionitis or the findings of unevenly accelerated villous maturation, which is a marker for low uteroplacental blood flow. Low uteroplacental blood flow is a well-established cause of spontaneous preterm birth.[107,108] It therefore seems likely that infection and low uteroplacental blood flow, rather than an overdistended uterus, are the most frequent causes of preterm birth with multiple fetuses.[108]

Preventing Acute Chorioamnionitis

To date, no fully effective means have been discovered to prevent acute chorioamnionitis, but it may be possible to prevent some of its complications. Giving antibiotics to mothers who have an oral temperature of 38° C or higher during labor has been reported to reduce the incidence of neonatal sepsis.[52,53] Preventing chorioamnionitis or controlling it before it initiates labor is a far bigger challenge. Once the infection has started labor, tocolytic agents, rest, and hydration are ineffective in stopping labor.[117] Discontinuing coitus or using a condom to keep sperm out of the vagina might reduce the frequency of acute chorioamnionitis if ways could be found to identify the pregnancies that are vulnerable to coitus-initiated chorioamnionitis (see Figs. 22-3 and 22-4). Unexplained cervical dilation is both a well-known risk for acute chorioamnionitis and a consequence of the infection. Because a number of days sometimes pass between the time the cervix begins to dilate and the onset of labor, some preterm deliveries might be prevented if antibiotics were given when cervical dilation is first noted. In one study, administering antibiotics when the cervix had already dilated lengthened from 17 days to 30 days the interval between the recognition of cervical dilation and delivery.[101]

Listeriosis

Infection by the gram-positive bacillus *Listeria monocytogenes* is an often unrecognized cause of preterm delivery and perinatal death. A minimum of clinical symptoms in the gravida can be followed by a high frequency of perinatal mortality and morbidity. This mortality has been reported to be as high as 71 percent.[38] Usually maternal symptoms are vague and nonspecific and are often interpreted as influenza. As a result the diagnosis is rarely made before labor and delivery, and most often the disorder is not recognized until the placenta is examined The few times the diagnosis has been made before delivery have been the result of cervical or maternal blood cultures that were prompted by uterine irritability, a dilating cervix, or a reduction in fetal movements.[60,79]

Listeriosis is mainly a disease that develops in individuals with altered immunity, which includes pregnancy. It has been estimated that *L. monocytogenes* infects one in 20,000 pregnant women.[157] Sporadic fetal infections have been reported from many nations, and occasional epidemics have been reported in hospitals, suggesting that the agent can be transmitted by interpersonal contacts during or after birth. In epidemics food is the most frequent vehicle of transmission. These foods have included milk, cheese, poorly cooked sausage, chicken, and prepacked salads.[21] The organism can multiply in household refrigerators, so food that might be contaminated must be recooked after refrigeration to be safe for consumption. The agent has been found in the soil and many times in human feces. In the majority of sporadic infections, the source of the infection is not identified. Maternal infection in the first trimester reportedly leads to abortion.[131] Infection in the second or third trimesters usually results in either stillbirth or a preterm birth that is followed by pneumonia and neonatal sepsis.[69,71] Only a few healthy children have been reported after the infection was diagnosed and treated during pregnancy.[30] Some of the survivors have been brain damaged.[21]

Clinically the infection often presents with a high maternal blood leukocyte count, fetal tachycardia, and neonatal sepsis. [7] A flulike illness in the mother usually starts only a few hours before delivery takes place, so the infection is almost never diagnosed in time to initiate therapy. Boucher and Yonekura have reported that the combinations of a high maternal leukocyte count, fetal tachycardia, decreased fetal heart rate variability and the absence of intrapartum fetal heart rate accelerations raise the possibility of fetal listerial sepsis.[17] However, these findings are not specific for a listerial infection. They are also seen in some cases of acute chorioamnionitis caused by a variety of virulent bacteria. A quick rise in maternal serum levels of antilisteriolysin-0 after the start of the infection is a more certain indicator of the diagnosis.[15]

Placental findings include a necrotizing villitis that often reaches the abscess stage and affects one side of the villus more than the other (Fig. 22-20). Sometimes the abscesses extend into adjacent villi. Acute funisitis and severe acute chorioamnionitis are often visible in the umbilical cord and chorionic plate of the placenta. The organism can often be demonstrated by Gram's stain. The affected fetuses are usually born preterm, and the infected neonates often have a rash, pneumonia, and hepatosplenomegaly. Gram's stains on smears of gastric contents, cultures of the placenta, and the skin lesions

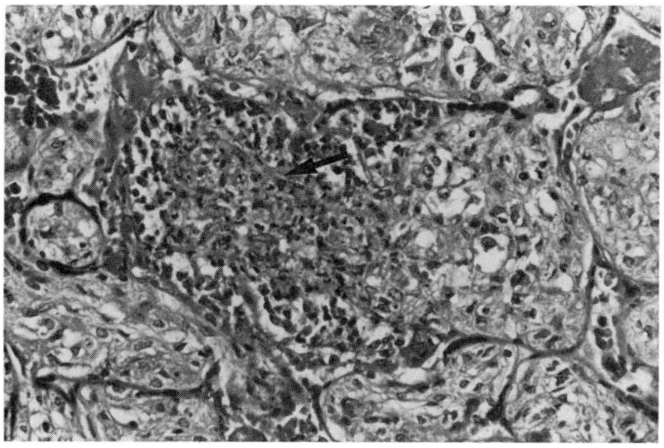

Figure 22-20 Listeriosis; necrotizing villitis has almost reached the abscess stage (arrow) (hematoxylin and eosin; original magnification ×240).

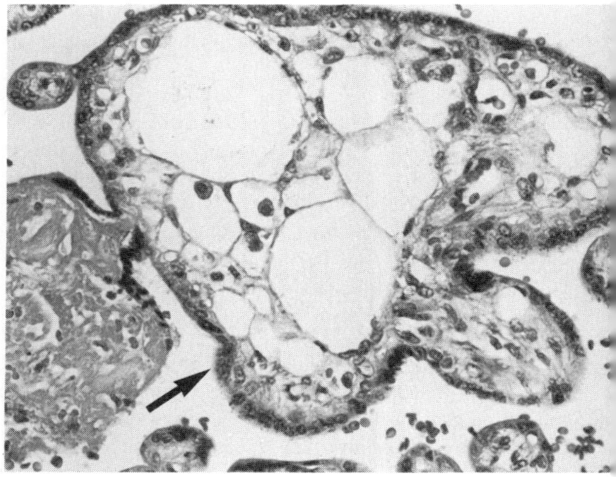

Figure 22-21 Congenital syphilis; a villus appears immature for gestational age and is very edematous (arrow) (hematoxylin and eosin; original magnification ×600).

often confirm the diagnosis. The organism can be difficult to culture. The liver is often massively infiltrated by granulomas in the infants who die. Smaller numbers of granulomas are sometimes present in the brain and other organs. Brain lesions are usually most severe in the pons and medulla. A number of cases have been treated antenatally and scars of the old abscesses identified in the placenta.[14] An infection with *Campylobacter* can produce placental lesions that closely resemble those produced by *Listeria,* so the diagnosis of a listerial infection cannot be made with certainty without a specific identification of the organism.[23]

Syphilis

Prenatal infection by *Treponema pallidum* is a major cause of stillbirth and neonatal death in many Third World nations, and it is now becoming more frequent in North America. In one African nation congenital syphilis was reportedly present in 5 to 8 percent of all neonates.[140]

First-trimester infections by *T. pallidum* occur but are difficult to recognize because the embryo is too immature to mount a tissue reaction to the spirochete.[64] Lesions in the fetus that are recognizable as syphilis usually first appear in the fifth month of gestation. The placenta and fetus can be infected during the primary and secondary stages of the maternal infection but not during its tertiary stage. The later the fetus is infected during the course of the maternal disease, the better the infant's chance of survival. Appropriate treatment of the mother during the first 4 months of pregnancy usually ensures that the neonate will not be infected.

The spirochete often spreads to multiple fetal organs and produces enough damage to cause stillbirth or neonatal death. When the fetus is macerated, the diagnosis can usually be made by radiologic examination of the long bones and a dark-field examination of the amniotic fluid for spirochetes.[176] Some neonates are asphyxiated as the result of severe placental villous edema (Fig. 22-21). Such edema has been much more frequent in the infected placentas of African than of U.S. neonates that we have examined. In the absence of neonatal clinical findings of antenatal hypoxia, the earliest sign of infection in the neonate is usually a rhinitis followed by a maculopapular rash with sloughing of the epithelium on the palms and soles and about the mouth of the recently born infant. Neonatal mortality is high when these desquamative lesions are present. Granulomatous lesions are present in the liver, lungs, and pancreas of some newborns with the disease. They have been much more frequent in the organs of the African than of U.S. neonates that we have examined.

The syphilitic placenta is typically enlarged, often exceeding 800 g, while the neonate is often growth retarded.[85,86] Individual peripheral villi are usually larger than normal, which partially explains the large size and immature appearance of some syphilitic placentas. The previously mentioned intracellular villous edema is another factor that often increases the weight of the syphilitic placenta (Fig. 22-21). When such edema is diffuse and severe, the infants are either stillborn or have neonatal clinical evidences of severe antenatal hypoxia. The result is neonatal respiratory distress, decreased renal function, and sometimes necrotizing enterocolitis and hypoxic brain damage. The spirochete can be identified in some infected placentas by use of the Warthin-Starry stain. In a few infected placentas, concentric layers of collagen surround the arteries in stem villi, and in rare cases endarteritis is present (Fig. 22-22). Focal plasma cell and lymphocyte infiltrates, giant cells, and fibrosis are sometimes present in placental villi.[14,134] Unfortunately, many syphilitic placentas do not have microscopic findings that are diagnostic of the disease, even when stains are employed to identify the spirochetes. As a result, placental examination fails to identify many cases of congenital syphilis.

Necrotizing funisitis is occasionally present in congenital syphilis. In a recent study 16 of 35 umbilical cords of neonates with congenital syphilis reportedly had such funisitis.[42] The lesion was described as often having

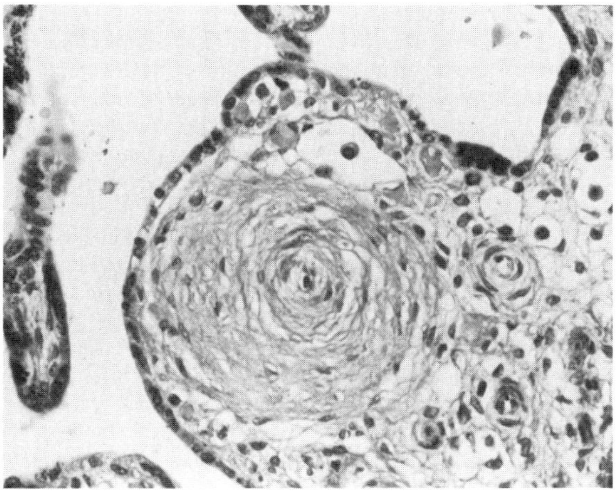

Figure 22-22 Concentric layers of collagen have nearly obliterated an artery in a stem villous of a syphilitic placenta (hematoxylin and eosin; original magnification ×600).

the gross appearance of a barber pole in which red and pale blue zones alternated with chalky white streaks in a spiral distribution. In cross-section the walls of the umbilical vessels were white and greatly thickened. Focal thrombosis of the umbilical vein was reported to be frequent. Microscopic examination reportedly showed an abscesslike necrosis centered around the umbilical vessels in Wharton's jelly. Of the scores of syphilitic placentas I have examined, only two or three of the associated umbilical cords had these necrotizing lesions. Syphilis is not the only or even the most frequent cause of necrotizing funisitis.[14]

Leprosy

Infections with *Mycobacterium leprae* reportedly produce no diagnostic lesions in the placenta.[35] Specifically, no acid-fast bacilli or acid-fast bacillary granules have been visible by microscopic examination, electron microscopy, or immunologic analyses. However, many of the placentas have reportedly been small because of the small size of their parenchymal cells.[35] This last description originated in Ethiopia, where I have examined more than a thousand placentas from women who did not have leprosy. Many of these placentas were subnormal in size because the gravidas were short in stature, thin, and had low pregnancy weight gains that were due to undernutrition. Thus undernutrition must be considered as a possible explanation for the small size of the placentas from the Ethiopian gravidas with leprosy.[35,108] The fetal undergrowth that has also been reported with leprosy might also be due to undernutrition.[35,108]

Lyme Disease *(Borrelia burgdorferi)*

The effects of *Borrelia burgdorferi* (Lyme disease) infections during pregnancy has received attention during recent years. Untreated, some of the pregnancies end in abortion, stillbirth, or liveborn infants with cardiac malformations.[82] These outcomes are rare enough that not all physicians agree that treatment for the disorder is necessary in pregnancy when the antibody titer is negative.[82] Unfortunately, there has not always been an increase in the maternal gestational antibody titer to the agent in cases in which the spirochete was subsequently identified in the tissues of the fetus or neonate.[82]

Group B Streptococcal Infections

Group B streptococcal (GBS) infections are a major life-threatening disorder in newborn infants. There is no convincing evidence that group B streptococci cross intact fetal membranes or very often reach the fetus via transplacental spread, so placental findings are not a very important feature of the disorder. The placenta is affected only when the disorder is acquired during the interval between membrane rupture and delivery. In this interval the organism can enter the uterine cavity and produce a severe acute chorioamnionitis. All five serotypes of GBS have been isolated in such cases. Adding such cases to the infections acquired during passage through the birth canal, the frequency of resulting fetal and neonatal infections ranges from 1.1 to 3.7 per 1,000 live births with case fatality rates sometimes exceeding 75 percent.[10,39]

The neonates characteristically exhibit respiratory distress, bacteremia, septic shock, and a persistent fetal circulation. Meningitis is present in about one in five cases. More than half of the affected children are sick within 6 hours of birth, and nearly half have low Apgar scores.[9] The origin of the bacteria is the maternal, cervical, vaginal, or anorectal flora.[10] Heavy fetal and neonatal GBS colonization, but not necessarily a heavy maternal colonization, predisposes to the disorder.[125] A low transfer of anti-GBS antibodies from mother to fetus appears to increase the susceptibility of the fetus and neonate to the infection.[19]

Fungal Infections

Candida Albicans

Candida albicans usually reaches the amniotic fluid and fetus by way of local infections in the extraplacental membranes adjacent to the cervical os. The membranes in such cases are sometimes studded with very small yellow-white nodules. The organism can disseminate to many fetal organs, but it is most often limited to the umbilical cord, skin, mucous membranes, and lungs.[178] The lesions appear on the surface of the umbilical cord as small clusters of sharply defined, flat, yellowish plaques varying in diameter from 2 to 5 mm.[45] The hyphae are easily identified in these lesions, admixed with neutrophils and occasional plasma cells just beneath the amnion. The acute inflammatory cells often can be seen migrating through the walls of nearby umbilical arteries or the umbilical vein toward the localized area of infection. Infections have been recognized in fetuses as early as the start of the second trimester of gestation.

Those born with the infection often develop skin lesions in intertriginous areas. These skin lesions are usually vesicles with red bases that sometimes evolve into pustules. Lesions in the oral cavity characteristically appear as shallow ulcers covered by a white plaque. When the infection disseminates, microabscesses can develop in the kidneys, liver spleen, heart, and brain. *Candida albicans* infections have occasionally been associated with the use of intrauterine contraceptive devices.[156]

Coccidioides immitis

Less than 100 cases of *coccidioidomycosis* during pregnancy have been reported. Several have included descriptions of placental infarcts with spherules of *C. immitis* and associated inflammation.[170,171] Only a few newborns have been infected, and it may be that some of the transmissions occurred during delivery rather than during pregnancy.[155]

Viral Infections

Cytomegalovirus Infection

The fetus is more often infected by cytomegalovirus (CMV) than by any other virus.[167] The reported rate of transmission to the fetus after a primary maternal infection is between 20 and 50 percent.[128,159] An infected fetus has about a 10 percent risk of being damaged.[125] The gravidas appear usually to acquire the virus from an older child in the family or through a close, usually sexual contact with another adult.[31,124,167] The maternal infection produces only vague, flulike signs and symptoms. Three percent of the women in one prospective study developed a primary cytomegalovirus infection during pregnancy, a third of which were transmitted to their fetuses.[159] It appears that the fetus can be infected and damaged by a recurrent as well as by a primary maternal infection.[141,181]

Ninety percent of the infections are asymptomatic in the neonate. The only fetal infections that produce long-term handicaps appear to be those that are acquired before midgestation;[129,159] some of these children are stillborn. There are many preterm births and many neonates with microcephaly, hepatomegaly, chorioretinitis, jaundice, and thrombocytopenia. Twenty to thirty percent of the neonates with clinical evidences of infection die, and 90 percent of the survivors of clinically evident neonatal infections have severe long-term handicaps including mental retardation, behavioral disorders, sensorineural hearing defects, and in a few instances cerebral palsy.[144] Hearing defects are reportedly the most frequent adverse outcome of the fetal infections.[144]

There is evidence that the placenta may sometimes be a host for a CMV infection that is acquired early in gestation but only begins to damage fetal organs at a much later stage of pregnancy (Fig. 22-23).[3,56] Placental lesions are often most severe in preterm infants, probably because the majority of such infants are infected earlier in gestation than are most infected full-term infants.[104] In most instances routine placental examination discloses a chronic villitis with lymphocytes, plasma cells, fibrosis, and sometimes necrosis of villi.[48] Some authors have

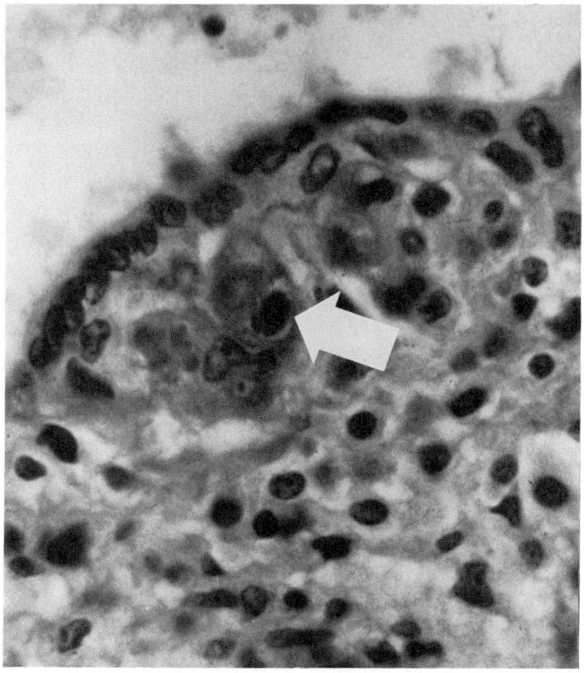

Figure 22-23 Villus of a 22-week gestation placenta. A cell with a typical cytomegalic nuclear inclusion is visible (arrow) (hematoxylin and eosin; original magnification ×2,000).

claimed that a heavy infiltration of plasma cells is strong evidence of a CMV infection (Fig. 22-24). Finding such plasma cells is helpful, but more than half of CMV-infected placentas do not have large numbers of these cells. When present, plasma cells usually secrete IgM and IgG. Other cells that infiltrate the villi usually include Hofbauer cells and T lymphocytes. B lymphocytes are usually absent. Intervillositis, calcification, and cells with intranuclear or cytoplasmic inclusions are found in association with villitis in some infected placentas.[48,104] When present, owl's eye nuclear inclusions are usually evidence of cytomegalic infections (see Fig. 22-23).[14]

As term approaches, cytomegalic inclusions become scarce in the placenta, but a proliferative villitis usually persists. Focal infiltration of the villi by lymphocytes is the most frequent finding in late gestation. When plasma cells are present, there is a good chance that cytomegalic inclusions can be found.[103] In those few instances when fetuses are hydropic, the placenta is usually very heavy because of villous edema.[48,103] Otherwise, CMV-infected placentas are usually normal or subnormal in weight. The use of immunofluorescent antibodies sometimes identifies infections in the placenta in which cytomegalic inclusions are absent.[2,48] In such cases the virus can often be grown from tissue taken from the placenta and amnion.

The diagnosis of congenital CMV infection usually depends on a combination of urine examination, rising antibody titers, virus isolation, and placental examination. Most recently viral culture of the amniotic fluid has been recommended as an adjunct to the other diagnostic procedures.[59] Because of recent advances in monoclonal antibody techniques, such cultures can be interpreted in from 1 to 3 days.

Most neonates with antenatally acquired CMV infections are normally grown.[104] However, early gestational CMV infections are apt to retard fetal and placental growth.[97,159] Organs of these neonates often have a subnormal number of cells, presumably as the result of cellular destruction by necrosis.[104] Fetal growth retardation is much less frequent with CMV than with rubella infections.

Herpes Simplex

Herpes simplex virus (HSV) genital infections are at an epidemic level in the United States with about 300,000 new cases diagnosed in women each year.[22] Transmission is by genital contact with individuals who are shedding the virus, with or without clinically evident lesions.[139] The infection can be acquired at any time during pregnancy.[20,99,154] If this is a primary infection, specific herpetic lesions will appear in the genital tract after about 6 days. Inguinal lymphadenopathy, fever, and myalgia usually accompany the genital lesions. Recurrences from latent infections are also frequent, particularly during pregnancy. Unlike the primary infections, recurrences often have only minor local manifestations and no systemic signs or symptoms.

A primary HSV infection poses a threat to the fetus.[22] Recurrent maternal infections are much less of a threat because maternal antibodies have been passed to the fetus.[22] The primary infections are high risk for abortion, preterm delivery, and an infected neonate.[22,116] Infection that takes place during organogenesis often produces serious organ damage.[66] More than 90 percent of infants with transplacental HSV infections present within 72 hours of birth with herpetic lesions in the skin.[66] Over 70 percent have had chorioretinitis and microphthalmia, and half have been reported to have microcephaly, hydranencephaly, or brain atrophy. Two-thirds of the infected neonates are symptomatic by 1 week of age and most of the rest by 3 weeks of age.[74] Four-fifths have seizures and serious neurologic abnormalities (Fig. 22-25).[74] Fetal growth retardation is frequent. The death rate exceeds 80 percent when the internal organs are involved. There is a much lower mortality rate when only the skin, eye, or mouth is infected.[177]

Herpes virus spread to the fetus in such cases is presumably hematogenous, but a few ascending infections have been reported.[14] A variety of lesions have been found in the placenta. They include necrosis of the amnion without inflammation, mononuclear cell infiltrates, coagulative necrosis, and villous edema.[1,62] Two placentas have reportedly had funisitis with infiltrating

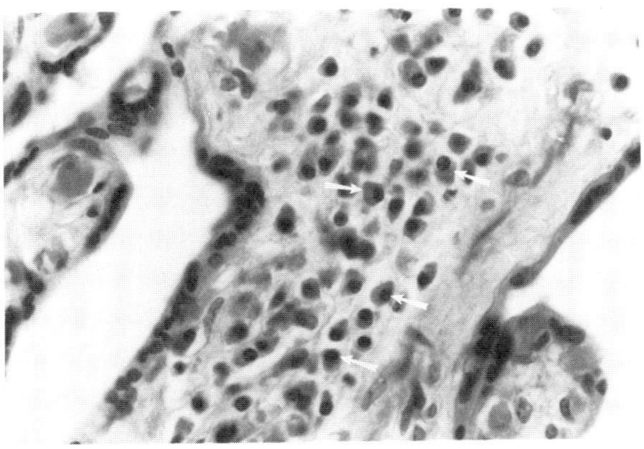

Figure 22-24 Many plasma cells (arrows) are infiltrating a placental villus in a case of congenital cytomegalovirus infection (hematoxylin and eosin; original magnification × 1,200).

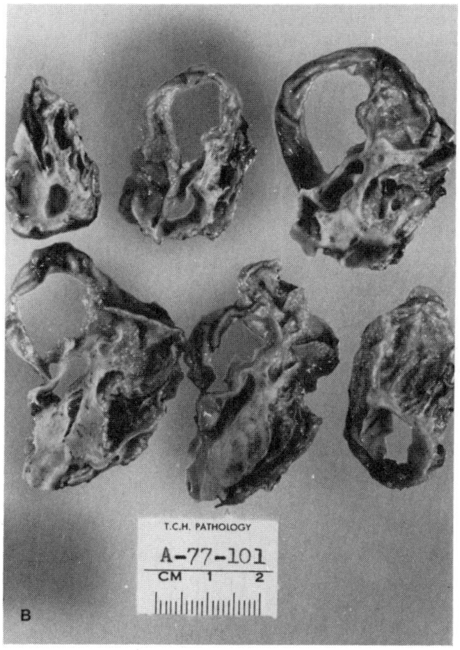

Figure 22-25 Extensive cortical atrophy is visible in the brain of this 7-week-old male who died of disseminated herpes virus infection. (From Naeye and Tafari, 1983.[114])

lymphocytes, plasma cells, and typical herpetic inclusion bodies in amniotic cells. In these two cases umbilical vessels had areas of necrosis, medial fibrosis, severe proliferative endovasculitis, and dystrophic calcification. Benirschke and Kaufmann reported a case with necrotizing chorioamnionitis that included a blister on the surface of the placenta.[14] Very large numbers of plasma cells were present, which is a rare finding. The diagnosis of herpes virus infection can often be confirmed by viral culture or by fluorescent antibody examination of the amnion and placenta.[135]

Rubella

The rubella virus disseminates throughout the placenta when mothers are infected during the first trimester of pregnancy, but only about 60 percent of the embryos and fetuses are infected.[98] The infections often persist through fetal life and sometimes for a year or longer after birth. Serious malformations and growth retardation are sometimes produced by the infection. During the first 2 months of gestation, maternal infections lead to abortion or produce serious malformations in about half of the embryos that are present. About a third of fetuses are similarly affected by a maternal infection during the third month of gestation. The risk drops to 10 percent during the fourth month and thereafter disappears, except for an occasional case of deafness with an infection that occurs until the twentieth week of gestation.[87] In addition to deafness, the most frequent manifestations of congenital rubella are cataracts, glaucoma, myopia, congenital heart disease, mental retardation, childhood diabetes mellitus, and occasionally a progressive encephalopathy that resembles subacute sclerosing panencephalitis.[166]

Growth retardation is frequent but not inevitable, and the degree to which individual organs are growth retarded varies greatly from one fetus to another (Fig. 22-26).[109] Cellular necrosis is one explanation for the growth retardation, but an even more important mechanism is the mitotic inhibitor that is released from infected cells.[126] Most of the organ malformations that are associated with congenital rubella are the apparent consequence of this virus-induced mitotic inhibition.[109,126]

Placentas infected during early gestation by the rubella virus have often had multiple foci of villitis with accompanying severe vasculitis. Late gestational placentas have had suppurative villitis and villous fibrosis of varying severity.[16] In most reported cases the villitis is nonspecific with an infiltration of lymphocytes and a few plasma cells. In such cases rubella villitis resembles the villitis seen with several other viral infections. Inclusions are often hard to find, but they have been identified in the trophoblast, the villous stroma, and the endothelial cells of infected placentas. A necrotizing endarteritis in villous vessels has been reported with recent infection.[18] In term placentas villi have reportedly had a greater than normal variation in size, presumably because the infection interferes with villous budding. This has produced a marked reduction in the number of terminal villi with a resulting low ratio of terminal to stem villi.[49]

Varicella (Chickenpox)

Only a few placentas infected with varicella have been described in the literature. Severe necrotizing and obliterative villitis and intervillitis have been reported.[47] The most complete descriptions are those of Blanc.[16] None of four placentas that he examined had gross abnormalities. All had multiple foci of subacute villitis with trophoblastic necrosis, a fusing of adjacent villi, lymphocytic infiltrates, occlusion of some villous vessels, and tuberculoid giant cells. A fifth placenta had a more chronic infection with plasma cell infiltrates and calcifications in peripheral villi.

Smallpox, Vaccinia

In the days when smallpox was an active disease, the virus often crossed the placenta and produced abortions and stillbirths. Several cases of placental infection with vaccinia were reported. Benirschke and Kaufmann described extensive necrosis of the trophoblast, intervillous fibrin deposits, and focal villous calcification with the infection.[14]

Mumps

The most complete report of placental findings with mumps is from three infections that terminated in the first trimester of pregnancy.[50] A diffuse, proliferative, necrotizing villitis was present with severe vasculitis. Cytoplasmic viral inclusions were present in the decidua.

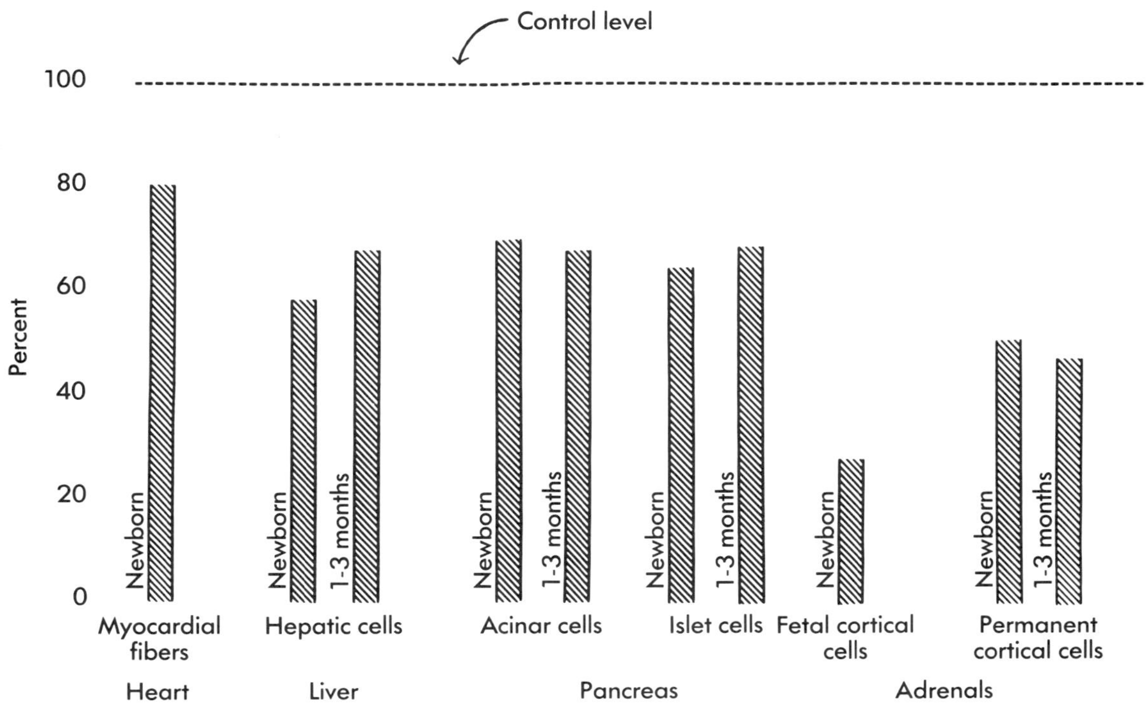

Figure 22-26 The growth retardation of most organs in newborns with congenital rubella is due to a subnormal number of cells in the affected organs. (From Naeye and Tafari, 1983.[114])

Hepatitis

Transplacental infections of hepatitis B virus (HBV) have been reported. They can result from both an acute maternal hepatitis B infection and from the chronic maternal asymptomatic carrier state. Between 70 and 90 percent of gravidas who have high hepatitis B surface antigen titers transmit HBV to their fetuses, and as many as 90 percent of the infected neonates become chronic carriers.[160] A few of the children reportedly have subsequent elevated blood levels of alanine amino transferase, presumably as the result of transmission of the disease across the placenta or at the time of birth.[175] The long-term outcome of these children is currently unclear. Mothers who have chronic non-A, non-B hepatitis during pregnancy reportedly do not experience any deterioration in liver function.[175]

Several placentas have been carefully examined, and the only finding has been the presence of large amounts of bilirubin in Hofbauer cells and in chorionic membrane macrophages.[14] There has been no inflammation or necrosis in the villi of the affected placentas.

Human Immunodeficiency Virus

Human immunodeficiency virus (HIV) infections produce a spectrum of immunodeficiency disorders, of which the acquired immunodeficiency syndrome (AIDS) is the end point. It has been estimated that about one in four maternal HIV infections are transmitted to the fetus via the placenta, but it is possible that some of these infections are transmitted during delivery.[69] At times the infected child becomes symptomatic with AIDS while the mother is still completely well and unaware of her infection. Most of the mothers have been intravenous drug abusers or have had sexual contact with drug abusers.

Both trophoblastic cells and placental endothelial cells appear to synthesize the HIV receptor, CD4. Maury and colleagues have shown that this receptor is present and sometimes infected with the virus in the first trimester of pregnancy.[89] Other modes by which the virus is presumably transmitted include the transplacental passage of infected maternal lymphocytes to the fetal circulation, exposure to maternal blood or other fluids during delivery, and the ingestion of breast milk.

Infected mothers who do not transmit the virus to their infants before or after birth appear to confer some immunologic protection against the virus to their offspring by way of a high-affinity antibody to gp120 epitope.[55] Children who acquire the infection in the perinatal period are usually symptomatic by 1 year of age and have a mean survival of about 3 years.[148] Clinical manifestations in children of antenatally acquired infections are in part the result of damage to the immune system with consequent defects in T and B lymphocytes. The most frequent consequences are a failure to grow and meet neurodevelopmental milestones (encephalopathy), chronic diarrhea, recalcitrant *Candida* esophagitis, recurrent bacterial infections, and lymphoid interstitial pneumonia.[148]

Pregnancy outcome appears to depend on the status of the infection in the gravida. Taking cigarette smoking, alcohol, drug abuse, and demographic factors into consideration, gravidas who are seropositive for HIV but do not have AIDS do not produce neonates who are growth retarded or have any other neonatal abnormality.[94] This report is in contrast to an African study in which neonates of seropositive gravidas were growth retarded.[143] This difference may be due to the higher frequency of debilitating AIDS in the African than in the U.S. gravidas. This favorable short-term outcome of the U.S. pregnancies occurred despite a small increase in the frequency of opportunistic infections in the U.S. gravidas.

Many presumably HIV-infected placentas have been examined, but only a few reports of placental findings have been published.[68,118] Acute chorioamnionitis and malarial parasites have been reported to be increased in frequency.[118] These findings suggest that they are secondary disorders rather than primary manifestations of the HIV infection. Their high frequencies could either be the consequence of HIV impairments in defense mechanisms or the result of the life-style of those infected with HIV. Gravidas who are seropositive for HIV and have CD4 (helper cell) counts under 300 cells per cubic millimeter are at a high risk for serious opportunistic infections during pregnancy.[95] Villitis, the lesions that is characteristic of other viral infections, has not been reported in HIV-infected placentas. It remains to be seen if the hypercellular villi reported in some presumably HIV-infected placentas are the result of HIV infection. Retrovirus-like particles have been claimed to be present in several of these placentas. This may not be a definitive finding because it is difficult to establish the identity of many viruslike particles that are seen in the placenta. Lewis and coworkers have demonstrated the presence of HIV by immunocytochemistry and by in situ hybridization in trophoblastic cells, Hofbauer cells, and embryonic blood cell precursors of aborted embryos.[77]

Parvovirus (Erythema Infectiosum)

Erythema infectiosum (fifth disease) is an infectious disorder caused by a single-stranded DNA virus known as parvovirus B19. It is transmitted by respiratory secretions and produces a febrile illness that lasts about a week and is accompanied by a reduced number of reticulocytes in the peripheral blood.[146] In another week a distinctive rash develops that produces a reddish flush on the cheek and a red, lacy appearance on the extremities and trunk. Many of the infections are asymptomatic. Recovery is uneventful without anemia unless the individual has a preexisting hemolytic disorder, in which case an aplastic crisis sometimes develops about a week after the clinical onset of the illness.[146] About half of the adults in the general population have antibodies against the agent and are not susceptible to reinfection.

There are many documented cases of abortion and fetal hydrops with the infection, apparently because the virus causes fetal anemia and heart failure. These disorders usually develop 4 to 6 weeks after the onset of the acute infection and are most frequent during or before midgestation. A few anemic newborns have been reported after third-trimester infections. The risk of embryonic or fetal death in women infected before midgestation has been estimated to be 3 to 9 percent.

The placentas of infected infants are large and pale because they are edematous. Microscopically, diffuse villous edema is present with eosinophilic intranuclear inclusion bodies in circulating normoblasts.[4] In some cases the villi are necrotic.[84] Livers of the infants who die have large amounts of hemosiderin, a reflection of the intense hemolysis that can take place before death.[84]

Parasitic Infections

Malaria

Malaria is a disorder that characteristically exists in a setting in which there are multiple other influences that also adversely affect women and their fetuses. Gravidas who are young and poorly nourished and receive very little antenatal medical care are most often affected by the parasite because they have the least immunity to it. Under these circumstances it is difficult to separate the placental findings of malaria from the findings of other adverse influences. Gravidas who have no immunity to malaria are often anemic after a malarial attack, and this anemia may be the reason why their placentas are sometimes very heavy. Maternal anemia is a well-known cause of placental hypertrophy.[108]

The chief microscopic finding in malarial infected placentas is the presence of plasmodial parasites in the intervillous blood.[106] Sometimes these parasites are in very large numbers. Other reported placental findings include chronic intervillositis with macrophages and brown pigment in the intervillous space.[174] In areas where malaria is endemic, gravidas normally have more plasmodial parasites in their blood than nonpregnant women.[90] This enhanced parasitemia and the other placental findings just mentioned are not usually associated with poor pregnancy outcomes for the gravida, the fetus, or the neonate.[90,106] In one study maternal anemia, which is a good marker for malarial infection, explained only 1 percent of birth weight variance in a population with endemic malaria.[132] The fetal growth retardation that has been reported with malaria is most likely the result of maternal undernutrition and malnutrition.[90] Most studies that have reported heavy parasitemia in placental blood have also found parasites in the blood of the associated newborns.[90] Very few of these newborns have had clinical evidences of malaria, presumably because they received antiplasmodial antibodies from their mothers before birth.

Nonimmune gravidas who contract malaria, particularly *Plasmodium falciparum,* sometimes have very poor pregnancy outcomes. In such gravidas the infection often leads to rapid hemolysis, severe anemia, and a high fever. This combination presumably accounts for the high rates of maternal mortality, abortions, stillbirths, and preterm deliveries that have occurred in malarial epidemics in nonimmune populations.[93]

Trypanosomes

It is not known how frequently the various trypanosomes infect embryos, fetuses, and placentas. *Trypanosoma cruzi* (Chagas' disease) produces microscopic findings in the placenta that include villitis and parasites that are both outside and inside macrophages in the villi, in the umbilical cord, and in the chorionic plate of the placenta.[6] The parasites can be present without any associated inflammatory reaction, so the acute chorioamnionitis that is found in some placentas with *T. cruzi* is almost certainly of bacterial or mycoplasmal origin. Several neonates who acquired *T. cruzi* before birth have had myocarditis, a granulomatous encephalitis, and a spread of the parasite to other organs, including the skin.[80] Some placentas with trypanosomes are reported to be larger than normal.[6] It remains to be seen whether this is related to the parasite or to coexisting disorders.

Toxoplasma Gondii

The cat is the definitive host for this intracellular parasite, which is capable of invading any cell in almost every warm-blooded animal. Because cats are ubiquitous throughout the world, *T. gondii* is present in almost all populations. The organism has a sexual cycle in the cat's intestinal mucosa, which produces oocytes that pass with the feces into the soil. Rodents ingest the oocytes and are infected, and the cycle is completed when the rodents are eaten by cats. Cats that hunt their own food are particularly dangerous souces of the infection.[161] Children are most often infected when they ingest infected soil during play. Pregnant women are at risk for the infection when they eat contaminated unwashed raw vegetables, fruit, and raw or undercooked meat.[44]

The antibodies associated with a chronic maternal infection protect the fetus. New maternal infections can spread to the embryo as early as the seventh week of gestation. It has been estimated that about 17 percent of such maternal infections that occur between the seventh and fourteenth weeks of gestation are transmitted to the embryo.[32] The lesions in early infected embryos and fetuses are very destructive, often leading to hydranencephaly, hydrops, stillbirth, and occasionally spontaneous abortion. The frequency of transmission progressively increases throughout pregnancy to reach 60 percent by the third trimester.[33] Infections acquired late in gestation are less destructive than those acquired in early gestation, but the lesions acquired at any gestational age can be disabling when they include cerebral periaqueductal and periventricular vasculitis and necrosis.

The first signs of the congenital infection can first appear at any time between the neonatal period and adult life. Most infected infants do not have obvious signs of their infection at birth. From follow-up studies it is known that most children with these latent infections subsequently develop clinical manifestations of their infection. In one study 11 of 13 children who had no signs of infection at birth had clinical manifestations of the disease at 8 years of age, even though some had received specific chemotherapy soon after birth.[179] Their first manifestation of the infection was usually chorioretinitis, which appeared at 3 to 4 years of age. Common late clinical manifestations of the disease include blindness, strabismus, encephalitis, hydrocephalus, intracranial calcifications, microcephaly, a nonfebrile seizure disorder, psychomotor impairments, jaundice, anemia, and thrombocytopenia (Figs. 22-27 and 22-28).[73]

There is a high correlation between *T. gondii* infection in the placenta and transmission of the parasite to the fetus, so the usual route of transmission to the fetus is presumably through the placenta. An occasional infection may be acquired during labor and delivery because a few of the infected infants have not had an elevated serum level of IgM at birth. The avidity-ELISA test can identify infections of recent origin.[75] Infected placentas are often markedly enlarged and show lesions that resemble the characteristic findings of erythroblastosis fetalis. The villi are markedly enlarged and edem-

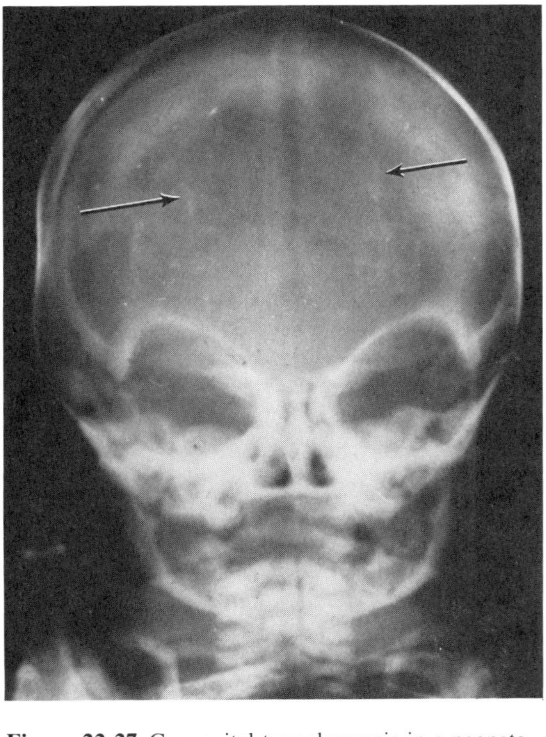

Figure 22-27 Congenital toxoplasmosis in a neonate with calcifications in the walls of the ventricles (arrows). (From Naeye and Tafari, 1983.[114])

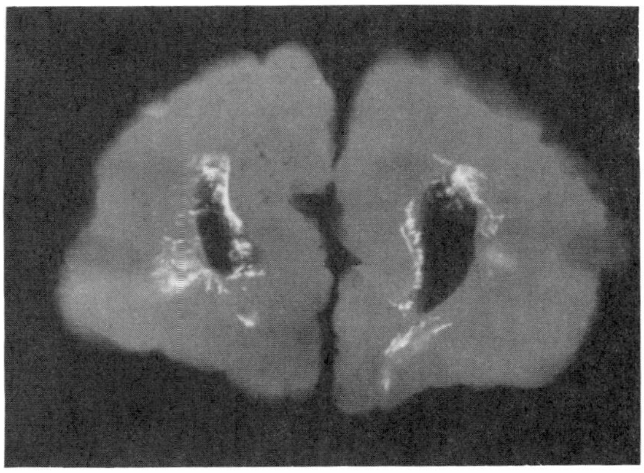

Figure 22-28 Postmortem x-ray through the frontal lobes of the brain of the same neonate shown in Figure 22-27. Arrows indicate heavy deposits of calcium in the walls of the ventricles. (From Naeye and Tafari, 1983.[114])

atous and often appear immature for their gestational age. They also usually have normoblasts in their blood vessels.[13] Foci of proliferative and necrotizing villitis have been observed in some cases. Sometimes the villitis is evidenced by the presence of lymphocytes, plasma cells, and fibrosis. The diagnosis is made by identifying the characteristic intracellular organisms. The organisms are difficult to find in the placenta, but when they are present they are usually found in typical cysts in the chorion or in the subchorionic tissue. Identification is sometimes difficult because degenerated syncytium can mimic the cysts.[14] It is often necessary to inject tissue homogenate into the abdominal cavity of mice and then identify the infection in their organs to be certain of the diagnosis.

References

1. Altshuler G. Pathogenesis of congenital herpesvirus infection: case report including a description of the placenta. Am J Dis Child 1974; 127:427–429.
2. Altshuler G. Placental infection and inflammation. In: Perrin EVDK, ed. Pathology of the placenta. New York: Churchill Livingstone, 1984:150–152.
3. Amirhessami-Aghili N, Manalo P, Hall MR, et al. Human cytomegalovirus infection of human placental explants in culture: histologic and immunohistochemical studies. Am J Obstet Gynecol 1987; 156:1365–1374.
4. Anand A, Gray ES, Brown T, et al. Human parovirus infection in pregnancy and hydrops fetalis. N Engl J Med 1987; 316:183–186.
5. Appelbaum PC, Holloway Y, Ross SM, Dhupelia I. The effect of amniotic fluid on bacterial growth in three population groups. Am J Obstet Gynecol 1977; 128:868–871.
6. Azogue E, LaFuente C, Darros C. Congenital Chagas disease in Bolivia, epidemiologic aspects and pathologic findings. Trans R Soc Trop Med Hyg 1985; 79:176–180.
7. Azzarelli B, Lafuze J. Amniotic basement membrane: a barrier to neutrophil invasion. Am J Obstet Gynecol 1987; 156:1130–1136.
8. Azziz R, Cumming J, Naeye R. Acute myometritis and chorioamnionitis during cesarean section of asymptomatic women. Am J Obstet Gynecol 1988; 159:1137–1139.
9. Baker CJ. Early onset group B streptococcal disease. J Pediatr 1978; 93:124–125.
10. Baker CJ, Edwards MS. Group B streptococcal infections. In Remington JS, Klein JO, eds. Infectious diseases of the fetus and newborn infant. Philadelphia: WB Saunders, 1983:820–881.
11. Bejar R, Curbelo V, Davis C, Gluck L. Premature labor: II. bacterial sources of phospholipase. Obstet Gynecol 1981; 57:479–782.
12. Benirschke K, Altschuler G. The future of perinatal physiopathology. In: Abramson H, ed. Symposium on the functional physiopathology of the fetus and neonate. St Louis: CV Mosby, 1971:158–168.
13. Benirschke K, Driscoll SG. The pathology of the human placenta. New York: Springer-Verlag, 1967.
14. Benirschke K, Kaufmann P. Pathology of the human placenta. New York: Springer-Verlag, 1990.
15. Berche P, Reich KA, Bonnichon M, et al. Detection of anti-listeriolysin O for serodiagnosis of human listeriosis. Lancet 1990; 335:624–627.
16. Blanc W. Pathology of the placenta, membranes, and umbilical cord in bacterial, fungal and viral infection in man. In: Naeye RL, Kissane JM, Kaufman N, eds. Perinatal diseases. Baltimore: Williams & Wilkins, 1981:67–132.
17. Boucher M, Yonekura ML. Perinatal listeriosis (early onset): correlation of antenatal manifestations and neonatal outcome. Obstet Gynecol 1986; 68:593–597.
18. Boyd PA. Placenta and umbilical cord. In Keeling JW, ed. Fetal and neonatal pathology. London: Springer-Verlag, 1987:45–76.
19. Boyer KM. Perinatal group B streptococcal infections: clinical significance and preventive strategies. In: Bellisario R, Mizejewski GJ, eds. Transplacental disorders: perinatal detection, treatment and management. New York: Alan Liss, 1990:141–167.
20. Brown ZA, Vontver LA, Benedetti J, et al. Effects on infants of a first episode of genital herpes during pregnancy. N Engl J Med 1987; 317:1246–1251.
21. Buchdahl R, Hird M, Gamsu H, et al. Listeriosis revisited: the role of the obstetrician. Br J Obstet Gynaecol 1990; 97:186–189.
22. Centers for Disease Control: Genital herpes infection, United States, 1966-1984. MMWR 1986; 35:402–404.
23. Coid DR, Fox H. Short review: campylobacters as placental pathogens. Placenta 1983; 4:295–306.
24. Confino E, Friberg J, Silverman S, et al. Penetration of bacteria and spermatozoa into bovine cervical mucus. Obstet Gynecol 1987; 70:134–136.
25. Cooperman NR, Kasim M, Rajashekaraiah KR. Clinical significance of amniotic fluid, amniotic membranes, and endometrial biopsy cultures at the time of cesarean section. Am J Obstet Gynecol 1980; 137:536–541.
26. Cooperstock M, England JE, Wolfe RA. Circadian incidence of premature rupture of the membranes in term and preterm births. Obstet Gynecol 1987; 69:936–941.
27. Cooperstock M, England JE, Wolfe RA. Circadian incidence of labor onset hour in preterm birth and chorioamnionitis. Obstet Gynecol 1987; 70:852–855.
28. Cox SM, McDonald PC, Casey ML. Cytokines and prostaglandins in amniotic fluid of preterm labor pregnancies: decidual origin in response to bacterial toxins. Paper presented at the thirty-sixth annual meeting of the Society of Gynecologic Investigation, San Diego, March 1989 (abstract).
29. Cox SM, Williams ML, Leveno KJ. The natural

history of preterm ruptured membranes: what to expect of expectant management. Obstet Gynecol 1988; 71:558–562.
30. Cruikshank DP, Warenski JC. First-trimester maternal *Listeria monocytogenes* sepsis and chorioamnionitis with normal neonatal outcome. Obstet Gynecol 1989; 73:469–471.
31. Dehner LP, Askin FB. Cytomegalovirus endometritis: report of a case associated with spontaneous abortion. Obstet Gynecol 1975; 45:211–214.
32. Desmonts G, Couvreur J. Toxoplasmosis, epidemiologic and serologic aspects of perinatal infection. In: Krugman S, Gershon AA, eds. Infections of the fetus and newborn: progress in clinical and biologic research. New York: Alan Liss, 1975:115.
33. Desmonts G, Couvreur J. Congenital toxoplasmosis: a prospective study of the outcome of pregnancy in 542 women with toxoplasmosis acquired during pregnancy. Ann Pediatr (Paris) 1984; 31:805–809.
34. Dong Y, St Clair PJ, Ramzy I, et al: A microbiologic and clinical study of placental inflammation at term. Obstet Gynecol 1987; 70:175–182.
35. Duncan ME, Fox H, Harkness RA, Rees RJW. The placenta in leprosy. Placenta 1984; 5:189–198.
36. Edwards LE, Barrada MI, Hamann AA, Hakanson EY. Gonorrhea in pregnancy. Am J Obstet Gynecol 1978; 132:637–641.
37. Ernest JM, Meis PJ, Moore ML, Swain M. Vaginal pH: a marker of premature rupture of the membranes. Obstet Gynecol 1989; 74:734–738.
38. Evans JR, Allen AL, Bortolussi R, et al. Follow-up study of survivors of fetal and early onset neonatal listeriosis. Clin Invest Med 1984; 7:329–334.
39. Ferrieri P. GBS infections in the newborn infant: diagnosis and treatment. In: Christensen KK, Christensen P, Ferrieri P, eds. Neonatal group B streptococcal infections. Basel: Karger, 1985:211–224.
40. FitzSimmons J, Callahan C, Shanahan B, Jungkind D. Chlamydial infections in pregnancy. J Reprod Med 1986; 31:19–22.
41. Flood B, Naeye RL. Factors that predispose to premature rupture of the fetal membranes. Journal of Obstetric and Gynecological Nursing 1984; 13:119–122.
42. Fojaco RM, Hensley GT, Moskowitz L. Congenital syphilis and necrotizing funisitis. JAMA 1989; 261: 1788–1790.
43. Fox CA, Meldrum SJ, Watson BW. Continuous measurement by radio-telemetry of vaginal pH during human coitus. J Reprod Fertil 1973; 33:69–75.
44. Frenkel JK. Toxoplasmosis: mechanisms of infection, laboratory diagnosis and managment. Current Topics of Pathology 1971; 54:28–75.
45. Friedman EA: Obstetric infections in labor. In Charles D, Finland M, eds. Obstetric and perinatal infections. Philadelphia: Lea & Febiger, 1973:501–516.
46. Fujimura M, Takeuchi T, Kitajima H, Nakayama M. Chorioamnionitis and serum IgM in Wilson-Mikity syndrome. Arch Dis Child 1989; 64:1379–1383.
47. Garcia AGP. Fetal infection in chickenpox and alastrim, with histopathologic study of the placenta. Pediatrics 1963; 32:895–901.
48. Garcia AGP, Fonseca EF, Marques RLS, Lobato YY. Placental morphology in cytomegalovirus infection. Placenta 1989; 10:1–18.
49. Garcia AGP, Marques RLS, Lobato YY, et al. Placental pathology in congenital rubella. Placenta 1985; 6:281–295.
50. Garcia AGP, Pereira JMS, Vidigal N, et al. Intrauterine infection with mumps virus. Obstet Gynecol 1980; 56:756–759.
51. Gibbs RS, Gassell GH, Davis JK, St Clair PJ. Further studies on genital mycoplasmas in intra-amniotic infection: blood cultures and serologic response. Am J Obstet Gynecol 1986; 154:717–726.
52. Gibbs RS, Disnmoor MJ, Newton ER, Ramamurthy RS. A randomized trial of intrapartum versus immediate postpartum treatment of women with intra-amniotic infection. Obstet Gynecol 1988; 72:823–828.
53. Gilstrap LC, Leveno KJ, Cox SM, et al: Intrapartum treatment of acute chorioamnionitis: impact on neonatal sepsis. Am J Obstet Gynecol 1988; 159:579–583.
54. Gilstrap LC. Leveno KJ, Cunningham FG, et al. Renal infection and pregnancy outcome. Am J Obstet Gynecol 1981; 141:709–716.
55. Goedert JJ, Mendez H, Drummond JE, et al. Mother-to-infant transmission of human immunodeficiency virus type 1: association with prematurity or low Anti-gp120. Lancet 1989; 2:1351–1354.
56. Goff E, Griffith BP, Booss J. Delayed amplification of cytomegalovirus infection in the placenta and maternal tissues during late gestation. Am J Obstet Gynecol 1987; 156:1265–1270.
57. Goodlin RC, Schmidt W, Creevy DC. Uterine tension and fetal heart rate during maternal orgasm. Obstet Gynecol 1972; 39:125–127.
58. Gravett MG, Nelson HP, DeRouen T, et al. Independent associations of bacterial vaginosis and *Chlamydia trachomatis* infection with adverse pregnancy outcome. JAMA 1986; 256:1899–1903.
59. Grose C, Weiner CP. Prenatal diagnosis of congenital cytomegalovirus infection: two decades later. Am J Obstet Gynecol 1990; 163:447–450.
60. Grundy HO, Dannar C. *Listeria monocytogenes*, a cause of unexplained death in low-risk patients? Mo Med 1988; 85:149–150.
61. Hager WD, Pauly TH. Fetal tachycardia as an indicator of maternal and neonatal morbidity. Obstet Gynecol 1985; 66:191–194.
62. Hain J, Doshi N, Harger JH. Ascending transcervical herpes simplex infection with intact fetal membranes. Obstet Gynecol 1980; 56:106–109.
63. Hanna NF, Taylor-Robinson D, Kalodiki-Karamanoli M, et al. The relation between vaginal pH and the microbiological status in vaginitis. Br J Obstet Gynaecol 1985; 92:1267–1271.
64. Harter CA, Benirschke K. Fetal syphilis in the

first trimester. Am J Obstet Gynecol 1976; 124:705–711.
65. Hiller SL, Martius J, Kronn M, et al. A case-controlled study of chorioamnionitis infection and histologic chorioamnionitis in prematurity. N Engl J Med 1988; 319:972–978.
66. Hutto C, Arvin A, Jacobs R, et al. Intrauterine herpes simplex virus infections. J Pediatr 1987; 110:97–101.
67. Ismail MA, Yang SL, Abusharif AN, Moawad AH. Immunoglobulins in prolonged ruptured membranes. Am J Obstet Gynecol 1985; 153:390–393.
68. Jauniaux E, Nessmann C, Imbert MC, et al. Morphological aspects of the placenta in HIV pregnancies. Placenta 1988; 9:633–642.
69. Katz SL, Wilfert GM. Human immunodeficiency virus infection of newborns. N Engl J Med 1989; 320:1687–1689.
70. Kelly CS, Gibson JL. Listeriosis as a cause of fetal wastage. Obstet Gynecol 1972; 40:91–97.
71. Kessel SS, Villar J, Berendes HW, Nugent RP. The changing pattern of low birth weight in the United States, 1970-1980. JAMA 1984; 251:1978–1982.
72. Khong TY, Frappell JM, Steel HM, et al. Perinatal listeriosis: a report of six cases. Br J Obstet Gynaecol 1986; 93:1083–1087.
73. Koppe JG, Loewer-Sieger DH, de Roever-Bonnet H. Results of 20-year follow-up of congenital toxoplasmosis. Lancet 1986; 1:254–256.
74. Koskiniemi M, Happonen JM, Jarvenpaa AL, et al. Neonatal herpes simplex virus infection: a report of 43 patients. Pediatr Infect Dis J 1989; 8:30–35.
75. Koskiniemi M, Lappalainen M, Hedman K. Toxoplasmosis needs evaluation. Am J Dis Chlid 1989; 143:724–728.
76. Lauweryns J, Bernat R, Lerut A, Detournay G. Intrauterine pneumonia, an experimental study. Biol Neonate 1973; 22:301–318.
77. Lewis SH, Reynolds-Kohler C, Fox HE, Nelson JA. HIV-1 in trophoblastic and villous Hofbauer cells and haematological precursors in eight-week fetuses. Lancet 1990; 335:565–568.
78. Lindner JGEM, Plantema FHF, Hoogkamp-Korstanje JAA. Quantitative studies of the vaginal flora of healthy women and of obstetric and gynaecological patients. J Med Microbiol 1978; 11:233–241.
79. Liner RI. Intrauterine *Listeria* infection: prenatal diagnosis by biophysical assessment and amniocentesis. Am J Obstet Gynecol 1990; 163:1596–1597.
80. Lisboa AC. On congenital Chagas' disease, anatomic-pathological study of six cases. Rev Inst Med Trop Sao Paulo 1960; 2:319–334.
81. Lou HC, Lassen NA, Friis-Hansen B. Impaired autoregulation of cerebral blood flow in the distressed newborn infant. J Pediatr 1979; 94:118–121.
82. MacDonald AB. Gestational Lyme borreliosis, implications for the fetus. Rheum Dis Clin North Am 1989; 15:657–677.
83. Madan E, Meyer MP, Amortegui AJ. Isolation of genital mycoplasmas and *Chlamydia trachomatis* in stillborn and neonatal autopsy material. Arch Pathol Lab Med 1988; 112:749–751.
84. Maeda H, Shimokawa H, Satoh S, et al. Nonimmunologic hydrops fetalis resulting from intrauterine human parovirus B-19 infection: report of two cases. Obstet Gynecol 1988; 72:482–485.
85. Malan AF. Special infections in the newborn (syphilis, tetanus, tuberculosis). In: Stern L, Vert P, eds. Neonatal medicine. New York: Masson, 1987:622–636.
86. Malan AF, Woods DL, Van Der Elst CW, Meyer MP. Relative placental weight in congenital syphilis. Placenta 1990; 11:3–6.
87. Marshall WC. Rubella: current problems and recent developments. Br J Clin Pract 1976; 30:56–59.
88. Martius J, Krohn MA, Hillier SL, et al. Relationships of vaginal *Lactobacillus* species, cervical *Chlamydia trachomatis,* and bacterial vaginosis to preterm birth. Obstet Gynecol 1988; 71:89–95.
89. Maury W, Potts BJ, Rabson AB. HIV-1 infection of first-trimester and term human placental tissue: a possible mode of maternal-fetal transmission. J Infect Dis 1989; 160:583–588.
90. McGregor IA. Epidemiology, malaria and pregnancy. Am J Trop Med Hyg 1984; 33:517–525.
91. McGregor JA, French JI, Richter R, et al. Antenatal microbiologic and maternal risk factors associated with prematurity. Am J Obstet Gynecol 1990; 163:1465–1473.
92. McShane PM, Heyl PS, Epstein MF. Maternal and perinatal morbidity resulting from placenta previa. Obstet Gynecol 1985; 65:176–182.
93. Menon R. Pregnancy and malaria. Med J Malaysia 1972; 27:115–119.
94. Minkoff HL, Henderson C, Mendez H, et al. Pregnancy outcomes among mothers infected with immunodeficiency virus and uninfected control subjects. Am J Obstet Gynecol 1990; 163:598–604.
95. Minkoff HL, Willoughby A, Mendez H, et al. Serious infections during pregnancy among women with advanced human immunodeficiency virus infection. Am J Obstet Gynecol 1990; 162:30–34.
96. Mitchell M. Causes of preterm labour. Paper presented at the symposium in honor of Professor Sir Alexander Turnbull, CBE, Oxford 30 June 1990.
97. Monif GRG, Egan EA, Held B, Eitzman DV. The correlation of maternal cytomegalovirus infection during varying stages in gestation with neonatal involvement. J Pediatr 1972; 80:17–20.
98. Monif GFG, Sever JL, Schiff GM, Traub RG. Isolation of rubella virus from products of conception. Am J Obstet Gynecol 1965; 91:1143–1146.
99. Montgomery JR, Flanders RW, Yow MD. Congenital anomalies and herpesvirus infection. Am J Dis Child 1973; 126:364–366.
100. Morales WJ. The effect of chorioamnionitis on the developmental outcome of preterm infants at one year. Obstet Gynecol 1987; 70:183–186.

101. Morales WJ, Angel JL, O'Brien WF, et al. A randomized study of antibiotic therapy in idiopathic preterm labor. Obstet Gynecol 1988; 72:829–833.
102. Moretti M, Sibai BM. Maternal and perinatal outcome of expectant management of premature rupture of membranes in the midtrimester. Am J Obstet Gynecol 1988; 159:390–396.
103. Mostoufi-Zadeh M, Driscoll SG, Biano SA, Kundsin RB. Placental evidence of cytomegalovirus infection of the fetus and neonate. Arch Pathol Lab Med 1984; 108:403–406.
104. Naeye RL. Cytomegalic inclusion disease, the fetal disorder. Am J Clin Pathol 1967; 47:738-744.
105. Naeye RL. Coitus and antepartum haemorrhage. Br J Obstet Gynaecol 1981; 88:765–770.
106. Naeye RL. Antenatal malarial infections. In: Scarpelli DG, Migaki G, eds. Transplacental effects on fetal health. New York: Alan R Liss, 1988:165–173.
107. Naeye RL. Pregnancy hypertension, placental evidences of low uteroplacental blood flow and spontaneous preterm delivery. Hum Pathol 1989; 20:441–444.
108. Naeye RL. Disorders of the placenta, fetus and neonate, their diagnosis and clinical significance. St Louis, Mosby-Year Book, 1991.
109. Naeye RL, Blanc WA. Pathogenesis of congenital rubella. JAMA 1965; 194:1277–1283.
110. Naeye RL, Maisels MJ, Lorenz RP, Botti JJ. The clinical significance of placental villous edema. Pediatrics 1983; 71:588–594.
111. Naeye RL, Peters EC. Causes and consequences of premature rupture of fetal membranes. Lancet 1980; 1:192–194.
112. Naeye RL, Ross SM. Amniotic fluid infection syndrome. Clin Obstet Gynecol 1982; 9:593–607.
113. Naeye RL, Ross SM. Coitus and chorioamnionitis: a prospective study. Early Hum Dev 1982; 6:91–97.
114. Naeye RL, Tafari N. Risk factors in pregnancy and diseases of the fetus and newborn. Baltimore: Williams & Wilkins, 1983.
115. Naeye RL, Tafari N, Judge D, Maraboe CC. Twins: causes of perinatal death in 12 United States cities and one African city. Am J Obstet Gynecol 1978; 131:267–272.
116. Naib ZM, Nahmias AJ, Josey WE, Wheeler JH. Association of maternal genital herpetic infection with spontaneous abortion. Obstet Gynecol 1970; 35:260–263.
117. Nazir MA, Pankuch GA, Botti JJ, Appelbaum PC. Antibacterial activity of amniotic fluid in the early third trimester. Am J Perinatol 1987; 4:59–62.
118. Nelson AM, Anderson V, Ryder R. Placental pathology as a predictor of perinatal HIV infection in infants born to HIV positive women in Kinshasa, Zaire. Paper presented at the fourth international conference on AIDS, Stockholm, 6 June, 1988 (abstract 6585).
119. Newton ER, Clark M. Group B streptococcus and preterm rupture of membranes. Obstet Gynecol 1988; 71:198–202.
120. Newton ER, Prihoda TJ, Gibbs RS. Logistic regression analysis of risk factors for intra-amniotic infection. Obstet Gynecol 1989; 73:571–575.
121. Novak RW, Platt MS. Significance of placental findings in early-onset group B streptococcal neonatal sepsis. Clin Pediatr (Phila) 1985; 24:256–258.
122. Pankuch GA, Cherouny PH, Botti JJ, Appelbaum PC. Amniotic fluid leukotaxis assay as an early indicator of chorioamnionitis. Am J Obstet Gynecol 1989; 161:802–807.
123. Pass MA, Gray BM, Khare S, Dillon HC Jr. Prospective studies of group B streptococcal infections in infants. J Pediatr 1979; 95:437–443.
124. Pass RF, Little EA, Stagno S, et al. Young children as a probable source of maternal and congenital cytomegalovirus infection. N Engl J Med 1987; 316:1366–1370.
125. Peckham CS, Logan S. Cytomegalovirus infection in pregnancy. In: Cosmi EV, DiRenzo GC, eds. Proceedings of the 11th European congress of perinatal medicine. Chur, Switzerland: Harwood, 1988 255–260.
126. Plotkin SA, Vaheri A. Human fibroblasts infected with rubella virus produce a growth inhibitor. Science 1967; 156:659–661.
127. Preece PM, Ades A, Thompson RG, Brooks JH. *Chlamydia trachomatis* infection in late pregnancy: a prospective study. Paediatr Perinat Epidemiol 1989; 3:268–277.
128. Preece PM, Blount JM, Glover J, et al. The consequences of primary cytomegalovirus infection in pregnancy. Arch Dis Child 1983; 58:970–975.
129. Preece PM, Pearl KN, Peckham CS. Congenital cytomegalovirus infection. Arch Dis Child 1984; 59:1120–1126.
130. Quinn PA, Butany J, Chipman M, et al. A prospective study of microbial infection in stillbirths and early neonatal death. Am J Obstet Gynecol 1985; 151:238–249.
131. Rappaport F, Rabinovitz M, Toaff R, Krochick N. Genital listeriosis as a cause of repeated abortion. Lancet 1960; 1:1273–1275.
132. Reinhardt MC. The African newborn in Abidjan, maternal and environmental factors influencing the outcome of pregnancy. In: Abei H, Whitehead R, eds. Maternal nutrition during pregnancy and lactation. Bern: Hans Huber, 1980:132.
133. Rhoads GG, Jackson LG, Schlesselman SE, et al. The safety and efficacy of chorionic villus sampling for early prenatal diagnosis of cytogenetic abnormalities. N Engl J Med 1989; 320:609–617.
134. Ricci JM, Fojaco RM, O'Sullivan MJ. Congenital syphilis: the University of Miami/Jackson Memorial Medical Center experience, 1986-1988. Obstet Gynecol 1989; 74:687–693.
135. Robb JA, Benirschke K, Barmeyer R. Intrauterine latent herpes simplex virus infection: I. spontaneous abortion. Hum Pathol 1986; 17:1196–1209.

136. Romero R, Oyarzun E, Mazor M, et al. Meta-analysis of the relationship between asymptomatic bacteriuria and preterm delivery/low birth weight. Obstet Gynecol 1989; 73:576–582.
137. Romero R, Scharf K, Mazor M, et al. The clinical value of gas-liquid chromatography in the detection of intra-amniotic microbial invasion. Obstet Gynecol 1988; 72:44–50.
138. Romero R, Sirtori M, Oyarzun E, et al. Prevalence, microbiology, and clinical significance of intraamniotic infection in women with preterm labor and intact membranes. Am J Obstet Gynecol 1989; 161:817–824.
139. Rooney JF, Felser JM, Ostrove JM, Straus SE. Acquisition of genital herpes from an asymptomatic sexual partner. N Engl J Med 1986; 314:1561–1564.
140. Rosenbert MJ, Schulz KF, Burton N. Sexually transmitted diseases in sub-saharan Africa. Lancet 1986; 2:152–153.
141. Rutter D, Griffiths P, Trompeter RS. Cytomegalic inclusion disease after recurrent maternal infection. Lancet 1985; 2:1182.
142. Ryan GM, Abdella TN, McNeeley SG, et al. *Chlamydia* trachomatic infection in pregnancy and effect of treatment on outcome. Am J Obstet Gynecol 1990; 162:34–39.
143. Ryder RW, Nsa W, Hassig SE, et al. Perinatal transmission of the human immunodeficiency virus type 1 to infants of seropositive women in Zaire. N Engl J Med 1989; 320:1637–1642.
144. Saigal S, Lynyk O, Bryce-Larke RP, Chernesky MA. The outcome in children with congenital cytgomegalovirus infection: a longitudinal follow-up study. Am J Dis Child 1982; 136:896–901.
145. Salafia CM, Mangam HE, Weigl CA, et al. Abnormal fetal heart rate patterns and placental inflammation. Am J Obstet Gynecol 1989; 160:140–147.
146. Samra JS, Obhrai MS, Constantine G. Parvovirus infection in pregnancy. Obstet Gynecol 1989; 73:832–834.
147. Schoonmaker JN, Lawellin DW, Lunt B, McGregor JA. Bacteria and inflammatory cells reduce chorioamniotic membrane integrity and tensile strength. Obstet Gynecol 1989; 74:590–596.
148. Scott GB, Hutto C, Makuch RW, et al. Survival in children with perinatally acquired human immunodeficiency virus type 1 infection. N Engl J Med 1989; 321:1791–1796.
149. Sibille Y, Lwebuga-Mukasa JS, Polomski L, et al. An in vitro model for polymorphonuclear-leukocyte-induced injury to an extracellular matrix. Am Rev Respir Dis 1986; 134:134–140.
150. Silver HM, Sperling RS, St Clair PJ, Gibbs RS. Evidence relating bacterial vaginosis to intraamniotic infection. Am J Obstet Gynecol 1989; 161:808–812.
151. Silver RK, Gibbs RS, Castillo M. Effect of amniotic fluid bacteria on the course of labor in nulliparous women at term. Obstet Gynecol 1986; 68:587–592.
152. Smith LG, Summers PR, Miles RW, et al. Gonococcal chorioamnionitis associated with sepsis: a case report. Am J Obstet Gynecol 1989; 160:573–574.
153. South M, Sever JL. Teratogen update: the congenital rubella syndrome. Teratology 1985; 31:297–307.
154. South MA, Tompkins WAF, Morris CR, Rawls WE. Congenital malformation of the central nervous system associated with genital type (type 2) herpesvirus. J Pediatr 1969; 75:13–18.
155. Spark RP. Does transplacental spread of coccidioidomycosis occur? Report of a neonatal fatality and review of the literature. Arch Pathol Lab Med 1981; 105:347–350.
156. Spaun E, Klunder K. *Candida* chorioamnionitis and intrauterine contraceptive device. Acta Obstet Gynecol Scand 1986 65:183–184.
157. Spencer JAD. Perinatal listeriosis. Br Med J 1987; 295:349.
158. Spiegel CA, Amsel R, Eschenbach D, et al. Anaerobic bacteria in nonspecific vaginitis. N Engl J Med 1980; 303:601–607.
159. Stagno S, Pass RF, Cloud G, et al. Primary cytomegalovirus infection in pregnancy. JAMA 1986; 256:1904–1908.
160. Stevens CE Toy PT, Tong MJ, et al. Perinatal hepatitis B virus transmission in the United States: prevention by passive-active immunization. JAMA 1985; 253:1740–1745.
161. Swartzberg JE, Remington JS. Transmission of *Toxoplasma*. Am J Dis Child 1975; 129:777–779.
162. Sweet RL, Landers DV, Walker C, Schachter J. *Chlamydia trachomatis* infection and pregnancy outcome. Am J Obstet Gynecol 1987; 156:824–833.
163. Tafari N, Ross SM, Naeye RL, et al. Failure of bacterial growth inhibition by amniotic fluid. Am J Obstet Gynecol 1977; 128:187–189.
164. Taylor J, Garite TJ. Premature rupture of membranes before fetal viability. Obstet Gynecol 1984; 64:615–620.
165. Thomas GB, Sbarra AJ, Feingold M, et al. Antimicrobial activity of amniotic fluid against *Chlamydia trachomatis, Mycoplasma hominis,* and *Ureaplasma urealyticum*. Am J Obstet Gynecol 1988; 158:16–22.
166. Townsend JJ, Baringer JR, Wolinsky JS, et al. Progressive rubella panencephalitis: late onset after congenital rubella. N Engl J Med 1975; 292:990–993.
167. Unsigned. Screening for congenital CMV. Lancet 1989; 2:599–600.
168. Vadillo-Ortega F, Gonzalez-Avila G, Karchmer S, et al. Collagen metabolism in premature rupture of amniotic membranes. Obstet Gynecol 1990; 75:84–88.
169. Vaes G. Cell-to-cell interactions in the secretion of enzymes of connective tissue breakdown, collagenase and proteoglycan-degrading neutral proteases: a review. Agents Actions 1980; 10:474–485.
170. VanBergen WS, Fleury FJ, Cheatle EL. Fatal maternal disseminated coccidioidomycosis in a nonendemic area. Am J Obstet Gynecol 1976; 124:661–664.

171. Vaughan JE, Ramirez H. Coccidioidomycosis as a complication of pregnancy. California Medicine 1975; 74:121–125.
172. Vintzileos AM, Campbell WA, Nochimson DJ, Weinbaum PJ. Preterm premature rupture of the membranes: a risk factor for the development of abruptio placentae. Am J Obstet Gynecol 1987; 156:1235–1238.
173. Wahl LM, Wahl SM, Mergenhagen SE, Martin GR. Collagenase production by endotoxin-activated macrophages. Proc Natl Acad Sci U S A, 1974; 71:3598–3601.
174. Walter PR, Garin Y, Blot P. Placental pathology changes in malaria, a histologic and ultrastructural study. Am J Path 1982; 109:330–342.
175. Wejstal R, Norkrans G. Chronic non-A, non-B hepatitis in pregnancy: outcome and possible transmission to the offspring. Scand J Infect Dis 1989; 21:485.
176. Wendel GD, Maberry MC, Christmas JT, et al. Examination of amniotic fluid in diagnosing congenital syphilis with fetal death. Obstet Gynecol 1989; 74:967–970.
177. Whitley R, Arvin A, Prober C, et al. Predictors of morbidity and mortality in neonates with herpes simplex virus infections. N Engl J Med 1991; 324:450–454.
178. Whyte RK, Hussain Z, deSa D. Antenatal infections with *Candida* species. Arch Dis Child 1982; 57:528–535.
179. Wilson CB, Remington JS, Stagno S, Reynolds DW. Development of adverse sequelae in children born with subclinical congenital *Toxoplasma* infection. Pediatrics 1980; 66:767–774.
180. Yoder PR, Gibbs RS, Blanco JD, et al. A prospective controlled study of maternal and perinatal outcome after intra-amniotic infection at term. Am J Obstet Gynecol 1983; 145:695–701.
181. Yow MD. Congenital cytomegalovirus disease: a NOW problem. J Infect Dis 1989; 159:163–167.

CHAPTER 23

Surgical Infections in Obstetric Practice

Hein Odendaal, M.D.
David Charles, M.D.

In pregnancy suppurative septic processes affecting organs outside the genital tract are almost exclusively limited to the gastrointestinal tract. The majority of acute abdominal conditions in the nongravid state can be readily appraised if the requisite history is acquired and clinical examination is repeated. Patients with an existing chronic condition such as Crohn's disease may become pregnant or need advice regarding the desirability of pregnancy. Difficult clinical problems can also evolve during or immediately after pregnancy. It is therefore essential for the physician to cover all contingencies and leave nothing to chance. It is mandatory that the obstetrician freely discuss such enigmas with surgical colleagues, but at the same time both should remember that the zeal for finite diagnosis must not supersede their responsibility for the patient's care and safety. In addition, we must realize that *tempus fugit,* and in many instances procrastination may seriously affect the prognosis. The obstetrician who does not deem it necessary to transfer the patient to the surgeon's care may eventually have to decide that with suitable precautions the best and safest method of obtaining the diagnosis may be by exploratory laparotomy.

Many patients seen by obstetricians for prenatal or postnatal care complain of one or more of the following: nausea, vomiting, constipation, abdominal distention, and, less frequently, pelvic pain. The majority of such symptoms can be readily explained on a physiologic basis. However, it cannot be emphasized too strongly that the diagnosis of a surgical complication in pregnancy may be fraught with needless and hazardous delay because the physician and frequently the patient misinterpret the presenting complaints. Certain symptoms of pregnancy may in fact be deterrents to the recognition of major disease entities.

For example, vomiting may be attributed to the pregnancy rather than to mechanical obstruction of the intestinal tract. Depending on the duration of pregnancy, lower abdominal pain may be considered to originate from either a threatened abortion or desultory labour, but one should always consider the possibility of an extragenital lesion. Again, it must be emphasized that accurate diagnosis depends on the appropriate assessment of subjective or objective findings, and no symptom or sign should be ignored or considered out of context. Similarly, one must be cognizant that pregnancy can modify the manifestations of surgical conditions, but all too frequently the obstetrician fails to accept the possibility of a dual diagnosis.

As previously stated, the obstetrician should always be willing to ask for consultative aid when it is required. To practice first-rate medicine, one must always be prepared to seek the opinion and judgment of those whose experience is greater. Even if the medical necessity does not exist, the obstetrician should be alert to anxiety and restiveness in the patient and family and respond by suggesting that the fresh viewpoint of a surgical consultant be obtained. To furnish maximum value, the obstetrician and surgical colleague should meet and discuss the problem. Consultations conducted through an exchange of notes are of very little value. Although a surgeon's advice and suggestions may be advantageous, the unfamiliarity of many general surgeons with the physiologic and physical changes that occur during pregnancy may preclude a proper interpretation of the clinical picture. Preferably the obstetrician must recognize the acute episode, utilize obstetric experience, and blend it with that of the surgeon. In the best interest of the patient, the obstetrician must think as a surgeon and the surgeon think as an obstetrician.

It is important to recognize that the physician in charge of a patient cannot abdicate responsibility for the care and management of the clinical problem. Management of a patient by a committee of consultants never ensures that the best opinion is brought to bear on the problem. A systematic physical examination must be performed, and it should include the routine evaluation of a pregnant patient as well as that of a patient who has a suspected acute abdominal lesion. The blood pressure should be recorded, and urine analysis is mandatory because it may help considerably in the differential diagnosis.

Temperature elevation induced in early pregnancy by progesterone is well recognized, but it may be overlooked in considering a diagnosis of acute appendicitis. The same applies to the slight leukocytosis normally associated with the gravid state. Unless the leukocytosis is marked, its value is not as significant in the pregnant patient in differentiating a possible inflammatory lesion and therefore can be relied upon only if it is markedly elevated or shows rises with successive counts.

Urinary tract infection, as exemplified by acute pyelonephritis, may be associated with marked abdominal pain, distention, and symptomatology that could easily simulate any acute abdominal catastrophe. Acute pyelonephritis may be associated with severe vomiting and dehydration. The pain may not be limited to the costovertebral angle but radiate along the course of the ureter. One must also consider the possibility of excessive abdominal distention from uterine, intestinal, or other causes because rigidity in a particular area may aid in the attainment of a correct diagnosis. In all pregnant women who present with acute abdominal symptoms, one must not neglect to examine the hernial orifices.

Abdominal auscultation is important in assessing the state of bowel and can aid in discriminating between obstruction and peritonitis. This part of the examination should be repeated at frequent intervals if any doubt exists. Accentuated bowel sounds simply denote excessive intestinal activity, which may be caused by any irritant or stimulant. After varying periods of time, increased peristalsis may be succeeded by atony, which is typical of peritonitis. Intermittent bowel sounds may be heard over distended and paralyzed gut; likewise, breath and cardiac sounds may be transmitted to the lower abdomen. If there is any suspicion that the pain could be of uterine origin as the result of premature labor or abortion, the pattern of uterine contractions can be discerned by palpation. Contraction is first felt by the hand placed on the uterine fundus, with pain noted a little later by the patient. Subsequently, cessation of subjective pain and relaxation of the uterus are noted. Deviation from this normal sequence, as when the patient complains more or less of constant pain, should lead one to entertain a diagnosis of abnormal uterine action. The close association between the visceral nerve supply to the lower colon and uterus may result in pain being felt mainly in the bowel.

Occasionally, within a few hours of parturition, a woman may complain of lower abdominal pain and pass into a state of shock not commensurate to any difficulty or bleeding encountered at the time of delivery. If pain is the main complaint, the diagnosis of acute appendicitis must be entertained. In contrast to uterine contractions associated with completion of the third state of labor, the pain will be continuous. If shock is present, it is essential to exclude internal hemorrhage from uterine rupture, and exploration of the uterus is necessary. A pelvic mass may be found, and the differential diagnosis again will include a possible inflammatory mass, volvulus, or a broad-ligament hematoma.

Later in the postpartum course, a lower abdominal mass associated with fever and signs of peritoneal irritation must be ascribed to acute appendicitis or postpartum infection. Because accurate diagnosis is the key to appropriate treatment, we shall confine ourselves more to the diagnostic problems than to surgical therapy, which usually becomes standard once an acute diagnosis is established, although therapy at times needs to be modified because of the presence of a gestation.

Appendicitis

Changes During Pregnancy

From about the sixteenth week of gestation, the uterus encroaches on the abdominal cavity and thereby displaces both the small and the large intestine. Radiologic studies have revealed that as pregnancy advances the appendix is gradually displaced from the right iliac fossa to the level of the iliac crest.[6] Such anatomic alterations modify the physical signs of acute appendicitis. Furthermore, because of the topographic changes, the omentum cannot be a successful guardian against peritoneal spread by an inflammatory process affecting the appendix. Likewise, the physiologic changes such as elevated cortisol levels may interfere with the peritoneal response to inflammation.

Prevalence

The prevalence of acute appendicitis during pregnancy is approximately 1 in 1,500 to 2,500.[5,27,58] Most of the patients present in the second trimester. Very few cases present in the first trimester.[46] Appendicitis may also occur in the newborn. Even in utero perforation of the appendix has been described.[45,52]

Maternal Mortality

Maternal mortality was 24 percent in 1908 but declined to 0.01 percent in 1976.[5] Mortality is rarely encountered today.[27,46]

Perinatal Mortality and Morbidity

Fetal loss in 1908 was 40 percent and, in the presence of peritonitis, rose to 79 percent. Since then it decreased to 8.7 percent in patients with simple appendicitis and 35.7 percent when peritonitis occurred.[5,27] Preterm labor occurs in 17 percent of the patients.[46] Perinatal mortality rises to 20 percent in perforated appendicitis, whereas it is only 3 percent when a laparotomy is performed for uncomplicated appendicitis.[48]

Clinical Features

Abdominal pain, particularly in the right lower quadrant, is considered as the most reliable symptom of appendicitis during pregnancy. However, this warning may be absent or minimal in 42 percent of patients at the initial examination.[46] Nausea and vomiting occur in 86 and 90 percent of patients, respectively.[46] Rebound tenderness is not present in a large number of patients and may not be elicited in patients with a retrocecal appendix. Other studies, however, report that 68 percent of patients have guarding and 77 percent rebound tenderness.[27] Diagnosis of acute appendicitis occurring during the first 6 months of pregnancy is usually not difficult. In the third trimester, however, diagnosis is more difficult. Diagnosis is also difficult postoperatively or in patients with abortion.[69] Although it is usually assumed that the diagnosis of acute appendicitis is more difficult during pregnancy, a recent case-control study shows that the diagnosis of acute appendicitis is not more difficult in the gravid state.[59]

Confirmation of Diagnosis

Pregnant patients with appendicitis demonstrate a wide range of white cell counts, with 23 to 70 percent having a white cell count of more than 15.0×10^9 per liter.[48] Ultrasound may also be helpful in the diagnosis. Schwerk and associates[60] found a positive predictive value of 95 percent of uncomplicated cases of acute appendicitis in the nonpregnant patient. They found that the ultrasound patterns consist of a hypoechoic fluid-distended lumen; a hyperechoic inner ring, representing the mucosa and submucosa; and an outer hypoechoic ring representing the muscularis extera. Ultrasound may also be helpful to diagnose a periappendicular abscess.[13,35] Laparoscopy can be used in early pregnancy if the disease cannot be established clinically.

Management

As an increase in mortality and morbidity is found in patients with a delay in diagnosis, immediate surgery is indicated when appendicitis is suspected in the pregnant woman.[19] It is important to keep rare causes of acute appendicitis, such as deciduosis or schistosomiasis, in mind.[50,65] Although prophylactic appendectomy does not seem to add to the risk of elective cesarean section, it is not recommended because of the increase in operating time and hospital stay.[55]

The type and location of the incision is determined by the gestational age and the certainty of the diagnosis. When the diagnosis is certain in early pregnancy, a muscle-splitting incision is acceptable. In the difficult case, a midline incision gives better exposure. It also gives sufficient exposure to evacuate a gravid uterus if necessary and for antepartum tubal ligation if indicated. A culture should be taken when pus is present. In these cases pelvic toilet using adequate amounts of lukewarm normal saline is essential. Postoperative antibiotics are necessary in cases of perforation, peritonitis, or abscess formation.

Ulcerative Colitis

Ulcerative colitis is an inflammatory disease of the colon and rectum. The etiology is unknown, but stress, infection, drugs, and psychological factors play a role in many cases.

Prevalence

Because the greatest incidence of the disease is between 30 and 40 years, it is not uncommon in pregnancy.

Maternal Morbidity and Mortality

Complications are numerous and diverse. The most common are perforation of the colon, acute colonic di-

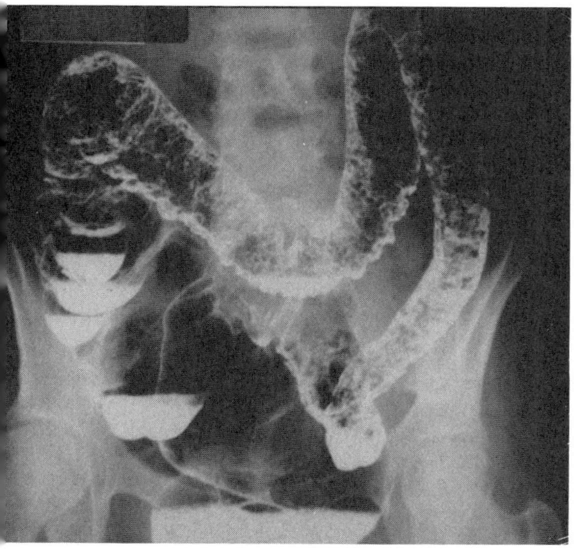

Figure 23-1 The features of note on this double-contrast barium enema are the severe continuous mucosal granularity and irregularity, the "thumbprinting" due to mucosal edema, and the mucosal ulcers. There is loss of haustration in the sigmoid and transverse colon. The rectosigmoid region appears relatively spared, which might be as a result of steroid enemas.

lation, hemorrhage, and carcinoma. Other complications are conjunctivitis, uveitis, ulceration of the mouth, erythema nodosum, arthritis, and hepatic dysfunction. Mortality is influenced by the severity of the first attack. The majority of attacks are mild and carry a low mortality. Patients with severe attacks have a mortality of 26 percent.[11] Excess mortality, when compared to the expected, is 9 percent at 5 years and increases to 23 percent at 25 years' duration of the disease. A case-control study found no significant influence of ulcerative colitis on the outcome of pregnancy.[56]

Perinatal Mortality

In an overview of 10 studies, reporting on 1,308 pregnancies, Miller[49] found that 85 percent of babies were normal. Only 1 percent had congenital abnormalities and 1 percent stillbirths. Spontaneous abortions occurred in 7 percent of cases.

Clinical Features

Diarrhea is the most common symptom and is usually of sudden onset. Stools contain blood and mucopus. Abdominal pain and tenderness are also present. Diarrhea causes dehydration, malnutrition, hypoproteinemia, anemia, and weight loss. There are many remissions, which may last for weeks, months, or years.

Confirmation of Diagnosis

The diagnosis is made on sigmoidoscopy and rectal biopsy. X-ray examination should be avoided during pregnancy, but certain complications may require three-way films of the abdomen or even contrast studies (Fig. 23-1).[20]

Effect of Pregnancy on Ulcerative Colitis

Patients who wish to start a family should preferably do so during a remission. However, the effects of the pregnancy are probably minimal as changes in the course of the disease would likely have occurred in the absence of pregnancy.[11,20,30] Exacerbations of ulcerative colitis are most likely to occur during the first trimester.[39,40] It seems that in patients with active disease roughly 45 percent get worse, about a quarter improve, and a quarter remain unchanged.[49]

Treatment

Management of pregnant patients is exactly the same as that of nonpregnant patients. Anemia should be prevented, and a high-protein, low-residue diet prescribed. There are no contraindications to the use of prednisolone or sulfasalazine.[11,20,40,49] Complications should be treated specifically. Colectomy has been performed for the fulminant case in late pregnancy and the puerperium. In these cases three of the five fetuses survived.[3,67]

Acute Cholecystitis and Cholelithiasis

Physiologic Changes

As a consequence of progesterone-mediated resistance to cholecystokinin activity, gallbladder activity appears to decrease in pregnancy. Calculi are subsequently allowed to grow. Gallbladder size in pregnancy is increased, and emptying is incomplete.[63]

Prevalence

The prevalence of gallstones is higher among women than men, and it increases with the number of pregnancies.[8] The rate in pregnancy is 0.6 to 8 cases in 10,000 births.[25,41,62] Asymptomatic cholelithiasis in pregnancy has a prevalence of 2.5 to 3.5 percent.[12,63] Although very rare, cholelithiasis can also occur in fetuses, children, and adolescents.[1,33]

Maternal Mortality

Operative mortality of cholecystectomy is 0.7 percent.[61]

Perinatal Mortality

Dixon and colleagues[18] found a 23 percent incidence of spontaneous or induced abortions. The total perinatal mortality associated with cholecystectomy is approximately 5 percent.[57]

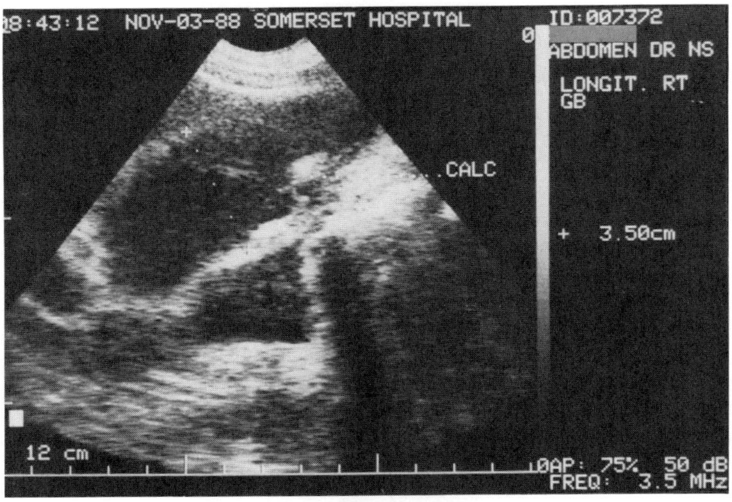

Figure 23-2 There is a hyperechoic gallstone present in the body of the gallbladder, which casts an acoustic shadow. The triangular hypoechoic region adjacent to the gallbladder represents postoperative intraperitoneal fluid.

Clinical Features

Symptoms are usually nausea and vomiting, right upper quadrant or epigastric pain, and abdominal tenderness.[32] The pain is of sudden onset and is frequently described as colicky or stabbing. Indigestion or intolerance of certain foods, especially fatty foods, may occur. The gallbladder is usually not palpable unless obstruction is present. Jaundice is an uncommon finding. Care should be taken not to confuse the clinical diagnosis of cholecystitis with other conditions such as the HELLP syndrome, which is characterized by hemolysis, elevated liver enzymes, and low platelet counts. It is one of the rare complications in patients with severe preeclampsia or eclampsia. Right upper quadrant pain in these patients should alert one to exclude the HELLP syndrome.[66]

Confirmation of Diagnosis

Labortaory results are usually nonspecific, reflected by mild elevations in the white cell count.[32] With the availability of sophisticated equipment such as ultrasound and experienced operators, the diagnostic accuracy of cholelithiasis is likely to approach 100 percent (Fig. 23-2).[24,25] During pregnancy, cholangiography is contraindicated, but operative cholecystography is fortunately effective in excluding gallstones in the common duct.[44]

Treatment

The correct method of treatment is still controversial as there are supporters of an immediate surgical approach on the one hand and those of a more conservative approach on the other hand by limiting surgery to the patients who truly failed medical management.[32,41] A conservative approach is usually effective in 80 percent of patients.[61] Total parenteral infusion has even been suggested to allow postponement of surgery until after pregnancy.[43] Dixon and coworkers,[18] to the contrary, found that surgery in the third trimester substantially reduced the duration of hospitalization. Gallstones causing pancreatitis is a different problem. It has been shown that delaying operative treatment is associated with recurrent gallstone pancreatitis with numerous admissions to hospital as well as increased fetal mortality and maternal morbidity.[10]

Regional Enteritis (Crohn's Disease)

The etiology of regional enteritis is unknown. Although it resembles ulcerative colitis in some respects, there are pathologic differences. Where ulcerative colitis is limited to the mucosa and submucosa, regional enteritis occurs throughout the bowel wall.

Prevalence

Fertility is reduced in patients with Crohn's disease, as demonstrated in a recent case-control study involving 200 patients.[47] It is therefore difficult to determine an accurate prevalence.

Maternal Mortality

Pregnancy is usually normal and without risks.[53] Modern technology enables one to attain a low maternal mortality. Perforation of the bowel, however, carries a risk, as demonstrated by a study of 33 cases of perforation in which two deaths occurred.[38]

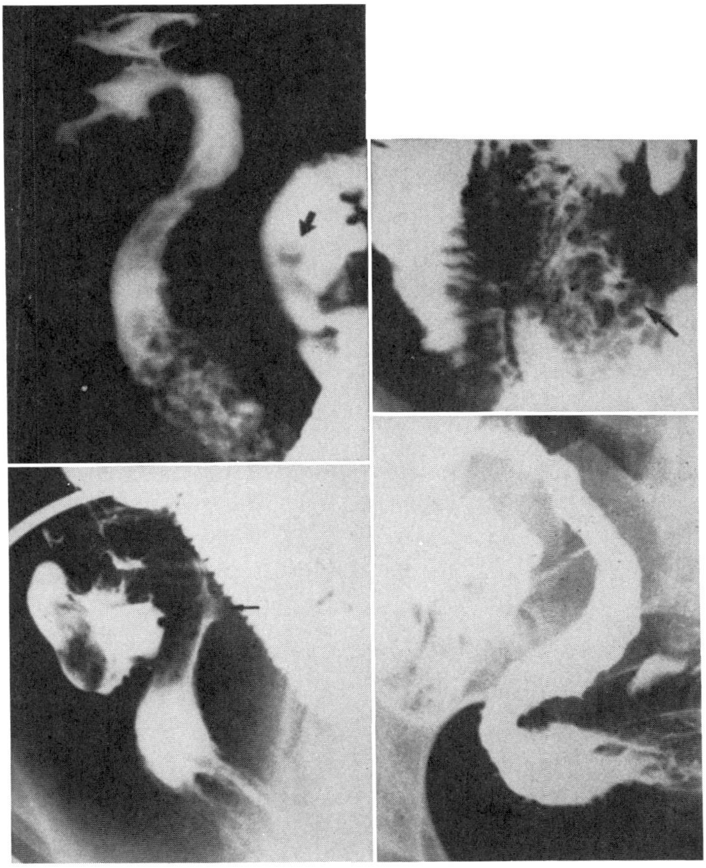

Figure 23-3 **A**, The classical appearance of an apthoid ulcer (arrow) in the distal small bowel. Apthoid ulcers are the earliest sign of Crohn's disease involving the terminal ileum and colon. **B**, Multiple apthoid ulcers (arrow) involving terminal ileum. **C**, The black arrow indicates an ulcer seen in profile. The four smaller arrows indicate a thickened swollen mucosal fold. Note the distorted cecum. **D**, The arrow indicates a collar button or collar stud ulcer, which is a submucosal ulceration.

Perinatal Mortality

Women with inflammatory bowel disease have about the same overall chance of giving birth to a normal living infant as do healthy women.[20,30] Increased risks of spontaneous abortion and preterm labor are reported by other workers, but this increased risk is associated with exacerbation of the enteritis and bowel resection during pregnancy.[53]

Clinical Features

Disease of the small bowel may present as a subacute inflammation of the terminal ileum and may imitate acute appendicitis. The terminal ileum becomes red and thickened with enlarged mesenteric lymph nodes. Chronic disease, however, is associated with recurrent abdominal pain, borborygmi, diarrhea, anemia, and weight loss. Colonic Crohn's disease is clinically similar to ulcerative colitis. The two conditions are distinguished only on histologic grounds.

Confirmation of Diagnosis

Pregnant patients should certainly undergo sigmoidoscopic examinations, rectal mucosal biopsies, and the necessary stool examinations. Unnecessary radiologic examinations should be avoided in pregnancy but they may be indicated when complications occur (Fig. 23-3).[21]

Effect of Pregnancy

When Crohn's disease is not active at the time of conception, it is likely to remain inactive during the pregnancy. If the disease is activated, it is more likely to do so during the third trimester.[39] Miller[49] reviewed five publications on Crohn's disease in pregnancy and found an overall recurrence rate of 27 percent. Other reviews found a lack of prospective studies, and consequently it was not feasible to predict the effect of pregnancy on the disease. Nielsen and associates[53] could not find any increased risk of exacerbation.

Treatment

Treatment usually consists of sulfasalazine and corticosteroids. These drugs do not influence the course of pregnancy or the frequency of neonatal jaundice or malformations. Pregnant women with Crohn's disease should therefore by given the same medical treatment as others. General therapy consists of a low-residue diet, antidiarrheal medication, the correction of anemia, a high-calorie, high-protein diet, and vitamin supplements. Extensive bowel resection is sometimes necessary in pregnancy. Maintenance of pregnancy in such cases necessitates parenteral nutrition.[26,54]

Acute Pancreatitis

Physiologic Changes

Possible mechanisms that predispose a pregnant patient to acute pancreatitis are the predilection to develop gallstones and atony of the biliary tract with subsequent stasis and reflux.[17] Underlying hypertriglyceridemia with a further rise in the triglycerides during pregnancy may also play a role.[15]

Prevalence

Acute pancreatitis develops once in 1,066 to 3,800 pregnancies.[17] Despite the low incidence of acute pancreatitis in pregnancy, there is indirect evidence that the gravid state predisposes patients to this entity.

Maternal Mortality

Maternal mortality is high. In the past it has been as high as 20 percent but declined with modern therapy.[22]

Perinatal Mortality

Fetal loss is about 10 percent.[17]

Clinical Features

Patients with milder forms may present with only pain and nausea. The pain begins in the epigastrium or in the right hypochondrium and radiates to the back and left flank. Nausea and vomiting commonly occur, and a low-grade fever is usually present.

Examination of the abdomen reveals tenderness, guarding, and abdominal distention. Occasionally the inflammatory reaction or abscess formation in the omentum may produce localized swellings.

Severe hemorrhagic pancreatitis is characterized by profound shock, hypotension, and marked hypovolaemia. Other features of severe pancreatitis are ecchymoses, pleural effusions, adult respiratory distress syndrome, ascites, and paralytic ileus.

Confirmation of Diagnosis

Specific tests employed to substantiate a diagnosis of acute pancreatitis rely on measurements of pancreatic enzymes, especially amylase. Although a rise in serum amylase is known to occur in most cases, false-negative results will be recorded if the blood is taken 24 to 72 hours after the acute episode or in cases with acute hemorrhagic pancreatitis and massive necrosis.

Strickland and associates have found that serum amylase levels may reach 150 IU per liter in normal gravid women, and such values are unrelated to duration of pregnancy and unaccompanied by a rise in serum amylase isoenzyme, as in normal women. They imply that the serum amylase activity remains the single most useful diagnostic test for pancreatitis in pregnant and nonpregnant women.[64]

Ultrasonographic demonstration of gallstones may point to underlying pancreatitis.

Management

The aims are to rest the pancreas and bowel and to prevent complications. Pain should be relieved, shock treated, and the electrolyte and fluid imbalance corrected. No specific therapy exists. Total parenteral nutrition may be necessary in the malnourished patient.

In a 22-year study, Block and Kelly[10] found 21 women with acute pancreatitis during or shortly after a pregnancy. Operation during the acute attack was required in only two cases. As gallstones were always the cause of pancreatitis, they recommended surgical treatment of gallstones in the second trimester and in the puerperium. Patients in whom the acute pancreatitis deteriorates should undergo surgery in whatever trimester they present.

Volvulus

Physiologic Changes

During pregnancy, the rapidly enlarging uterus displaces the abdominal viscera, thereby predisposing to the occurrence of volvulus.

Prevalence

The prevalence of intestinal obstruction in pregnancy is one in 2,500 to 3,500.[14] Volvulus accounts for 44 percent of cases of obstruction in pregnancy.[7] It is most frequently encountered during the later stages of pregnancy or in the puerperium following abdominal delivery.[23,28] In order of frequency, volvulus of the large bowel involves the sigmoid colon, the cecum, and the transverse colon.[39] It has even been discovered at fetal necropsies.[4] Fetal volvulus may present as fetal distress during labour.[68]

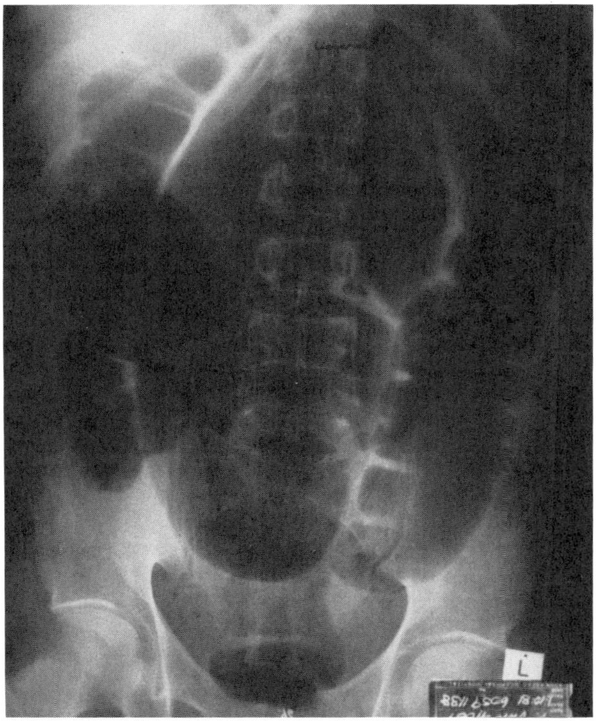

Figure 23-4 The features are those of a sigmoid volvulus, with a dilated loop of bowel arising out of the pelvis and extending up into the left hypochondrium above T10, overlapping the liver.

Maternal Mortality

Review of the world literature revealed 112 cases.[37] The maternal mortality rate is 21 percent but rises to 43 percent when it occurs postpartum.[31]

Perinatal Mortality

Very few studies mentioned their perinatal mortality rate. In a small study, Hamlin and Palermilno[29] reported two stillbirths in five cases.

Clinical Features

Patients with volvulus may present as an acute abdominal emergency. Diagnosis during pregnancy may be difficult because of the obscuring minor complaints in pregnancy such as constipation, abdominal distention, vomiting, or abdominal discomfort. The presence of cramps and vomiting should alert the physician to the possibility of bowel obstruction. A preoperative diagnosis is seldom made merely on the history.

Confirmation of Diagnosis

A flat plate of the abdomen may show gaseous distention and fluid levels. Repeated films are frequently required before positive evidence can be attained. The finding of enormously dilated loops of bowel alerts the physician to the possibility of volvulus (Fig. 23-4).

Management

Early operative intervention is essential to prevent perforation of the bowel. Treatment should include derotation, decompression, and resection of devitalized segments. The surgery required may therefore be relatively simple or rather extensive. Delay in diagnosis and therapy are associated with a high mortality.

Intestinal Obstruction

Prevalence

Intestinal obstruction in pregnancy is uncommon. The reported prevalence is 1 in 3,600 to 66,431 deliveries.[2]

Clinical Features

Intestinal obstruction during pregnancy is often difficult to diagnose. This is mainly due to the uterus causing abdominal distention with displacement of the bowel laterally and posteriorly and the systemic effects, which may mimic the main symptoms of pregnancy. Approximately 60 percent of cases are due to adhesions.[2,20,34]

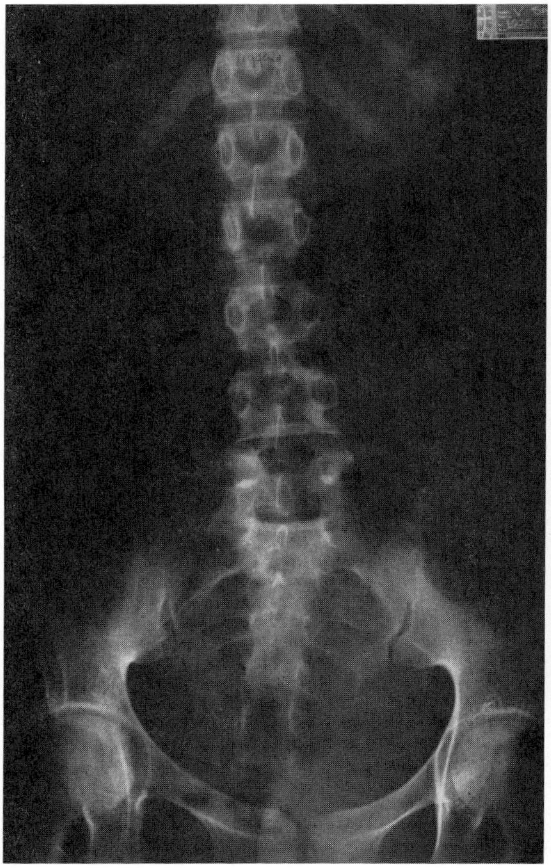

Figure 23-5 The abdominal x-ray demonstrates obstructed dilated loops of small bowel, with multiple air fluid levels on the erect film. There is an abnormal gas pattern in the right iliac fossa with the appearance of a mass lesion. This is the typical appearance of an obstructive lesion of the terminal ileum. At laparotomy, the obstructive lesion was resected and proved histologically to be secondary to tuberculosis.

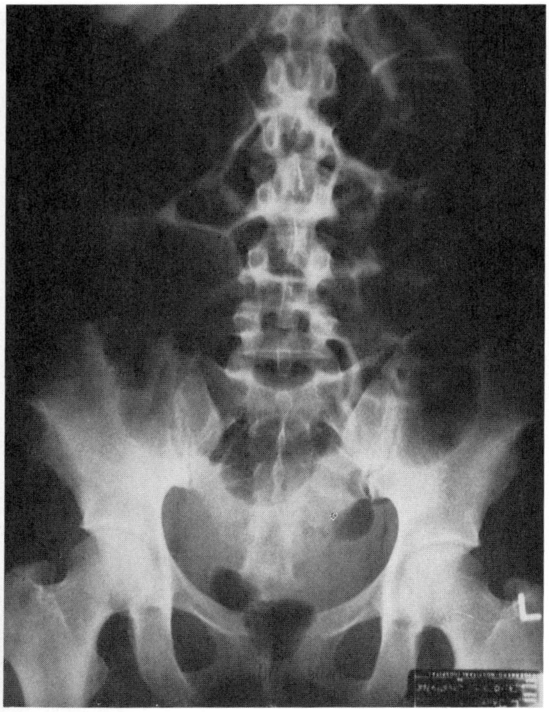

Figure 23-6 The abdominal x-ray demonstrates dilation of both small and large bowel. Final diagnosis was ileus secondary to acute pelvic inflammatory disease.

Other causes are volvulus, intussusception, extrinsic uterine pressure, and hernias. Mugati[51] reported a higher incidence in the puerperium, contrary to the accepted higher incidence during gestation. The predominant symptoms are pain, vomiting, distention, and constipation.

Confirmation of Diagnosis

If intestinal obstruction is being considered, radiologic examination of the abdomen is extremely valuable, as distended loops of bowel and the limits of the distended areas may be readily defined. It is frequently stated that fluid levels are diagnostic of obstruction, but this is not invariably the case. Radiologic findings need to be correlated with the clinical history and picture (Fig. 23-5). The radiation dosage required to take two abdominal films is approximately 0.1 Gy, which is very low indeed.

Measurement of the white cell count does not help in making the diagnosis.[20]

Fetal Complications

The prevalence of fetal death or preterm labor is 35 to 50 percent in the third trimester.[36]

Management

Insertion of a nasogastric tube to reduce the risks of aspiration at the time of induction of anesthesia is essential. Prophylactic antibiotics are recommended in the case where perforation or strangulation is suspected. A vertical incision is preferable to a transverse one. At term a cesarean section may be required in order to gain access to the site of obstruction. Routine abdominal delivery, however, is not advisable.

Puerperal Paralytic Ileus

Mild paralytic ileus may be caused by rough handling of the bowel during surgery or by peritoneal contamination by amniotic contents (Fig. 23-6). Exposure to the atmosphere with subsequent drying of the intestines may also play a role. Severe ileus may be caused by retroperitoneal hemorrhage[42] or peritonitis. Initial therapy is usually conservative with proper attention to fluid and electrolyte balance. Laparotomy is indicated when intra-abdominal pathology is suspected.

Pelvic Inflammatory Disease During Pregnancy

Several cases of acute salpingitis or pelvic inflammatory disease have been described in pregnancy.[9,16] The most common cause for the infection is transcervical bacterial transport via the uterus, which does not become totally occluded prior to the twelfth week of pregnancy. Other causes for the infection are by direct transfer or hematogenous or lymphatic spread. Exacerbation of an acute infection may also occur.

Symptoms vary from patient to patient. The most common symptoms are abdominal pain, anorexia, nausea, and vomiting. Low-grade fever occurs in 50 percent of patients.

Conservative treatment is preferable, but a precise diagnosis of this rare condition prior to laparotomy is not always easy. Acute salpingitis is sometimes encountered at laparotomy performed for presumed acute appendicitis. Removal of the normal appendix in these cases is not recommended, as this may increase the risk of abortion. Fetal wastage is approximately 50 percent in pregnancy complicated by acute or chronic pelvic inflammatory disease.[9]

Summary

Once the decision is made to operate on any pregnant woman with an acute abdomen, the question arises as to the preoperative use of tocolytic agents. It has been shown that preterm labor is rare before the third trimester, even in the presence of severe peritonitis.[34] It occurs more often in late pregnancy. These patients should therefore be very carefully observed for early signs of preterm labor to ensure timely administration of tocolytics.

Early recognition of surgical conditions during pregnancy is essential because prompt institution of appropriate therapy reduces morbidity and mortality. The obstetrician must be alert to the early and occult signs of these problems and must differentiate them from the confusing abdominal symptoms of the accompanying pregnancy. As delay in diagnosis may jeopardize the patient's life, exploratory laparotomy is essential when an acute surgical condition cannot be excluded.[9]

References

1. Abbitt PL, McIlhenny J. Prenatal detection of gallstones. JCU 1990; 18:202–204.
2. Allen JC. Sigmoid volvulus in pregnancy. J R Army Med Corps 1990; 136:55–56.
3. Anderson JB, Turner GM, Williamson RC. Fulminant ulcerative colitis in late pregnancy and the puerperium. J R Soc Med 1987; 80:492–494.
4. Ashworth TG. Fetal volvulus of the small intestines. J Clin Pathol 1988; 41:594–595.
5. Babaknia A, Hossein P, Woodruff JD. Appendicitis during pregnancy. Obstet Gynecol 1977; 50:40–44.
6. Baer JL, Reis RA, Arans RA. Appendicitis in pregnancy with changes in position and axis of the normal appendix in pregnancy. JAMA 1932; 98:1359–1364.
7. Ballantyne GH. Review of sigmoid volvulus. Dis Colon Rectum 1982; 25:823–830.
8. Barbara L, Sama C, Labate AMM, et al. A population study on the prevalence of gallstone disease: the Sirmione study. Hepatology 1987; 7:913–917.
9. Blanchard AC, Partorek JG, Weeks T. Pelvic inflammatory disease during pregnancy. South Med J 1987; 80:1363–1365.
10. Block P, Kelly TR. Management of gallstone pancreatitis during pregnancy and the postpartum period. Surg Gynecol Obstet 1968; 168:426–428.
11. Broström O. Prognosis in ulcerative colitis. Med Clin North Am 1990; 74:201–218.
12. Chesson RR, Gallup DG, Gibbs RL, et al. Ultrasonographic diagnosis of asymptomatic cholelithiasis in pregnancy. J Reprod Med 1985; 30:920–922.
13. Coady DJ, Snyder JR, Subramanyam BJ. Appendiceal abscess in pregnancy: diagnosis by ultrasound. JCU 1986; 14:70–71.
14. Davis MR, Bohon CJ. Intestinal obstruction in pregnancy. Clin Obstet Gynecol 1983; 26:833–838.
15. De Chalain TM, Michell WL, Berger GM. Hyperlipidemia, pregnancy and pancreatitis. Surg Gynecol Obstet 1988; 167:469–473.
16. De Kock M, Odendaal HJ. Acute salpingitis in pregnancy. S Afr Med J 1972; 46:21–22.
17. De Swiet M. Medical conditions in pregnancy. London: Blackwell Scientific, 1989:496–499.
18. Dixon NP, Faddis DM, Silberman H. Aggressive management of cholecystitis during pregnancy. Am J Surg 1987; 154:292–294.
19. Doherty DM, Lewis FR. Appendicitis: continuing diagnostic challenge. Emerg Med Clin North Am 1989; 7:537–553.
20. Donaldson DR, Parkinson DJ. Intestinal obstuction in pregnancy. J R Coll Surg Edinb 1985; 30:372–374.
21. Donaldson RM. Inflammatory bowel disease. N Engl Med J 1985; 312:1616–1619.
22. Faintuch J, Sobrado JCW, Trinconi AF, et al. The management of acute pancreatitis in pregnancy—the coadjuvant of parenteral feeding. Rev Hosp Clin Fac Med Sao Paolo 1989; 44:76–79.
23. Farming J, Cross BC. Post-cesarean section cecal volvulus. Am J Obstet Gynecol 1988; 158:1200–1202.
24. Fleischer AC, Shah DM, Entman SS. Sonographic evaluation of maternal disorders during pregnancy. Radiol Clin North Am 1990; 28:51–58.
25. Friley MD, Douglas G. Acute cholecystitis in pregnancy and the puerperium. Am Surg 1972; 38:314–317.
26. Gatenby SJ. Maintenance of pregnancy in Crohn's disease by parenteral nutrition: a case study. Human Nutrition and Applied Nutrition 1987; 345–349.

27. Gomez A, Wood M. Acute appendicitis during pregnancy. Am J Surg 1979; 137:180–183.
28. Graubard Z, Graham KM, van der Merwe FJ, Koller AB. Caecal volvulus in pregnancy. S Afr Med J 1988; 73:188.
29. Hamlin CH, Palermilno DA. Volvulus associated with pregnancy: report of 5 cases. Am J Obstet Gynecol 1966; 94:1147–1148.
30. Hanan IM, Kirsner JB. Inflammatory bowel disease in the pregnant woman. Clin Perinatol 1985; 12:669–682.
31. Harer WB Jr, Harer WB Sr. Volvulus complicating pregnancy or puerperium. Obstet Gynecol 1958; 12:399–406.
32. Hiatt JR, Hait JC, Williams RA, Klein SR. Biliary disease in pregnancy: strategy for surgical management. Am J Surg 1986; 151:263–265.
33. Holcomb GW Jr, Holcomb GW 3d. Cholelithiasis in infants, children and adolescents. Pediatr Rev 1990; 11:268–274.
34. Hunt MG, Martin JN, Martin RW, et al. Perinatal aspects of abdominal surgery for nonobstetric disease. Am J Perinatol 1989; 6:412–417.
35. Jaffe R, Gruber A, Abramowicz J, et al. Sonographic diagnosis of periappendicular abscess in pregnancy. Am J Obstet Gynecol 1985; 153: 623–624.
36. Kammerer WS. Non-obstetric surgery during pregnancy. Med Clin North Am 1979; 63:1157–1164.
37. Kantor HM. Midgut volvulus in pregnancy: a case report. J Reprod Med 1990; 35:577–580.
38. Katz S, Schulman N, Levin L. Free perforation in Crohn's disease: a report of 33 cases and review of the literature. Am J Gastroenterol 1986; 81: 38–43.
39. Kerry RI, Ramson HK. Volvulus of the colon: etiology, diagnosis and treatment. Arch Surg 1969; 99:215–222.
40. Korelitz BI. Pregnancy, fertility and inflammatory bowel disease. Am J Gastroenterol 1985; 80:365–370.
41. Landers D, Carmona R, Combleholme W, Lim R. Acute cholecystitis in pregnancy. Obstet Gynecol 1987; 69:131–133.
42. Leiberman JR, Mazor M, Dreval D. Puerperal adynamic ileus. Int J Gynaecol Obstet 1988; 26:285–290.
43. Lockwood C, Stiller RJ, Bolognese RR. Maternal total parenteral nutrition in chronic cholecystitis, a case report. J Reprod Med 1987; 32:785–788.
44. Machi J, Sigel B, McGarth EC, et al. Operative ultrasonography in the biliary tract during pregnancy. Surg Gynecol Obstet 1985; 160:119–123.
45. Martin LW, Glen PM. Prenatal appendiceal perforation: a case report. J Pediatr Surg 1986; 21:73–74.
46. Masters K, Levine BA, Gaskill HV, Sirinek KR. Diagnosing appendicitis during pregnancy. Am J Surg 1984; 148:768–771.
47. Mayberry JF, Weterman IT. European survey of fertility and pregnancy in women with Crohn's disease: a case control study by European collaborative group. Gut 1986; 27:821–825.
48. McGee TM. Acute appendicitis in pregnancy. Aust N Z J Obstet Gynaecol 1989; 29:378–385.
49. Miller JP. Inflammatory bowel disease in pregnancy: a review. J R Soc Med 1986; 79:221–225.
50. Moore GR, Smith CV. Schistosomiasis associated with rupture of the appendix in pregnancy. Obstet Gynecol 1989; 74:446–448.
51. Muguti GI. Intestinal obstruction during pregnancy and the puerperium at Mpito Central Hospital. J R Coll Surg Edinb 1988; 33:156–158.
52. Narasimharao KL, Mitra SK, Pathak IC. Antenatal appendicular perforation. Postgrad Med J 1987; 63:1001–1003.
53. Nielsen OH, Andreasson B, Bondesen S, et al. Pregnancy in Crohn's disease. Scand J Gastroenterol 1984; 19:724–732.
54. Nugent WF, Rajala M, O'Shea RA, et al. Total parenteral nutrition in pregnancy: conception to delivery. J Parenter Enterol Nutr 1987; 11:424–427.
55. Parsons AK, Sauer MV, Parsons MT, et al. Appendectomy at cesarean section: a prospective study. Obstet Gynecol 1986; 68:497–482.
56. Porter RJ, Stirrat GM. The effects of inflammatory bowel disease on pregnancy. A case-controlled retrospective analysis. Br J Obstet Gynaecol 1986; 93:1124–1131.
57. Printen KJ, Ott RA. Cholecystectomy during pregnancy. Am Surg 1978; 44:432–434.
58. Punnonan R, Aho AJ, Grönroos M, Liukko P. Appendectomy during pregnancy. Acta Chir Scand 1979; 145:555–558.
59. Richards C, Daya S. Diagnosis of acute appendicitis in pregnancy. Can J Surg 1989; 32:358–360.
60. Schwerk WB, Wichtrup B, Rothmund M, Rüschoff J. Ultrasonography in the diagnosis of acute appendicitis: a prospective study. Gastroenterology 1989; 97:630–639.
61. Simon JA. Biliary tract disease and related surgical disorders during pregnancy. Clin Obstet Gynecol 1983; 26:810–821.
62. Sparkman R. Gallstones in young women. Ann Surg 1957; 145:813–823.
63. Stauffer RA, Adams A, Wygol J, et al. Gallbladder disease in pregnancy. Am J Obstet Gynecol 1982; 144:661–664.
64. Strickland DM, Hauth VC, Widdish J, et al. Amylase and iso amylase activities in serum of pregnant women. Obstet Gynecol 1984; 63:389–391.
65. Suster S, Moran CA. Deciduosis of the appendix. Am J Gastroenterol 1990; 85:841–845.
66. Watson CJ, Thomson HJ, Calne R. HELLP: it's not cholecystitis. Br J Surg 1990; 77:539-540.
67. Watson WJ, Gaines TE. Third-trimester colectomy for severe ulcerative colitis. J Reprod Med 1987; 32:869–872.
68. Witter FR, Molteni RA. Intrauterine intestinal volvulus with hemoperitoneum presenting as fetal distress at 34 weeks' gestation. Am J Obstet Gynecol 1986; 155:1080–1081.
69. Wright EA. A case of acute appendicitis in pregnancy. Aust N Z J Obstet Gynaecol 1987; 27:256–257.

CHAPTER 24

Anti-Infective Chemotherapy in Obstetrics and Gynecology

Roger E. Bawdon, Ph.D.

In this chapter, the mechanism of action, Food and Drug Administration (FDA) category in relation to maternal and fetal toxicity, teratogenic effect, and placental transfer of various antimicrobial compounds are discussed.

Drug Classes and Pregnancy Categories

The FDA requires that all prescription drugs be labeled with information concerning their teratogenic or nonteratogenic effects.[12] The FDA has established five categories (A, B, C, D, X) to indicate teratogenic potential during pregnancy and the short- and long-term effects of these drugs on the mother and child (Tables 24-1 and 24-2).

Category A drugs are those for which well-controlled studies conducted in pregnant women have failed to show a risk to the fetus.

Category B drugs are those that have not demonstrated a fetal risk in animal studies, but for which there have been no adequate studies in women, or for which some risks have been discovered in animal studies, although studies in women have not established these risks.

Category C drugs are those for which there are no controlled studies in women or animals, or for which there are adverse effects in animal studies and no reported studies in women.

Category D drugs are those that have been proven to have had an adverse effect on the human fetus, However, even with this potential risk, the drugs may be administered to pregnant women if the clinical benefits exceed the risk of birth defects.

Category X drugs have a definite risk of fetal birth defects, and the risk of the use of the drugs far outweighs the benefits.

Antibacterial Agents

Beta-Lactam Antibiotics

With biosynthetic modifications, many penicillin antibiotics have been developed that have characteristics such as acid stability and penicillinase resistance that extend their antimicrobial spectra. Although these penicillins vary in their antimicrobial spectra, they still exhibit similar mechanisms of action in that they penetrate outer membranes of gram-negative bacteria and are selective for various penicillin-binding proteins. All penicillins are category B antibiotics and may be used in pregnancy.[4]

Another class of beta-lactam antibiotics is the cephalosporins, which are closely related to the penicillin antibiotics. Both penicillins and cephalosporins have the beta-lactam ring; the difference is that the cephalosporins contain a six-membered dihydrometathiazine ring, and the penicillins contain a five-membered tetrahydrothiazole ring. With the isolation and identification of the basic structure, the chemical synthesis of numerous cephalosporins has become possible. Based on antimicrobial spectra, cephalosporins have been classified as first, second, or third generation. All cephalosporins are

Table 24-1 Definition of FDA Pregnancy Categories*

Pregnancy Category	Definition
A	Adequate studies in pregnant women have not demonstrated a risk to the fetus in the first trimester of pregnancy and there is no evidence of risk in later trimesters.
B	Animal studies have not demonstrated a risk to the fetus but there are no adequate studies in pregnant women; or animal studies have shown an adverse effect, but adequate studies in pregnant women have not demonstrated a risk to the fetus during the first trimester of pregnancy and there is no evidence of risk in later trimesters.
C	Animal studies have shown an adverse effect on the fetus, but there are no adequate studies in humans, and the benefits from the use of the drug in pregnant women may be acceptable despite its potential risks; or there are no animal reproduction studies and no adequate studies in humans.
D	There is no evidence of human fetal risk, but the potential benefits from the use of the drug in pregnant women may be acceptable despite its potential risks.
X	Studies in animals or humans or adverse reaction reports or both have demonstrated fetal abnormalities; the risk of use in a pregnant woman clearly outweighs any possible benefit.

*Regardless of the designated pregnancy category or presumed safety, no drug should be administered during pregnancy unless it is clearly needed.[12]

category B antibiotics. Most of these compounds have been utilized in obstetrics and gynecology without any detrimental effects.

There are several additional beta-lactam antibiotics. The substitution of the sulfur atom in the penicillin ring with a carbon atom results in compounds called *carbapenems;* imipenem is one example. Another class of beta-lactams is the monobactams. An example of a monobactam is aztreonam.

Other compounds that belong to the beta-lactams are the beta-lactamase inhibitors, which structurally are fused beta-lactam rings. These compounds have virtually no antibacterial activity yet bind irreversibly to most of the common beta-lactamase enzymes responsible for the inactivation of many of the penicillins and cephalosporins. They are used in combination with penicillins and cephalosporins to prevent inactivation by beta-lactamases and thereby increase the antibacterial activity of these drugs. Two of these compounds, sulbactam and clavulanic acid, are in current clinical use.

Tetracyclines

The tetracycline compounds, first introduced in 1948, include chlortetracycline, oxytetracycline, tetracycline, minocycline, and doxycycline. They share a broad spectrum of activity for both gram-positive and gram-negative bacteria and in addition include *Chlamydia, Mycoplasma, Rickettsia,* some mycobacteria, and *Amoeba.*[11] Their mechanism of action is inhibition of protein synthesis by binding to the bacterial 30s ribosomes, and prevention of tRNA from combining with microbial messenger RNA.[8] The tetracyclines are all closely related and differ mainly in their half-lives and suitability for parenteral administration. Most have the same toxicities. Microbial resistance is shared by all tetracyclines.

Soon after their introduction into clinical practice, it was observed that large doses of tetracycline, 8.0 g per day orally or 2.0 g or more per day intravenously, resulted in hepatotoxicity that could be fatal. Subsequently, fetal hepatotoxicity was recognized in pregnant women who received the usual recommended dosages of tetracycline, 2.0 g per day orally. The metabolism of tetracycline is modified in pregnancy and associated with resultant retention and excessive blood levels.

The tetracyclines also are not recommended during pregnancy because they bind to calcium and are deposited in bones. In animal studies, administration during pregnancy has resulted in inhibition of bone growth and impaired osteogenesis. Because of these toxicities they are category D antibiotics.[5] The binding of tetracyclines to calcium forms a calcium-tetracycline-orthophosphate complex and is responsible for the brown discoloration in teeth of children up to the age of 5 years. Of the tetracyclines only two—tetracycline and doxycycline—are generally used in obstetrics and gynecology, for the treatment of sexually transmitted disease.

Chloramphenicol

Another antimicrobial used extensively for the last 35 years is chloramphenicol. Chloramphenicol is in a class by itself, and its chemical structure consists of a nitrobenzene complex, which is combined with dichloroacetic acid.

Chloramphenicol is probably most noted for its toxicity, which includes aplastic anemia, thrombocytopenia, and granulocytopenia. In addition, as a result of excessive dosages administered to neonates in whom hepatic clearance mechanisms had not matured, deaths occurred. The condition was designated the "gray baby syndrome." Chloramphenicol is consequently a category C antibiotic because of the possibility of gray baby syndrome.[7]

Table 24-2 FDA Pregnancy Categories for Various Classes of Drugs

Class of Drugs	Specific Drug	FDA Pregnancy Category
Penicillins		B
Cephalosporins		B
	Moxalactam	C
Carbapenim	Imipenem-cilastatin	C
Monobactam	Aztreonam	B
Aminoglycosides		D
Tetracyclines	Doxycycline	D
		D
Erythromycin		B
Clindamycin		(B)*
Vancomycin		C
Fluoroquinolones		C
Chloramphenicol		(D)*
Metronidazole		(B)*
Trimethoprim-sulfamethoxazole		C
Ketoconazole		C
Fluconazole		C
Isoniazid		(B)*
Rifampin		(B)*
Ethambutol		C
Pyrazinamide		?
Amantadine		C
ddI 2′3′ dideoxyinosine ? FDA caloquine		B
Acyclovir		C
Ganciclovir		C
Zidovudine		C
Quinine		X
Mefloquine		C
4-Aminoquinolones	Chloroquine	(C)*
8-Aminoquinolones	Primaquine	(C)*
Mebendazole		C
Praziquantel		B

*Parentheses indicate that safety in pregnancy has not been established but no reports of congenital defects are known. *(B)* = similar to B; *(C)* = similar to C; *(D)* = similar to D; *?* = unknown, insufficient experience to categorize.

Erythromycin

Erythromycin is a hydroxylated macrocyclic lactone, one of the macrolide antibiotics. There are a number of macrolide and more recently azalide antibiotics. The macrolides act by binding to the 50s ribosome and inhibiting the translocation step in protein synthesis.[6] Although the drug binds to both gram-positive and gram-negative bacteria, it is more effective against gram-positive bacteria because of better penetration into the cell membrane of these microorganisms.

Erythromycin has been used in obstetric and gynecologic infections primarily for the treatment of syphilis in the penicillin-allergic patient and for chlamydial and mycoplasmal infections. Erythromycin is a category B antibiotic.

Clindamycin

Another drug used in obstetrics and gynecology is clindamycin. Clindamycin has broad anaerobic coverage, including *Bacteroides fragilis* and other *Bacteroides* spp. and is used in obstetrics and gynecology for infections in which anaerobes are suspected. In addition, it is active against *Streptococcus pyogenes* (groups A, B, C, G) and some strains of *Staphylococcus aureus*.[21] Clindamycin is a category B antibiotic.

Quinolones

The fluoroquinolone compounds have recently been introduced into clinical practice.

The mechanism of action of all quinolones is related to DNA replication. During the replication process, the double-helix DNA strand must be separated into two strands to permit transcription. Because of the length of the strands, they tend to tangle or overwind, and the bacterial enzyme DNA gyrase is responsible for prevention of overwinding, raveling, and breaking of DNA strands. The quinolones block the action of the bacterial DNA gyrase. Because humans do not have DNA gyrase, quinolones do not influence human DNA replication.

The quinolones have antimicrobial activity against most gram-positive and aerobic gram-negative bacteria, although activity against streptococci is marginal. The currently available agents are not active against anaerobes. In addition, the quinolones are effective against *Chlamydia trachomatis, Neisseria gonorrhoeae,* and *Ureaplasma urealyticum*. They are not active against *Treponema pallidum*. Quinolone compounds are category C antibiotics.

Aminoglycosides

The aminoglycoside antibiotics are a unique class of antibiotics that were discovered in 1944. Streptomycin was the first of many antibiotics with the common structural formula containing aminoglycoside-aminocyclitol frequently referred to as aminoglycoside antibiotics. The more common aminoglycoside antibiotics used in the United States are streptomycin, neomycin, kanamycin, gentamicin, tobramycin, amikacin, netilmicin, and spectinomycin. This group of antibiotics is active against aerobic gram-negative bacilli, except that streptomycin, neomycin, kanamycin, and spectinomycin are not active against *Pseudomonas aeruginosa*. They are active against *Mycobacterium tuberculosis* and some strains of *Staphylococcus aureus*.

Streptomycin, kanamycin, and tobramycin are category D drugs because of eighth cranial nerve toxicity to both the mother and the fetus. The other aminoglycosides are category C antibiotics because of their ototoxicity and nephrotoxicity.

Vancomycin

Vancomycin is a unique complex tricyclic glycoprotein antibiotic that is the agent of choice against methicillin-resistant *S. aureus*.[17] Vancomycin is a category C antibiotic.

Sulfonamides

Sulfonamides are in category B because of the risk of malformation. However, because they predispose to the development of kernicterus if given near term, they are included in category D.

Trimethoprim was synthesized in 1956 and has a broad spectrum of antibacterial action that is synergistically enhanced when used in combination with sulfonamides. The most frequent combination is that of trimethoprim-sulfamethoxazole.[20] Trimethoprim is a category C drug because it inhibits folic acid metabolism. Fortunately, there is little placental transfer of the drug. Placebo-controlled studies have failed to reveal an increase in fetal anomalies.

Rifampin

Rifampin has antimicrobial activity against most gram-positive bacteria, *Mycobacterium tuberculosis, M. leprae,* and some gram-negative bacteria. Although the drug is active against many bacteria, the development of resistance is a common problem with rifampin. In addition to its key role in the treatment of tuberculosis, it is often used in combination with other agents such as nafcillin in the treatment of systemic infections. Rifampin is a category C drug because of a higher-than-usual incidence of congenital anomalies in pregnant patients.

Antituberculosis Agents

The drugs used for treatment of tuberculosis include isoniazid, rifampin, ethambutol, *p*-amino salicylic acid (PAS), pyrazinamide, and cycloserine. All these drugs are category C drugs with the exception of ethambutol, which is a category B drug.

Antifungal Agents

There are essentially two classes of antifungal agents: those used for superficial or topical infections and those used for systemic infections. However, there is some overlap in the use of these compounds, as some may be used for either superficial infections or systemic infections.

Among the most widely used systemic antifungal agents is amphotericin B, which is one of the polyene macrolide antibiotics. It is active against dimorphic fungi including *Histoplasma capsulatum, Blastomyces dermatitidis, Paracoccidioides brasiliensis, Coccidioides immitis, Aspergillus* spp., *Candida* spp., and *Cryptococcus neoformans*.

Amphotericin B is a category B antifungal agent and has not caused congenital anomalies in infants of mothers given the drug during all trimesters of pregnancy. These were well-controlled studies involving thousands of patients.

The imidazoles and triazoles are another class of antifungal agents, some of which may be used for both systemic and topical administration.[2] Clotrimazole, miconazole, and ketoconazole are the imidazoles most frequently used for treatment of *Candida albicans* vaginitis. For systemic infections, the imidazoles are effective against *C. albicans*. Clotrimazole is a category B drug, and miconazole is a category C drug, whereas oral ketoconazole probably should not be used during pregnancy because of its possible maternal toxicity.[3] Fluconazole has a mechanism of action like that of imidazoles, has broad-spectrum antifungal activity, and is used only for oral therapy. Fluconazole is a category C drug.

Antiviral Agents

The effectiveness of antiviral agents has left a lot to be desired when compared to the effectiveness of antibacterial and antifungal agents. The reason for this lack of effectiveness relates to viral dependence on nucleic acids and metabolites of the host cell for its replication and metabolic activity. Because of this utilization, antiviral compounds are also toxic to the host cell.

The more commonly used antiviral compounds are acyclovir, amantadine, azidothymidine, ganciclovir, idoxuridine, and vidarabine.

Azidothymidine (AZT) was developed for the purpose of anti-HIV therapy. The drug does not eliminate the virus from the infected individual. However, the drug has been responsible for improving the quality of life for many months. One important use of AZT may be the improvement of maternal health until the fetus can be delivered. Preliminary data from our laboratory suggest that there is little embryotoxicity or teratogenic effect in rats given 10 times the therapeutic dose of AZT.[16] In addition, we have shown that AZT is rapidly transported to the fetal circulation and into placental tissues when infused into the maternal circulation in an in vitro human placenta model.

The mechanism of action is against viral RNA dependent DNA polymerase, which interferes with chain elongation during DNA chain elongation.[23] AZT has some synergistic activity when used in combination with other antiviral compounds including interferon, acyclovir and, didanosine. The drug is active but not clinically useful against Epstein-Barr virus. It is not effective against the herpes virus or varicella zoster virus.

Acyclovir is an anti–herpes simplex virus compound, which chemically is 9-[(Z-hydroxylthoxy) methy] guanine. The compound inhibits viral replication by inhibition of DNA chain termination and replication.[10] The drug is effective in systemic viral infections when prescribed early on and is frequently used to prevent recurrent herpes type 1 and type 2 infections. The drug has been used in pregnant patients with recurrent herpes to reduce viral shedding and to prevent neonatal herpes infection. Acyclovir is also active against varicella zoster infections.

Ganciclovir is chemically very similar to acyclovir. The mechanism of action of ganciclovir is similar to acyclovir, but it has a somewhat longer half-life and appears to be more toxic than acyclovir. Ganciclovir is used in the treatment of cytomegalovirus (CMV) retinitis, a condition that uniformly leads to blindness. It is classified as category C with mutagenicity and teratogenicity in laboratory animals. It is a prototype category C agent; use in pregnant women may be acceptable despite its potential risks, given the indication for which it is administered.

Didanosine (ddI) has recently been licensed as an anti-HIV agent. Its mechanism of action is similar to that of zidovudine (AZT). It is being used in patients who are intolerant of zidovudine for reasons of sick effects or toxicity and in patients who have shown progressive clinical deterioration on zidovudine. Regimens being studied include alternating courses of zidovudine and didanosine. It is classified as category B.

Vidarabine and idoxuridine are used topically for herpes simplex keratoconjunctivitis.

Amantadine is an effective prophylactic and therapeutic agent in combating influenza A infections. The mode of action of amantidine is possible interference with cell penetration and uncoating of the virus.[19] Amantadine is not generally used in pregnant women; however, it may be useful in women who develop life-threatening influenza A with hypoxemia, which may be lethal to the fetus.

Antiparasitic Agents

Parasitic infections in pregnant women in the United States are uncommon. The exceptions to this are *Trichomonas vaginalis* and *Toxoplasma gondii*. Toxoplasmosis is the most important parasitic infection in obstetrics in the United States, where the infection rate is about 2 to 5 percent of all pregnancies, with about 2 to 5 percent of these infections resulting in fetal involvement. Vaginitis caused by the protozoan *Trichomonas vaginalis* is common.

Pyrimethamine in combination with a short-acting sulfonamide is used for the treatment of *Toxoplasma gondii*. Pyrimethamine is in a class of compounds that act by inhibition of folate metabolism. Pyrimethamine is a category C drug; however, the use of the drug during pregnancy has not resulted in congenital malformations.[14,15]

Metronidazole is an important antiparasitic drug because of its effectiveness against *T. vaginalis, Entamoeba histolytica,* and *Giardia lamblia*. The drug is also unique in that it is also effective against many anaerobic bacteria, including *Bacteroides fragilis*. Metronidazole is a category B drug; however, there are conflicting data as to the first-trimester use of the drug. Although some studies have shown teratogenic risk factors when this compound is prescribed in the first trimester, other studies have shown no effect. It is recommended that it not be used in the first trimester. Second- and third-trimester use has not been shown to cause congenital malformations.[18]

Placental Transfer

The transfer of organic and inorganic compounds and ions across the placenta range from simple diffusion to complicated transport systems (see Chapter 25). Before a discussion of placental drug transfer can be attempted, the types of transfer must be elucidated. The transfer of all materials fall into five basic categories: simple diffusion, facilitated diffusion, active transport, pinocytosis, and leakage.[19]

Most simple molecules, including oxygen, carbon dioxide, urea, and some drugs, are transported across the placenta by simple diffusion, which is related to the concentration gradient in the maternal and fetal unit and to the flow rate of the uteroplacental and umbilical blood.

Facilitated diffusion (as opposed to simple diffusion) is a much more rapid mechanism for the transport of compounds across the placenta that cannot be accounted for by Fick's equation for diffusion. According to the Fick's equation, diffusion can be predicted by knowing a number of values and constants such as flux (flow rate), thermal diffusion coefficient, and the coefficient of thermal conductivity when applied to the thermal energy.[1] Similar results are obtained with simple compounds, as a decrease from an area of high concentration to an area of low concentration is recorded on the maternal side, whereas in the fetal compartment, there is a proportional increase in drug concentration. Compounds up to a molecular weight of 5,000 are included in this category, as well as glucose, erythritol, and sucrose.

Active transport is responsible for the high concentration of some compounds such as amino acids, vitamins, and nucleosides. It is important to note that the D-isomers are not transported as actively as the L-forms.[22]

Complex compounds such as IgG, fat particles, and perhaps viral particles are transported across the placenta by pinocytosis. Pinocytosis is similar to phagocytosis except pinocytosis is the engulfment of liquid. In this case, the pseudopodial projects of the syncytiotrophoblastic layer engulfs or surrounds small amounts of maternal plasma. Little is known about this transfer mechanism, but electron microscopy has demonstrated that it does exist.

Material may be transported across the placenta by breaks in the placental membrane. Although the frequency with which these breaks occur has not been established, they obviously do happen. Maternal sensitization to fetal red blood cell Rh antigens is exemplified by this mechanism.

Most drugs are transported across the placenta by simple diffusion. The assumption that all drugs in a particular class are transported across the placenta at an equal rate is incorrect, as is evident from studies of the cephalosporin antibiotics. Ceftizoxime is transported across the placenta at a much higher rate than cefoperazone. The transport of ceftizoxime is probably related to its molecular structure.[13]

References

1. Atkins PW. Molecules in motion—the kinetic theory of gases. In: Physical chemistry. San Francisco: WH Freeman, 1978; 24:804–818.
2. Bennett J. Antifungal agents. In: AG Gilman, TW Rall, Nies AS, Taylor R, eds. The pharmacological basis of therapeutics. Ed 8. Elmsford NJ: Pergamon Press, 1990: 50:1169–1171.
3. Bennett J. Antifungal agents. In: AG Gilman, TW Rall, Nies AS, Taylor R, eds. The pharmacological basis of therapeutics. Ed 8. Elmsford, NY: Pergamon Press, 1990:50:1168–1169.
4. Briggs GG, Freeman RK, Sumner JY. Penicillin G on drugs in pregnancy and lactation. In: Butler JP, ed. Ed 3. Baltimore: Williams & Wilkins, 1990:482–483.
5. Briggs GG, Freeman RK, Sumner JY. Tetracycline on drugs and pregnancy and lactation. In: Butler JP, ed. Ed 3. Baltimore: Williams & Wilkins, 1990:593–597.
6. Brisson-Noël A, Trieu-Cuot P, Courvalin P. Mechanism of action of spiramycin and other macrolides. J Antimicrob Chemother 1988; 22:S13–18.
7. Burns LE, Hodgman JE, Cass AB. Fatal circulatory collapse in premature infants receiving chloramphenicol. N Engl J Med 1959; 261:1318–1321.
8. Chopra I, Howe TGB. Bacterial resistance to the tetracyclines. Microbiol Rev 1978; 42:707–724.
9. Davies WL, Grunert RR, Hoff RF, et al. Antiviral activity of 1-adamantanamine hydrochloride. Science New York 1964; 144:862–863.
10. Douglas RG. Antiviral agents. In: Gilmar AG, Rall TW, Nies AS, Taylor R, eds. The pharmocological basis of therapeutics. Ed 8. Elmsford, NY: Pergamon Press, 1990:51:1184–1186.
11. Duggar BM. Aureomycin: product of continuing search for new antibiotics. Ann N Y Acad Sci 1948; 51:177–180.
12. Food and Drug Administration: Pregnancy categories for prescription drugs. FDA Drug Bulletin 1979; Sept:23–24.
13. Fortunato SJ, Bawdon RE, Maberry MC, Swan KF. Transfer of ceftizoxime surpasses that of cefaperzone by the isolated human placenta perfused in vitro. Obstet Gynecol 1990; 75:830–833.
14. Hengst VP. Investigations of the teratogenicity of doroprim (pyrimethomine) in humans. Zentralbl Gynakol 1972; 94:551–555.
15. Lee RV. Parasites and pregnancy: the problem of malaria and toxoplasmosis. Clin Perinatol 1988; 15:351–363.
16. Little BB, Bawdon RE, Christmas JT, et al. Pharmacokinetics of azidothymidine during late pregnancy in Long-Evans rats. American Journal of Obstetrics and Gynecology 1989; 161:732–734.
17. McCormick MH, Stark WM, Pittenger GE, Pittenger RC, McGuire JM. Vancomycin a new antibiotic: I. chemical and biologic properties. Antibiotics Annual 1955: 606–610.
18. Morgan IFK. Metronidazole treatment in pregnancy. Int J Gynaecol Obstet 1978; 15:501–502.

19. Moya F, Thorndike V. Passage of drugs across the placenta. Am J Obstet Gynecol 1962; 84:1778–1798.
20. Roth B. '5-benzyl-2,4-diaminopyrimidines as antibacterial agents: I. synthetic and antibacterial activity in vitro. J Med Pharm Chem 1962; 5:1103–1107.
21. Sande MA, Mandell GL. Antimicrobial agents. In: Gilman AG, Rall TW, Nies AS, Taylor P, eds. The pharmocological basis of therapeutics. Ed 8. Elmsford, NY Pergamon Press, 1990:1135–1137.
22. Schneider H, Panigel M, Dancis J. Transfer across the perfused placenta of antipyrine, sodium, and leucine. Am J Obstet Gynecol 1972; 114:822–828.
23. Yarchoan R, Mitsuya H, Broder S. Clinical and basic advances in the antiretroviral therapy of human immunodeficiency virus infection. Am J Med 1989; 87:191–200.

CHAPTER 25

Placental Transmission of Antimicrobial Agents

David Charles, M.D.

Advances in perinatal medicine can often be derived from the application of knowledge gleaned from former eras rather than as a result of startling new information. Preterm labor is the major cause of perinatal morbidity and mortality. The majority of low-birth-weight infants result from a reduction in the duration of the pregnancy rather than intrauterine growth retardation. Several decades ago many physicians were convinced that if all premature births could be eliminated the stillbirth and neonatal death rate would be more than halved. At that time the common causes of preterm birth were considered to be due to the following conditions:

1. Maternal ill health as a result of malnutrition, hypertensive disorders, or antepartum hemorrhage
2. Multiple pregnancy
3. Fetal abnormalities

Despite progress in improving the general health of pregnant women, prematurity remains the leading cause of perinatal morbidity and mortality. A predisposing cause cannot be elicited in most cases, and as a result prevention has been difficult. However, an increasing assemblage of information suggests that infection is a major etiologic factor for preterm birth.

Obstetricians in the first half of the century were so imbued with the prevention of puerperal sepsis that they failed to address the possibility of an infectious etiology for preterm labor. The prevention of prematurity is of great importance, but in view of the fact that in approximately 40 percent of cases it is impossible to discover the cause one cannot be too sanguine of the results of prophylaxis by nutritional supplements and enhanced prenatal care. Such measures did have a major effect in reducing the prematurity rate initially, but the incidence of preterm births has not decreased in the United States during the past 40 years.

Perinatal Infections

At the same time it has long been recognized that infections of the newborn were among the most important and dangerous problems of the neonatal period. The fetus and premature newborn are physiologically disadvantaged because they are relatively immunodeficient by reason of their immaturity and are thus prey to endogenous microbes harbored in the birth canal and to exogenous microbes colonizing their immediate environment after birth. Such infections are dangerous not only because of the mortality of affected infants but more particularly because of the risk to which every infant in the perinatal unit is exposed, however healthy. The incidence of infections in the neonate exceeds that at all other ages.

Despite all measures adopted to date, the preterm delivery rate remains at approximately 7 percent of deliveries. The etiology of preterm birth is only partially understood, as multiple factors may play a role either alone or in unison. The mechanism for the initiation of both term and preterm labor remains to be determined. During the past decade burgeoning evidence has indicated that genital tract infections frequently play a role in premature rupture of the membranes and preterm labor. Russell[34] has presented evidence that clinical and histologic chorioamnionitis occurs more frequently in association with preterm deliveries. Naeye and Peters[25] from their studies found that intra-amniotic infection was two to three times more common when the membranes ruptured just prior to the onset of preterm labor compared to amniorrhexis just after the initiation of labor. They considered that infection may initiate premature labor. A proportion of patients with premature labor with intact membranes and no fever have bacterial amnionitis. In such cases fetal tachycardia precedes maternal tachycardia and fever. It is well recognized in obstetrics that more mothers and infants are liable to early-onset infectious sequelae after a preterm delivery compared with one at term.

Current research suggests that chorioamnionitis is often the result of an ascending infection caused by cervicovaginal pathogens. Improved methodology for the isolation of anaerobes has underscored their importance in intra-amniotic infections. Pure cultures of *Bacteroides bivius, B. fragilis,* or *Peptostreptococcus* may be isolated in cases of neonatal sepsis or postpartum endometritis as a sequel to chorioamnionitis.

Preterm Labor

Bobitt and Ledger[3] were the first to use direct sampling of amniotic fluid by means of amniocentesis to demonstrate the presence of pathogenic organisms in patients with preterm labor. Bobitt and associates[2] reported that bacteria may be present in approximately 25 percent of amniotic fluid samples in patients in preterm labor or premature rupture of the fetal membranes compared with about 2 percent of samples from patients in late pregnancy with no such complications. Romero and associates[33] from their studies estimate that at least 25 percent of preterm deliveries occur in women with an intra-amniotic infection and conclude that although such an infection may be subclinical in nature it is a major factor in the etiology of preterm labor.

Bacterial Vaginosis

The most common cause of vulvovaginitis in women during reproductive life is bacterial vaginosis (BV). Although the specific cause of BV remains to be determined, it is characterized by a lack of lactobacilli in the vaginal flora and a predominance of anaerobic species. It has been suggested that BV may be the result of either a change in the vaginal flora or endogenous infection. *Gardnerella vaginalis,* which has been implicated in BV, has been shown by Wood and coworkers[39] in in vitro studies to interfere with the adherence of lactobacilli to vaginal epithelial cells. Rabe and coworkers[32] have reported an association between facultative viridans group streptococci and BV in gravid women. Eschenbach and associates[11] conclude from their studies that lactobacilli may not be able to protect a patient against BV unless the organisms can produce hydrogen peroxide. This is in accord with the view that BV reflects a suppression of hydrogen peroxide–producing lactobacilli, which in women without this entity are the predominant species in the vaginal flora. Evidence has been accumulating that links BV with preterm delivery. Gravett and associates[18] studied the relationship between prematurity, selected cervicovaginal bacteria, and 30 demographic, socioeconomic, and obstetric variables. They found that preterm labor at less than 36 weeks' gestation occurred in 25 percent of the patients with BV and in 13 percent of women without BV in a univariate analysis. Furthermore, preterm labor of less than 34 weeks, premature amniorrhexis, birth weight of less than 2,500 g, and amniotic fluid infection were also associated with BV in their analysis. Martius and associates[24] in a case-control study reported that BV was present in 34 percent of the gravid patients who delivered before 37 weeks' gestation and in 18 percent of the control group who were delivered at term. Hillier and coworkers[19] in a case-control study of chorioamniotic infection in relation to prematurity found that such an infection is strongly related to histologic chorioamnionitis and may be a cause of preterm birth. By means of multiple regression analysis controlling for confounding variables, they found that the intrapartum diagnosis of BV was associated with recovery of organisms between the chorion and amnion in both term and preterm gestations. These investigators demonstrate in a succinct manner that if 20 percent of gravid patients have BV then treatment of this entity could have a major effect on the prevention of preterm labor in their clinic.

Intra-amniotic Infection

Intra-amniotic infection is a well-recognized risk factor for neonatal sepsis. Likewise, there is no doubt that bacterial infections play a role in preterm labor and amniorrhexis. It is therefore not surprising that antimicrobial therapy is being increasingly prescribed to women in late pregnancy. Consequently, a knowledge of the placental transfer of antimicrobial agents from mother to fetus is essential to all who deal with the gravid patient because infection in its many guises appears to play a significant role in preterm labor and perinatal problems. Because intra-amniotic infection is a recognized risk as regards neonatal sepsis antibiotic therapy is frequently instituted prior to parturition. Support for such an approach comes from a randomized trial of patients with intra-amniotic infection conducted by Gibbs and associates,[17] who showed that neonatal sepsis was significantly reduced when antimicrobial therapy was initiated during labor rather than after parturition. This study underlines the importance of collecting data pertaining to the transfer of antibiotics from mother to fetus following labor.

It is now well-nigh half a century since Eastman[10] wrote:

Only when the factors causing prematurity are clearly understood can any intelligent attempt at prevention be made.

Fetal Drug Exposure

The administration of any therapeutic agent to gravid women must be equated with the physiologic changes and modifications in the pharmacokinetic and pharmacodynamic disposition of drugs that transpire in pregnancy. Moreover, clinicians must be alert to possible untoward effects of drugs on the fetus. The thalidomide disaster warned society that any pharmacologic agent that traverses the placenta may have detrimental effects on the biologic systems of the fetus. Thalidomide also drew attention to species differences in drug effects. To assess potential drug toxicity in the fetus in various mammalian species, it is necessary to ascertain both the relevant equilibration kinetics between the maternal organism and fetus and the disposition of the drug in the fetus. Theoretically these parameters can be determined in animals by repeated analyses of biologic fluids and tissues from both mother and fetus. Although such studies are feasible in animals, the data obtained cannot be readily extrapolated to humans.

Consequently, the administration of any drug to a gravid patient should be positively justified. Unfortunately, information on the effects of most drugs during pregnancy is either minimal or anecdotal and often not available to the clinician. Drugs prescribed during pregnancy may impair morphogenesis, inhibit embryonic development, and result in congenital anomalies that often simulate those observed in genetic disorders. As the vast majority of the antimicrobial agents pass from mother to fetus, it is important that the clinician appreciates that rapid equilibration takes place between the maternal and fetal circulations and consequently fetal exposure to therapeutic agents may be far more extensive than is generally realized. In fact, it is advisable that any fetus exposed in utero to any drug prescribed to the mother be evaluated at intervals during the first 7 years of life. The latter is warranted as certain drugs may have delayed effects on the fetus that may not be apparent in the neonate. Furthermore, certain drug effects persist for a longer time in the fetus than in the mother. Conversely, although the fetus may be exposed to a drug, the concentration achieved may not be adequate to attain any therapeutic effect, much less harm.

Physiologic Changes of Pregnancy

The progressive physiologic alterations that accompany pregnancy can have a marked effect on drug disposition. The changes in the maternal organism include an increase in body water, fat, and weight. In addition, there is an expansion of the plasma volume, a reduction in serum albumin concentration, and a variation in other plasma protein values, as well as marked alterations in steroid hormone levels. These changes accompany increased cardiac output, renal plasma flow, and glomerular filtration. Such physiologic alterations are likely to influence the pharmacokinetics of many therapeutic agents prescribed during pregnancy.

Cardiovascular Changes

The increase in cardiac output and blood volume are important for maternal as well as fetal homeostasis. These adaptations are initiated before the end of the first trimester. They are accompanied by a reduction in uterine vascular resistance and augmentation of uterine blood flow, which during late pregnancy is about 20-fold that observed in the nongravid subject. The alteration in blood volume results in a reduction of serum proteins, particularly albumin, which is apparent by the eighth week of gestation. Likewise, there is a reduction in the maternal plasma concentration of solutes.

Water Storage

The total body water increases about 8 L during the course of pregnancy. The major portion is distributed between the conceptus, maternal tissues, and vascular compartment. Approximately 2.5 L of water is sequestered in the interstitial space. Adaptations in osmotic relationships in the extracellular compartment affect both the transfer and retention of water. Although a reduction in colloid osmotic pressure compatible with the transfer of water to the extravascular compartment is evident, this is not substantiated as a determinant for the fluid retention that occurs during pregnancy. Furthermore, the neonate has a greater proportionate extracellular volume and total body water than the adult. In the premature infant, water makes up 86 percent of its body weight, and in the term neonate it comprises only 70 percent of body weight. It can thus be assumed that such variations in body water in the pregnant patient and fetus can influence the distribution of drugs.

Fetal Hemodynamics

A further facet of drug transfer to the fetus relates to fetal hemodynamics. The cardiac output in an infant at the time of birth is about 200 ml per kilogram body weight per minute, which is about two to five times that in the adult, although the stroke volume and the weight of the left ventricle are approximately the same per kilogram of body weight in the fetus and adult. The high fetal heart rate is important in sustaining cardiac output. The high cardiac output is interpreted as compensation for the fact that the organization of the placental vascular channels is not particularly efficacious for gaseous exchange. Consequently, in order to satisfy fetal oxygen requirements, a large volume flow is necessary via the placenta in both the maternal and fetal compartments.

Because much of umbilical venous blood bypasses the fetal liver via the ductus venosus and the lungs by way of the ductus arteriosus, a higher drug concentration is delivered to the fetal heart and central nervous system. Such complexities of drug distribution in the fetal compartment may mean that a specific amount of a drug may be safe for the mother but result in toxic levels in the fetus, especially if the drug has a narrow therapeutic index. This has clinical relevance as the purpose of antimicrobial therapy is to achieve effective and nontoxic steady-state blood and tissue concentrations. As most of the antibiotics prescribed during pregnancy are for maternal infections, it must be stated that in respect to the fetus we have minimal information pertaining to their therapeutic efficacy and toxicity. Moreover, the pattern of fetal defects associated with any specific agent may vary as the gestation progresses to term, and any noxious compound can influence fetal growth and invoke congenital pathologic entities.

Drug Equilibration

The dynamics of equilibration between maternal and fetal blood have not been thoroughly evaluated. In many studies concerning the placental transmission and fetal equilibration of various substances, it is frequently presupposed that placental and fetal tissues are homogeneous. Such assumptions are not necessarily true, and in the fetus drug equilibration cannot be reconciled with a simple exponential equation.[4] Many of the mathematical models utilized in placental transfer studies have regarded the placenta as a mixing chamber of finite volume in which the umbilical and maternal blood are equipoised, despite the fact that there is no physiologic data to support this concept. At any particular time only small fractions of the maternal and fetal blood volume are in close proximity to each other. The actual placental volume in early pregnancy is greater than that of the fetus and remains thus until after the seventeenth week of gestation. Because of the physiologic adjustments that occur during the course of pregnancy, the pharmacokinetic data derived from studies in nongravid women for any drug cannot be applied to gravid subjects. Physicians should realize that noxious effects of drugs on the fetus may not be recognized until early childhood. For example, it is possible that drugs administered to a mother in late pregnancy may affect fetal cerebral development. At present, little is known as regards fetal exposure to any specific drug on the chemical processes in the brain. In fact, the aftereffects of drug exposure by the fetus in utero on cerebral function have barely been examined, but some information derived from postnatal behavioral tests suggests that the later phases of fetal cortical development may be modified.

Mechanics of Placental Transfer

Therapeutic agents such as antibiotics enter the fetal compartment primarily by diffusion, and the transfer rate across the placenta is governed by such physicochemical factors as the available surface area, membrane thickness, lipid solubility, the degree of ionization, molecular size, and concentration gradient. Nonionized, lipophilic molecules readily diffuse across the placenta. Although the gradient across the placenta is primarily a function of the amount of drug administered to the mother, it can be affected by the volume of drug distribution in the maternal and fetal extracellular space, uterine blood flow, and maternal and fetal drug excretion, as well as the plasma protein-binding propensity of the drug. Protein binding is rarely the rate-limiting step in drug transfer because the change between the bound and unbound states generally occurs more rapidly than placental perfusion or transmission. In the fetus, sustaining a normal water-to-solute balance is complicated because of the constant interchange that takes place between the amniotic fluid compartment and the fetus. The available data on fetal renal function are incomplete. The fetal kidneys are capable of a degree of function by the twentieth week of gestation, which can be correlated with changes in the chemical composition of the amniotic fluid. The major route for drug transfer to the amniotic fluid is via the placenta and the fetal circulation. Water-soluble drugs are excreted in the fetal urine. Lipid-soluble compounds may, however, diffuse across the fetal membranes interposed between the maternal circulation and amniotic fluid, as well as fetal mucous membranes and immature skin. Lipid membranes basically comprise bound cellular plasma membranes forming a continuous lipid layer. Water-soluble molecules, with a molecular weight of about 100 daltons, readily diffuse across such membranes. Lipid-soluble molecules rapidly traverse lipid membranes as long as their molecular weight does not exceed 600 daltons, whereas those with molecular weights greater than 1,000 are impeded. This is not entirely correct, as some studies have demonstrated that colistin, which has a molecular weight in excess of 1,000 daltons, can be rapidly transferred via the placenta to the fetus from the maternal circulation.[4]

Protein Binding

In regard to the placental transfer of antibiotics, it is necessary to discuss the role of plasma proteins as they represent ligands for antimicrobial agents. The relevance of protein binding and the clinical importance of antibiotic tissue levels are frequently alluded to by pharmacologists as well as physicians involved in the therapy of infectious diseases. The role of protein binding in the determination of tissue concentrations and the direct chemotherapeutic properties of the agent have been incompletely evaluated. *Protein binding* can be defined as the rapid and reversible affinity of a drug by ionic bonding with protein. Albumin is the predominant protein involved in this process. The binding affinities and number of binding sites on various proteins for a given antibiotic undoubtedly differ, but the influence of alterations in the total concentrations of specific proteins on the binding of drugs has not been completely evaluated. The degree to which an antibiotic can be bound, however, is affected by many factors. For example, when the concentration of a protein is reduced, the extent of binding is reduced. It is well recognized that drugs can compete for binding sites and result in the displacement of various compounds. The latter is exemplified by the increase of free bilirubin produced by sulfonamides and by this means exposes a fetus or neonate to the hazard of kernicterus.

As far as antimicrobial therapy is concerned, protein binding can have a direct effect on antimicrobial activity. The free drug concentrations in the blood, which is the unbound moiety, are more closely allied to drug effect than is the combination of bound and unbound concentrations. The latter is in accord with the fact that only the unbound antibiotic can act against bacteria. This implies that a compound that is 50 percent protein bound has one-half of the in vitro activity of a compound that is minimally bound. As only the free fraction can pass into the tissues, it is assumed that alterations in protein binding affect tissue distribution. This is an overexemplified view, as the tissues into which the antimicrobial agent diffuses also contain albumin and associated binding sites. Numerous experiments employing in vitro and mathematical models demonstrate differences in drug concentrations in extravascular compartments. They could be explained by the variation in protein binding of therapeutic agents. The degree of protein binding of drugs can vary from essentially no binding for antibiotics like amikacin or kanamycin to a high affinity in the case of dicloxacillin, ceftriaxone, and cefaperazone. Many different models have been used to investigate the penetration of antibiotics into the extravascular tissues and indirectly the effects of protein binding upon drug distribution. It is considered that the free concentration mediates a drug's pharmacologic activity. The total (bound plus free) drug concentration is measured when plasma levels are utilized in clinical practice for the adjustment of dosage. The relationship between the free and total drug concentration is normally consistent within individuals. The dislodgment of a compound from plasma protein by another can change the equilibrium between the free and total concentration and make interpretation more difficult. Under circumstances in which binding to a protein by a therapeutic agent is highly variable, estimation of the total drug levels may be deceptive, and serious underdosing or overdosing may ensue when such values are used as therapeutic guidelines.

In addition to binding reversibly to proteins, antibiotics are capable of binding to various tissue constituents. For example, the aminoglycosides bind to nucleic acids and liposomes, and many penicillins bind to hemoglobins and fatty acids. The clinical relevance of such observations is poorly understood. The affinity of aminoglycosides for liposomes in the renal tubular cells and their subsequent destruction are considered to be of importance in the evolution of the nephrotoxicity associated with this particular group of antibiotics. The whole problem is not quite as simple as originally believed because the degree of uptake from the tubular lumen to the cell does not equate with toxicity, as netilmicin has a greater uptake than gentamicin yet is less nephrotoxic. These factors must always be considered in addition to the changes in the plasma binding of drugs in pregnancy in order to define the effect of pregnancy on drug distribution, placental transfer, and potential danger to the fetus.

Placenta

The placenta has a multiplicity of functions, and consequently there is no simple way of assessing its total activity. In all probability, there is no other tissue involved in so many diverse biologic processes. It is derived from the chorion frondosum and the decidua basalis. Consequently, the placental trophoblastic tissue is unique in that it comprises the junction between two genetically dissimilar organisms. It is the interface between mother and fetus, and its maternal surface is the site of important transport mechanisms. The placental participation in a variety of cytochemical processes betokens the complexity and diversity of its activity. The maternal aspect of the syncytiotrophoblast is composed of an intricate system of functional units.

Early Gestation

The earlier view that the placenta was merely a sieve for the exchange of nutrients and certain metabolites between the mother and fetus was too facile. The circulation of maternal and fetal blood through the placenta is finely attuned to allow for the efficient transmission of nutrients for the sustenance of the developing conceptus. The fluctuations in the maternal and fetal circulations do not, however, compromise the economy of either party. After the third week of gestation, the development and vascularization of the chorionic villi and the enlargement of the uterine vessels and their apposition to the fetal villi permit diffusion of compounds from the maternal to the fetal circulation. By the end of the first trimester, intercellular pores are apparent, and they permit the transmission of relatively large lipophilic and hydrophilic molecules. The progressive vascularization and attenuation of the interface between mother and fetus that occurs increase the available membranous area and consequently decrease the distance required for the diffusion of compounds. The hemochorial placenta as exhibited in humans has always been regarded as the form of chorioallantoic placenta that is in closest proximity to the fetal vasculature because the trophoblast is in direct contact with maternal blood.

Late Gestation

The human placenta increases in weight during pregnancy, although the rate is reduced in the latter weeks. Placental development and growth necessitate a stage of active cell replication followed by minimal cell division accompanied by an increase in protoplasmic mass and cellular size. The hyperplastic growth phase of the human placenta is complete by the thirty-sixth week of gestation. The morphologic changes involve continuous proliferation of the chorionic villi and an expansion of the fetomaternal interface, which in late pregnancy is approximately 12 square meters. As pregnancy progresses, marked functional alterations take place in the placenta, as evidenced by its competency to transfer nutrients and other compounds to the fetal compartment. Throughout pregnancy the placenta retains the capacity for selective permeability for the transmission of compounds between mother and fetus.

Regardless of the physical nature and transfer rate of any drug through the placenta, transmission is governed by the concentration gradient that exists across the cell membranes and the interaction between the solute and ligand as it moves from plasma water through the placenta.

Pathology

Pathologic changes in the placenta, as seen in association with essential hypertension, diabetes mellitus, or pregnancy-induced hypertension, may affect placental permeability. Placental transmission of drugs may be modified by abnormalities of the umbilical cord such as absence of one umbilical artery or a velamentous insertion.

Pharmacokinetics

Structurally, antibiotics fall into several distinct chemical classes. Although characteristics peculiar to antimicrobial agents allow for their measurement by discrete chemical and bioassay techniques, one should be acquainted with the fact that the various chemical classes include amino acids, polypeptides, and glycosides. Furthermore, all solutes traverse multicellular membranes through aqueous channels and/or the plasma component of the cellular layer.

Pharmacokinetics have frequently been applied to the study of antibiotics. The ultimate value of pharmacokinetics to the patient is data useful for individualizing the dosage. Such information can readily be derived from animals and nongravid humans and is necessary for dosage selection to treat an infection. Such data can be beneficial in dosage selection as in vitro assays of bacterial susceptibility furnish only an approximate level for effective therapy, and pharmocokinetic data permit the calculation of the dosage required to attain an efficacious concentration.

Whereas the physiologic changes that accompany pregnancy must alter the value of certain pharmacokinetic parameters of drug disposition, the magnitude of the differences that may be observed in the gravid compared to nongravid women remains to be established. The difficulties of obtaining such data for gravid patients is due to the fact that such studies must obviously be quite limited and confined to agents for which there is a clinical need, so that standardization of conditions is infrequently attained. In addition, there are difficulties in obtaining corresponding data from an adequately matched group of nonpregnant females for comparison.

Drug Distribution

Most of the data available relate to studies conducted either in the last weeks of pregnancy, during labor, or at delivery. In general, drug transference from one compartment to another can be elucidated by first-order kinetics, as, for example, the rate of drug transfer from the plasma to the urine is directly proportional to the plasma drug concentration. The specific rate constant is generally the proportional constant between the transfer rate and plasma drug concentration. Drug distribution, which implies transference of the compound to extravascular fluids, is often a rapid process with a relatively large constant. The volume of distribution in single-compartment pharmacokinetics may be calculated by dividing the dose by the peak serum concentration attained after a single intravenous bolus. As a result, an alteration in the volume of distribution affects the peak serum concentration after a given dose. Furthermore, the volume of distribution has a direct effect on the half-life of a drug, which is the time required to reduce the drug concentration by one-half.

Intravenous Administration

In the nongravid patient, many therapeutic agents are rapidly distributed following intravenous administration; consequently, only elimination processes require consideration in delineating the alteration in body fluid of plasma drug concentrations as a function of time. After a fixed dose has been administered, the time course of an agent in the plasma may vary markedly among individuals. This applies to both gravid and nongravid subjects. The variability subsequent to the intravenous administration of a drug is caused by differences among patients as well as the apparent volume of distribution and half-life of the drug. The basis of the difference among individuals may be genetic in origin or related to disease entities.

Oral Administration

The variability may be more pronounced after oral administration, as the absorption rate of a drug from the gastrointestinal tract varies with the rate of gastric emptying and the time of drug administration in relationship to meals, formulation, and dosage. In the nongravid subject, drugs are on occasion incompletely absorbed after oral administration, and this may be increased in gravid patients because of decreased gastric motility. The delayed gastric emptying time in pregnancy could be responsible for a reduction in a drug's therapeutic efficacy as well as serum concentration. Oral drug therapy in pregnancy may be adversely affected on account of nausea and vomiting, which are frequently associated with the gravid state and in turn predispose to patient noncompliance. Philipson[27] compared the serum levels of ampicillin in the same patients during and subsequent to pregnancy after oral and intravenous administration of the antibiotic. It is obvious from such comparative studies that the optimal data are those derived from women who are their own nonpregnant controls. These studies showed that the mean plasma levels of ampicillin, whether administered by mouth or systemically, were significantly lower during pregnancy than in the nongravid state. Other studies have revealed that the oral administration of erythromycin to pregnant women resulted in reduced serum concentrations in comparison with those found in nonpregnant subjects.[29]

Fetal Pharmacokinetics

It is difficult to elucidate the pharmacokinetics of the human fetus, as it is not feasible to obtain sequential serum drug concentrations simultaneously in mother and fetus over a prolonged period of time. By the use of a series of different patients who receive an antibiotic at various time intervals prior to delivery, one can acquire a fetal blood sample from each infant at birth and achieve a pharmacokinetic analysis. Despite such studies, the information is suspect as many involve few patients and frequently the conclusions are derived without due consideration of the time interval between the administration of the antibiotic to the parturient and collection of maternal and fetal blood samples. Moreover, fetal concentrations of a therapeutic agent when derived from umbilical cord blood analyses do not depict the true levels in either the fetal vascular or extravascular compartments. Very few studies have considered placental size relative to that of the fetus in dynamic studies of maternal-fetal drug relationships, although the effect of placental tissue volume on the time constant for equilibration is small in late pregnancy because of disparity in size between placenta and fetus. The effects of changes in maternal-placental and fetal-placental blood flow are, however, relatively greater during the latter weeks of pregnancy than in the second trimester. The significance of maternal blood flow has not been taken into account in studies involving the placental transfer of drugs during parturition. The maternal blood flow into the intervillous space is modified by alterations in intrauterine pressure on account of myometrial activity, and this requires due note in studies conducted in parturients. Similarly, the process of drug equilibration in the mature fetus can be derived only by determination of both the umbilical arterial and venous drug concentrations. The venous value reflects the concentrations in the fetal vascular or tissue compartments. Urine samples collected from infants at birth in conjunction with serum data would enable one to calculate the biologic half-life, the apparent volume of distribution, and the urinary clearance of an antimicrobial agent in the term fetus. Such data would permit comparison of compounds with similar therapeutic properties with respect to their time course in the fetus. Furthermore, it is possible to analyze at the same time the rate of drug elimination by the mother and compare it with that of the fetus. From such quantifiable pharmacokinetic parameters, it should be possible to design dosage regimens of therapeutic agents for the gravid patient and decrease the risks of fetal toxicity. At a more fundamental level, it is recognized that the interactions among antibiotic, pathogenic organism, and host are complex, and a comprehensive approach to this problem necessitates detailed evaluation of the individual components of the chain of events. Such studies during pregnancy are difficult because of the complex of physiologic changes in the material organism and those evolving in the conceptus, as well as the predicament of acquiring appropriate samples for analysis.

Calculation of Dosage

Because of the limited value of the information obtained from a single-dose regimen in respect of placental transfer, studies have been carried out during labor utilizing a continuous infusion technique for antibiotic administration subsequent to an initial loading dose. The justification for this approach is the assumption that when a drug is administered by continuous infusion, the serum concentration gradually increases with time until a steady-state concentration is attained. The steady-state concentration *(C)* is considered to be proportional to the dose of the drug delivered over a specific period of time *(D/t)* and inversely proportional to the volume *(V)* of distribution and the overall elimination constant *(k)* for the drug. The latter can be expressed in the following manner:

$$C = \frac{D/t}{kV}$$

By utilizing the values of serum half-life and distribution volume available in the literature for a specific antibiotic, a dosage schedule can be computed so that a steady state can be attained. A bolus dose *(B)* can be equated with this formula so that:

$$B = \frac{D/t}{k}$$

By utilizing this formulation, the steady-state concentration in the maternal serum for various antimicrobial agents is below the predicted value. A rapid increase in fetal serum and amniotic fluid concentrations has been observed, but they fail to correlate with the maximum and minimum maternal serum levels. A positive correlation is noted, however, between the cord serum and amniotic fluid concentrations.

Drug Equilibration in Fetus

In any discussion pertaining to the assessment of drug equilibration in the fetal circulation, one must take into account the distribution differences of the therapeutic agent between the amniotic fluid and the fetal gastrointestinal tract. The fetal and placental tissues are not homogeneous, and, as has already been mentioned, drug equilibration in the fetus is not a simple exponential function of time. It is thus obvious that antibiotic distribution and disposition in the maternal and fetal compartments reflect a complex integrated series of pharmacodynamic processes. The two systems are interdependent, and consequently multiple kinetic events occur simultaneously.[4]

Reduction in Half-Life

Cummings, in a review of published results of pharmacokinetic studies conducted in pregnant and nonpregnant women, was unable to note any overall trend in the parameters listed. Furthermore, he failed to elicit any generally applicable alterations in the disposition of the drugs as a result of pregnancy.[8] Philipson has, however, noted a reduced half-life for a number of antibiotics during pregnancy.[28] It is suggested that drugs with reduced half-lives in pregnancy are those agents that normally have rapid rates of excretion, minimal metabolism, and direct renal excretion, as exemplified by ampicillin. Likewise, Philipson and Stiernstedt attributed the lower plasma concentrations of cefuroxime in pregnancy to increased renal clearance.[30]

Variables Affecting Placental Transfer

At present our knowledge of placental transfer is grossly inadequate, particularly with regard to quantitative kinetic data that would permit calculation of transfer rates. The latter specifically applies to detailed systemic measurements made at various stages of pregnancy because it is well recognized that the tissue layers interposed between the fetal capillaries and maternal blood become progressively reduced as the gestation proceeds. The amount and time course of fetal absorption of antibiotics are difficult to predict because of the many variables that can affect placental transmission of the agents. The time course of maternal antibiotic concentration and subsequent transfer to the fetal compartment depends on the antibiotic dosage prescribed. Both the amplitude and duration of maternal serum levels affect the amount of antibiotic transmitted. The amount of drug reaching the placenta is increased in women with impaired urinary output, and excess dosage in patients with no impairment of renal funtion likewise results in increased drug transfer to the fetus. The antibiotic concentrations in the fetus, especially for those agents with only a narrow range between the therapeutic and toxic levels, are unavailable. Peak levels, in addition to the duration they are maintained in the fetal compartment, are important when one considers agents such as some of the aminoglycosides that have the potential to be nephrotoxic and ototoxic. The amount of data available is small and often merely deals with a few subjects. Furthermore, there are some anomalous or ambiguous results in the literature stemming from inappropriate pharmacokinetic calculations, wide-ranging values in healthy nongravid controls, or the utilization of data from inappropriately chosen controls.[5]

Crossover Studies

Philipson indicated that the optimal method of procuring pharmacokinetic parameters of an antibiotic in pregnancy is by the utilization of crossover studies, with every woman acting as her own nonpregnant control.[27] This investigator has used this approach as the prototype to study the pharmacokinetics of ampicillin[27] and cefuroxime,[30] as well as cephadrine and cefazolin.[31] In all instances the plasma antibiotic concentrations were lower in pregnancy than in the nongravid state. The majority of studies do not utilize this model approach, and consequently there are many discrepancies in the literature pertaining to pharmacokinetic studies in pregnancy.[5,26]

Use of In Vitro Placental Perfusion

Because of the difficulties already alluded to regarding placental transfer studies in women, it is not surprising to note than an in vitro perfusion system has been utilized for this purpose. Placentas obtained immediately on completion of the third stage of labor are used. An appropriate placental lobule is selected, and independent maternal and fetal circulations established. The perfusates for such studies are composed of Earle's buffered salt solution supplemented with glucose and a mixture of amino acids in physiologic concentrations. The technique and instrumentation have been utilized for numerous placental transfer studies.[35,36] The transfer rates across the placenta are most accurately quantitated when neither perfusate is recirculated because by such a step a constant level of substrate can be maintained in the donor circulation with minimal backflow from the recipient circulation.

By the use of this experimental model, it has been shown that cefoperazone and sulbactam, a beta-lactamase inhibitor, readily traverse the placenta by simple diffusion.[14] The studies failed to demonstrate any active transport mechanisms for these compounds. These investigators had previously reported that higher concentrations of ceftizoxime were achieved in cord blood and amniotic fluid than in the maternal blood after the parturient had received 2 g of the antibiotic every 8 hours for more than three doses.[16] In view of these findings they utilized the in vitro perfusion system to compare the placental transfer of ceftizoxime with cefoperazone.[15] They demonstrated that ceftizoxime had a transfer rate superior to cefoperazone. Such studies indicate that different antimicrobial agents of the same family may show marked disparity in respect to placental transmission.

Similar studies have demonstrated that azidothymidine (AZT), a nucleoside analogue used as an antiviral agent in the therapy of the acquired immunodeficiency syndrome (AIDS), is readily transmitted across the placenta by an energy-dependent transport mechanism.[22] This observation is endorsed by the fact that dipyridamole, which inhibits nucleoside transport, when added to the perfusate on the maternal aspect of the placental cotyledon results in a reduction in AZT transfer. Little and associates[23] reported that in the rat AZT rapidly traverses the placenta and appears to be concentrated in the fetoplacental compartment. They consider that the significant levels attained in the fetal compartment could be ascribed to fetal hepatic immaturity or that the drug is actively transported to the fetal compartment. From their studies they concluded that the teratogenic propensity of this compound in rats born after exposure to several times the usual human dose is small. Shepard [37] has, however, found that rodent animal models are unsatisfactory for predicting the potential of a drug to be teratogenic in humans.

In Vitro Studies of Antiviral Agents

Watts and associates,[38] in a report of three gravid patients who received AZT 200 mg orally every 4 hours in the second half of their pregnancies, noted no persistent adverse effects of the therapy in the women or their babies.

Umbilical cord serum levels of AZT ranged from 113 percent to 127 percent of the maternal levels. Amniotic fluid levels of AZT were several times higher than simultaneous umbilical cord serum levels, which indicates that the fetal kidneys are capable of excreting the drug. The elimination half-life of AZT in the infants was 9 to 18 times that in the mothers. These investigators underscore the fact that the impact of the longer elimination half-life and high amniotic fluid levels of the drug on perinatal transmission is unknown. Larger studies are therefore required to establish the safety, efficacy, and dosage regimens of AZT in the gravid patient.

Studies have been conducted using the in vitro perfusion system to ascertain whether pentamidine isethionate can be transferred from mother to fetus.[13] This therapeutic agent is used in the therapy of *Pneumocystis carinii* pneumonia, which is the most common major opportunistic infection in AIDS patients and may be the presenting problem in such patients. Such patients often demonstrate adverse reactions to drugs. Approximately 60 percent of AIDS patients treated with trimethoprim-sulfamethoxazole (TMP-SMX) for this infection develop a rash, leukopenia, or some other adverse effect. For such individuals pentamidine therapy is prescribed because of the critical status of these patients, despite the fact that this drug causes hypoglycemia, hyperglycemia, and nephrotoxicity. Studies with the in vitro perfusion model show that significant concentrations of the drug are present in the placenta, but minimal transfer occurs from the maternal to fetal side. Despite a paucity of available data on the effects of this drug on the fetus, the in vitro studies imply minimal fetal exposure.

Chow and Jewesson,[6] in their review of the pharmacokinetics and safety of antimicrobial agents in pregnancy, emphasized that data on these topics were sparse and all such compounds should be critically evaluated for potential teratogenicity. In this respect it is well to remember that work of Paul Ehrlich, the father of modern chemotherapy. He thought of chemotherapeutic agents in terms of their ability to react with chemoreceptors on or in the pathogenic organism. Ehrlich concentrated on changing the structure of toxic compounds to avoid damage to the cells of the host and thereby achieve a favorable therapeutic index. Such concepts are essential in circumventing any potential damage to the intrauterine patient.

Discrepancies in Pharmacokinetic Studies

In reviewing the recent literature on antibiotic concentrations in amniotic fluid, cord blood, and placental membranes, one finds a marked variation in antibiotic dosage as well as in patient selection. Some studies involve patients who are receiving therapy for intrapartum infections; others use patients who are prescribed antibiotic therapy subsequent to premature rupture of the membranes. The majority of the studies involve only a limited number of observations, but all confirm placental transfer to the fetus of the antibiotics prescribed. Data pertaining to maternal and fetal serum and amniotic fluid concentrations of various antibiotics have been adequately documented in recent reviews.[5,26] They underscore discrepancies in the interpretation of the data. Even when the same antibiotic has been utilized, inconsistant maternal serum concentrations have been reported. Bergogne-Berenzine and associates[1] found that the level of cefuroxime after intramuscular administration of the compound in a dosage of 750 mg to be lower in the maternal serum than in nongravid subjects. The serum antibiotic concentration was measured by a microbiologic agar diffusion method. Craft and colleagues,[7] utilizing similar methodology and an identical dosage for cefuroxime, reported that the serum levels and half-lives attained in their patients were comparable with the normal range for the nongravid patient.[1] Philipson and Stiernstedt[30] reported a crossover study in which seven women were given an intravenous injection of 750 mg of cefuroxime during pregnancy and again several months postpartum and discovered that the plasma concentrations were significantly reduced in pregnancy. They attributed the lower plasma levels to an increase in renal clearance, which is in accord with their finding that the recovery of the antibiotic in the urine and its clearance were significantly higher in the gravid state. These investigators also reported that the pharmacokinetic data obtained at parturition and late pregnancy differed from those observed in the first half of pregnancy. They concluded that values obtained at parturition may not be representative of pregnancy per se. These studies stress the importance of well-designed pharmacokinetic investigations in the evaluation of antibiotics in the gravid patient.

It has been established that the variability in serum erythromycin levels is greater in gravid women than in nonpregnant women or males. The mean and peak serum concentrations of erythromycin were unrelated to age, weight, or duration of pregnancy.[29] When the major phase of drug absorption and distribution has equilibrated, the serum concentration is presumed to reflect the drug level at its site of action in the tissues. Erythromycin was the antibiotic of choice for the treatment of syphilis in gravid women who are allergic to penicillin. The marked patient-to-patient variation in maternal serum concentration of erythromycin after oral administration would account for infants born with the stigmata of congenital syphilis whose mothers who had received erythromycin therapy during pregnancy.

Risks of Adverse Effects on Fetus

In some sections of the community, not only is AIDS encountered in the gravid patient but also there is a recrudescence of tuberculosis. The indications for chemotherapy and the management of the pregnant woman with tuberculosis do not differ from those prescribed for the nonpregnant patient. Treatment should be initiated with two agents prescribed at standard dosage, and the duration of therapy should not be modified on account of the gravid status of the patient. Six of the chemotherapeutic agents used in tuberculosis therapy have been shown to be transmitted across the placenta. The drugs with documented transplacental passage are isoniazid, rifampin, ethambutol, cycloserine, kanamycin, and streptomycin. The most appropriate therapy if the disease is not extensive is the combination of isoniazid and ethambutol. Both these agents attain comparable blood levels in the mother and fetus. If a third agent is required during the second half of pregnancy because of extensive or severe disease, rifampin can be prescribed. Fetal concentrations attained are only 20 to 30 percent of the maternal levels. Streptomycin ototoxicity appears to affect a relatively large number of fetuses exposed, and approximately one in six have a degree of vestibular defects or impaired hearing.[20] Consequently, this aminoglycoside should not be used in pregnancy. There is no available data pertaining to the placental transfer of the other agents used in the treatment of tuberculosis. The gastrointestinal side effects of para-aminosalicylic acid and the central nervous system effects of cycloserine make their use in pregnancy undesirable. Little is known about the use of pyrazinamide, capreomycin, viomycin, or thiacetazone in pregnancy. A teratogenic propensity has been attributed to ethionamide, and therefore use of this agent is proscribed in pregnancy.[21]

Studies of Drug Safety in Pregnancy

The benefits of any pharmacologic agent prescribed in pregnancy must be carefully assessed before the fetus is exposed to any inherent risks associated with such therapeutic measures. The ever-increasing knowledge of the clinical effects of drugs used in pregnancy on the fetus and neonate demands that any such use be positively justified by clearly identified benefits that outweigh the risks. Of paramount importance to the study of drug safety in pregnancy is the ability to define and record maternal drug usage. Documented drug exposure of the fetus has increased during the past 25 years. The average number of drugs ingested in pregnancy in the 1960s, according to Forfar and Nelson,[12] was 4; in the 1970s, according to Doering and Stewart,[9] the number stood at 11. The latter investigators did a careful study of a large series of patients and discovered that some of the women had ingested more than 20 different pharmacologically active agents. More than 80 percent of the drugs had not been prescribed for the particular patients. Consequently, it must be pointed out that mere reliance on chart reviews or pharmacy data may miss a great many instances of drug exposure. Thousands of fetuses each year are exposed to a complex assortment of drugs that vary in their propensity to produce adverse reactions. Therefore, in many instances assignment of a cause-effect relationship between an adverse fetal effect and drug exposure is impossible. The most comprehensive approach is through the utilization of prospective data collection techniques. Few studies have been concerned with the epidemiology of antibiotic usage in pregnancy. For the majority of antimicrobial agents, there is insufficient information concerning risks to the fetus from administration of drugs to gravid patients. This lack of information cannot be construed to imply that a specific agent is harmful or that it is safe. Stated simply, the information is just not available. No antimicrobial agent currently available has to date been positively implicated as a teratogen in humans.

Future

The only way to achieve a correct approach in every individual obstetric patient is by therapeutic drug monitoring. Such a measure should not be regarded as experimentation but considered an integral part of the therapeutic intervention. Only by such an undertaking will we be able to circumvent therapeutic failures, eschew iatrogenic disease in the intrauterine patient, and depart from empiricism in the direction of precise tabulation of pharmacologic and clinicopharmacologic effects.

References

1. Bergogne-Berezine E, Pierre J, Even P, et al. Placental transfer of cefuroxime in late pregnancy. Future Trends in Chemotherapy 1981; 4:215–219.
2. Bobitt JR, Hayslipp CC, Damato JD. Amniotic fluid infection as determined by trans-abdominal amniocentesis in patients with intact membranes in premature labor. Am J Obstet Gynecol 1981; 140:947–951.
3. Bobitt JR, Ledger WJ. Amniotic fluid analysis: its role in maternal and neonatal infection. Obstet Gynecol 1978; 51:56–62.
4. Charles D. Placental transmission of antibiotics. Obstetrics and Gynecology Annual 1979; 8:19–86.
5. Charles D, Larsen B. Placental transfer of antibiotics in antimicrobial therapy. In: Rustuccia AM, Cunha BA, eds. Antimicrobial Therapy New York: Raven Press, 1984:519–533.
6. Chow AW, Jewesson PJ. Pharmacokinetics and safety of antimicrobial agents during pregnancy. Rev Infect Dis 1985; 7:287–313.
7. Craft I, Hullinger BM, Kennedy MRK. Placental transfer of cefuroxime. Br J Obstet Gynaecol 1981; 88:141–145.
8. Cummings AJ. A survey of pharmacokinetic data from pregnant women. Clin Pharmacokinet 1983; 8:344–354.
9. Doering PL, Stewart RB. The extent and character of drug consumption during pregnancy. JAMA 1978; 239:843–846.
10. Eastman NJ. Prematurity from the viewpoint of the obstetrician. Am Pract Dig Treat 1947; 1:343–352.
11. Eschenbach DA, Davick PAR, Williams BL, et al. Prevalence of hydrogen peroxide–producing *Lactobacillus* species in normal women and women with bacterial vaginosis. J Clin Microbiol 1989; 27:251–256.
12. Forfar JO, Nelson MM. Epidemiology of drugs taken by pregnant women: drugs that may affect the fetus adversely. Clin Pharmacol Ther 1973; 14:632–642.
13. Fortunato SJ, Bawdon RE. Determination of pentamine transfer in the in vitro perfused human cotyledon with high-performance liquid chromatography. Am J Obstet Gynecol 1989; 160:759–761.
14. Fortunato SJ, Bawdon RE, Baum M. Placental transfer of cefoperazone and sulbactam in the isolated in vitro perfused human placenta. Am J Obstet Gynecol 1988; 159:1002–1006.
15. Fortunato SJ, Bawdon RE, Maberry MC, Swan KF. Transfer of ceftizoxime surpasses that of cefoperazone by the isolated human placenta perfused in vitro. Obstet Gynecol 1990; 75:830–833.
16. Fortunato SJ, Bawdon RE, Welt SI, Swan KF. Steady-state cord and amniotic fluid ceftizoxime levels continuously surpass maternal levels. Am J Obstet Gynecol 1988; 159:570–573.
17. Gibbs RS, Dinsmoor MJ, Newton ER, Ramamurthy RS. A randomized trial of intrapartum versus immediate postpartum treatment of women with intra-amniotic infection. Obstet Gynecol 1988; 72:823–828.

18. Gravett MG, Nelson HP, DeRouen TA, et al. Independent association of bacterial vaginosis and *Chlamydia trachomatis* infection with adverse pregnancy outcome. JAMA 1986; 256:1899–1903.
19. Hillier SL, Martius J, Krohn M, et al. A case-control study of chorioamnionic infection and histologic chorioamnionitis in pregnancy. N Engl J Med 1988; 319:972–978.
20. Holdiness MR. Transplacental pharmacokinetics of the antituberculosis drugs. Clin Pharmacokinet 1987; 13:125–129.
21. Holdiness MR. Teratology of the antituberculosis drugs: a review. Early Hum Dev 1987; 15:61–74.
22. Liebes L, Mendoza S, Wilson D, Dancis J. Transfer of zidovudine (AZT) by human placenta. J Infect Dis 1990; 161:203–207.
23. Little BB, Bawdon RE, Christmas JT, et al. Pharmacokinetics of azidothymidine during late pregnancy in Long-Evans rats. Am J Obstet Gynecol 1989; 161:732–734.
24. Martius J, Krohn MA, Hillier SL, et al. Relationships of vaginal *Lactobacillus* species, cervical *Chlamydia trachomatis*, and *bacterial vaginosis* to preterm delivery. Obstet Gynecol 1988; 71:89–95.
25. Naeye RL, Peters EC. Causes and consequences of premature rupture of the membranes. Lancet 1980; 1:192–194.
26. Nau H. Clinical pharmacokinetics in pregnancy and perinatology, 11 penicillins. Dev Pharmacol Ther 1987; 10:174–198.
27. Philipson A. Pharmacokinetics of ampicillin during pregnancy. J Infect Dis 1977; 136:370–376.
28. Philipson A. Pharmacokinetics in antibiotics in pregnancy and labour. Clin Pharmacokinet 1979; 4:297–309.
29. Philipson A, Sabath LD, Charles D. Erythromycin and clindamycin absorption and elimination in pregnant women. Clin Pharmacol Ther 1976; 19:68–77.
30. Philipson A, Stiernstedt G. Pharmacokinetics of cefuroxime in pregnancy. Am J Obstet Gynecol 1982; 142:823–828.
31. Philipson A, Stiernstedt G, Ehrnebo M. Comparison of the pharmacokinetics of cephadrine and cefazolin in pregnant and non-pregnant women. Clin Pharmacokinet 1987; 12:136–144.
32. Rabe LK, Winterscheid KK, Hillier SL. Association of viridans group streptococci from pregnant women with bacterial vaginosis and upper genital infection. J Clin Microbiol 1988; 26:1156–1160.
33. Romero R, Sirtori M, Oyarzun E, et al. Infection and labor: V. prevalence microbiology and clinical significance of intraamniotic infection in women with preterm labor and intact membranes. Am J Obstet Gynecol 1989; 161:817–824.
34. Russell P. Inflammatory lesions of the human placenta: I. clinical significance of acute chorioamnionitis. Am J Diag Gynecol Obstet 1979; 1:127–137.
35. Schneider H, Huch A. Dual in vitro perfusion of an isolated lobe of human placenta: method and instrumentation. Contr Gynecol Obstet 1985; 13:40–47.
36. Schneider H, Panigel M, Dancis J. Transfer across the perfused human placenta of antipyrine, sodium and leucine. Am J Obstet Gynecol 1972; 114:822–828.
37. Shepard TH. Human teratogenicity. Adv Pediatr 1986; 33:225–268.
38. Watts DH, Brown ZA, Tartaglione T, et al. Pharmacokinetic disposition of zidovudine during pregnancy. J Infect Dis 1991; 163:226–232.
39. Wood JR, Sweet RL, Catena A, et al. In vitro adherence of *Lactobacillus* species to vaginal epithelial cells. Am J Obstet Gynecol 1985; 153:740–743.

CHAPTER 26

Use and Abuse of Antibiotics in Obstetric Practice

William J. Ledger, M.D

Physicians usually elect a therapeutic strategy with antibiotics that falls between two extremes. One course is based on a reluctance to prescribe any antibiotics because of the dangers to the mother and the fetus. In many instances this is a real, not a theoretical concern. Pregnant women with pyelonephritis died of liver failure following excessive intravenous doses of tetracycline.[54] The mistaken hypothesis for this high intravenous dosage strategy was that if a good outcome could be achieved with normal doses of tetracycline, a higher rate of cure could be gained with higher doses. The deaths were the tragic result of this flawed logic. Physician concerns about the toxicity of antibiotics in pregnancy are not limited to the mother. Hyperbilirubinemia has been reported in the premature newborns of mothers who received a long-acting sulfa drug before delivery,[37] and staining of the teeth of newborns whose mothers received tetracycline during pregnancy has been noted.[33] Because of such reports, most obstetricians have eliminated members of these two families of antibiotics from their therapeutic planning. The resulting caution among physicians in the consideration of antibiotics for pregnant women is further reinforced by the FDA's insert labeling for antibiotics. Except for penicillin and erythromycin, antibiotic package inserts have the admonition that the safety of this drug for pregnant women has not been established. This labeling reinforces some physicians' reluctance to use antibiotics in pregnant women.

At the other extreme is the compunction felt by many obstetricians to prescribe antibiotics for most high-risk obstetric patients. As physicians do microbiologic screening for more and more organisms, they feel the pressure to eliminate the antepartum carriage of "pathogens" in the vagina and the bladder. They are single-minded in their belief that antibiotic interventions will prevent premature labor and premature rupture of membranes. Because prematurity accounts for most neonatal morbidity and mortality, their zeal to intervene is understandable. What is not clear is whether this therapeutic aggressiveness actually prevents premature labor. For most physicians, reality lies somewhere between these two extremes. Antibiotics should be prescribed in the antepartum period when there is a clear therapeutic indication.

Pregnant women who need antibiotics pose difficult therapeutic decisions for physicians. The potential toxicity of antibiotics for the mother and the fetus must be acknowledged. Just as important in the treatment strategy is the problem of antibiotic dosing for pregnant women. Lower serum levels of antibiotics are achieved in pregnant women, when compared to nonpregnant women of the same weight.[48] This lower maternal level occurs whether the antibiotics are given orally, intramuscularly, or intravenously. One factor in this observed result is related to maternal blood volume expansion during pregnancy. Another is the formation of a separate compartment, the placenta and the fetus, which draws off antibiotics from the maternal intravascular space. For the clinician, this diminished antibiotic level in the maternal serum is further reflected by lower levels of antibiotics in important tissue compartments. For the mother, this means lower antibiotic levels in the central nervous system than in the nonpregnant state; for the fetus, serum levels are usually lower than those recorded in the mother. Knowledge of the mean inhibitory concentration (MIC) of antibiotics for the organisms involved in the infection is another need of the clinician to determine the dosages needed. These are all-important considerations for the physician when antibiotics are prescribed for symptomatic pregnant women.

Classes of Antibiotics Available to Obstetricians

Penicillins

The penicillins are one of the two groups of antibiotics for which admonitions about the safety of these drugs for pregnant women are not carried on the drug insert. The other antibiotic so characterized is erythromycin.

Penicillins are a remarkably useful family of antibiotics for the obstetrician. They are usually well tolerated, and large doses can be prescribed for pregnant women if necessary. There is not a narrow range of therapeutic levels that are safe, as is true with other classes of antibiotics. In addition, they are "cidal" antibiotics, and modifications in structure have given them an increasingly broad spectrum of antibacterial activity. When penicillins were first introduced into clinical practice in the 1940s, their original target was the gram-positive aerobes. The emergence of resistance of the coagulase-positive staphylococci in the 1950s led to the development of semisynthetic penicillins, which again made this organism susceptible. Broader-spectrum penicillins introduced in the 1960s, 1970s, and 1980s have extended penicillin's coverage to gram-negative aerobes as well as gram-positive and gram-negative anaerobes and to *Chlamydia trachomatis*. The addition of a beta-lactamase inhibitor extends the spectrum of activity of these antibiotics. They are the family of antibiotics of choice for many of the infections seen in antepartum patients. The most serious shortcoming of this family of antibiotics is that some women are allergic to penicillin, but even these women have the option of desensitization if penicillin is the drug of choice, as it is in the case of syphilis.[9]

Erythromycin

Erythromycin is another antibiotic with no warning on the drug insert about its safety in pregnancy. Despite this benefit, it has limited usefulness for the obstetrician. It is not a well-tolerated oral antibiotic for a pregnant woman. Standard oral dosing produces abdominal bloating and gastrointestinal distress in many women. Although a safe antibiotic, it also achieves low blood levels in the fetus. Because of this shortcoming, it is no longer recommended as a treatment alternative for the pregnant woman who has syphilis.[9] It effectively treats maternal syphilis but does not always eliminate the spirochete from the fetus.

Cephalosporins

Although not recommended for use in pregnancy, the cephalosporins are widely used by obstetricians. They share with the penicillins low toxicity and a wide range of antibacterial activity. In some instances they have specific advantages over penicillin G, ampicillin, amoxicillin, carbenicillin, ticarcillin, mezlocillin, and piperacillin in the treatment of organisms, such as the coagulase-positive staphylococci, *Neisseria gonorrhoeae,* and *Klebsiella*. Patients allergic to penicillin can have a concomitant reaction to the cephalosporins, so there is a subpopulation of women who are not candidates for their prescription.

Aminoglycosides

Aminoglycosides have limited usefulness for the obstetrician. The major concern has been the toxicity of these drugs for the fetus, particularly eighth-nerve damage. This adverse fetal result has been reported with infrequent dosing with streptomycin for the long-term treatment of tuberculosis.[11] Obviously, this causes a reluctance to prescribe aminoglycosides in pregnancy. In addition, it is difficult to achieve therapeutic levels with standard doses of aminoglycosides; peak and trough levels often have to be measured to see if therapeutic doses have to be modified.[34] The main therapeutic usefulness of aminoglycosides is against gram-negative aerobes. Fortunately, most of these infections in pregnant women are limited to the urinary tract, and there are many alternative antibiotics for the treatment of urinary tract infections.

Aztreonam

Aztreonam is an antibiotic with an antibacterial spectrum similar to the aminoglycosides. It provides excellent coverage for gram-negative aerobes. The advantages over aminoglycosides are the lack of renal and eighth-cranial-nerve toxicity. Blood testing for antibiotic levels is not required. The biggest disadvantage is the expense of the drug. To date, studies of infection in pregnant women with this antibiotic have not been done.

Clindamycin

Clindamycin is an effective drug against anaerobes, and it also has activity against *C. trachomatis*. Despite this, it has limited usefulness for obstetricians. Anaerobic infections are uncommon in the antepartum course. The most frequent situation in which clindamycin is considered for antepartum treatment is the discovery of lower genital carriage of *C. trachomatis*. The two alternative antibiotics available are erythromycin and amoxicillin. Although the safety of this antibiotic in pregnancy has not been established, no adverse fetal effects have been reported to date. Diarrhea can occur when this antibiotic is prescribed. Pseudomembranous enterocolitis due to *Clostridium difficile* is a rare complication, but the presence of this toxin should be searched for in the woman with diarrhea.

Metronidazole

Metronidazole is an effective drug against anaerobes and the protozoan *Trichomonas vaginalis*. Anaerobic infections are uncommon during the antepartum period, but trichomonas vaginitis does occur with some frequency in pregnant women. This may have some significance for obstetricians in the future, for a higher incidence of preterm labor has been noted in patients with vaginal carriage of trichomonas.[26] There are concerns about the safety of metronidazole for pregnant women. It has a mutagenic effect on some strains of bacteria[62] and a carcinogenic effect in animals.[53] Despite this, no serious problems have been attributed to its use in pregnant women to date. I have prescribed this antibiotic for patients with symptomatic trichomonas vaginitis after the first trimester of pregnancy.

Quinolones

The quinolones have particularly good activity against gram-negative aerobes, and members of this family are active against *C. trachomatis*. The major problem with this antibiotic has been the prolongation of the half-life of caffeine in the blood stream when it has been used.[58] It can disturb the sleep patterns of unaware patients. Although the safety of this class of drugs has not been established for pregnant women, it is another option for a pregnant woman with a urinary tract infection or vaginal colonization with *C. trachomatis*.

Use and Misuse of Preventive Antibiotics for Asymptomatic Pregnant Women

I believe much of the infectious disease focus upon possible etiologies of premature labor has been misguided. There has been wave after wave of microbiologic observations that maternal carriage of organisms in the vagina or the urinary tract is associated with premature labor. In part, this scientific approach was dictated by the research technology available. Infectious disease investigators were able to use microbiologic techniques to isolate and identify organism colonization in the vagina or the bladder. They then determined that colonization was associated with an increased incidence of premature labor. A number of important questions have to be raised about the significance of this investigative approach. Is colonization by these organisms the cause of premature labor? If so, then antibiotic intervention that eliminates maternal carriage should have a beneficial effect. In fact, as we will note, in one example after another, the antibiotic strategies employed to date have not consistently improved pregnancy outcomes. Our information in this area is still incomplete. Perhaps some of the species of a particular isolate are more virulent than others so that colonization alone is not the key. It is also possible that individual host responses to these colonizing organisms varies from one pregnant woman to another and makes some women more likely to have preterm labor than others. Finally, and most appealing as a theory to me, the presence of these organisms may only be a marker for sexual activity, poverty, or age, which may be more important than colonization as a cause of premature labor and delivery. These questions remain unanswered at present. With this as a background, let us examine some of the colonization correlations and antibiotic treatment strategies to prevent premature labor.

Asymptomatic Bacteriuria

The concept of asymptomatic bacteriuria was an important infectious disease breakthrough of the 1950s. Its scientific basis was a statistical analysis of colony counts of clean voided urine samples. The studies demonstrated that a colony count of 10^5 or greater of a single species of bacteria per milliliter of urine correlated well with the presence of bacteria in the bladder. Because urine is a good culture medium, this technique required careful preparation by the patient to get a clean voided urine sample and immediate transport of the specimen by the physician to the laboratory, or, if this was not possible, storage in the refrigerator until the laboratory could process the specimen. An immediate and important impact on clinical practice was the realization that this technique eliminated the necessity for the use of a catheter in women for the diagnosis of urinary tract bacterial colonization and infection. There is a risk of subsequent infection when a catheter is used, so this was a beneficial diagnostic advance.

Widespread first-trimester transfer screening of pregnant women with this noninvasive diagnostic technique yielded an important correlation. Those women with asymptomatic bacteriuria were more likely to have premature labor and delivery.[45] This was an exciting finding that offered the hope that noninvasive screening followed by antibiotic intervention could improve perinatal mortality figures by reducing the frequency of premature labor. Unfortunately, the initial high hopes were dashed by the results of subsequent studies. Antibiotic intervention in these pregnant women with asymptomatic bacteriuria did not lower the incidence of premature labor.[20] Despite this, there are benefits to pregnant women for urine screening and antibiotic treatment for those with high colony counts. Women with asymptomatic bacteriuria in the first trimester have a higher than expected incidence of pyelonephritis later in pregnancy that can be reduced by antibiotic treatment before the patient is symptomatic to eliminate bacteriuria.[27] A number of antibiotics can be used. The most popular choices are oral penicillins, such as ampicillin 500 mg four times a day before meals for 10 days, or oral cephalosporins, such as cephalexin 500 mg four times a day before meals for 10 days. For the penicillin-allergic patient, nitrofurantoin (Macrodantin) 50 mg four times a day after meals for 10 days can be prescribed.

Mycoplasma

Mycoplasma became another important focus as a cause of premature labor in the 1950s and 1960s. Exciting early observations stirred interest in this as a possibility. The first was the discovery that maternal vaginal carriage of *Mycoplasma* identified a population with a higher than expected rate of prematurity, with a mean weight of the babies from this population of women significantly lower than controls.[41] Even more intriguing was an antibiotic intervention study of patients with asymptomatic bacteriuria.[20] Although the study showed no improvement in the prematurity rate with antibiotic treatment for asymptomatic bacteriuria, control patients without bacteriuria who received tetracycline, an antibiotic effective against *Mycoplasma,* had a lower incidence of prematurity.[20] Could it be that this resulted from the treatment of women who were asymptomatic vaginal carriers of *Mycoplasma?* There are a number of problems in the interpretation of the role of *Mycoplasma* in premature labor. Many more pregnant women are colonized with this organism than have premature babies. Studies have shown more than 50 percent of pregnant women colonized with one or more strains of *Mycoplasma* with no difference in the gestational ages of those women colonized and those who were not.[41] Although the use of erythromycin did improve some parameters of fetal outcome, many successfully treated patients remained culture positive for *Mycoplasma*. This lack of correlation with *Mycoplasma* carriage casts doubt on this hypothesis.[41] Further doubt comes from the discovery that antepartum culture for *Ureaplasma urealyticum* was not useful in predicting preterm labor or premature rupture of the membranes.[7]

Neisseria Gonorrhoeae

There are no controlled studies about the impact on prematurity of *Neisseria gonorrhoeae* colonization of the genital tract of pregnant women. This is understandable. Women with premature labor and premature rupture of the membranes have been noted to be culture positive for *Neisseria gonorrhoeae*.[21] How long these women have been colonized with this pathogen before the onset of symptoms is not known. Screening in the first trimester for this organism has always dictated treatment when the patient is culture positive because this is a known pathogen for men, women, and newborns. As a result, no untreated control group of pregnant women is available for evaluation. Because the eyes of the newborn can become infected during labor and delivery, this organism should be screened for in pregnancy and treatment initiated in those women who are culture positive. Over the years, penicillin has been the treatment of choice. In the past decade, particularly in urban centers, there has been a tremendous increase in the number of penicillin-resistant strains of *Neisseria gonorrhoeae*. Because of this, a cephalosporin is a better choice than penicillin. Some possible choices include cefoxitin or cefotetan 2 g intramuscularly plus 1 probenecid orally or ceftriaxone 250 mg intramuscularly.[10]

Chlamydia Trachomatis

Chlamydia trachomatis has been closely evaluated as a pathogen for pregnant women. Some clear correlations between maternal carriage and newborn infection have been noted. Newborns of pregnant women colonized with this organism are at greater risk for developing conjunctivitis and pneumonia.[59] In contrast, an association of *C. trachomatis* colonization and premature labor has not been established to my satisfaction. One early study showed this relationship,[39] but a subsequent study showed a correlation only with women who had IgM present to *C. trachomatis,* suggesting a recent infection with a systemic maternal response.[28] To date, there is no convincing evidence that early detection and treatment of women colonized with *C. trachomatis* decreases the prematurity rate.

These findings should guide antibiotic interventions for pregnant women. First-visit and third-trimester pregnancy screening for *C. trachomatis* is done by some American obstetricians and those women who are culture positive, are treated with either oral erythromycin or oral amoxicillin.[14] This is appropriate treatment for a sexually transmitted pathogen for men and women, but I do not believe this antibiotic intervention lowers the prematurity rate. I favor screening in the early third trimester for *C. trachomatis* with antepartum treatment because there have been failures of postpartum antibiotic ointment application on the newborn to prevent chlamydial conjunctivitis[14] and because *C. trachomatis* pneumonia can occur. The options for antepartum treatment are an oral erythromycin 500 mg four times a day for 10 days or oral amoxicillin 500 mg four times a day for 10 days. Unless the patient is allergic to penicillin, I favor the amoxicillin treatment, for it is better tolerated by pregnant women.

Group B Beta-Hemolytic Streptococcus

The group B beta-hemolytic streptococcus is an organism of great concern for the obstetrician. It can be a source of significant morbidity and mortality for newborns, and it is a frequent cause of difficulty. With an attack rate of two to four cases per 1,000 live births, it is a problem for obstetricians 20 times more frequent than the more familiar herpes, syphilis, and rubella.

As is the case with *C. trachomatis,* there are many unanswered questions about the group B streptococcus pathologic role in pregnancy. One study noted a correlation between first-trimester colonization and a subsequent increased incidence of premature rupture of membranes, premature labor, and delivery.[51] Although this correlation was noted, to date there have been no reports that first-trimester antibiotic treatment for vaginal group B streptococcal colonization has improved newborn outcomes. Maternal colonization with the group B beta-hemolytic streptococcus is high, more than 20 percent of some obstetric populations.[3] It is possible that maternal vaginal carriage is an insensitive marker for the risk of prematurity. Another study has suggested that colonization of the urinary tract is a more sensitive sign for the risk of prematurity.[44] Confirmation of the relationship of group B streptococcal colonization and pre-

Table 26-1 Clinical Characteristics of Group B Beta-Hemolytic Streptococcus Disease in the Newborn

Characteristics	Early Onset	Late Onset
Mean age of onset	20 hours	24 days
Incidence of prematurity	Increased	Not increased
Obstetric problems	Frequent (60%)	Uncommon
Common manifestations	Septicemia (30-40%) Meningitis (30%) Pneumonia (30-40%)	Meningitis (85%) Bacteremia without focus Bone or joint infection
Serotypes isolated	Ia, Ib, Ic 30% II 30% III (40% nonmeningeal; 80% meningeal isolates)	III 93%
Mortality rate	55%	23%

mature labor has been suggested by one study,[51] and we await the results of the NIH cooperative study of this. I am not convinced that early pregnancy screening and antepartum treatment of maternal colonization with this organism will lower the incidence of premature delivery.

The group B beta-hemolytic streptococcus does have a serious impact on the newborn. It is estimated that 12,000 to 15,000 newborn infants are infected each year in the United States. There is a clinical pattern to the disease seen in these babies. Group B streptococcus disease in the newborn is classified as early-onset and late-onset disease. The clinical and microbiologic characteristics are noted in Table 26-1.[4] As noted in the table, there are both a high mortality rate and residual morbidity in some of the survivors with meningitis who are successfully treated. This is a disease of vertical transmission; that is, the mother is colonized in the lower genital tract and the fetus becomes infected. The problem for the obstetrician is that many more pregnant women are colonized than there are newborns who become infected. The ratio of maternal colonization rate to newborn attack rate is 20:1 to 100:1.[2] In addition, there is evidence that treatment for the premature baby begun in the newborn period is ineffective in early-onset problems.[49] This spectrum of clinical difficulties makes it difficult to formulate an effective preventive therapeutic strategy.

To reduce morbidity and mortality due to the group B beta-hemolytic streptococcus, the focus has been on predelivery treatment of the mother. This timing has had better outcomes than treatment limited to the newborn.[6,43] Fortunately, the group B streptococcus remains very susceptible to penicillin. There are still many questions about the timing for screening and antibiotic intervention. Screening for vaginal colonization and antibiotic treatment has not been universally employed for two reasons: It has not been demonstrated to improve pregnancy outcome, and in many cases recolonization with the group B streptococcus occurs at the time of delivery.[24] Other alternatives for antepartum screening and treatment have more popularity. One championed by Boyer and Gotoff includes obtaining cultures of the vagina and rectum at 26 to 28 weeks using selective culture media. Culture-positive patients who subsequently present with premature labor or prolonged rupture of the membranes are given intrapartum ampicillin, 2 g intravenously, followed by 1 g every 4 hours until delivery.[6] An alternative approach has been suggested by Mead and Minkoff.[43] They advocate that a vaginal culture be obtained from women in premature labor or with premature rupture of the membranes, with ampicillin treatment given for those who are culture positive or who continue to labor with cervical dilation before laboratory results are available.[43] For those women who are penicillin allergic, intravenous erythromycin or clindamycin can be given. Neither of these strategies will eliminate all cases of newborn infection due to the group B beta-hemolytic streptococcus.

Bacterial Vaginosis

A new correlation between maternal colonization and prematurity is the increased rate of newborn problems in women with bacterial vaginosis. Bacterial vaginosis is an enigma to me. The name identifies a recognizable symptomatic clinical entity in women who complain of a foul-smelling vaginal discharge and who have no microscopic evidence of an inflammatory response, that is, few or no white blood cells, hence the term *vaginosis*, not *vaginitis*. A specific microbiologic pathogen is not known, although the symptoms are probably caused by an overgrowth of anaerobic bacteria. In addition to this confused microbiologic etiology, the clinical diagnosis is a soft measure, depending upon the presence of three or four of the following signs: (1) a homogeneous vaginal discharge, (2) an alkaline vaginal pH, (3) a "fishy" odor when a drop of vaginal secretions is added to 10 percent potassium hydroxide (KOH), and (4) more than 20 percent of the epithelial cells observed microscopically are stipled with bacteria (clue cells).[1] The next step of etiologic investigation has been to apply these criteria in a screening technique in pregnant women who have not volunteered any symptoms. In this setting, there has been a correlation with "bacterial vaginosis" and a higher incidence of premature rupture of the membranes and premature labor and delivery.[40] How well this will guide therapy is not known. One study of antibiotic intervention with amoxicillin did not eliminate vaginosis and did not reduce the prematurity rate.[16]

There are other correlations between microbiologic isolates and premature labor. These include *Trichomonas vaginalis*[26] and *Bacteroides* species.[32] No antibiotic intervention studies to see if there was an improvement in outcome have been reported to date.

Antibiotics for Pregnant Women with Infection

There is a belief among physicians that pregnant women are more susceptible to infection. Much of the evidence for this stems from studies in the preantibiotic era. It was observed that morbidity and mortality were higher in pregnant women with *Streptococcus pneumoniae* pneumonia.[23] This is not unexpected because the immune-suppressing mechanisms that allow a pregnant woman to maintain a foreign protein graft, the placenta and the fetus, would also be expected to diminish the pregnant woman's response to infecting pathogenic bacteria. Awareness of this possibility should be part of antibiotic planning when the physician prepares to treat infections in pregnant women.

Urinary Tract Infections

The most common site of infection in the antepartum period is the urinary tract. This is not unexpected. Women in the childbearing age group have a greater susceptibility to urinary tract infection, and pregnancy increases that risk. Urine is an excellent culture medium, and pregnancy is associated with more urinary collecting system stasis, as urine transit from the kidney to bladder slows, the renal collecting system dilates, and bladder capacity increases. Urinary tract infections are common clinical problems.

One major therapeutic focus has been prevention of pyelonephritis. There is solid evidence that antepartum screening for asymptomatic bacteriuria in the first trimester of pregnancy identifies a population at much higher risk to develop pyelonephritis later.[27] A population for preventive treatment is identified. There are many alternative antibiotic regimens that are effective for this task. The most popular is ampicillin or amoxicillin 500 mg orally four times a day before meals for 10 days. Other effective regimens particularly useful for the penicillin-allergic patient are nitrofurantoin (Macrodantin) 100 mg orally four times a day after meals for 10 days and ciprofloxacin 500 mg orally twice a day for 10 days. Although many obstetricians recoil from this, I have used sulfisoxazole (Gantrisin) 500 mg four times a day before meals for 10 days in pregnant women with asymptomatic bacteriuria, with the caveat to stop the medication if there is any suggestion of labor. All of the medications, with the exception of penicillin, are not advocated for use in pregnancy, but I believe they are safe for pregnant women for this preventive therapeutic study purpose.

Despite all of these preventive efforts, some pregnant women will present to the obstetrician with pyelonephritis. This is a common antepartum problem. Some experts estimate it occurs in 1 to 2 percent of antepartum patients.[15] In addition to being a frequent disorder, it can be serious. Bacteremia is a frequently associated phenomenon. Endotoxemia can also occur. Although sustained hypotension is rare, endotoxin-mediated problems that may be encountered include transient renal dysfunction, pulmonary injury (adult respiratory distress syndrome), and anemia.[13] Such patients can present serious therapeutic problems.

The diagnosis of pyelonephritis is usually not difficult for the obstetrician. These patients often present with flank pain, urinary frequency and dysuria, a fever, and nausea and vomiting. Costovertebral angle tenderness can be elicited easily, and a clean voided urine sample should be sent for culture to identify the organism and determine antibiotic susceptibilities.

Antibiotic selection is only one part of the treatment equation. These patients require adequate intravenous fluid hydration to make up for fluid losses associated with the fever and vomiting. In addition, they must be monitored closely to be sure there is no evidence of renal dysfunction or pulmonary distress.

The antibiotic of choice for pyelonephritis has been ampicillin or amoxicillin, given 1 g intravenously every 6 hours until the patient has been afebrile for at least 24 hours and is tolerating oral feedings, when either ampicillin or amoxicillin can be given orally four times a day before meals to complete 10 days of therapy. There is controversy about the care of these patients for the remainder of the pregnancy. I have been influenced by Harris and continue antibiotic prophylaxis with nitrofurantoin (Macrodantin) 100 mg daily for the rest of the pregnancy.[27] Investigators from the Los Angeles County–University of Southern California obstetric service disagree. They favor continued surveillance of these patients for bacteriuria, with antibiotic intervention if bacteriuria is detected, instead of prolonged antibiotic prophylaxis.[36] There is controversy about the use of a penicillin as initial treatment in these patients. One recent report analyzed the antibiotic susceptibilities of organisms isolated from patients with pyelonephritis.[18] There was a high incidence of resistance to ampicillin of the gram-negative organisms isolated from the urine of these pregnant women with pyelonephritis. This was a study with interesting findings. In contrast to an earlier surveillance study of obstetric infection, the incidence of resistance to ampicillin was much higher.[35] In addition, the treatment results with a cephalosporin were quite good. What is not known is the significance of the laboratory findings of resistance for the treatment of patients with pyelonephritis. Ampicillin is cleared through the urinary tract, and the concentration in the urine is many times greater than that achieved in the serum. Organisms resistant at serum levels can be susceptible at the high concentration achieved in the urine. The relative effectiveness of a penicillin versus a cephalosporin will only be established by a future prospective study. My own inclination for the initial selection of cephalosporins is related to the frequency of the recovery of *Klebsiella* on a particular service. If *Klebsiella* is frequently isolated, then cephalosporins are a good choice. Aminoglycosides are infrequently used in these patients. They are usually reserved for the critically ill patient with pyelonephritis who has hypotension, renal dysfunction, and adult respiratory distress syndrome[13] or for the patient who is allergic to penicillin. Aztreonam is perhaps a better choice in this clinical situation because of its lack of renal toxicity, although its safety in pregnancy has not been established.

Lower urinary tract infection, cystitis, follows none of the diagnostic rules for either asymptomatic bacteriuria or pyelonephritis. There is correlation between the finding of *Escherichia coli* in the bladder of symptomatic women, using suprapubic aspiration, with colony counts much lower than the 10^5 standard used for asymptomatic bacteriuria or pyelonephritis.[56] The clinician evaluating a patient with symptoms of cystitis should note on the laboratory request that any isolate of *E. coli* has significance and antibiotic susceptibility studies should be conducted. In addition, there is no evidence that first-trimester screening and treatment has any impact on the frequency of cystitis in pregnancy.[27] This observation is difficult to explain. Asymptomatic bacteriuria identifies women at risk for pyelonephritis but not cystitis. How is the bladder bypassed in these cases of upper urinary tract infection? These questions will be the subject of future investigations.

The treatment of women with cystitis is straightforward. They are usually not seriously ill and can be treated with an oral antibiotic as an outpatient. Some alternative regimens include ampicillin or amoxicillin 500 mg before meals for 10 days; cephalexin 500 mg four times a day before meals for 10 days; nitrofurantoin (Macrodantin) 100 mg twice daily afterwards for 10 days; ciprofloxacin 500 mg twice daily for 10 days; and sulfisoxizole 500 mg four times a day before meals for 10 days. A post-treatment culture should be obtained to be certain the bacteria have been cleared from the urinary tract. If *E. coli* was the initial isolate, any number of colonies of *E. coli* has significance.

Sexually Transmitted Diseases

Patients with urinary tract symptomatology of urgency, frequency, or burning can have urethritis instead of cystitis. Cultures for *N. gonorrhoeae* and *C. trachomatis* should be obtained in these women. If the culture is positive for *N. gonorrhoeae,* the treatment of choice is cefoxitin or cefotetan 2 g intramuscularly plus 1 g orally of probenecid or a single intramuscular injection of 250 mg of ceftriaxone.[10] If the culture is positive for *C. trachomatis,* the treatment of choice is amoxicillin 500 mg orally four times a day before meals for 10 days.[14] For the penicillin-allergic patients, erythromycin 500 mg orally before meals four times a day for 10 days can be given.

Syphilis is an uncommon but serious disease for the pregnant women and the fetus. Although rare, the frequency in the United States has increased in recent years, particularly in urban centers in New York, Florida, Texas, and California.[8] Most of these patients are asymptomatic, and the diagnosis is made by a positive screening antibody reagin test, confirmed by a specific antibody test for *Treponema pallidum.* This spirochete is very susceptible to penicillin and replicates slowly, approximately once a day. As a result, low doses of penicillin need to be maintained in the serum and at body sites for long periods of time. This is the rationale for the use of penicillin benzathine. The treatment is one intramuscular injection of 2.4 million units of penicillin benzathine if the disease has been acquired within the last year or three intramuscular injections of 2.4 million units of penicillin at weekly intervals if the infection was acquired more than 1 year ago at an unknown time.[9] There are concerns about this proposed therapy regimen. The low levels of penicillin benzathine may not be sufficient for the spirochete load in the body tissues of pregnant patients with secondary syphilis. A daily injection of procaine penicillin for 10 days could be a better choice for a long-term cure. In addition, a violent systemic response, the Herxheimer reaction, is frequently seen in pregnant women with either a chancre or secondary syphilis.[31] Uterine activity and fetal heart rate decelerations have been noted as well in these women. For this reason, I believe these antepartum patients should be admitted and hydrated with intravenous fluids, with the mother and fetus carefully monitored while receiving daily injections of procaine penicillin. Because erythromycin given to the pregnant women does not achieve high levels in the fetus, it is no longer recommended for treatment during pregnancy.[9] These patients should be desensitized and treated with penicillin.

Chorioamnionitis

The next most common antepartum infection problem facing the obstetrician is the patient who develops chorioamnionitis. There are two categories. Although most of these cases follow rupture of the membranes with no immediate odor, transplacental passage of bacteria secondary to maternal bacteremia has been noted, with the subsequent development of chorioamnionitis with intact membranes. This has been noted in patients with infections from the group B beta-hemolytic streptococcus,[19] *Listeria monocytogenes,*[47] and *Haemophilus influenzae.*[63] In these situations, an accurate microbiologic diagnosis is important to guide the selection of antibiotics. It can be secured by amniocentesis with Gram's stain and culture of the amniotic fluid. Although past teaching has been that the uterus should be emptied when chorioamnionitis has been diagnosed, there have been frequent instances of successful intravenous treatment with antibiotics without immediate delivery. The most recent example was successful intrauterine treatment of a patient with a *L. monocytogenes* infection.[29] Intravenous antibiotics treat the mother and cross the placenta to treat the fetus as well. For each of these organisms, the drug of choice is intravenous ampicillin 2 g four times a day. Some strains of *H. influenzae* are resistant to ampicillin.[55] This frequency of ampicillin resistance varies on a regional basis in the United States. If ampicillin resistance to *H. influenzae* is a problem, based on laboratory findings, then intravenous chloramphenicol can be prescribed, 1 g every 6 hours. If the patient with these infections is allergic to penicillin, a variety of alternative antibiotics can be given. Intravenous clindamycin 900 mg every 8 hours should be effective for the group B beta-hemolytic streptococcus and *L. monocytogenes.* Intravenous chloramphenicol can be given for the penicillin-allergic patient with a laboratory-confirmed *H. influenzae* infection.

The vast majority of patients developing chorioamnionitis are diagnosed following premature rupture of the membranes. Although the frequency of intrauterine infection increases with the length of time the membranes are ruptured, some cases of chorioamnionitis can be seen shortly after the membranes rupture.[42] Of those patients with premature rupture of membranes, more frequent infections are seen when this event occurs before the thirty-fourth week of pregnancy. There has been an increasing trend toward maintaining the pregnancy in these women. In those women with a preterm fetus, the hope is that more maturity for the newborn will be gained by more time in utero,[17] whereas there is increasing evidence that lack of intervention at term is associated with a good maternal and fetal outcome.[30] Following this strategy puts some women at risk for infection. There have been a number of attempts to identify early the small number of women who subsequently will develop chorioamnionitis. These efforts include measuring maternal C-reactive protein.[22] An elevated measure identifies a group at high risk to develop infection. Another study equated decreased amniotic fluid volume as determined by ultrasound examination with infection,[61] but the specificity of this relationship was challenged in a subsequent study.[25] Finally, transabdominal amniocentesis has been employed to obtain amniotic fluid,[64] but this process is impossible in women with little fluid who are a higher risk for infection. None of these screens is sensitive enough to ensure the identification of all patients at high risk for infection. The major therapeutic concerns of the obstetrician in these situations are the organisms that can cause newborn sepsis and death. These include the group B beta-hemolytic streptococcus, *E. coli, H. influenzae,* and *L. monocytogenes*. Prior to specific identification of the organism, the regimen of choice would be either ampicillin or amoxicillin given intravenously to the mother, 2 g every 6 hours until delivery. For the penicillin-allergic patient, a combination of clindamycin intravenously 900 mg every 8 hours and gentamicin 1.5 mg per kilogram every 8 hours provides good alternative coverage. If *H. influenzae* has been specifically identified in a penicillin-allergic woman, intravenous chloramphenicol 1 g intravenously every 6 hours can be given. In addition to this focus on the newborn, there is a risk of maternal infection after delivery that is further increased many times if a cesarean section is required.[60] Gram-negative anaerobes are important in these maternal infections; either intravenous cefoxitin 2 g every 8 hours, cefotetan 2 g every 12 hours, or the aforementioned combination of intravenous clindamycin and gentamicin can be prescribed. A similar strategy to treat maternal infections should be followed in those febrile patients with a pregnancy loss before 20 week's gestation.

Respiratory Tract Infections

Respiratory tract infections are frequently seen during pregnancy, particularly during the winter months. A sore throat or bronchitis is often seen. These women should have cultures obtained for the presence of a group A beta-hemolytic streptococcus. If the physician suspects a group A beta-hemolytic streptococcal infection because the patient is febrile with an inflammed oropharynx or if the culture is positive, then an oral penicillin, ampicillin 500 mg four times a day before meals, can be given. Pregnant outpatients receiving these drugs are at risk for developing *Candida albicans* vaginitis. They can be given vaginal antifungal treatment on a preventive base. The majority of pregnant women with an upper respiratory infection have no bacterial etiology. In this situation, it is appropriate to withhold antibiotics until a culture report demonstrates the presence of the group A beta-hemolytic streptococcus.

Pneumonia is an uncommon disease among pregnant women. In one review of an urban poor population of 89,219 women, 39 (.04 percent) were admitted to the hospital with a diagnosis of pneumonia.[5]

Despite the small number of pregnant women seen with this disease, it can be a serious problem. Death occurred in one-third of pregnant women with this respiratory disease in the preantibiotic era.[23] Death is a rarity today because of the availability of antibiotics and ventilatory aids, but many of these patients are seriously ill.

The choice of antibiotics is dependent upon the identification of the pathogen involved. Unlike soft-tissue pelvic infections, there is usually a single pathogen involved. Clinical and laboratory findings can be used to guide the choice of antibiotics. The most common cause of a community-acquired pneumonia in the winter months is *Streptococcus pneumoniae*. In the febrile patient with lobar consolidation on chest roentgenogram examination and gram-positive diplococci present on microscopic examination of the expectorate, confirms the diagnosis. Penicillin is the drug of choice for these women, 2 million units intravenously every 6 hours. For the penicillin-allergic patient, erythromycin is an alternative choice, 500 mg intravenously every 6 hours. Other organisms can be involved in these pneumonias. A group A beta-hemolytic streptococcus should be suspected if the patient has an associated empyema. Intravenous penicillin is the drug of choice. Pneumonia due to coagulase-positive staphylococci can occur as a complication of influenza.[52] This diagnosis should be considered in a woman with pneumonia when "flu" is a common clinical problem and clumps of gram-positive cocci are seen on microscopic examination of a Gram's stain of the expectorate. An intravenous first-generation cephalosporin should be prescribed, either cephalothin 2 g every 6 hours or cefazolin 2 g every 8 hours. If the patient is allergic to penicillin, intravenous vancomycin 0.5 g every 6 hours can be given. *Haemophilus influenzae* should be suspected if gram-negative rods are seen on Gram's stain. Intravenous ampicillin 2 g every 6 hours is the antibiotic of choice. Rarely, ampicillin-resistant *H. influenza* will be encountered.[55] If this occurs, intravenous chloramphenicol, 1 g every 6 hours can be given. There are other atypical pneumonias, less commonly seen, in which bacteria are not seen on Gram's stain of the expectorate. When this occurs, the differential diagnosis should include Legionnaires' disease and mycoplasma pneumonia. A polymerase chain reaction (PCR) test can be done on the expectorate to confirm the diagnosis of *Legionella;* cold agglutinins can be done on blood to confirm the diagnosis of *Mycoplasma*. The antibiotic of choice for both pathogens is intravenous erythromycin 500 mg every 6 hours. Finally, in an urban poor population, *Mycobacterium tuberculosis* and *Pneumocystis carinii* are possibilities. Tuberculosis should be strongly considered if apical changes are seen on roentgenogram examination. An expectorated specimen should be obtained for smear and culture. Combination antibiotic therapy with isoniazid and ethambutol should be given. If isoniazid is given, supplemental pyridoxine should be given. *Pneumocystis carinii* pneumonia should be part of the differential diagnosis in any woman with diffuse alveolar changes on roentgenogram and physical examination. The diagnosis can be confirmed by microscopic examination of a brochoscopic aspirate. The treatment of choice is the combination of trimethoprim and sulfamethoxazole. In each of the last two diagnoses, HIV testing should be offered to the patient.

Lyme Disease

Lyme disease has new relevance for obstetricians. It is a new disease, just described in 1975, and it is an increasing source of queries to obstetricians from patients who are afraid they have the disease or have been in areas where ticks are endemic. This is particularly true in the Northeast, the Midwest, and in the West, where the incidence of Lyme disease is higher than in other parts of the country.[57] The concerns arise from the fact that, in addition to maternal infection, transplacental infection can occur with intrauterine fetal death or subsequent impairment of newborn cerebral function.[38] Clinically the disease can be suspected if a red macule or papule appears at a site where a tick bite could occur and then spreads. Parallel with this the patient notes malaise, fatigue, headache, chills, and fever. Blood can be drawn for IgM antibodies and treatment begun with antibiotics. Because tetracycline is contraindicated for a pregnant woman, the antibiotic of choice is penicillin phenoxymethyl 500 mg four times a day orally for at least 10 days. For the penicillin-allergic patient, erythromycin 500 mg orally four times a day for at least 10 days can be prescribed. Patients should be treated for a longer period of time if symptoms persist.

Gastrointestinal Disease

The presence of the pregnant uterus and the lowered sensitivity of the peritoneum make it difficult to diagnose the site of infection in the gastrointestinal tract during pregnancy.

Acute cholecystitis is one of the more common gastrointestinal problems during pregnancy because of the increased frequency of gallstone formation. New imaging equipment makes the diagnosis much easier in the patient with nausea, vomiting, and right upper quadrant pain. The antibiotic of choice for these patients is either intravenous ampicillin 2 g every 6 hours or intravenous cefazolin 2 g every 8 hours. For the penicillin-allergic patient, intravenous erythromycin 500 mg every 6 hours can be given. Occasionally the imaging reveals a liver abscess, usually an amebic abscess that will respond to intravenous metronidazole 1 to 2 g every 12 hours.

Appendicitis is frequently missed in pregnancy because the women are often afebrile, without leukocytosis, and have right midquadrant rather than right lower quadrant tenderness.[50] Operative care is essential for cure, but antibiotics are an important adjuvant. Intravenous ampicillin 2 g every 6 hours or intravenous cefazolin 2 g every 8 hours usually suffices because the numbers of gram-negative anaerobes are usually not high in this site. For the penicillin-allergic patient, a combination of intravenous clindamycin 900 mg every 8 hours and gentamicin 1.5 mg per kilogram every 8 hours can be given.

Diarrhea is a common clinical problem for the obstetrician, but bacterial diarrhea is rare. Stool cultures should be obtained, particularly for the patient whose symptoms persist more than 24 hours. Some of the bacterial isolates that have been implicated in diarrhea include *E. coli, Campylobacter, Yersinia enterocolitica, Salmonella,* and *Shigella*. The diagnosis should be based on a positive culture result. Antibiotics can be prescribed for the patient who remains symptomatic, and the choice can be based upon antibiotic susceptibility studies. They are commonly prescribed for *Shigella* and *Campylobacter* infections but are probably not indicated for *Salmonella* infections unless there is a suspected extraintestinal infection such as chorioamnionitis.

Primary peritonitis is a rare condition in pregnant women. The diagnosis can be confirmed by paracentesis, and the usual pathogens include the gram-positive organisms *S. pneumoniae* and the group A beta-hemolytic streptococci. The treatment of choice is intravenous penicillin 2 million units every 6 hours. For the penicillin-allergic patient, intravenous erythromycin 500 mg every 6 hours can be given.

Meningitis

Bacterial meningitis is a rare but serious infection in a pregnant woman. Bacterial identification is critical for care, and this requires a spinal tap in any febrile patient who presents with a headache, nausea, vomiting, and nuchal rigidity. The spinal fluid should have a Gram's stain, culture, and chemical studies performed on it. The most common organisms seen in adults are *Neisseria meningitidis,* manifested by gram-negative cocci on Gram's stain, and *S. pneumoniae,* which show up as gram-positive diplococci. *Haemophilus influenzae,* a gram-negative rod, is rarely seen in adults. *Listeria monocytogenes* can be confusing because bacteria are not usually seen on Gram's stain and the CSF glucose is normal. The diagnosis is usually confirmed by culture. For all of these patients, the antibiotic of choice is intravenous ampicillin 2 g every 6 hours. In the case of *Listeria,* intravenous gentamicin 1.5 mg per kilogram every 8 hours should be added to the regimen. For penicillin-allergic patients, intravenous chloramphenicol 1 g every 6 hours is an acceptable alternate choice.

Bacterial Endocarditis

Bacterial endocarditis is a rare infection in pregnant women. A study in 1983 reported an incidence of 1 in 4,000 deliveries,[46] and another in 1988 reported an incidence of 1 per 16,500 deliveries.[12] In my own obstetric service in New York City, I am not aware of a single case in the past decade, during which more than 30,000 deliveries occurred. This disease is more common among urban poor, particularly those who are intravenous drug users. This diagnosis should be considered in any febrile patient with localizing signs of infection who is lethargic. The most specific diagnostic clinical sign is a changing heart murmur, and ultrasound is helpful in confirming the presence of vegetations on the heart valves. At least three blood cultures 30 to 60 minutes apart should be obtained to identify the organism involved. In most patients, a combination of intravenous penicillin 2 million units every 4 hours and intravenous gentamicin 1.5 mg per kilogram every 8 hours suffices. If *Staphylococcus aureus* is recovered, intravenous cephalothin 2 g every 6 hours or intravenous cefazolin 2 g every 8 hours should be given instead of the penicillin. For the penicillin-allergic patient, intravenous vancomycin 0.5 g every 6 hours should be prescribed.

Conclusion

This is the picture of the antibiotic treatment of infection during pregnancy. Antibiotics should be prescribed with caution, after a clinical diagnosis has been made and appropriate cultures obtained. Most patients respond to the initial selection of antibiotics, but the culture can be invaluable in guiding therapy for the patient who remains febrile and has failed to respond to the prescribed treatment.

References

1. Amsel R, Totten PA, Spiegel CA, et al. Non-specific vaginitis: diagnostic criteria and microbial and epidemiologic association. Am J Med 1983; 74:14–22.
2. Anthony BF, Okada DM. The emergence of Group B streptococci in infections of the newborn infant. Annu Rev Med 1977; 28:355–369.
3. Anthony BF, Okada DM, Hobel CJ. Epidemiology of the group B streptococcus: maternal and nosocomial sources for infant acquisitions. J Pediatr 1979; 95:431–436.
4. Baker CJ, Edwards MS. Group B streptococcal infections. In: Remington JS, Klein JD, eds. Infectious diseases of the fetus and newborn infant. Ed 3. Philadelphia: WB Saunders, 1990.
5. Benedetti TJ, Valle R, Ledger WJ. Antepartum pneumonia in pregnancy. Am J Obstet Gynecol 1982; 144:413–417.
6. Boyer KM, Gotoff SP. Prevention of early onset neonatal group B streptococcal disease with selective intrapartum chemoprophylaxis. N Engl J Med 1986; 314:1665–1669.
7. Carey JC, Blackwelder WC, Nugent RP, et al. Antepartum cultures for *Ureaplasma urealyticum* are not useful in predicting pregnancy outcome. Am J Obstet Gynecol 1991; 164:728–733.
8. Centers for Disease Control: Congenital syphilis: United States 1983-1985. JAMA; 256:3206.
9. Centers for Disease Control: Guidelines for the prevention and control of congenital syphilis. MMWR 1988; 37:S1–S13.
10. Centers for Disease Control: Pelvic inflammatory disease: guidelines for prevention and treatment. MMWR 1991; 40:1.
11. Conway MN. Streptomycin in pregnancy: effect on the fetal ear. Br Med J 1965; 2:260–263.
12. Cox SM, Hankins GDV, Leveno KJ, Cunningham FG. Bacterial endocarditis. J Reprod Med 1988; 33:671–674.
13. Cox SM, Shelburne P, Mason R, et al. Mechanisms of hemolysis and anemia associated with acute antepartum pyelonephritis. Am J Obstet Gynecol 1991; 164:587–590.
14. Crombleholme J, Schachter J, Grossman M, et al. Amoxicillin therapy for *Chlamydia trachomatis* in pregnancy. Obstet Gynecol 1990; 75:752–756.
15. Duff P. Pyelonephritis in pregnancy. Clin Obstet Gynecol 1984; 27:17–31.
16. Duff P, Lee ML, Hillier SL, et al. Amoxicillin treatment of bacterial vaginosis during pregnancy. Obstet Gynecol 1991; 77:431–435.
17. Druzin M, Toth Ml, Ledger WJ. Non-intervention in premature rupture of the amniotic membranes. Surg Gynecol Obstet 1986; 163:5–10.
18. Dunlow S, Duff P. Prevalence of antibiotic-resistant uropathogens in obstetric patients with acute pyelonephritis. Obstet Gynecol 1990; 76:241–244.
19. Eickhoff TC, Klein JO, Daly AK, et al. Neonatal sepsis and other infections due to group B hemolytic streptococci. N Engl J Med 1964; 271: 1221–1228.
20. Elder HA, Santamarina BAG, Smith SA, Kass EH. The natural history of asymptomatic bacteriuria during pregnancy: the effect of tetracycline on the clinical course and the outcome of pregnancy. Am J Obstet Gynecol 1971; 111:441–462.
21. Elliott B, Brunham RC, Laga M, et al. Maternal gonococcal infection is a preventible risk factor for low birth weight. J Infect Dis 1990; 161:531–536.
22. Evans MI, Hajj SN, Devve LD, et al. C-reactive protein as a predictor of infectious disease morbidity with premature rupture of the membranes. Am J Obstet Gynecol 1980; 138:648–652.
23. Finland M, Dublin JD. Pneumococcal pneumonias complicating pregnancy and the puerperium. JAMA 1939; 122:1027–1032.
24. Gardner SW, Yow MD, Leeds LJ, et al. Failure of penicillin to eradicate group B streptococcal colonization in the pregnant woman. Am J Obstet Gynecol 1979; 135:1062–1065.
25. Gonik B, Bottoms SF, Cotton DB. Amniotic fluid volume as a risk factor in preterm premature rupture of the membranes. Obstet Gynecol 1985; 65:456–459.
26. Hardy PH, Hardy JB, Nell EE, et al. Prevalence of six sexually transmitted disease agents among pregnant inner-city adolescents and pregnancy outcome. Lancet 1984; 2:333–337.
27. Harris RE. The significance of eradication of bacteriuria during pregnancy. Obstet Gynecol 1979; 53:71–73.
28. Harrison HR, Alexander ER, Weinstein L, et al. The epidemiology and effects of cervical *C. trachomatis* and mycoplasmal infections in pregnancy. JAMA 1983; 250:1721–1727.

29. Kalstone C. Successful antepartum treatment of listeriosis. Am J Obstet Gynecol 1991; 164: 57–58.
30. Kappy KA, Cetrulo CL, Knuppel RA, et al. Premature rupture of the membranes: a conservative approach. Am J Obstet Gynecol 1979; 134:655–661.
31. Klein VR, Cox SM, Mitchell MD, Wendel GD Jr. The Jarisch-Herxheimer reaction complicating syphilis therapy in pregnancy. Obstet Gynecol 1990; 75:375–380.
32. Krohn MA, Hillier SL, Lee ML, et al. Vaginal *Bacteroides* species are associated with an increased rate of preterm delivery among women in preterm labor. J Infect Dis 1991; 164:88–93.
33. LeBlanc AL, Perry JE. Transfer of tetracycline across the human placenta. Texas Journal of Reproductive Biology and Medicine 1967; 25:541–545.
34. Ledger WJ. Aminoglycosides in gynecologic infections. Am J Med 1986; 80:216–221.
35. Ledger WJ, Reite AM, Headinton JT. A system for infectious disease surveillance on an obstetric service. Obstet Gynecol 1971; 37:769–778.
36. Lenke RR, Van Dorsten JP, Schifrin BS. Pyelonephritis in pregnancy: a prospective randomized trial to prevent recurrent disease evaluating suppressive therapy with nitrofurantoin and close surveillance. Am J Obstet Gynecol 1983; 146:953–957.
37. Lucey JF, Driscoll JJ. Hazards to newborn infants of administration of long-acting sulfonamides to pregnant women. Pediatrics 1959; 24:498.
38. Markowitz LF, Steere AC, Benach JL. Lyme disease during pregnancy. JAMA 1986; 255:3394.
39. Martin DH, Koustsky L, Eschenbach DA, et al. Prematurity and perinatal mortality in pregnancies complicated by maternal *Chlamydia trachomatis* infection. JAMA 1982; 247:1585–1588.
40. Martius J, Krohn MA, Hillier SL, et al: Relationships of vaginal *Lactobacillus* species, cervical *Chlamydia trachomatis,* and bacterial vaginosis to preterm birth. Obstet Gynecol 1988; 71:89–95.
41. McCormack WM, Rosner B, Lee Y-H, et al. Effect on birth weight of erythromycin treatment of pregnant women. Obstet Gynecol 1987; 69:202–207.
42. Miller JM, Pupkin MJ, Hill GB. Bacterial colonization of amniotic fluid from intact fetal membranes. Am J Obstet Gynecol 1980; 136:796–804.
43. Minkoff H, Mead P. Approach to the prevention of early onset group B beta hemolytic streptococcal sepsis. Am J Obstet Gynecol 1986; 154:973–977.
44. Moller M, Thomsen AC, Borch K, et al. Rupture of fetal membranes and premature delivery associated with group B streptococci in urine of pregnant women. Lancet 1984; 2:69–70.
45. Norden CW, Kass EH. Bacteriuria of pregnancy: a critical appraisal. Annu Rev Med 1968; 19:431.
46. Pastorek JG, Plauche WC, Faro S. Acute bacterial endocarditis in pregnancy: a report of three cases. J Reprod Med 1983; 28:611.
47. Petrilli ES, D'Ablaing G, Ledger WJ. *Listeria monocytogenes* chorioamnionitis: diagnosis by transabdominal amniocentesis. Obstet Gynecol 1980; 55:S5–S8.
48. Phillipson AEL. Pharmacokinetics of antibiotics in the pregnant woman. In: Antibiotics in obstetrics and gynecology. Boston: Martinus Nijhoff, 1982.
49. Pyati SP, Pildes RS, Jacobs NM, et al. Penicillin in infants weighing two kilograms or less with early onset group B streptococcus disease. N Engl J Med 1983; 308:1383–1389.
50. Reed C, Killackey M. The acute surgical abdomen in pregnancy. Infection in Surgery 1982; 1:26.
51. Regan JA, Chao S, James SL. Premature rupture of membranes, preterm delivery, and group B streptococcal colonization of mothers. Am J Obstet Gynecol 1981; 141:184–186.
52. Robertson L, Caley JP, Moore J. Importance of *Staphylococcus aureus* in pneumonia in the 1957 epidemic of influenza A. Lancet 1958; 2:233.
53. Rustia M, Shubik P. Induction of lung tumors and malignant lymphomas in mice by metronidazole. J Natl Cancer Inst 1972; 48:721.
54. Schultz JC, Adamson JS, Workman WW, Norman TD. Fatal liver disease after intravenous administration of tetracycline in high dose. N Engl J Med 1963; 269:999–1004.
55. Smith AL. Current concepts: Antibiotics and invasive *Haemophilus influenzae.* N Engl J Med 1976; 294:1329.
56. Stamm WE, Counts GW, Running KR, et al. Diagnosis of coliform infection in acutely dysuric women. N Engl J Med 1982; 307:463–468.
57. Steere AC, Malawiota SE. Cases of Lyme disease: location correlated with distribution of *Ixodes dammini.* Ann Intern Med 1979; 91:730.
58. Stille W, Harder S, Mieke S, et al. Decrease in caffeine elimination in man during co-administration of 4-quinolones. J Antimicrob Chemother 1987; 20:729.
59. Sweet RL, Landers DV, Walker C, Schacter J. *Chlamydia trachomatis* infection and pregnancy outcome. Am J Obstet Gynecol 1987; 156:824–833.
60. Sweet RL, Ledger WJ. Puerperal infections morbidity: a two year review. Am J Obstet Gynecol 1973; 117:1093–1100.
61. Ventzileos AM, Campbell WA, Nochimson DJ, et al. Qualitative amniotic fluid volume versus amniocentesis in predicting infection in preterm premature rupture of the membranes. Obstet Gynecol 1986; 67:579–583.
62. Voogd CE, Vanderstel JJ, Jacobs JJ. Mutagenic action of metronidazoles: I. metronidazole, nimorazole, dimetridazole, ionidazole. Mutat Res 1974; 26:483.
63. Wallace RJ Jr, Baker CJ, Quinones FJ, et al. Nontypable *Haemophilus influenzae* (biotype 4) as a neonatal, maternal, & genital pathogen. Rev Infect Dis 1983; 5:123–136.
64. Yeast JD, Garite TJ, Dorchester W. The risks of amniocentesis in the management of premature ruptures of the membranes. Am J Obstet Gynecol 1984; 149:505–508.

PART III

The Neonate

CHAPTER 27

Infections in the Newborn Infant

Jerome O. Klein, M.D.

Infectious disease presenting in the newborn infant may be acquired by one of five routes: in utero, at the time of delivery, in the nursery, in the household after discharge from the nursery, and as a result of an underlying anatomic or physiologic disability. Although signs in the neonate may be common to one or more routes of acquisition, each is characterized by different microbial agents that require different strategies of management. For the purpose of this review, my discussion focuses on infectious diseases that present during the first 4 weeks of life. More information is available in a textbook on infections in the fetus and newborn infant.[28]

Microbiology and Pathogenesis

Infections Acquired in Utero

In utero infection occurs via the placenta and may result in resorption of the embryo, abortion, stillbirth, malformation, intrauterine growth retardation, prematurity, and signs of local or multisystem disease in the newborn infant.

Microbiology

The pregnant woman is subject to the various systemic, respiratory, and gastrointestinal illnesses of all adults. Most infections remain localized without effect on the developing fetus. A relatively small number of microorganisms may invade the blood stream and infect the placenta or fetus. The organisms of particular concern include those identified in the acronym TORCH: *Toxoplasma gondii,* rubella virus, cytomegalovirus (CMV), and herpes simplex virus (HSV). However, a new acronym is needed to include the other well-described causes of in utero infection: syphilis, enteroviruses, varicella-zoster viruses (VZV), and human immunodeficiency virus (HIV). In selected areas, *Plasmodium* and *Trypanosoma cruzi* are responsible for in utero infection. Recently recognized agents such as parvovirus B19 and *Borrelia burgdorferi* may cause harm to the fetus.

Efficiency of transmission of organism from mother to fetus

The efficiency of transmission from the infected mother to the fetus varies among microbial agents and may also vary with the trimester of pregnancy. In the cases of rubella and toxoplasmosis, in utero transmission occurs only as a result of primary infection, whereas in utero transmission of CMV has been described for recurrent infections as well as the primary episode.

The risk of congenital rubella infection in children exposed to mothers with symptomatic rubella was high in the first trimester (90 percent before 11 weeks gestation), declined gradually to a low of 25 percent at 23 to 26 weeks, and then rose to 67 percent after 31 weeks' gestation. The proportion of infants with congenital defects was 100 percent for nine infants whose mothers had symptomatic rubella before 11 weeks' gestation and none after 16 weeks' gestation.[16]

In contrast, the frequency of stillbirth and clinical and subclinical congenital toxoplasmosis among offspring of 500 women who acquired toxoplasma infection during pregnancy was least in the first trimester (14 percent), increased in the second trimester (29 percent), and was highest in the third trimester (59 percent).[10]

The efficiency of transmission is more difficult to describe in CMV infection because congenital infection may result from both primary and recurrent infections. Based on studies in Birmingham, Alabama, and other centers, Stagno[29] estimated the maternal risk of primary and recurrent CMV infections during pregnancy: 1 to 4 percent of women have primary infection during pregnancy; 40 percent of these women transmit the infection to the fetus, of whom 5 to 15 percent develop sequelae; congenital infection due to recurrent CMV (intrauterine infection in the presence of humoral immunity) is 0.5 to 1 percent; and none to 1 percent of the infants have clinically apparent disease or sequelae.

The rate of transmission of HIV from the mother to the fetus in the United States and Europe is 25 to 35 percent but the data are insufficient to identify efficiency of transmission of the virus by trimester. Infants at risk appear to be those born to symptomatic women who have more advanced disease and who have low maternal T-4 lymphocyte counts.[24]

Pathogenetic Mechanisms

Teratogenesis. Cytomegalovirus, rubella virus, coxsackieviruses B3 and B4, and VZV are teratogens and cause disruption of organogenesis. The mechanisms for tissue damage in utero due to these microorganisms remain uncertain but include cell death, alterations in cell growth, and chromosomal damage. The specific causes of cellular damage during the period of organogenesis are poorly understood. Preblud and Alford[27] reviewed the pathogenesis of fetal rubella infection and considered as possible causes of cell damage vascular insufficiency, chromosomal breaks, interference with mitosis, and reduced cellular multiplication time. Some viruses and mycoplasmata cause chromosomal damage in tissue culture.[1] Varicella-zoster virus[2] induces chromosomal breaks in vitro and in vivo, but the relationship of these effects to the unique teratogenesis of VZV (hypoplastic limb abnormalities) remains unknown.

Developmental Abnormalities. Widespread structural abnormalities that result in developmental abnormalities contrast with teratogenesis, the interruption of organogenesis. Maldevelopment of formed organs is characteristic of congenital syphilis, toxoplasmosis, and transplacental herpes simplex virus infection. The inflammatory reaction, tissue damage, and scarring due to these infections are responsible for the signs of disease apparent in the congenitally infected infant. Thus the hydrocephalus or microophthalmia due to intrauterine *T. gondii* is a result of a necrotizing process in the developing organ.

Premature Birth. *Premature birth* is defined as birth of a viable infant before the thirty-seventh week of gestation and may result from almost all microorganisms capable of establishing fetal infection including *T. gondii,* CMV, HSV, *Treponema pallidum, Listeria monocytogenes, Mycobacterium tuberculosis,* and coxsackievirus B; HIV and *Plasmodia* are also likely agents responsible for prematurity. The reason that some women have premature labor remains uncertain. A promising area of research was suggested by studies of phospholipids in placental membranes by Bejar and colleagues.[4] The investigators suggest that labor is initiated by the activation of an enzyme, phospholipase A_2, which hydrolyzes phospholipids in the placental membranes, resulting in an increase in free arachidonic acid and an increased synthesis of prostaglandins. Various bacteria that are normally present in the maternal genital tract have phospholipase activity. Premature labor may be stimulated by endocervical or intrauterine infection due to organisms with phospholipase A_2 activity. These studies have yet to be confirmed or extended.

Intrauterine Growth Retardation. Low birth weight, less than 2,500 g or "small for date," suggesting intrauterine growth retardation, is associated with many maternal infections, but there is definite evidence to establish a causal relationship only for rubella, CMV, and toxoplasmosis. The small size may be a result of a decreased number of morphologically normal cells,[18,19] as occurs in rubella and CMV. Noninfectious causes such as maternal toxemia or placental deficiences appear to cause small size because of the reduced amount of cytoplasm in the cells.

Infections Acquired During Delivery

The fetus is protected from the microbial flora of the maternal genital tract until microscopic or gross disruption of the fetal membranes occurs. If delivery is delayed, the organisms may ascend and produce inflammation of the placenta, umbilical cord, and fetal membranes. Infection of the fetus may also result from aspiration of infected amniotic fluid. In the absence of prolonged rupture of membranes prior to delivery, the infant is colonized during passage through the birth canal. At first the infant is colonized on the skin and mucosal surfaces, where the organisms may multiply without harm to the neonate. In a few infants, invasion of the blood stream occurs from foci in the upper respiratory tract, skin wounds or abrasions, or devitalized tissues of the umbilical cord.

Microbiology

The microorganisms responsible for disease in the neonate acquired during delivery are those present in the maternal genital tract. Although the list of organisms in the maternal genital flora is long, relatively few are significantly associated with neonatal disease (Table 27-1). They include bacteria (group B streptococci [GBS], *Escherichia coli,* and *Neisseria gonorrhoeae*), viruses (hepatitis B, CMV, HSV, and possibly HIV), chlamydia *(C. trachomatis),* mycoplasmata (*Ureaplasma urealyticum* and *Mycoplasma hominis*), and fungi *(Candida albicans).*

Pathogenesis

Specific mechanisms relating to invasive disease for the neonate while still in the womb or during the delivery process remain obscure. Many infants are colonized on the skin or respiratory tract, but only a small number proceed to invasive disease. Among those who do develop invasive disease, some infants die or have severe sequelae, whereas other infants with invasive disease have good outcomes with few or no sequelae. Although the pathogenetic mechanisms for invasiveness and outcome remain enigmatic (as for older infants and children who develop bacteremia or meningitis), clinical and epidemiologic experience provides data about features associated with infants who develop invasive disease and who have a poor prognosis.

Infants who develop sepsis from organisms resident in the maternal microbial flora usually have one or more risk factors. The most significant risk factors are low birth weight and premature delivery. Other risk factors

Table 27-1 Microbiology of Infectious Disease in the Newborn Infant

Microorganism	Route of Infection: IN UTERO	DURING DELIVERY	NOSOCOMIAL	HOUSEHOLD
Bacteria				
Group A streptococci		±	±	
Group B streptococci		+	±	
N. gonorrhoeae		+		
Staphylococcus aureus			+	
S. epidermidis			+	
E. coli		+		
L. monocytogenes	+	+		
Pseudomonas aeruginosa			+	
B. burgdorferi	±	±		
T. pallidum	+			
Viruses				
Influenza (and other respiratory viruses)			+	+
Enteroviruses	+		±	±
Cytomegalovirus	+	+		
Herpes simplex	+	+		
Varicella-zoster	+			
Rubella	+			
Parvovirus	±			
Hepatitis B	±	+		
HIV	+	±		
Mycoplasmata				
U. urealyticum		±		
M. hominis		±		
Fungi				
C. albicans		+		
Chlamydia				
C. trachomatis		+		
Protozoa				
T. gondii	+			
Plasmodia	+			

+ = major cause of fetal or neonatal disease; ± = occasional or uncertain cause of fetal or neonatal disease.

of importance include premature rupture of membranes, septic or traumatic delivery, fetal anoxia, and chorioamnionitis or other signs of maternal peripartum infection. The data about risk factors for invasive bacterial disease are most completely described for group B streptococcal infections and include high colony counts of GBS in genital cultures, GBS bacteriuria during pregnancy, prolonged rupture of membranes for more than 18 hours, delivery at less than 37 weeks' gestation, and intrapartum fever.[3]

The virulence of the invading microorganism has been identified as a factor in the K1 strains of *E. coli* and selected phage types of *Staphylococcus aureus*.

Infections Acquired in the Nursery

The neonate may be infected in the nursery by organisms transmitted from human sources (medical and nursing personnel, other infants, mothers), by contaminated materials (solutions for the skin or nebulization reservoirs), and by procedures that break the barrier of the skin (heel sticks) or mucous membranes (urinary catheters or endotracheal tubes) or are inserted in blood vessels (intravascular catheters). Blood used for transfusion may be unknowingly contaminated, and breast milk from the mother or banked from a surrogate mother may contain pathogens. The use of disposable materials, the attention paid to infection control, and the careful testing of blood prior to transfusion have diminished but not eliminated the threat of nosocomial infections in the nursery.

Microbiology

Staphylococcus aureus and *S. epidermidis* remain a common cause of infection in the nursery. Of particular concern are strains that are resistant to methicillin and other beta-lactam antistaphylocccal antibiotics.

The common respiratory viruses may be spread by caretakers and may occur in epidemic form. Severe illness may result from infection with respiratory syncytial virus; infants with underlying cardiac or pulmonary disease are at most risk.

Hepatitis B antigen, CMV, HIV, HSV, *S. aureus*, GBS, and *Salmonella* spp. have been identified in mother's milk and infection may be transmitted via this route. Oxtoby reviews data about another retrovirus, human T-cell leukemia virus (HTLV-1), which is endemic in areas of Japan and the West Indies. She suggests that breast feeding may be the predominant mode of transmission of HTLV-1 from mother to infant.[23]

Solutions used in nebulization equipment, room humidifiers, and bathing solutions may be contaminated by Pseudomonads, *Serratia marcescens*, and *Flavobacterium* spp., organisms that multiply in aqueous environments at room temperature.

Blood used for replacement or exchange transfusion in neonates may be a source of infection for hepatitis B antigen, HIV, CMV, and in malarious areas *Plasmodium* spp.

Pathogenesis and Transmission

Important factors in the pathogenesis of infection acquired in the nursery are the changes in the newborn populations (increased survival of very-low-birth-weight and premature infants), the use of invasive procedures for maintaining and monitoring the infants, and the prolonged stays required to nurture in the intensive care unit.

Catheterization of the umbilical vein and artery has been associated with sepsis, umbilical cellulitis, and abscesses. Intravenous alimentation is discussed later.

Respiratory agents may spread to neonates by droplets from the respiratory tract of adults or other newborn infants or on the hands of parents or caretakers. Spread of staphylococcal and streptococcal infections to infants may be associated with asymptomatic carriers, but outbreaks have often resulted when a caretaker has had a suppurative lesion.

Parenteral Feeding and Infection

Intravenous alimentation has been an important advance in nutritional support for the very-low-birth-weight infant, but a high incidence of bacteremia, usually caused by coagulase-negative staphylococci, has been associated with the procedure.

The results of recent studies provide insight into the association of parenteral feeding and neonatal sepsis caused by coagulase-negative staphylococci. Strains of staphylococci isolated from infected ventricular shunts or intravascular catheters produce a slime, or glycocalyx, that promotes the adherence and growth of microcolonies on the surfaces of synthetic polymers used in the manufacture of catheters.

The sequence of events in infants with sepsis who receive lipid emulsions through intravenous catheters was described by Freeman and colleagues:[11] colonization of the skin and mucosa by coagulase-negative staphylococci; adherence to the outside of the percutaneous intravascular catheter by the organisms, which then gain access to the interior of the catheter through cutaneous or hematogenous routes; development of microcolonies of staphylococci protected by the slime layer within the catheter; and rapid growth of bacteria following introduction of the intravenous lipid, leading to invasion of the blood when the organisms reach a sufficient number.

Breast Milk and Infection

In most instances when an organism has been cultured from mother's milk, no harm comes to the infant. The risk to the infant from banked milk may be higher than from maternal milk because the infant lacks antibody to the infecting organism that would have been passively transferred from the mother. Banked human milk has been associated with outbreaks of disease in neonates due to *E. coli, Klebsiella pneumonia*, and *Salmonella* spp. The infectious risks of human breast milk are discussed by Ogra and Fishaut.[21]

The role of breast milk in transmission of HIV is of concern because of the importance of breast feeding in providing nutrition and immunologic protection in the first year of life, particularly in developing countries. Breast milk has been documented to be a source of transmission of HIV in case reports of mothers who were transfused with HIV-infected blood after the child's delivery or developed disease postpartum through heterosexual contact.[23] Oxtoby suggests that these circumstances of acute infection need to be differentiated from the usual event in which the mother is infected throughout pregnancy. Infection during the acute period occurs before development of antibody and may be a time when breast milk has a higher titer of transmissible virus.[24] Bcause of the importance of breast feeding in the nutrition of infants in the developing world, the World Health Organization suggests that in those areas women be encouraged to breast-feed even if they are known to be HIV infected.[37] In contrast, in the United States and Western Europe, HIV-infected mothers are discouraged from breast feeding because other forms of nutrition are feasible.

Infection Acquired in the Household

The newborn infant is susceptible to the common respiratory and enteric pathogens that are transmitted to the new arrival by siblings, parents, and visitors. If an infant who is well when discharged from the nursery and has no significant risk factors associated with gestation and delivery develops signs of infectious disease after a period of well-being at home, a household-acquired infection is likely. Although the neonate possesses passively transferred antibody to some of the infectious agents, others including the common respiratory viruses and invasive bacterial pathogens may cause serious disease.

The congenitally infected infant may be a source of infection for members of the household. Rubella virus, HSV, or CMV may be shed in urine, pharyngeal secretions, or skin lesions for months to years after birth. Suppurative lesions due to *S. aureus* may be a source of infection for other members of the household.

Infants With Underlying Anatomic or Physiologic Disabilities

Genitourinary infection early in life may serve to identify an underlying anatomic or physiologic disability of the urinary tract. Similarly, otitis media in the first month of life may be an indication of underlying eustachian tube and middle ear system dysfunction.

Infants with underlying immune defects may not

Table 27-2 Clinical Manifestations of Neonatal Infection Acquired in Utero or at Delivery

	Microorganism					
Clinical Sign	RUBELLA VIRUS	CMV	*T. GONDII*	HSV	*T. PALLIDUM*	GROUP B *STREPTOCOCCUS* OR *E. COLI*
Hepatosplenomegaly	+	+	+	+	+	+
Jaundice	+	+	+	+	+	+
Pneumonitis	+	+	+	+	+	+
Petechiae or purpura	+	+	+	+	+	+
Vesicles	−	+	−	+ +	+	−
Maculopapular exanthema	−	−	+	+	+ +	−
Meningoencephalitis	+	+	+	+	+	+
Microcephalus	−	+ +	+	+	−	−
Hydrocephalus	+	+	+ +	+	−	−
Intracranial calcifications	−	+ +	+ +	−	−	−
Hearing deficits	+ +	+	−	−	+	−
Myocarditis	+	−	+	+	−	−
Congenital defects	+ +	−	−	−	−	−
Bone lesions	+ +	−	+	−	+ +	−
Glaucoma	+ +	−	−	−	+	−
Chorioretinitis or retinopathy	+ +	+	+ +	+	+	−
Cataracts	+ +	−	+	+	−	−
Optic atrophy	−	+	+	−	−	−
Uveitis	−	−	+	−	+	−
Keratoconjunctivitis	−	−	−	+ +	−	−

− = either not present or rare in infected infants; + = occurs in infants with infection; + + = has special diagnostic significance for this infection.

have systemic infections until passively acquired maternal antibody is dissipated. Because the half-life of immune globulin G is 23 days, such infectons are likely to occur after 3 months of age.

Clinical Signs

Clinical manifestations of infection acquired in utero, during delivery, or postnatally include common and nonspecific signs of systemic or local disease and some signs that are relatively specific to the microorganism (Table 27-2). A constellation of signs should suggest possible diagnoses (Table 27-3). The signs of congenital infection may be present at birth or appear months to years later.

Early- and Late-Onset Disease

Two patterns of disease, early onset and late onset, have been associated with systemic bacterial infections during the first month of life. Although best documented for infections caused by group B streptococci, the concept is also applicable to other invasive bacterial infections, including *L. monocytogenes*. The source of invasive organisms is the maternal tract for both patterns and in addition, for late-onset disease, the nursery and household. Early-onset disease presents as a multisystem illness during the first 4 days of life with a mortality in excess of 15 percent (and up to 50 percent if signs appear in the first 24 hours). The infants usually have one or more risk factors of the pregnancy and delivery, including premature delivery, low birth weight, chorioam-

Table 27-3 Syndromes in the Neonate Caused by Congenital Infections

Microorganism	Signs
Toxoplasma gondii	Hydrocephalus, diffuse intracranial calcifications, chorioretinitis
Rubella	Cardiac defects, sensorineural hearing loss, cataracts
Cytomegalovirus	Microcephalus and periventricular calcifications
Herpes simplex	Vesicular lesions, keratoconjunctivitis
Syphilis	Bullous, macular, and eczematous skin lesions involving the palms and soles, rhinorrhea, dactylitis and other signs of osteochondritis and periostitis
Varicella-zoster	Limb abnormalities, cicatricial lesions
Parvovirus	Diffuse edema (in utero, hydrops fetalis)
AIDS	Severe thrush, failure to thrive, recurrent bacterial infections, calcifications of the basal ganglia

nionitis, and other signs of peripartum maternal infection. Signs of late-onset disease have onset at 5 days to 2 months of age and are more likely to be slowly progressive with focal signs, the most important of which is meningitis, and a mortality of 10 to 20 percent. Included in late-onset disease are nosocomial infections that occur in infants who remain in the nursery for prolonged periods of time.

The concept of early and late infection is also applicable to infections acquired in utero. Each infection may have signs during the newborn period or signs that first appear months to years later.

Congenital toxoplasmosis may be manifested by chorioretinitis at birth or identifiable later in the first decade of life. In a prospective study of ophthalmologic outcome in children born with subclinical congenital toxoplasmosis, the age of onset of eye disease ranged from 1 month to 9 years.[36] Sensorineural hearing loss due to congenital rubella may not be appreciated by the parent and not detected until the child enters school. A progressive panencephalitis believed due to congenital rubella infection has been described in 11- to 14-year-old children.[32]

The signs of congenital HIV infection may be present at birth or appear months to years later. The average onset of AIDS acquired in utero is 5 to 10 months of life, but signs including interstitial pneumonitis, hepatosplenomegaly, and failure to thrive may appear earlier.

Nonspecific Signs

Nonspecific signs of in utero infection include premature delivery and/or low birth weight. Signs of a generalized systemic infection include purpura, jaundice, enlargement of the liver or spleen, and pneumonitis or meningoencephalitis. One or more of these signs are common to in utero infection due to rubella, CMV, HSV, coxsackievirus B, *T. gondii,* or *T. pallidum.* Most of these signs may also be present with infections acquired at delivery, including those due to enteroviruses, GBS, gram-negative enteric bacilli, and *L. monocytogenes.*

Nonspecific signs of particular concern in infants with bacterial sepsis or meningitis include hyperthermia or hypothermia, respiratory distress, apnea, cyanosis, vomiting, and lethargy or irritability.

Although all infants with invasive bacterial infection are not febrile, fever is a particularly important sign for approximately half of newborn infants with bacterial sepsis and meningitis. In a review of infants with bacterial sepsis and meningitis, 51 percent and 61 percent, respectively, had hyperthermia; 15 percent of infants with sepsis were hypothermic.[13] Three studies provide useful data about temperature and the association of this sign with systemic bacterial disease to guide management.[6,22,34] The following points about fever in the neonate may be taken from the cumulative results: temperature elevation in full-term infants is uncommon, temperature elevation is infrequently associated with systemic infection when only a single elevated reading occurs, temperature elevation that is sustained for more than 1 hour is frequently associated with infection, and temperature elevation without other signs of infection is infrequent.

Specific Signs

Skin and Mucous Membranes

Nonspecific signs include maculopapular rashes, petechiae, and purpura. Location of the rash appears to be of diagnostic significance only for the erythematous macular lesions on the palms and soles associated with congenital syphilis.

Cellulitis may be associated with streptococcal and staphylococcal infections and gram-negative enteric bacilli. Pustules and abscesses are usually due to staphylococcal infections. Bullous lesions may be due to congenital syphilis or infection due to *S. aureus.* Purulent or hemorrhagic lesions that rupture and leave a necrotic base (ecythyma gangrenosa) may be due to *P. aeruginosa.* Severe mucocutaneous candidiasis has been associated with AIDS. Vesicular lesions are usually associated with HSV infection but also occur with infection due to CMV and VZV. Cicatricial lesions may represent scars from the pox lesions of congenital VZV.

Central Nervous System

Central nervous system manifestations of congenital infection include meningoencephalitis, hydrocephalus and microcephalus, intracranial calcifications, paralyses, and hearing deficits. Meningoencephalitis is common to many congenital infections and is defined by focal neurologic findings and CSF signs of inflammatory response.

A survey of clinical signs in 255 newborn infants studied at six medical centers revealed that seizures were the most frequent sign of neurologic disease (40 percent). Other specific signs of disease were less common: bulging or full fontanelle (28 percent) and nuchal rigidity (15 percent).[13]

Microcephalus and hydrocephalus are common in congenital infections due to CMV, HSV, and *T. gondii*; microcephalus is usually associated with CMV, and hydrocephalus is most characteristic of toxoplasmosis.

Intracranial calcifications are found in congenitally infected infants with disease due to CMV and toxoplasmosis: CMV disease is associated with calcifications in periventricular areas; *T. gondii* disease is more likely to be scattered in the white matter.

Sensorineural hearing deficits are part of the congenital rubella syndrome but are also present in congenital infections due to CMV and syphilis.

A characteristic encephalopathy that may progress to dementia with focal neurologic signs and cerebral atrophy is seen in children with early-onset AIDS. Neurologic signs may be evident during the first month of life.

Lesions of the Extremities

Intrauterine growth retardation lines are apparent in roentgenograms of long bones and suggest infection due to congenital rubella. Osteochondritis and periostitis (often occurring as dactylitis) are found in infants with congenital syphilis.

A unique maldevelopment of the extremities that presents as hypoplasia of the limbs may result from congenital VZV. The lesions may be restricted to unilateral involvement of one limb and often associated with hypoplasia or absence of digits.

Eye Lesions

Conjunctivitis is most commonly associated with infections acquired at delivery from organisms present in the maternal birth canal, *N. gonorrhoeae* and *C. trachomatis*. Herpes simplex is associated with conjunctivitis or keratoconjunctivitis.

Glaucoma, chorioretinitis, or cataracts are part of the congenital rubella syndrome, and less commonly the latter two are associated with HSV. Chorioretinitis may be due to *T. gondii* and may be present at birth or years later.

Microophthalmia is associated with congenital rubella virus and toxoplasmosis.

Uveitis is a sequela of congenital syphilis or *T. gondii* infection.

Diagnosis

Prenatal Diagnosis

Clinical Diagnosis

Many infectious diseases with serious consequences for the fetus are difficult to diagnose in the mother on clinical grounds alone. Infections that invade the blood stream and may infect the fetus with few or nonspecific signs in the mother include rubella virus, CMV, *T. gondii*, HSV, and HIV. Only 50 percent of women infected with rubella have a rash, and fewer than 10 percent of women with toxoplasmosis have clinical evidence of disease. Primary CMV or toxoplasmosis should be suspected in pregnant women with signs and symptoms similar to those of infectious mononucleosis but who are heterophile negative. The genital lesions of HSV and syphilis may be without symptoms and go unrecognized.

Isolation and Identification of the Infectious Agent

Although direct isolation of the organism is the most specific mode of diagnosis and directs appropriate management, it is relatively infrequent among the important pathogens responsible for infections of the pregnant woman. Bacterial organisms can be isolated from body fluids such as blood, cerebrospinal fluid, and urine. Identification of organisms from the genital tract does not distinguish virulent from nonvirulent organisms.

Tests for the presence of hepatitis B virus surface antigen (HBsAg) are available. The U.S. Public Health Service now recommends universal screening of all pregnant women for HBsAg.[17]

Direct isolation of *T. gondii* from fetal blood has been accomplished with ultrasound guidance by Daffos and colleagues.[7] Fetal blood sampling for diagnosis of congenital rubella was demonstrated by the same investigators. The technique may be of value for diagnosis of other in utero infections as well as monitoring the pharmacokinetics of antimicrobial agents in the fetus.

Examination of desquamated cells and fluid obtained by amniocentesis is of value in diagnosis of viruses or bacteria shed from the placenta, skin, urine, or tracheal fluid of the infected fetus. Rubella virus,[8] CMV,[15] and HBsAg.[25] have been identified in amniotic fluid obtained from amniocentesis.

Chlamydia trachomatis is an obligate intracellular organism and is found in endocervical cells in the pregnant woman and in conjunctival scrapings in the infant. Cell culture is expensive and takes as long as 7 days for a confirmed negative result. Direct immunofluorescence, ELISA, and DNA probes circumvent these disadvantages of cell culture.

Cytology and Histology

Cell scrapings or smears from the cervix and vagina may reveal epithelial cells with multinucleated giant cells and intranuclear inclusions of value in diagnosis of VZV and HSV.

The urine sediment of the mother and child should be examined for the presence of epithelial cells with intranuclear inclusions indicative of CMV.

Serologic Diagnosis

Serologic diagnosis of specific infection in the pregnant woman requires demonstration of a significant rise in antibodies (IgG) or a high titer of early antibody (IgM). Although uncommonly available, the ideal circumstance is availability of the serologic status of the woman at the onset of pregnancy. If early serum is not available, a serum sample should be obtained as soon as possible after recognition of an infection and a second sample obtained 2 to 3 weeks later. A single serum test to measure IgM is available for *T. gondii* and rubella but not for the other organisms of concern to the fetus.

The diagnosis of syphilis in pregnancy depends on serologic detection of nontreponemal antibodies to cardiolipin (Venereal Disease Research Laboratory [VDRL] or rapid plasma reagin [RPR]) followed by confirmation by a specific treponemal antibody assay (fluorescent treponemal antibody absorption test [FTA-ABS]). The VDRL or RPR titers can be sufficiently high that the "prozone" effect leads to a false-negative result. This phenomenon is particularly likely in HIV seropositive women. Serial dilutions are necessary to detect the high titer. In areas with a high prevalence of syphilis and HIV, routine quantitative serologic assays should be performed. Programs for diagnosis of HIV infection rely on detecting the presence of anti-HIV antibody in the pregnant mother. Because of the presence of transplacental maternal antibodies, the presence of serum IgG antibody to HIV is not diagnostic until the infant is at least 15 months of age, when maternal antibodies are likely to have dissipated. The absence of antibodies in formerly seropositive infants does not rule out infection until the infant is older than 2 years of age because specific antibody synthesis may be delayed.[12]

Skin Tests

Tuberculin skin tests should be considered routine in the care of the pregnant patient. Use of the antigens for tuberculosis and mycobacteria may be administered to the mother without risk to the fetus.

Diagnosis in the Newborn Infant

Isolation and Identification of Microorganisms

Isolation of organisms from a significant body fluid or tissue such as blood, cerebrospinal fluid, urine, skin vesicle fluid, or a suppurative focus remains the most valid method of specific microbiologic diagnosis. In critically ill children, aspiration of the lung in pneumonia, middle ear fluid, or other foci of infection is warranted to provide specific microbiologic diagnosis. Organisms cultured from the skin, umbilicus, external ear, or stool indicate colonization and do not establish the etiology of the infectious disease.

A high incidence of parasitemia is present in infants with congenital toxoplasmosis with or without clinical signs; Desmonts and Couvreur[9] isolated *T. gondii* from the peripheral blood of 30 infants (43 percent of those sampled).

Spirochetes are present and may be visualized by dark-field examination from open skin and mucous membrane lesions of the neonate. Penicillin in recommended dosage causes a complete disappearance of viable treponemes from lesions within hours.[33]

Congenital infection is associated with prolonged shedding of the organisms. Rubella virus can be recovered from pharyngeal secretions, urine, conjunctival fluid, and feces for weeks to months after birth; at 1 year 2 to 20 percent of infants are still shedding virus from the pharynx.[5] Cytomegalovirus is isolated from the urine or saliva for up to 6 years following congenital or perinatal infection;[30] asymptomatic infants may excrete larger quantities of virus than severely ill older immunocompromised patients. Recurrent skin vesicles associated with congenital HSV contain virus and may be a source of infection for contacts.

Antigen detection in the form of latex agglutination and counterimmunoelectrophoresis for GBS, use of enzyme immunosorbent assay for *T. gondii,* and use of electron microscopy for diagnosis of CMV are now available. Molecular probes and amplification procedures will likely add to our abilities to identify specific organisms.

Cytology

Giemsa-stained conjunctival scrapings are useful for diagnosis of the gram-negative diplococci of *N. gonorrhoeae* and for identification of the inclusion bodies of inclusion conjunctivitis of the newborn caused by *C. trachomatis*.

Cerebrospinal Fluid Examination

Because meningitis may accompany sepsis, CSF examination should be a part of the diagnostic plan in infants with suspected invasive disease. The cell count and concentrations of protein and sugar differ in normal newborn infants when compared with older children and adults, differ in premature infants when compared to term infants, and change with postnatal age. A wide range exists for all subgroups in the first months of life. Meningitis is usually present in neonates with white blood cell counts higher than 50 per cubic millimeter, concentrations of protein higher than 150 mg per deciliter, and a glucose ratio CSF/serum less than 60 percent. A summary of results of selected studies of hematologic and chemical characteristics of CSF is provided by Klein and Marcy.[14]

Positive VDRL in cerebrospinal fluid indicates presence of syphilitic infection of the central nervous system.

Laboratory Aids

Routine laboratory methods now available are of minimal assistance in diagnosis of systemic infections in the newborn infant. The total white blood cell count is variable in bacterial sepsis and indicates an increased incidence of invasive disease if high (greater than 30,000 per cubic millimeter) or low (less than 5,000 per cubic millimeter).

Absolute elevation of number of eosinophils is of diagnostic assistance for respiratory infections due to *C. trachomatis* and *Bordetella pertussis*. Tipple and colleagues identified eosinophilia of 300 per cubic millimeter in 71 percent of infants with chlamydial pneumonitis.[31]

The importance of acute phase reactants remains uncertain but of continuing investigational interest. To varying degrees, they reflect inflammatory activity, but sensitivity and specificity for invasive bacterial disease are inconsistent among the studies. Erythrocyte sedimentation rate, serum fibrinogen, C-reactive protein, haptoglobin, alpha$_1$-acid glycoprotein (orosomucoid), and leukocyte enzyme activity, alone or in combination, may suggest risk for invasive bacterial disease but are of insufficient sensitivity and specificity to be clinically useful now. Philip and Hewitt provided data that suggested the proportion of bands over total neutrophils was the most sensitive assay and white blood cell count higher than 5,000 the most specific for bacterial sepsis.[26]

Immunology

Elevated levels of serum immunoglobulin, especially IgG and T-cell abnormalities, are identified in infants with AIDS. Elevated IgM and IgG concentrations are also associated with diagnosis of chlamydial pneumonia in infants.

Serology

Serologic studies should be performed in the neonate and mother to ascertain the presence of in utero or postnatal infection. Serologic tests are available for *T. gondii,* rubella, CMV, HSV, HIV, VZV, and syphilis. To distinguish passively transferred maternal antibody from antibody derived from infection in the neonate, it is necessary to obtain early and late blood specimens from the infant. Because the half-life of IgG is 23 days, the first sample is obtained soon after the presumptive diagnosis, and the second sample should be obtained at least two half-lives or more than 46 days later. Measurement of IgM antibody provides evidence of current infection in the neonate, but the only assays of value are for *T. gondii* and rubella. Delayed and defective anti-HIV response in infants has been detected.[12]

Radiologic Signs

Chest x-rays should be obtained for identification of pneumonitis. Although nonspecific, it may provide evidence for local or systemic involvement of all the major congenital infections.

Radiologic examination of the long bones may provide specific information about congenital infection due to rubella and syphilis. Bony radiolucencies that resolve after birth are identified in congenital rubella. Bony involvement in infants with congenital syphilis is widespread and includes not only long bones but also skull, spine, and ribs. Changes range from radiopaque bands to areas of radiolucency. Metaphyses and diaphyses are usually involved, including irregular demineralization and new bone formation.

Skull x-rays should be obtained. The pattern of calcification, if present, may provide clues to the diagnosis: diffuse calcifications are seen in congenital infection due to *T. gondii,* periventricular calcifications are characteristic of CMV infection, and calcification of the basal ganglia have been identified in children with AIDS.

Management

Prenatal Management

The most effective management of infectious diseases in the pregnant woman that threaten the fetus and newborn infant is prevention of the infections of importance.

Vaccines

Utilization of available vaccines in recommended schedules in childhood should provide durable protection against infections throughout the childhood years. Of particular importance is determining that appropriate rubella vaccination has been provided. Use of tetanus toxoid in areas where infection has significant risks for the newborn should be a priority for public health officials.

Cautions for the Pregnant Woman

Physicians should inform pregnant women about avoidance of contact with patients with specific communicable diseases. The pregnant woman should avoid intercourse with her sexual partner if he has a vesicular lesion on the penis that may be due to HSV or if he is known or suspected to be infected with HIV.

Pregnant women should avoid eating raw or undercooked lamb, pork, and beef because such products may contain *T. gondii*. Women should also avoid contact with cat feces, which are highly infectious if they contain the oocysts of *T. gondii*.

Chemotherapy

Chemotherapy is available for bacterial infections and many of the nonbacterial infections that are of concern for the developing fetus. Therapy should be instituted when there is a secure diagnosis in pregnancy of infection due to *T. gondii* or *T. pallidum*. Data are unavailable to assess the risk-benefit ratio of treatment during pregnancy in the woman who has symptomatic or asymptomatic HIV infection. Because of the possible teratogenicity of some antituberculous drugs, most experts believe it is preferable to wait for the end of pregnancy rather than institute therapy during pregnancy (if the clinical condition of the patient permits).

Chemoprophylaxis

With the most sensitive microbiologic methods for detection of group B streptococci in vaginal and anorectal mucosa, 15 to 40 percent of pregnant women are GBS positive. Vertical transmission results in asymptomatic colonization of about 70 percent of infants, and about 1 percent of newborn infants born to group B streptococcal carriers develop early-onset GBS sepsis. Because selective intrapartum maternal chemoprophylaxis using parenteral ampicillin has been demonstrated to prevent both GBS maternal disease and early-onset sepsis in the neonate, a protocol for its use has been suggested. Baker[3] recommends the following program:

1. Pregnant women should be screened for GBS at 26 to 28 weeks' gestation by culture of lower vaginal and anal secretions or by GBS antigen test at onset of labor or rupture of membranes.
2. Women who are GBS culture or antigen positive and have a risk factor for delivery of an infant with GBS sepsis should receive chemoprophylaxis.
3. Risk factors include gestation of less than 37 weeks, rupture of membranes for more than 12 hours, fever higher than 100.6°F during labor, or a history of GBS bacteriuria during pregnancy.
4. The antibiotic regimen demonstrated to be effective is intravenous ampicillin (2 g initially, followed by 1 g every 4 hours until delivery).

Immune Globulins

Human immune globulins are available for administration after exposure to selected virus infections of importance in pregnancy, including rubella, measles, VZV, and hepatitis A. Although these products may prevent or modify clinical signs, there are no data that they are of value in protecting the fetus of the susceptible woman against infection. The use of immune globulin after maternal exposure to rubella virus should be limited to those women to whom, in the event of documented infection during pregnancy, therapeutic abortion is unacceptable.

Special Issues Associated with HIV Infection

Dual infection with HIV and syphilis is common. At present, the optimal therapy for syphilis that protects the fetus in the HIV-infected pregnant woman is uncertain. Because of the uncertainty of the efficacy of treatment in patients with dual infections, some experts advocate retreatment of the infant after delivery in spite of prior maternal therapy.

Management of the Neonate

The infant with signs of sepsis at birth may have infection acquired in utero or at delivery. Among in utero infections, chemotherapy is available for toxoplasmosis, HSV, VZV, and syphilis. Every effort should be made to diagnose these infections and begin appropriate therapy when a specific microbial diagnosis is available.

Successful management of neonatal bacterial sepsis includes early diagnosis and prompt initiation of appropriate antimicrobial therapy and supportive measures. The strategy is similar to that for other infectious diseases: knowledge of the likely pathogens, studies of appropriate body fluids to identify the pathogen in the patient, choice of safe and effective antimicrobial agents based on knowledge of the presumed pathogens, and readjustment of the therapeutic plan when results of cultures are available and the clinical course indicates success or failure of initial therapy.

Chemotherapy

Currently most invasive disease in neonates in the United States and Western Europe is due to GBS and gram-negative enteric bacilli. A penicillin is the choice for GBS. Choice of therapy for gram-negative infections depends on the current pattern of antibiotic susceptibility in the local hospital but is likely to be an aminoglycoside such as gentamicin. The initial choice of antibiotics should be reevaluated when results of cultures and susceptibility tests become available. The duration of therapy depends on the initial response to the appropriate antibiotics but should be 7 to 10 days in most infants with sepsis, pneumonia, or minimal focal infections; the minimum duration of therapy for meningitis caused by gram-negative enteric bacilli or GBS is 21 days.

Antiviral therapies are now available for treatment of newborn infants infected with HSV (acyclovir and vidarabine), VZV (acyclovir), and respiratory syncytial virus (ribavirin). Investigations are now in progress to study the efficacy and safety of therapy for neonates born to women infected with HIV. A survey of Zidovudine (AZT) use in 43 pregnant women with HIV infection indicates the drug was well tolerated and not associated with malformations in the newborn, premature birth, or fetal distress.[28a]

The clinical pharmacology of antibiotics administered to the newborn is unique and cannot be extrapolated from the data of absorption, excretion, and toxicity in the adult. The safety of new antimicrobial agents is of particular concern because toxic effects, such as sensorineural nerve damage, may not be detected until years later.

Adjunctive Therapies

Because mortality and morbidity due to treatable diseases remains high, investigators have looked to adjunctive therapies to amplify and extend the efficacy of antimicrobial agents. Current programs are directed to replacing deficits in the host defenses of the infected neonate and include use of granulocyte transfusion, exchange transfusion, and standard and modified hyperimmune immunoglobulins.

Chemoprophylaxis

Ophthalmic preparations including erythomycin or silver nitrate are standard modes of prophylaxis for ophthalmitis due to *N. gonorrhoeae* and *C. trachomatis*. Other uses of chemoprophylaxis in the newborn period include isoniazid to reduce morbidity from tuberculosis in infants who are unavoidably in contact with infected persons and hexachlorophene baths to prevent staphylococcal disease.

Immune Globulins

Although many investigators have attempted to assess the value of intravenous immune globulin (IVIG) to prevent neonatal sepsis, the efficacy of the material in prevention of disease remains uncertain. In theory, IVIG should be of particular value to the premature infant who is born with low serum IgG concentrations and whose hypogammaglobulinemia is exacerbated during the first weeks of life. Deficiency of transplacentally acquired maternal antibody is a risk factor for invasive disease caused by group B streptococci and the K1 serotype of *E. coli*. Recent studies suggest efficacy of IVIG administered to premature infants to prevent sepsis but have been criticized for deficiencies in study design and statistical analysis.[20] These studies have prompted development of multicenter trials.

Human immune serum globulins are available for use in newborns for hepatitis A, hepatitis B, VZV, measles, tetanus, and agammaglobulinemia. Products and dosage schedules are reviewed by Wilson.[35]

Vaccines

Hepatitis B vaccine has been recommended for universal immunization of newborn infants by the U.S. Public Health Service. The specific schedules for administration of the vaccine are currently in discussion.

Bacille Calmette-Guérin (BCG) is used extensively in Scandinavia and Finland for neonates but is recommended only for selected infants in the United States. Usage is recommended when contact with tuberculous patients who are infectious is unavoidable.

Sepsis in the Newborn Infant Recently Discharged from Nursery

Signs of infection appearing in the first month of life after discharge from the nursery must be aggressively managed. The source of the infection may include late-onset congenital infection or infection acquired at delivery or in the nursery, or it may be the result of underlying anatomic, physiologic, or metabolic abnormalities.

Fever is relatively uncommon in the first weeks of life, but when it does occur the incidence of severe disease, including sepsis, meningitis, and pneumonia, is sufficiently high to warrant careful evaluation. Physical examination should seek to identify signs associated with congenital or late-onset infection. Culture of urine should be done if no other focus is identified, and cultures of blood and cerebrospinal fluid and a chest radiograph should be considered if the infant is believed to have systemic infection.

References

1. Allison AC, Paton GR. Chromosomal abnormalities in human diploid cells infected with mycoplasma and their possible relevance to aetiology of Down's syndrome (mongolism). Lancet 1966; 2:1229–1230.
2. Aula P. Chromosomes and viral infections. Lancet 1964; 1:720–721.
3. Baker CJ. Maternal chemoprophylylaxis for group B streptococcal sepsis. Report Pediatr Infect Dis 1991; 3:1–2.
4. Bejar R, Curbelo V, David C, Gluck L. Premature labor: II. bacterial sources of phospholipase. Obstet Gynecol 1981; 57:479–482.
5. Cooper LZ, Krugman S. Clinical manifestations of postnatal and congenital rubella. Arch Ophthalmol 1967; 77:434–439.
6. Craig WS. The early detection of pyrexia in the newborn. Arch Dis Child 1963; 38:29–35.
7. Daffos F, Forestier F, Capella-Pavlovsky M et al. Prenatal management of 746 pregnancies at risk for congenital toxoplasmosis. N Engl J Med 1988; 318:271–275.
8. Davis IE, Tweed GV, Chin IDV, et al. Intrauterine diagnosis of cytomegalovirus infection: viral recovery from amniocentesis fluid. Am J Obstet Gynecol 1971; 109:1217–1219.
9. Desmonts G, Couvreur J. Toxoplasmosis: epidemiologic and serologic aspects of perinatal infection. In: Krugman S, Gershon AA, eds. Infections of the fetus and the newborn infant. Progress in clinical and biological research. Vol 3. New York: Alan R Liss, 1975; 115–132.
10. Desmonts G, Couvreur J. Congenital toxoplasmosis: a prospective study of the offspring of 542 women who acquired toxoplasmosis during pregnancy. Pathophysiology of congenital disease. In: Thalhammer O, Baumgarten K, Pollak A, eds. Perinatal medicine, sixth European congress. Stuttgart: Georg Thieme, 1979; 51–60.
11. Freeman J, Goldmann DA, Smith NE, et al. Association of intravenous lipid emulsion and coagulase-negative staphylococcal bacteremia in neonatal intensive care units. N Engl J Med 1990; 323:301–308.
12. Gretano C, Scano G, Carbonari M, et al. Delayed and defective anti-HIV IgM response in infants Lancet 1987; 1:631 (letter).
13. Klein JO, Marcy SM. Bacterial sepsis and meningitis. In: Remington JS, Klein JO, eds. Infectious diseases of the fetus and newborn infant, Ed 3, Philadelphia: WB Saunders, 1990; p 620.
14. Klein JO, Marcy SM. Bacterial sepsis and meningitis. In: Remington JS, Klein JO, eds. Infectious diseases of the fetus and newborn infant, Ed 3, Philadelphia: WB Saunders, 1990;626.
15. Levin MJ, Oxman MN, Moore MG, et al. Diagnosis of congenital rubella in utero. N Engl J Med 1974; 290:1187–1188.
16. Miller E, Cradock-Watson JE, Pollock TM. Consequences of confirmed maternal rubella at successive stages of pregnancy. Lancet 1982; 2:781–784.
17. Recommendation of the Immunization Practices Advisory Committee. Prevention of perinatal transmission of hepatitis B virus: prenatal screening of all pregnant women for hepatitis B surface antigen. MMWR 1988; 37:341.
18. Naeye RL. Cytomegalic inclusion disease: the fetal disorder. Am J Clin Pathol 1967; 47:738–744.
19. Naeye RL, Blanc W. Pathogenesis of congenital rubella. JAMA 1965; 194:1277–1283.
20. Noya FJD, Baker CJ. Intravenously administered immune globulin for premature infants: a time to wait. J Pediatr 1989; 115:969–971.
21. Ogra PL, Fishaut M. Human breast milk. In: Remington JS, Klein JO, eds. Infectious diseases of the fetus and newborn infant. Ed 3. Philadelphia: WB Saunders Company, 1990:82–84.
22. Osborn LM, Bolus R. Temperature and fever in the full-term newborn. J Fam Pract 1985; 20:261.
23. Oxtoby MJ. Human immunodeficiency virus and other viruses in human milk. Pediatr Infect Dis J 1988; 7:825–835.
24. Oxtoby MJ. Perinatally acquired HIV infection. In: Pizzo PA, Wilfert CM, eds. Pediatric AIDS. Baltimore: Williams & WIlkins, 1991:12.
25. Papaevangelou G, Kremastinov T, Prevedourakis C, et al. Hepatitis B antigen and antibody in maternal blood, cord blood and amniotic fluid. Arch Dis Child 1974; 49:936–939.
26. Philip AGS, Hewitt JR. Early diagnosis of neonatal sepsis. Pediatrics 1980; 65:1036–1041.
27. Preblud SR and Alford CA, Jr. Rubella. In: Remington JS, Klein JO, eds. Infectious diseases of the fetus and newborn infant. Ed 3, Philadelphia: WB Saunders, 1990; 196–214.
28. Remington JS, Klein JO, eds. Infectious diseases of the fetus and newborn infant. Ed 3, Philadelphia: WB Saunders, 1990.

28a. Sperling RS, Stratton P, O'Sullivan MJ, et al. A survey of zidovudine use in pregnant women with human immunodeficiency virus infection. N Engl J Med 1992; 326:857–861.

29. Stagno S. Characteristics of CMV infection in pregnancy. N Engl J Med 1985; 313:1270–1274.
30. Stagno S, Pass RF, Dworsky ME, et al. Congenital and perinatal cytomegaloviral infections. Semin Perinatol 1983; 7:31–42.
31. Tipple M, Beem MO, Saxon E. Clinical characteristics of the afebrile pneumonia associated with *Chlamydia trachomatis* infection in infants less than 6 months of age. Pediatrics 1979; 63:192–197.
32. Townsend JJ, Baringer JR, Wolinsky JS, et al. Progressive rubella panencephalitis: late onset after congenital rubella. N Engl J Med 1975; 292:990–993.
33. Tucker HA, Robinson RCV. Disappearance time of *T. palladum* from lesions of early syphilis fol-

lowing administration of crystalline penicillin G. Bulletin of the Johns Hopkins Hospital 1947; 80:169–173.
34. Voora S, Srinivasan G, Lilien LD, et al. Fever in full-term newborns in the first four days of life. Pediatrics 1982; 69:40–44.
35. Wilson CB. Developmental immunology and role of host defenses in neonatal susceptibility. In: Remington JS, Klein JO, eds. Infectious diseases of the fetus and newborn infant. Ed 3. Philadelphia: WB Saunders, 1990.
36. Wilson CB, Remington JS, Stagno S, et al. Development of adverse sequelae in children born with subclinical congenital *Toxoplasma* infection. Pediatrics 1980; 66:767–774.
37. World Health Organization. Breast feeding/breast milk and human immunodeficiency virus (HIV). Wkly Epidemiol Rec 1987; 33:245–246.

Index

D

M

N